AF764335

Visceral Vessels and Aortic Repair

Yamume Tshomba
Domenico Baccellieri • Roberto Chiesa
Editors

Visceral Vessels and Aortic Repair

Challenges and Difficult Cases

Springer

Editors
Yamume Tshomba
Unit of Vascular Surgery
Fondazione Policlinico Universitario
A. Gemelli IRCCS, Università
Cattolica del Sacro Cuore
Rome
Italy

Unit of Vascular Surgery
San Raffaele Scientific Institute
Vita-Salute University
Milan
Italy

Domenico Baccellieri
Unit of Vascular Surgery
San Raffaele Scientific Institute
Milan
Italy

Roberto Chiesa
Unit of Vascular Surgery
San Raffaele Scientific Institute
Vita-Salute University
Milan
Italy

ISBN 978-3-319-94760-0 ISBN 978-3-319-94761-7 (eBook)
https://doi.org/10.1007/978-3-319-94761-7

Library of Congress Control Number: 2019932824

© Springer Nature Switzerland AG 2019
This work is subject to copyright. All rights are reserved by the Publisher, whether the whole or part of the material is concerned, specifically the rights of translation, reprinting, reuse of illustrations, recitation, broadcasting, reproduction on microfilms or in any other physical way, and transmission or information storage and retrieval, electronic adaptation, computer software, or by similar or dissimilar methodology now known or hereafter developed.
The use of general descriptive names, registered names, trademarks, service marks, etc. in this publication does not imply, even in the absence of a specific statement, that such names are exempt from the relevant protective laws and regulations and therefore free for general use.
The publisher, the authors, and the editors are safe to assume that the advice and information in this book are believed to be true and accurate at the date of publication. Neither the publisher nor the authors or the editors give a warranty, express or implied, with respect to the material contained herein or for any errors or omissions that may have been made. The publisher remains neutral with regard to jurisdictional claims in published maps and institutional affiliations.

This Springer imprint is published by the registered company Springer Nature Switzerland AG
The registered company address is: Gewerbestrasse 11, 6330 Cham, Switzerland

Contents

List of Videos

Movie 5.1	A case of infrarenal abdominal aortic aneurysm associated with right inferior polar artery originating from the aneurysm. Perfusion of cold crystalloid into the orifices of the right inferior polar artery was performed, the aorto-aortic bypass reconstruction and direct reimplantation of the inferior polar artery to the graft has been performed. Post-operative CT scan shows the correct patency of the both renal arteries and right inferior polar artery (MOV 228597 kb)
Movie 5.2	Infrarenal abdominal aortic aneurysm associated to Horseshoe Kidney treated with aorto-aortic bypass reconstruction behind the kidney with direct reimplantation of the renal artery to the graft (MOV 1055 kb)
Video 14.1	Midesophageal four-chamber view. Severe right ventricle dysfunction (WMV 1325 kb)
Video 14.2	Midpapillary transgastric view. Severe right ventricle dysfunction with left ventricle D-shape (WMV 1568 kb)
Video 14.3	Midpapillary transgastric view. Severe left ventricle dilation and systolic dysfunction (AVI 1916 kb)
Video 14.4	Mid-transgastric short-axis view. Empty left ventricle with papillary muscles "kissing" (AVI 14042 kb)
Movie 19.1	Video showing Gore Hybrid Vascular Graft (GHVG) deployment during TAAA open repair. The GHVG is gently placed into the artery for 2–3 cm. The stent is released and ballooned after deployment. The cold renal perfusion catheter is then immediately reinserted into the graft. Of note stiches for fixation of GHVG to the renal artery and device. Finally, the proximal anastomosis to the main aortic graft is completed (AVI 189508 kb)

Electronic supplementary material is available in the online version of the related chapter on SpringerLink: http://link.springer.com/

Part I

Introductory Remarks

1 Anatomical Overview and Imaging of the Aorta and Visceral Arteries

Gabriele Ironi, Giorgio Brembilla, Giulia Benedetti, and Francesco De Cobelli

1.1 Anatomy

The thoracic aorta extends proximally from the aortic annulus to the diaphragmatic crura distally. It is subdivided into three parts: the ascending aorta, the arch and the descending aorta. The ascending aorta comprises the aortic root and the tubular ascending aorta. The aortic root lies between the aortic annulus and the sinotubular junction. The sinuses of Valsalva arise from the aortic root. The tubular ascending aorta runs from the sinotubular junction to the brachiocephalic trunk. The coronary arteries are the only branches of the ascending aorta. The aortic arch begins at the brachiocephalic trunk and ends at the origin of the left subclavian artery. The isthmus extends from the left subclavian artery to the ligamentum arteriosum. Three branches usually arise from the aortic arch: the brachiocephalic trunk, the left common carotid artery and the left subclavian artery. The brachiocephalic trunk divides into the right common carotid artery and the right subclavian artery. In 6% of people, the left vertebral artery arises directly from the arch [1]. The bovine arch is another variant in which the left common carotid artery arises from the brachiocephalic trunk rather than the aorta [1]. Another arch variant is the ductus diverticulum, a focal bulge along the inner aspect of the isthmus representing a remnant of the ductus arteriosus. Traumatic aortic transection also occurs in this location and can occasionally be difficult to differentiate from a ductus diverticulum. However, the ductus diverticulum has smooth margins with obtuse angles relative to the adjacent aorta. Aortic transection has irregular margins with acute angles relative to the nearby aortic walls.

The descending thoracic aorta extends from the isthmus to the diaphragmatic crura. In contrast to the ascending aorta, the descending thoracic aorta has multiple branches, including the bronchial, intercostal, spinal and superior phrenic arteries and various small mediastinal branches.

The abdominal aorta starts immediately before the emergence of the superior adrenal arteries, approximately at the level of the T12 vertebral body. The juxtarenal abdominal aorta diameter normally measures less than 3 cm. The abdominal aorta supplies visceral and parietal arteries that arise in three vascular planes before it bifurcates to form the common iliac arteries at the L4.

The unpaired visceral arteries to the gastrointestinal tract include the celiac, superior mesenteric and inferior mesenteric arteries. These vessels arise in the midline anterior plane. Shortly

G. Ironi · G. Brembilla · G. Benedetti
F. De Cobelli (✉)
Department of Radiology and Experimental Imaging Center, San Raffaele Scientific Institute, Milan, Italy

Vita-Salute San Raffaele University, Milan, Italy
e-mail: ironi.gabriele@hsr.it; brembilla.giorgio@hsr.it; benedetti.giulia@hsr.it; decobelli.francesco@hsr.it

© Springer Nature Switzerland AG 2019
Y. Tshomba et al. (eds.), *Visceral Vessels and Aortic Repair*,
https://doi.org/10.1007/978-3-319-94761-7_1

after its origin, the celiac axis gives rise to three main branches: the left gastric, splenic and common hepatic arteries. The latter subsequently bifurcates into the proper hepatic artery and the gastroduodenal artery.

The paired visceral arteries include the renal, adrenal and gonadal arteries, which run through the lateral plane to supply the urogenital and endocrine abdominal organs. The subcostal, inferior phrenic and lumbar arteries are paired parietal arteries to the diaphragm and body wall, arising in the posterior oblique plane.

As the only unpaired parietal artery, the middle sacral originates posteriorly. The common iliac artery bifurcates at the pelvic brim to yield the hypogastric arteries, which subsequently divide into anterior and posterior branches.

Up to 30% of subjects have one or more accessory renal arteries on each side that most commonly supply the lower pole, usually arising from the mid-abdominal aorta but occasionally from the distal aorta or common iliac arteries [2, 3]. There are also numerous variations of celiac anatomy, most commonly accessory or replaced individual hepatic arteries, with numerous subtypes described in the Michels' classification [4].

1.2 Ultrasound

Ultrasonographic imaging (US) is characterized by widespread availability, low costs, a lack of ionizing radiation or the use of IV iodinated contrast. For these reasons, it is considered the screening examination of choice: the US Preventive Services Task Force recommended a one-time screening for AAA with US in men of 65–75 years of age who have a history of smoking and for men 65–75 years of age who do not have a history of smoking [5]. Moreover, it can be used in adjunction to conventional cross-sectional imaging studies (CT, MRI) in the preoperative evaluation and post-operative surveillance of visceral vessels potentially affected by aortic procedures. For example, evaluation of branch vessel stenosis with CT angiography can be limited by metallic artefact due to radiopaque markers used for correct deployment of the devices: in these cases, US Doppler findings are evaluated in conjunction with CTA for proper surveillance.

The possible drawbacks of US are operator dependency and technical limitation in the examination of obese patients and in the presence of bowel gas. Furthermore, US has limited reliability in detecting morphologic alterations such as stent fracture or migration, and it has inferior sensitivity and specificity in identifying endoleaks [6].

US examination is performed with the patient in a supine position; the C2–C5 curved transducer is commonly used, with frequency varying upon body habitus (2–4.5 MHz). The transducer is placed in the midline and the abdomen scanned in both longitudinal and sagittal planes. For Doppler evaluation, the smallest angle of insonation should be used and should always be <60°, as it affects the measurements of peak systolic velocity. It is of fundamental importance that the Doppler examination be performed so that it may be easily reproduced, in order to reliably compare results and not to attribute velocity variations between studies to disease progression.

In patients undergoing aortic surgery, US examination focuses on the abdominal aorta and renal/mesenteric vessels (i.e. celiac artery, superior mesenteric artery). The same principles for US evaluation apply both to preoperative evaluation and post-operative surveillance of stent grafts; it must be noted that stents are not always discretely identified, depending mainly on patient characteristics and vessel anatomy.

After anatomical and morpho-dimensional evaluation of vascular structures, the first step in US evaluation is the use of colour Doppler for the correct identification of the vessels and for sample volume placement in spectral Doppler analysis. Morphology of spectral Doppler waveform is then evaluated, and peak systolic velocity (PSV) and end-diastolic velocity (EDV) are measured. Doppler waveforms vary depending upon the type of visceral vessel investigated: celiac artery (CA), renal arteries (RA) and superior mesenteric artery (SMA) in the postprandial phase are low-resistance vessels (resistive index [RI] of 0.55–0.7, with wider normal ranges of 0.55–0.81 reported for hepatic artery), while SMA in fasting state and inferior mesenteric artery (IMA) are high-resistance vessels (RI >0.7). Celiac artery and SMA resistance may be affected also by anatomic variants, occurring in up to 20% of individuals: hepatic artery branch arising from SMA is the most common and may explain a low-resistance waveform in the SMA during fasting state.

1.2.1 Aorta

The abdominal aorta should be evaluated both in transverse and sagittal planes, in order to measure the external diameter (outer wall to outer wall) at its widest point; any thrombus apposition or calcification should be described. Then, spectral Doppler waveform is evaluated with PSV-EDV measurements using the smallest possible angle of insonation (always <60°), as previously mentioned.

1.2.2 CA, SMA and IMA

Celiac and mesenteric vessels arise from the anterior aspect of the aorta and are best imaged in the sagittal plane; conversely, hepatic artery (HA) and splenic artery (SA) are best evaluated in the transverse plane. For each vessel, spectral Doppler velocities should be sampled proximally, at the mid and distal tract.

Several velocity cut-offs have been proposed in scientific literature to diagnose arterial stenosis in native mesenteric vessels. PSV >275 cm/s for SMA and PSV >200 cm/s for CA can be used to accurately diagnose vessel stenosis >70% [7]. IMA is not routinely evaluated, as the presence of stenosis has generally limited clinical relevance; PSV >250 cm/s can be used to diagnose >50% stenosis and PSV >270 to predict >70% stenosis accurately [8]. Conversely, there are no accepted criteria to diagnose pathologic stenosis in aortic branches after surgery/interventional procedures, with evidence that the cut-off used to predict stenosis in native vessels overestimates stenosis in stented/prosthetic vessels. The most plausible explanation is that the stents may reduce vessel wall compliance and may alter velocities, even in the absence of true stenosis. Proposed criteria for post-operative stenosis are PSV >325 cm/s for >50% stenosis in stented SMA and PSV >274 cm/s in CA [9]. A valuable approach would be to evaluate changes over time by performing an examination soon after the surgical procedure in order to establish baseline parameters upon which to compare subsequent evaluations.

1.2.3 Renal Arteries

Correct evaluation of renal arteries can be difficult and time-consuming, even for experienced operators. RA usually arise 1–2 cm below the SMA, from the anterolateral (right RA) or posterolateral (left RA) aspect of the aorta. With an anterior approach, it could be difficult to obtain a correct angle of insonation for spectral Doppler analysis, as RA course parallel to the ultrasound beam; a lateral approach may thus be indicated. Accessory renal arteries, when present, can be missed due to their small size. Spectral Doppler analysis should be performed at the origin, proximal, mid and distal tract of the vessel to evaluate PSV, ESV and flow anomalies. In the presence of a stent, velocity measurements are obtained also within the stent.

Normal renal arteries are low-resistance vessels, with typical waveform and persistence of diastolic flow. Normal RA PSV is <180 cm/s; a cut-off velocity of >200 cm/s is generally accepted for diagnosis of RA stenosis >50%. Other clues to vessel stenosis are increased post-stenotic turbulent flow, increased aorto-renal ratio (RAR >3.5) with marked reduction of flow velocity at the distal segment and tardus-parvus pattern waveform in segmental arteries [10]. Other parameters that can be evaluated at this level are acceleration time, acceleration index and early systolic peak. Arterial velocities are usually combined with Doppler analysis of segmental arteries that allow evaluation of renovascular resistances; parenchymal damage with RI >0.8 is associated with fewer functional benefits after revascularization therapy [11].

Also for renal arteries, there are no accepted criteria for the diagnosis of stenosis in stented or prosthetic arteries. A proposed criterion for renal artery stenosis >60% in patients treated with fenestrated stent grafts consisted of PSV >280 cm/s and RAR >4.5 [12]. Again, the best approach would be to perform an early examination after the surgical procedure in order to establish baseline parameters upon which to compare subsequent evaluations.

1.2.4 Contrast-Enhanced Ultrasound (CEUS)

CEUS is an emerging technique that uses contrast agents to improve visualization of anatomic structures and characterization of focal lesions. There are several contrast agents available, consisting in microbubbles of gas stabilized by a shell (sulphur hexafluoride with a phospholipid shell [SonoVue-Lumason], octafluoropropane with a lipid shell [Definity-Luminity] and perfluorobutane with a phospholipid shell [Sonazoid]). In vascular surgery patient settings, CEUS is believed to improve the detection of endoleaks, and some authors in literature even claim its superiority over CTA [13]. However, at the time of writing, there are no indications of CEUS in vascular evaluation, as in 2016 the Food and Drug Administration approved Lumason only for the examination of the liver in adults and paediatric patients.

1.3 MDCT Angiography

Historically, diagnostic vascular imaging has been performed using digital subtraction angiography (DSA) by means of intravascular catheters. The development of multidetector computed tomography (MDCT) has radically transformed the role of CT in vascular investigation. MDCT angiography (MDCTA) allows high spatial resolution, including nearly isotropic submillimetre voxels and rapid single-breath-hold image acquisition. MDCTA yields inherent advantages over DSA, such as noninvasiveness, outstanding extravascular anatomic depiction, superior celerity, widespread accessibility, greater affordability and lower radiation dose for patients and staff, along with multiplanar post-processing for interventional planning. Thanks to these benefits, MDCTA has largely replaced DSA in routine clinical practice for the evaluation of a newly diagnosed dilatation of the aorta (Fig. 1.1), surveillance of known aortic aneurysms and follow-up after surgical or endovascular treatment [3]. Other disorders affecting the aortoiliac system may be evaluated

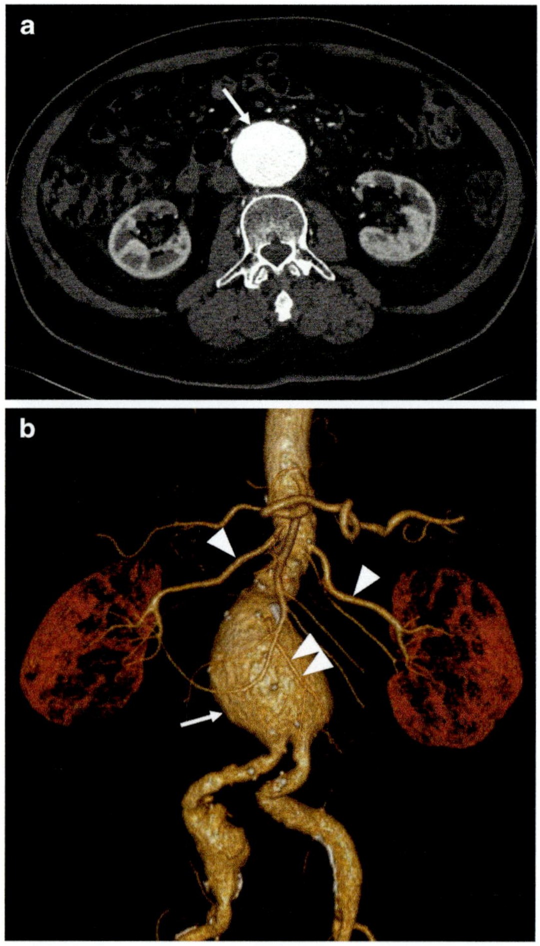

Fig. 1.1 Axial CT image (**a**) and volume-rendered 3D image (**b**) demonstrate a saccular infrarenal AAA (arrow). Note the distance between aneurysm sac and renal arteries (arrowhead). Double arrowhead IMA

by this technique, including atherosclerotic disease, dissection, intramural hematoma, penetrating ulcer, post-traumatic vascular injury and vasculitides.

Several technical issues are supposed to be considered when performing CTA. Inclusion of a non-contrast CT scan is mandatory for imaging suspected aortic syndrome since intramural hematomas are more evident without intra-arterial contrast enhancement. In the same way, calcifications are best depicted in non-contrast CT scan because of the high tissue contrast between calcium and the surrounding unenhanced tissue. Intravenous injection of iodinated contrast material is required for the intravascular opacification in CTA and has to be carefully optimized considering timing, amount and injection rate.

Injection rate actually concerns how fast the iodinated contrast agent is delivered to the vascular territory of interest. Visceral organ enhancement is relatively independent of flow rates; on the opposite, angiographic opacification heavily relies on contrast material flow and varies directly with flow rates [14]. CTA is usually performed with flow rates of 4–6 mL/s to balance a strong peak vascular enhancement with practical considerations regarding venous access, as flow rates above 5–6 mL/s become difficult to achieve with conventional peripheral cannulas [15]. Performing a flush with 20–30 mL of saline at the same injection rate as that of the contrast bolus pushes the latter from the upper extremity venous system into the central circulating blood volume. This procedure also increases the length of peak aortic enhancement and decreases the total amount of the injected contrast required for adequate aortic enhancement by 10–15 mL [14].

Due to the fact that each patient presents different circulatory times, there is a substantial risk of scanning the subject too early (with an insufficient amount of contrast material in the vessels) or too late (with undesirable venous opacification during the arterial phase) when using a fixed delay time. Therefore, synchronizing scan acquisition with contrast material delivery to the vascular territory of interest is another critical point of the CTA examination. Contrast appearance time is most commonly assessed by one of two methods. The arrival time of a test bolus of 10–20 mL administered at flow rates similar to the main contrast bolus used during MDCTA acquisition, such as 5–6 mL/s, can be assessed in order to accurately calculate the time-to-peak enhancement, so as to customize the delay time during the main contrast bolus. In the automated bolus tracking technique, a region of interest is placed over a certain location by the operator, so that the scan is initiated when the appropriate threshold for vascular enhancement is reached.

Another variable that affects contrast material administration is patient body weight. Indeed, if a fixed amount of contrast material is used, some subjects will receive an insufficient dose of contrast material (with inadequate opacification of the vessels), and at the same time, others will receive an excessive dose of contrast (which would be spared to reduce the cost of the CT examination). The overall contrast volume should be approximately equal to the injection rate (in mL/s) multiplied by the scan duration in second plus 5–10 s: typical contrast volumes range from 60 to 120 mL [16].

After the acquisition of the arterial phase, a portal venous phase is usually obtained with a 60–70 s delay time from the beginning of contrast material infusion in order to evaluate for late filling of potential false lumen in dissections, slow endoleaks in endovascular stent repair (Fig. 1.2), contrast extravasation from aortic rupture (Fig. 1.3) or inflammatory enhancement in vasculitides and infections.

Digital image post-processing of the acquired data is performed using various algorithms, including maximum intensity projection (MIP), volume rendering (VR) and multiplanar reconstruction (MPR) techniques (Fig. 1.4). VR provides us a topographic display of the aortoiliac system and visceral arterial branches, by means of an exquisite immersive visualization for browsing the 3D volume and displaying vascular pathology as well. MIP techniques are two-dimensional representations of three-dimensional data that yield angiography-like images with an excellent overview of vascular anatomy. They require viewing

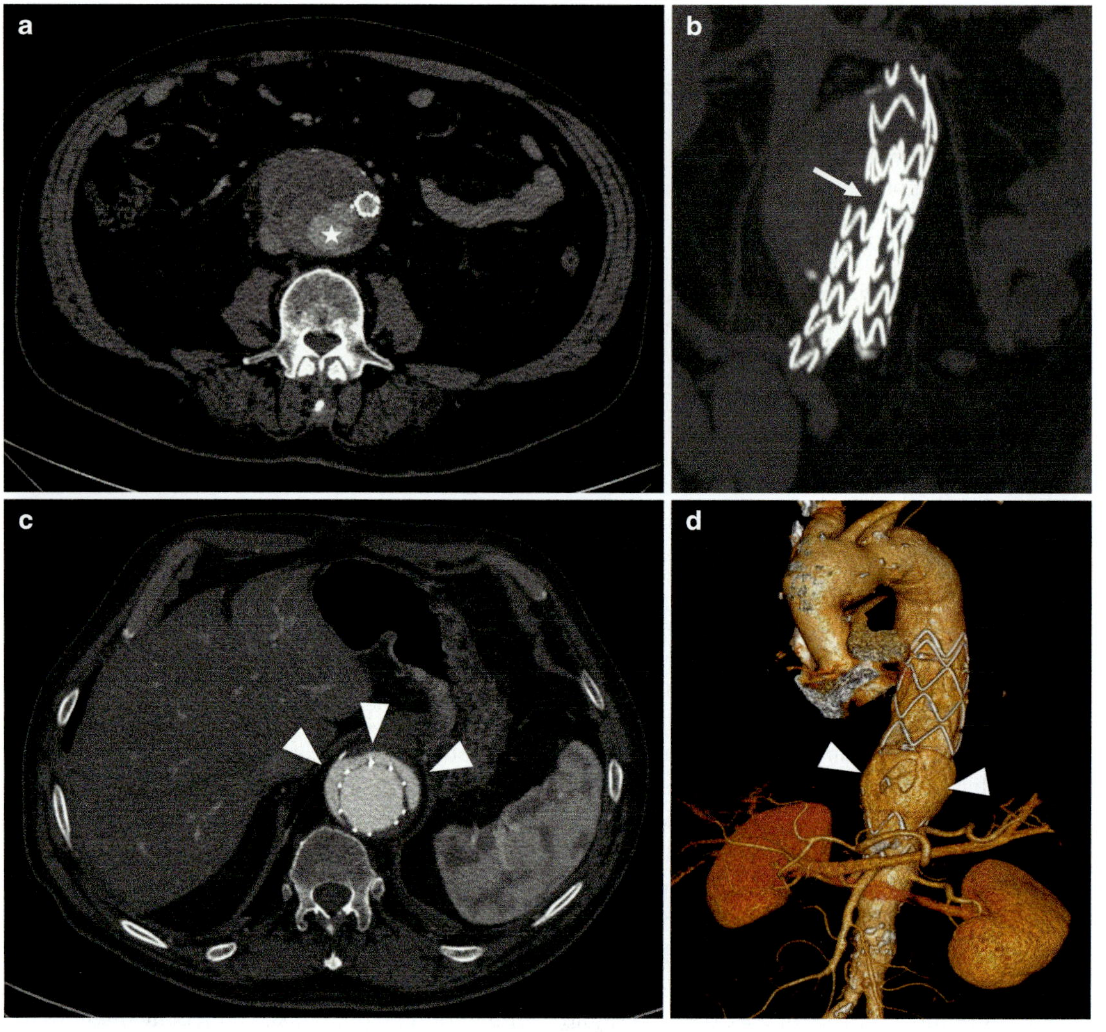

Fig. 1.2 (**a**, **b**) 80-year-old man with a progressively enlarging false lumen due to endoleak after endovascular aortic repair for AAA. Axial CT image (**a**) shows the enhancing false lumen (star) external to the stent graft at the level of the right iliac branch. MIP reconstruction (**b**) demonstrates discontinuity (arrow) of the metal prosthesis at the origin of the right iliac stent-graft branch. (**c**, **d**) 69-year-old man with endoleak after endovascular repair for TAAA. Axial CT image (**c**) and VR image (**d**) show contrast material accumulation (arrowheads) in the false lumen external to stent graft

from different angles for a three-dimensional perspective. MIP is limited in the evaluation of vascular stenosis because of the superimposition of high-attenuating vascular calcifications over the vessel lumen. In these circumstances, multiplanar reformations can display inner lumen and outer mural calcification and can accurately portray the degree of arterial stenosis. Ideally, the assessment of CTA datasets is best accomplished through a two-step process of standard axial image interpretation and subsequent 3D image review.

Many patients undergoing evaluation of the aorta will need serial imaging follow-up over many years for monitoring aneurysm size, extent of dissection and possible post-procedural complications. Multiple strategies have been introduced in MDCTA in an attempt to reduce patient radiation dose without degradation of image quality. With automatic tube current modulation, the tube current is by default reduced when scanning low-attenuating regions and increased for areas of higher atten-

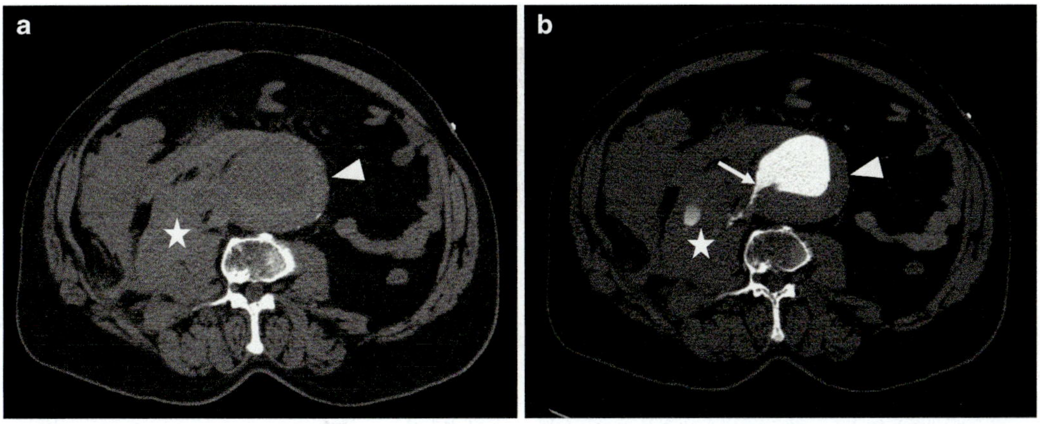

Fig. 1.3 Axial non-contrast image from CTA (**a**) demonstrates a large retroperitoneal hematoma (star) and AAA (arrowhead), compatible with ruptured AAA. Axial contrast-enhanced image (**b**) demonstrates irregularity along the right lateral wall of the aorta with active extravasation of contrast material into the hematoma (arrow), confirming exact site of AAA rupture

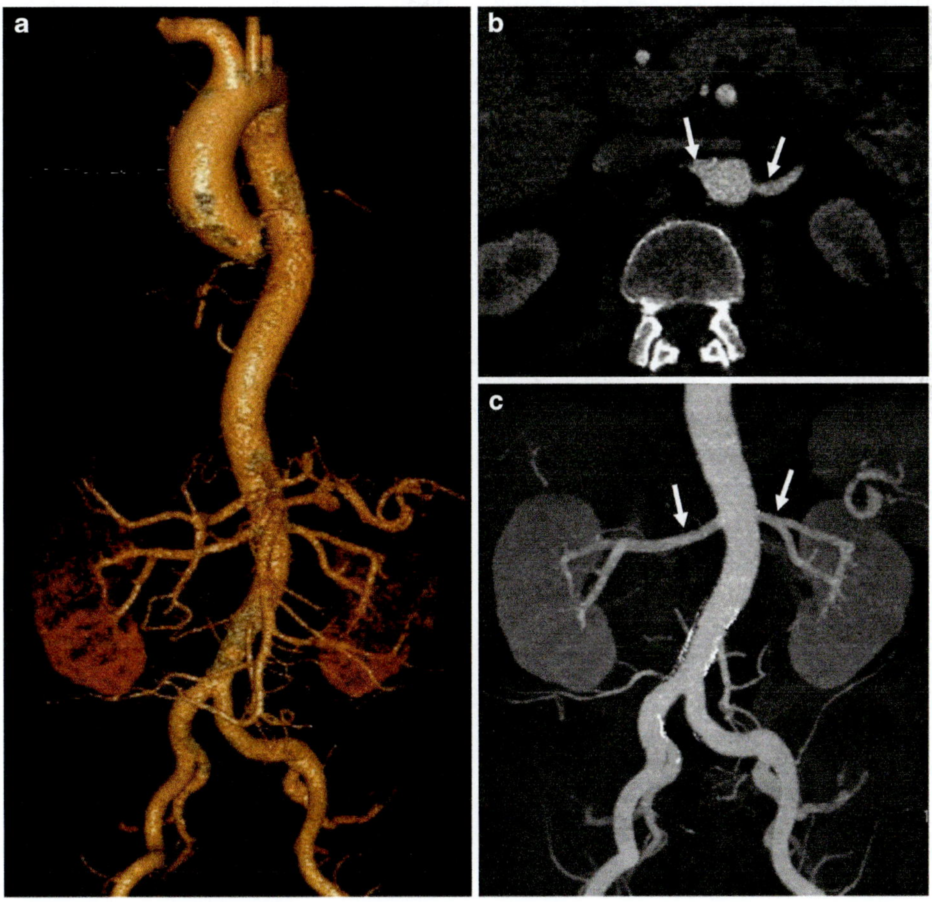

Fig. 1.4 (**a**) Volume-rendered 3D image in a coronal projection, after bone editing, shows the normal anatomy of the aorta and its branches. (**b**) Axial contrast-enhanced image shows the origin of renal arteries (arrows). (**c**) Coronal MIP rendering demonstrates a complete map of the renal arteries (arrows) in one image, but three-dimensional relationship is not maintained with MIP renderings. (**d**) MPR of the right renal artery: this technique is useful for elongating a tortuous structure in order to identify the location of maximal vessel dilation or narrowing

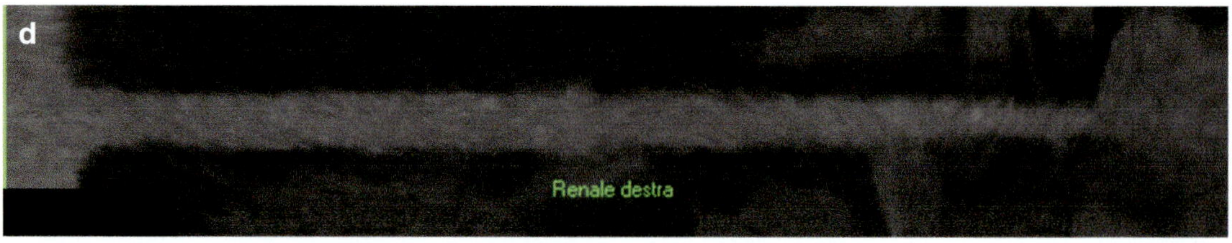

Fig. 1.4 (contineud)

uation. Iterative reconstruction algorithms allow for radiation dose reduction by improving the signal-to-noise ratio at lower tube current levels [17].

Thanks to its rapid acquisition of CT volumes during peak arterial enhancement and isotropic resolution, MDCTA permits the visualization of smaller arterial structures, such as abdominal visceral branches, becoming a useful tool to study normal and variant anatomy as well as pathologic conditions of the visceral vasculature (Figs. 1.5 and 1.6). For example, CT angiography is helpful in the evaluation of the renal arteries regarding stenosis, vascular mapping in healthy living renal donors and transplant recipients as well as vascular complications after renal transplantation. In this case, MDCT angiography especially focuses on renal artery anatomy with emphasis on possible variations that may hamper kidney transplantation, such as early branching or accessory renal arteries. These may arise from vessels as far distant as the common iliac artery, so that failure to detect such vessels may cause partial post-transplant infarction.

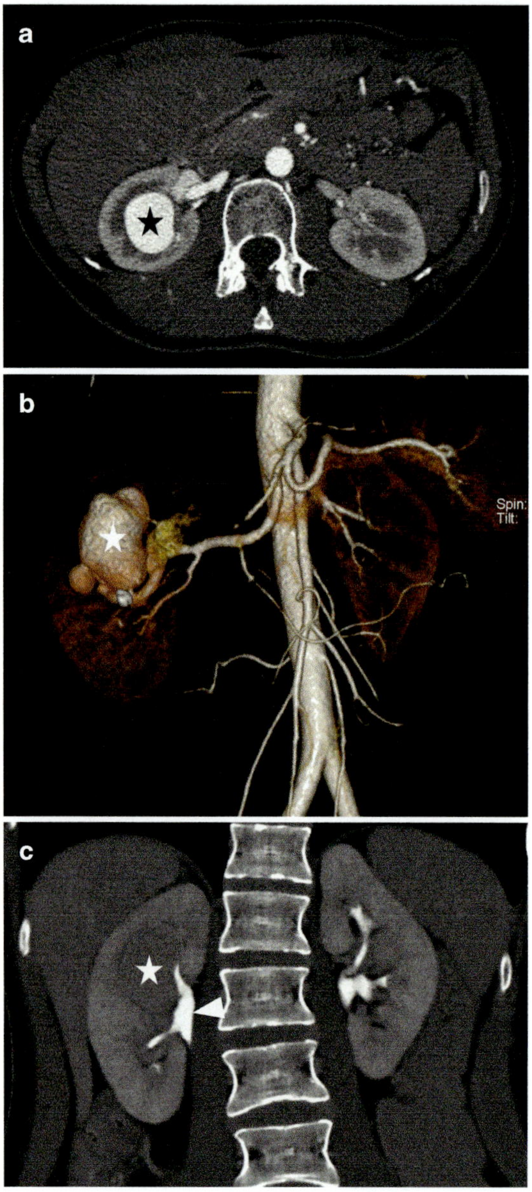

Fig. 1.5 Axial contrast-enhanced image (**a**) and VR image (**b**) show a big saccular aneurysm (star) arising from an intrarenal branch of the right renal artery. Delayed coronal CT image (**c**) delineates the relationship of the aneurysm sac (star) to the renal pelvis (arrowhead)

1.4 Magnetic Resonance Angiography

Nowadays, magnetic resonance angiography (MRA) has become a good alternative to the imaging modalities listed above, allowing a non-invasive depiction of blood vessels, with reasonable timing, mainly due to great technological developments (such as parallel imaging, phased-array coils and fast slew rate). Furthermore, MR angiography uses radiofrequencies combined with magnetic fields instead of ionizing radiations, which is safer for the patient [18].

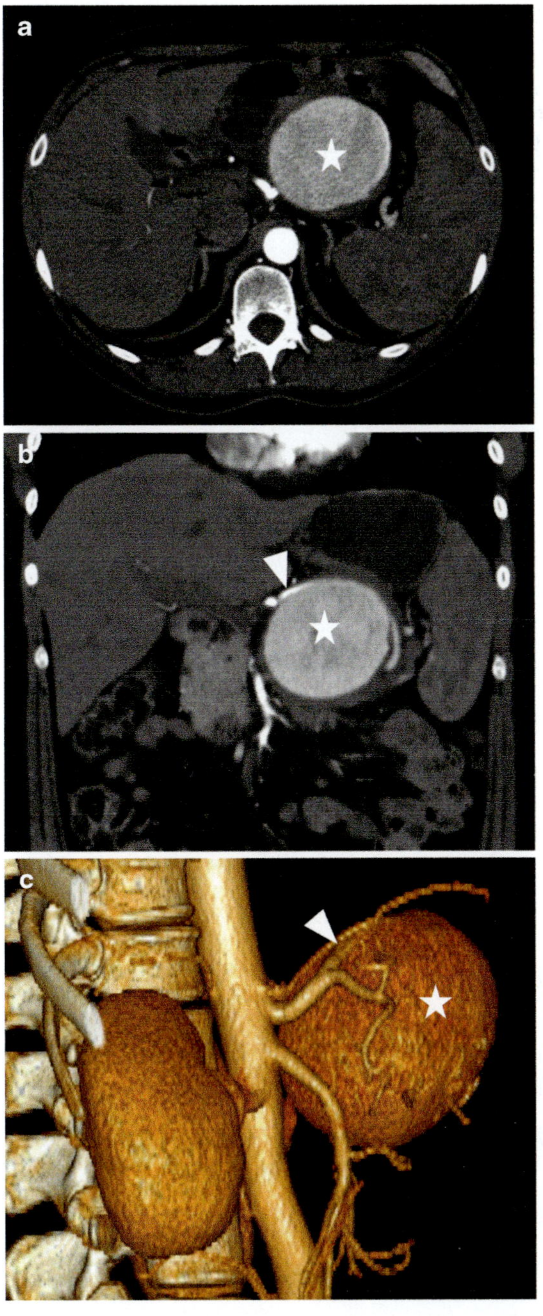

Fig. 1.6 Axial (**a**) and coronal (**b**) CT images show a large enhancing aneurysm (star) arising from the splenic artery (arrowhead). VR image (**c**) again shows the large splenic artery aneurysm (star) and better defines its relationship with splenic artery (arrowhead)

MR angiography also allows for the quantification of blood flows in terms of direction and velocity. Datasets can be acquired in 3D or as stacks of 2D images, containing all the vessels in the volume of interest. When 3D datasets are acquired, post-processing can obtain reconstruction in any projection.

MRA sequences are mainly divided into two groups: contrast and non-contrast MR angiography (Fig. 1.7). Acquiring MRA without the need for contrast injection is extremely useful, especially in patients with impaired renal function. Nevertheless, when contrast agent is used, it is usually a gadolinium chelate, always 'safer' compared to iodinated contrast agents.

MRA has the incredible added value of providing information about vessels, but not only: thanks to the MR imaging ability of characterizing tissues, detailed information can be obtained even regarding the vessel walls (Fig. 1.8) and thrombi and, in general, about surrounding tissues.

1.4.1 Non-contrast MR Angiography (Flow-Based MRA)

Blood flows often create artefacts which can influence and weaken image quality. On the other hand, these same artefacts can be used to develop noninvasive imaging techniques with no need for contrast agent injection [19]. There are few main 'flow effect' categories which must be cited because they can be advantageously used to obtain MRA sequences:

- 'Amplitude effect' or time of flight (TOF) takes advantage from blood proton flow inside a volume of interest, where surrounding static tissue have been saturated so that they cannot produce signal. Therefore, only moving protons, specifically, the protons of blood subject to a movement, will generate signal.

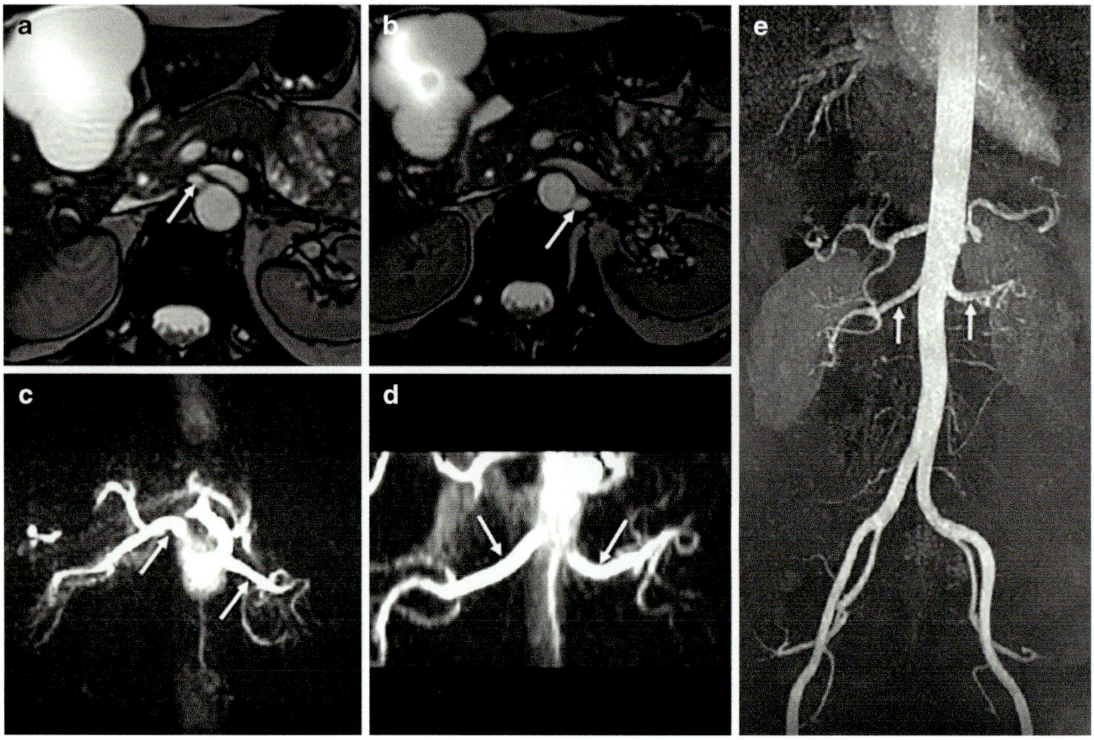

Fig. 1.7 Axial-balanced MR images (**a**, **b**) show the origin of the left and right renal arteries (arrow). Axial (**c**) and coronal (**d**) MIP reconstructions of phase-contrast images clearly depict both renal arteries without contrast medium administration. MIP reconstruction of images obtained during administration of contrast medium (**e**) renal arteries is indicated by arrows

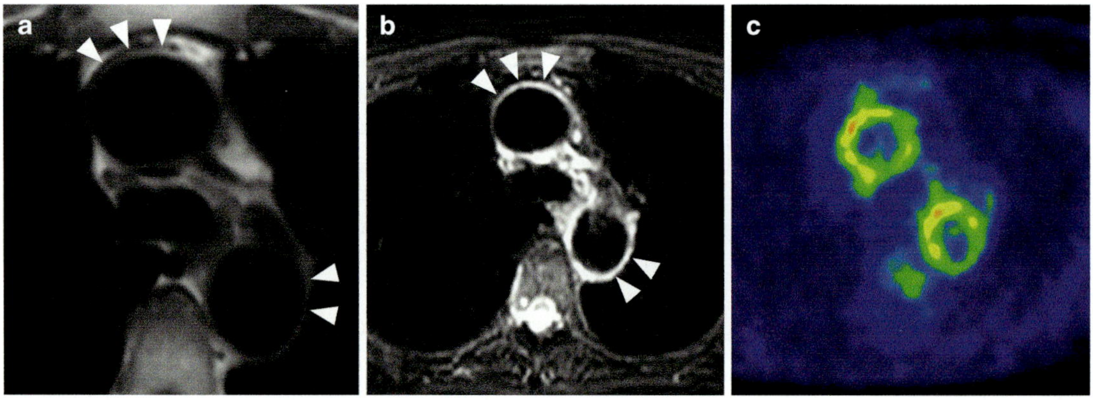

Fig. 1.8 50-year-old female with giant cell arteritis. Proton density (PD) image (**a**) shows arterial wall thickening (arrowheads). Arterial wall is hyperintense in STIR MR image (**b**) indicating the presence of oedema and inflammation. FDG-PET study (**c**) depicts increased metabolic activity of the vessel wall

- Phase-contrast effect (PC) takes advantage of the detection of changes in phase of the transverse magnetization of blood protons flowing along the direction of a magnetic field compared to stationary protons.
- The so-called signal void phenomenon is something to be aware of: it consists in the lack of signal from protons moving outside the field of view (which is the area we are studying). On the contrary, when blood flow is turbulent, protons can move back to the voxel where they originally were giving signal.

Different non-contrast MRA techniques are now listed:

1. Time-of-flight (TOF) MRA:

Usually consists of a gradient echo sequence, optimized to maximize signal of vascular structures compared to the one of other anatomical structures, saturating signal from surrounding stationary tissue. Fat saturation and selective water content saturation can also help to improve signal. TOF MRA takes advantage from the 'entry slice phenomenon', also known as 'inflow enhancement', which refers to the gain of signal coming from blood protons entering the voxel.

Signal intensity is directly proportional to flow velocity and is related to vessel length and orientation. Signal will be higher if the sequence is acquired perpendicular to the major axis of the vessel.

This sequence does not allow to differentiate arterial from venous flow; therefore, the two can sometimes appear overlapped. To selectively image venous or arterial flows, TOF MRA can take advantage from the opposite flow direction of these two vascular structures, which can be differentiated using added selective saturation pulses.

TOF MRA can be:

- 2D (sequential, multislice), which consists in the sequential acquisition of single thin sections. 2D is more sensitive to slow flows and useful for venous studies. 2D TOF can also overcome respiratory motion, allowing acquisition of single or few breath-held slices at a time. The main limit of these 2D sequences is their low spatial resolution due to medium-high slice thickness compared to 3D technique [20].
- 3D (volume slab) consists in the contemporary acquisition of data from a single volume, successively subdivided into several thin slices. 3D has good spatial resolution and good signal-to-noise ratio. 3D sequences also allow for the reconstruction of images in different planes, not only in the original acquisition plane. 3D is more sensitive to quick flows and small vessels. The main 3D TOF MRA limits are related to poor sensitivity to slow flows, high sensitivity to breathing artefacts and a long acquisition time [21].

TOF MRI has been widely used for vascular study of the head and neck, especially for carotids and the Willis circle.

2. Phase-contrast sequences are gradient echo sequences based on the detection of changes to the phase of moving protons inside the vessels under study, when under the effect of a bipolar gradient. The bipolar gradient generates different changes in phase, depending on whether spins are stationary or moving: when spins are stationary, their phase variation depends only on their position; when spins are moving, phase variation depends on their position, movement direction and velocity. It is therefore important to set the right parameters before acquiring these sequences, such as the right VENC (velocity encoded), to avoid artefacts related to a wrong codification of proton velocity.

The main advantage of PC is their ability to give information on position, direction and velocity of flows. To obtain a quantitative evaluation of a flow, the acquisition needs to be perpendicular to the flow direction; then, a time-resolved curve of flow velocity can be obtained. When both the time-resolved curve of flow velocity and the sectional area of the vessel are calculated, flow can be quantified [22].

3. 4D flows are the latest version of phase-contrast sequences: a 4D flow sequence is a PC with flow-encoding resolved relative to all three dimensions of space and to the dimension of time along the cardiac cycle (3D + time = 4D). 4D flows allow retrospective placement of analysis planes at any location within the acquisition volume and calculation of blood flow through any planes of interest across the 3D volume. They can be used to derive time-averaged 3D phase-contrast MR angiography (PC-MRA). PC can be 2D or 3D as well. PC plays an important role in the study of arterial and venous malformations, as well as cardiac valvular flows [23, 24].

4. Fast imaging with steady-state precession (TrueFISP): is a sequence with a very particular high blood signal, thanks to a mixed T2/T1 weight. These sequences are very quick and allow acquisition of breath-held 3D images, with prospective synchronization. They have been widely used for renal artery study. The limit is that not only blood but also fluids have high signal [25].

Main limits of non-contrast MRA are possible overlap of arterial and venous flows, multidirectionality of flows, turbulence, respiratory and cardiac movement artefacts and high fat signal.

1.4.2 Contrast MR Angiography

Constant improvement of hardware and software allows the development of contrast-enhanced magnetic resonance angiography (CE-MRA), which is based on intravenous administration of a bolus of paramagnetic extracellular contrast agent which significantly increases blood signal intensity during its first passage due to its ability of shortening the T1. Images are acquired during the first passage of the contrast into arteries. Vessels are imaged independently from flow type (i.e. laminar, turbulent) and velocity. CE-MRA is also unaffected by flow de-phasing, which often takes place in tortuous and stenotic vessels.

CE-MRA usually consists of a 3D gradient echo (FLASH) sequence, which is very quick and can image vessels in the arterial phase before significant venous enhancement (<30 s of acquisition length).

Of fundamental importance is the correct timing of CE-MRA acquisition: images need to be coordinated with contrast arrival in the vessel of main interest. Contrast agent dose should also be limited: the dose should be kept to the minimum necessary to obtain good opacification.

All CE-MRAs require the acquisition of a pre-contrast scan and the angiographic scan (during the higher peak of enhancement inside the vessels) [26, 27].

CE-MRA can be differentiated according to different ways of acquiring images in relation to contrast agent injection:

1. Test bolus MRA: The angiographic sequence is preceded by a dynamic sequence acquired every few seconds on the vessel of interest during the injection of a small amount of contrast agent. After the acquisition of this sequence, a ROI is drawn on the central part of the vessel of interest, through dedicated software, to obtain the time of arrival of contrast agent, so that it can be used as the right timing for the acquisition of the full sequence.
2. Fluoroscopic MRA is a real-time triggering CE-MRA. A real-time sequence, located on the vessel of interest, is acquired during contrast injection, to show the contrast arrival into the vessel so that the sequence can be manually started when preferred according to the vessel opacification.
3. Bolus track, also called 'automated bolus detection' technique, is another real-time triggering CE-MRA. A real-time sequence, located on the vessel of interest, is acquired during contrast injection, and a ROI is positioned in the centre of the vessel. The scan automatically measures the intensity of the pixel in the ROI, so that when the predefined threshold is reached, the scan will automatically start to acquire the main sequence.

Irrespective of the kind of sequence used, subtraction of pre- and post-contrast images should always be completed, to obtain pictures where filled vessels only are visualized. Several reconstructions are possible starting from CE-MRA.

CE-MRA has become very popular in several contexts: for evaluation of atherosclerotic pathology involving carotid arteries, thoracic and abdominal aorta, mesenteric vessels and upper and lower extremity vessels, pre-surgical planning for kidney donors and receivers, follow-up of patients undergoing surgery (i.e. bypass), study of arterial or venous malformation and study of congenital abnormalities such as aortic coarctation.

1.4.3 Contrast Agents

There are two main categories of contrast agents (CA) used for MRA: gadolinium (Gd)-based CA and iron oxide (IO)-based CA [28, 29].

1. Paramagnetic gadolinium-based CA

Gadolinium chelates are popular contrast agents, which are of main use in clinical routine considering high availability. They are paramagnetic, which means they shorten the T1 relaxivity of tissues where they are injected. They can be further subdivided according to the ability or inability to interact with intravascular proteins.

Specifically, gadolinium CA with no capacity for protein interaction are simply extracellular, interstitial and intravascular CA, excreted and unchanged through the kidneys. Examples of these CA are Gd-BDTPA (Magnevist), Gd-DOTA (Dotarem), Gd-DTPA-BMA (Omniscan) and Gd-BT-DO3A (Gadovist).

Gadolinium CA with weak protein interaction, such as the Gd-BOPTA (MultiHance) and Gd-EOB-DTPA, can weakly and transiently interact with serum proteins, specifically albumin. Therefore, they have higher T1 relaxivity which manifests as a greater intravascular signal intensity. They show good vessel enhancement up to 50–60 min after CA injection.

Finally, the so-called blood pool CA are Gd-derived CA with a prolonged and increased intravascular signal. They are composed of two types of molecules: Gd chelates with strong protein interaction, which allows them to stay for longer inside vessels, and Gd CA with macromolecular structures whose dimension limits their extravasation.

Gadolinium safety: gadolinium has been proven to be safe, especially at low doses. A possible concern is the occurrence of nephrogenic systemic fibrosis (NSF), which is a fibrosis of unexplained origin, which has been seen in patients with impaired renal function (eGFR <30). The gadolinium retention within the body following possible transmetalation and release of free gadolinium has been hypothesized as possible cause and concern. Allergic reaction to gadolinium is possible, even though very uncommon (occurrence reported between 0.005 and 0.7%) [30].

2. Superparamagnetic iron oxide-based CA

These CA are based on ultrasmall IO particles (e.g. USPIO or gadofosveset trisodium, Vasovist, the latter no more in use). They strongly shorten T1 relaxivity, but they also have T2* effect, generating possible artefacts, especially at high-contrast doses.

1.4.4 Multiparametric MRI: Complimentary Sequences

An important characteristic of MR imaging is the possibility of pairing other kinds of sequences to standard MRA sequences. For example, T2-STIR sequences can be added when studying vascular pathology, especially inflammatory pathology, such as arthritis. T2 sequences are highly sensitive to the presence of oedema, which appears as hyperintensity of signal within a structure. Proton density and T1 sequences may also help characterize pathologic tissues, when present (such as thrombi, ulcer or fibrotic changes).

1.4.5 Reconstruction

There are several ways to manipulate and reconstruct images to obtain the overall morphology and spatial relationship of anatomical structures:

- Multiplanar reconstruction or reformation (MPR) is the process of reformatting images from the original reconstruction plane into a different orientation, without altering the MRA voxels. They allow to visualize both vessels and surrounding structures within the same image. MPRs often consist of sagittal, axial and coronal images or images orientated according to the main axes of the vascular structure of interest. Reconstructions on oblique planes are sometimes feasible, as they are extremely useful for a proper analysis of tortuous vessels.
- Maximum intensity projection (MIP) is the most popular MRA image reconstruction, allowing a bi-dimensional representation of vessels. It produces images similar to those from conventional X-ray angiography. Firstly, the reconstruction orientation should be planned (i.e. vertical, horizontal, lateral), and then MIP are obtained casting parallel rays through the 3D dataset with each pixel of the projection image plane representing the maximum signal intensity encountered along the corresponding way. They are very useful for visualizing arterial phase of contrast-enhanced MRA. On the other hand, MIP can hide some anatomical details and spatial relationship of vessels with the surroundings. Overlapping of several structures could potentially hide or mimic a significant stenosis [31].
- Volume rendering (VR) allows the visualization of all 3D data of a volume into a single 2D projection. It works on voxel intensity, creating translucent rendering of the full volumetric dataset. Usually, the operator can manually select colour, opacity and luminosity corresponding to different voxel intensities. For VR, intensity values of different structural parts of the image are given to be classified as visible or non-visible (or with a specific colour or opacity).
- Virtual intraluminal endoscopy is used to evaluate the vascular wall from the inside. It combines the feature of endoscopic viewing and cross-sectional volumetric imaging, creating a series of perspective views calculated from points inside the vasculature. These views can then be reconstructed with surface or volume rendering. This technique is not routinely used, because of its poor diagnostic advantages, despite being an advanced technique.

References

1. Berko NS, Jain VR, Godelman A, Stein EG, Ghosh S, Haramati LB. Variants and anomalies of thoracic vasculature on computed tomographic angiography in adults. J Comput Assist Tomogr. 2009;33:523–8.
2. Liu PS, Platt JF. CT angiography of the renal circulation. Radiol Clin N Am. 2010;48:347–65.
3. Budovec JJ, Pollema M, Grogan M. Update on multidetector computed tomography angiography of the abdominal aorta. Radiol Clin N Am. 2010;48:283–309.
4. Ugurel MS, Battal B, Bozlar U, Nural MS, Tasar M, Ors F, Saglam M, Karademir I. Anatomical variations of hepatic arterial system, coeliac trunk and renal arteries: an analysis with multidetector CT angiography. Br J Radiol. 2010;83:661–7.
5. Guirguis-Blake JM, Beil TL, Senger CA, Whitlock EP. Ultrasonography screening for abdominal aortic aneurysms: a systematic evidence review for the U.S. preventive services task force. Ann Intern Med. 2014;160:321–9.
6. Raman KG, Missig-Carroll N, Richardson T, Muluk SC, Makaroun MS. Color-flow duplex ultrasound scan versus computed tomographic scan in the surveillance of endovascular aneurysm repair. J Vasc Surg. 2003;38(4):645–51.
7. Moneta GL, Lee RW, Yeager RA, Taylor LM, Porter JM. Mesenteric duplex scanning: a blinded prospective study. J Vasc Surg. 1993;17:79–86.
8. Pellerito JS, Revzin MV, Tsang JC, Greben CR, Naidich JB. Doppler sonographic criteria for the diagnosis of inferior mesenteric artery stenosis. J Ultrasound Med. 2009;28:641–50.
9. Aburahma AF, Mousa AY, Stone PA, Hass SM, Dean LS, Keiffer T. Duplex velocity criteria for native celiac/superior mesenteric artery stenosis vs in-stent stenosis. J Vasc Surg. 2012;55:730–8.

10. Olin JW, Piedmonte MR, Young JR, DeAnna S, Grubb M, Childs MB. The utility of duplex ultrasound scanning of the renal arteries for diagnosing significant renal artery stenosis. Ann Intern Med. 1995;122:833–8.
11. Radermacher J, Chavan A, Bleck J, et al. Use of Doppler ultrasonography to predict the outcome of therapy for renal-artery stenosis. N Engl J Med. 2001;344:410–7.
12. Mohabbat W, Greenberg RK, Mastracci TM, Cury M, Morales JP, Hernandez AV. Revised duplex criteria and outcomes for renal stents and stent grafts following endovascular repair of juxtarenal and thoracoabdominal aneurysms. J Vasc Surg. 2009;49:827–37.
13. Gürtler VM, Sommer WH, Meimarakis G, Kopp R, Weidenhagen R, Reiser MF, Clevert DA. A comparison between contrast-enhanced ultrasound imaging and multislice computed tomography in detecting and classifying endoleaks in the follow-up after endovascular aneurysm repair. J Vasc Surg. 2013;58:340–5.
14. Bae KT. Intravenous contrast medium administration and scan timing at CT: considerations and approaches. Radiology. 2010;256:32–61.
15. Fleischmann D. CT angiography: injection and acquisition technique. Radiol Clin N Am. 2010;48:237–47.
16. Scheske JA, Chung JH, Abbara S, Ghoshhajra BB. Computed tomography angiography of the thoracic aorta. Radiol Clin N Am. 2016;54:13–33.
17. Hara AK, Paden RG, Silva AC, Kujak JL, Lawder HJ, Pavlicek W. Iterative reconstruction technique for reducing body radiation dose at CT: feasibility study. Am J Roentgenol. 2009;193:764–71.
18. Schneider G, Prince MR, Meaney JFM, Ho VB. Magnetic resonance angiography. Berlin: Springer; 2005. p. 358.
19. Korosec FR, Mistretta CA. MR angiography: basic principles and theory. Magn Reson Imaging Clin N Am. 1998;6:223–56.
20. Keller PJ, Drayer BP, Fram EK, Williams KD, Dumoulin CL, Souza SP. MR angiography with two-dimensional acquisition and three-dimensional display. Work in progress. Radiology. 1989;173:527–32.
21. Laub GA, Kaiser WA. MR angiography with gradient motion refocusing. J Comput Assist Tomogr. 1988;12:377–82.
22. Laub G, Gaa J, Drobnitzky M. Magnetic resonance angiography techniques. Electromedica. 1998;66:68–75.
23. Dyverfeldt P, Bissell M, Barker AJ, et al. 4D flow cardiovascular magnetic resonance consensus statement. J Cardiovasc Magn Reson. 2015;17:72.
24. Vasanawala SS, Hanneman K, Alley MT, Hsiao A. Congenital heart disease assessment with 4D flow MRI. J Magn Reson Imaging. 2015;42:870–86.
25. Deshpande VS, Shea SM, Laub G, Simonetti OP, Finn JP, Li D. 3D magnetization-prepared true-FISP: a new technique for imaging coronary arteries. Magn Reson Med. 2001;46:494–502.
26. Lohan DG, Saleh R, Nael K, Krishnam M, Finn JP. Contrast-enhanced MRA versus nonenhanced MRA: pros and cons. Appl Radiol. 2007;36:3–15.
27. Lin J, Li D, Yan F. High-resolution 3D contrast-enhanced MRA with parallel imaging techniques before endovascular interventional treatment of arterial stenosis. Vasc Med. 2009;14:305–11.
28. Kirchin M, Runge V. Contrast agents for magnetic resonance imaging: safety update. Top Magn Reson Imaging. 2003;14:426–35.
29. Laurent S, Vander EL, Muller RN. Comparative study of the physicochemical properties of six clinical low molecular weight gadolinium contrast agents. Contrast Media Mol Imaging. 2006;1:128–37.
30. Runge VM. Safety of magnetic resonance contrast media. Top Magn Reson Imaging. 2001;12:309–14.
31. Calhoun PS, Kuszyk BS, Heath DG, Carley JC, Fishman EK. Three-dimensional volume rendering of spiral CT data: theory and method. RadioGraphics. 1999;19:745–64.

Ischaemic Preconditioning: The Rationale and Evidence-Based Outcomes

2

George Hamilton

2.1 Introduction

Reperfusion injury is a process well recognised and understood by vascular surgeons where return of arterialised blood flow to a previously ischaemic organ or tissue often results in a complex pathophysiological cascade ending in potentially irreversible cellular damage. The sequelae of this process are frequently seen in vascular surgery after reperfusion of a previously ischaemic lower limb. The resulting profoundly acute inflammatory syndrome gives rise to raised compartmental pressure within the muscles of the lower limb requiring fasciotomy. Reperfusion injury however can develop in several other surgical scenarios including coronary artery bypass grafting and other cardiac interventions, organ transplantation and major vascular surgery, in particular aortic aneurysm repair and carotid endarterectomy. Obviously in these scenarios, fasciotomy is not an option, and since the 1980s, there has been research into avoiding or at least mitigating reperfusion injury.

G. Hamilton (✉)
Royal Free London NHS Foundation Trust, London, UK

Great Ormond Street Hospital NHS Foundation Trust, London, UK

Medical School, University College London, London, UK
e-mail: g.hamilton@ucl.ac.uk

The initial focus was on treating reperfusion injury in coronary artery bypass grafting for myocardial ischaemia. This involved applying limited periods of ischaemia alternating with reperfusion before completion of a coronary artery bypass graft. This technique, known as ischaemic postconditioning, has been assessed in several clinical trials which have confirmed that infarct size can be reduced with this methodology [1]. A major drawback of this technique however is that it is highly invasive.

Following this discovery the possibility of preconditioning before the ischaemia-reperfusion insult to a target organ was explored. Remote ischaemic preconditioning was first shown to have a beneficial effect on other organs and tissues in the heart [2]. This finding generated a great deal of interest and research into the possible effects of remote preconditioning particularly as the methodology was inherently safe and non-invasive. There have been various protocols, but most commonly the remote preconditioning process involves inflation of a tourniquet or blood pressure cuff above systolic arterial pressure of the upper limb with alternating periods most commonly of 5 min of ischaemia followed by 5 min reperfusion. There have been many studies, both experimentally in animals and clinically with differing preconditioning protocols, indicating that the optimal preconditioning schedules may be different for the individual target organs.

© Springer Nature Switzerland AG 2019
Y. Tshomba et al. (eds.), *Visceral Vessels and Aortic Repair*,
https://doi.org/10.1007/978-3-319-94761-7_2

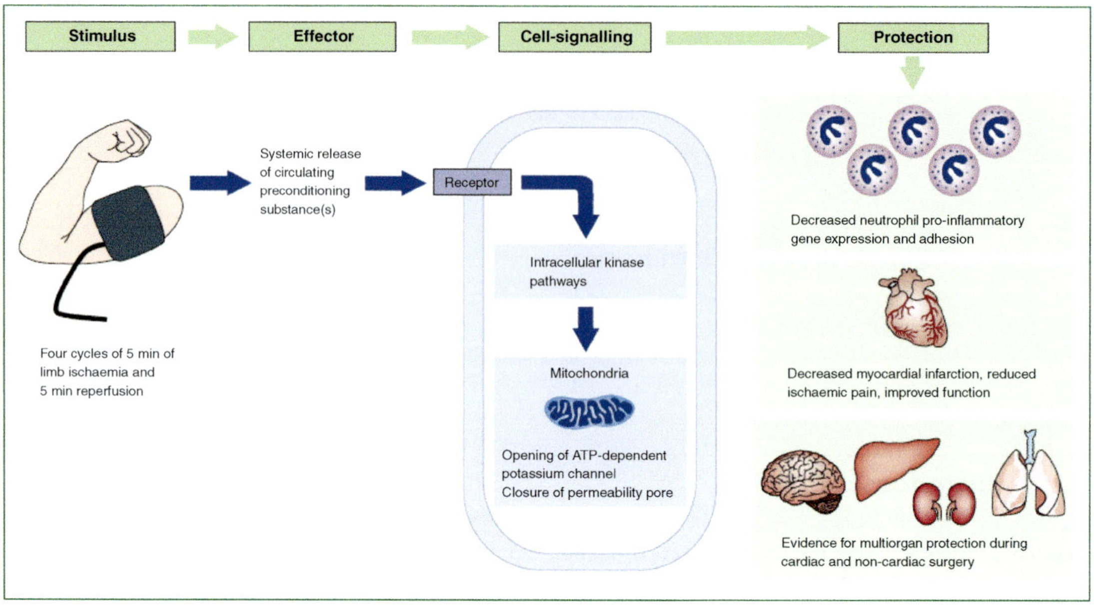

Fig. 2.1 Remote ischaemic preconditioning stimulates release of 'humoral' moieties into the circulation to modulate the potentially fatal effects of organs or tissues under prolonged ischaemia. Taken from [4]

2.2 Current Understanding of the Potential Protective Effects of Preconditioning

The pathophysiology of reperfusion injury is complex and will not be described in detail in this chapter. The central pathophysiological process is postulated to be an increase in mitochondrial permeability transition pore opening. This results in profound impairment of mitochondrial activity, ATP production and cell death. The end result of ischaemic preconditioning signalling is inhibition of this effect [3]. The protective effect of remote preconditioning implies that the molecules and mechanisms activated within the skeletal muscle of the preconditioned arm are transferred systemically to provide a similar protective effect across the body and its various organs. Two waves of effects have been identified, the first early preconditioning known as the early window of protection and the second happening over the days or weeks following known as the second window of protection.

Three major pathways have been confirmed to be involved in the early wave of protection, namely, the humeral route with release of active molecules, the neurogenic pathway with direct effects on nerve signalling on end organs and the immunological route by alteration of immune cells (Fig. 2.1). As a result of activation of the humeral and neurogenic pathways, kinase cascades are induced which will mitigate open mitochondrial permeability transition pores; the immune pathway probably works by modulation of gene and receptor expression on immune cells modulating the inflammatory response. The second window of protection also implicates release of iNOS and COX-2 [3].

2.3 Methods of Preconditioning

There are various methods described in clinical preconditioning. In cardiothoracic and vascular surgery, more invasive preconditioning techniques are possible, for example, temporary occlusion of a coronary artery in coronary artery bypass grafting or temporary occlusion of the iliac artery or other intra-abdominal arteries during open abdominal vascular surgery. With specific regard to the evidence base for vascular surgery, the immediate methodologies mostly involve clamping of one of the iliac arteries once the peritoneal cavity is opened and before the reconstructive procedure for either aneurysmal or occlusive disease takes place. A typical protocol would be clamping of the left common iliac artery for a period of 5 min with removal of the clamp and reperfusion for a further period of 5 min, and this cycle is repeated 3–5 times. An alternative is clamping of the supra-coeliac aorta with a similar schedule—obviously this requires more dissection and presents greater haemodynamic challenge to the vascular patient and the associated pathologies.

The preferred methodology involves inducing ischaemia-reperfusion cycles on the skeletal muscle most commonly of the arm or less commonly of the leg. This is achieved by placement of a tourniquet with inflation above systolic pressure. Typical schedules involve 5 min periods of occlusion followed by 5 min of reperfusion with repetition of the cycle between three and five times. In common to all of these remote preconditioning methodologies, this is performed before the definitive procedure takes place.

2.4 The Evidence for Ischaemic Preconditioning

2.4.1 Animal Studies

There is a very extensive literature on ischaemic preconditioning in animal models which are important in understanding the pathophysiology. Furthermore, the positive evidence from these animal studies is much more definitive and conclusive than that found in clinical studies. With specific regard to the effect of ischaemia-reperfusion on organs, the intestine is found to be more sensitive to the adverse effects than other internal organs [5]. Animal studies have focused on clarifying the various mechanisms involved in ischaemia reperfusion particularly focusing on neutrophilic activation of inflammatory mediators and cell apoptosis. Typical of these studies is a recent report from Gian Xi'an from China which found that ischaemic preconditioning by occlusion of the superior mesenteric artery in rats ameliorated intestinal injury. This was by attenuation of the neutrophil-endothelial adhesion cascade by reduction of ICAM-1 and VCAM-1 expression and also of the TNF-alpha-induced NF-κB signalling pathway [6].

Review of the experimental in vivo data shows an almost universal benefit for ischaemic preconditioning in all organs studied. These positive results continue to be a major driver for ongoing research to further unravel and understand the mechanisms involved.

2.4.2 The Clinical Evidence for Ischaemic Preconditioning

There is a considerable body of evidence based on clinical trials and series reporting looking primarily at its effects on the heart, brain and kidney as individual organs. There is also a respectable body of evidence with regard to its effects in vascular surgery, primarily focused on abdominal aortic aneurysm repair.

2.5 Cardiac Surgery

In common with studies in other organs, the early reports were based on measurement of surrogate markers. Since 2010 the focus is more on clinical outcomes. These primary end points were death, acute kidney injury or renal failure, stroke and non-fatal myocardial infarction. There have been several meta-analyses with the most recent reported in 2016 analysing a total of 5652 patients in 27 trials. In this meta-analysis, remote ischaemic preconditioning was found to reduce the risk of myocardial infarction from 12.6% to 10.2% (OR 0.72, 95% CI 0.52–1.00) and acute renal failure from 22.9% to 20.6% (OR 0.73, 95% CI 0.53–1.00). In addition to a reduction of composite all-cause mortality, myocardial infarction, stroke or acute renal failure from 43.2% to 39.2% (OR 0.60, 95% CI 0.39–0.90), there was also a significantly shorter stay in intensive care as well as total hospital stay. No differences were found however in mortality (OR 1.10, 95% CI 0.81–1.51) [7].

2.6 The Kidney

A recent review for the Cochrane database on "Ischaemic preconditioning for the reduction of renal ischaemia reperfusion injury" analyses all the up-to-date data. This exhaustive analysis looked at outcomes both primary and secondary with sub-analysis for the method of remote ischaemic preconditioning used and the type of surgical intervention (open abdominal vascular surgery, cardiothoracic surgery and transplantation) [3]. The outcomes identified were universally negative in the 28 studies identified. There was no protective effect for primary or secondary endpoints. In terms of the method for remote ischaemic preconditioning used, adverse effects were found in one study after invasive vascular clamping, but no adverse effects were found with cuff inflation to the arm or leg. A possible significant benefit was found in this review with a subgroup of patients who underwent invasive clamping of the arteries prior to the procedure which seemed to be more effective compared to the non-invasive cuff inflation. The review urges care in interpretation of this however since this finding was based on only three studies with one of them having a high degree of heterogeneity. This review came to the conclusion that based on up-to-date data, the routine use of remote ischaemic preconditioning in major surgery at the present time cannot be justified. The authors conclude however that further randomised controlled trials should take place with the recommendation that these should focus on surgery involving significant kidney ischaemia-reperfusion injury, in particular open abdominal aortic or kidney transplant surgery.

2.7 Vascular Surgery

There have been several clinical trials of remote ischaemic preconditioning in vascular surgery, most of which are randomised and blinded. Composite primary endpoints were used in the majority, namely, of mortality, myocardial infarction, stroke and renal and respiratory failure, in addition to measurement of troponin-1 values. The most recent studies in vascular surgery have been on an "all comers" basis including various vascular procedures such as open and endovascular abdominal aortic aneurysm repair, lower limb bypass surgery and carotid endarterectomy. A possibly important consideration in interpretation of the outcomes is the heterogeneity in the data with regard to general and anaesthetic protocols. In particular the use of propofol may have an inhibitory effect on the possible cardioprotective properties of remote ischaemic preconditioning [8].

Table 2.1 Lists of the trials specific to vascular surgery

Review of these trials universally shows no effect on myocardial injury, renal injury or clinical outcomes based on moderate to high level data with 7 out of the 11 trials being blinded prospective randomised comparisons [9–19].

There are a total of four meta-analyses of evidence for remote ischaemic preconditioning in vascular surgery [20] (Table 2.2).

The results show no benefit for either clinical outcomes or biomarkers, from remote ischaemic preconditioning for patients undergoing vascular surgery. This is true for patients having abdominal aortic aneurysm repair, carotid endarterectomy or peripheral revascularisation [21–24].

2.8 Summary

Virtually all of the available clinical evidence confirms that there is no clinically relevant benefit from remote ischaemic preconditioning for patients undergoing vascular surgery. This lack of benefit includes all of the end organs studied, namely, the heart, kidney, lungs and brain (the data for the lung and brain have not been included in this chapter) and specifically regarding any beneficial effect on the bowel or the end organs of the mesenteric circulation. There is an abundance of data however from animal studies showing significant beneficial effects of remote ischaemic preconditioning. From the animal data, we can conclude that there is a clear potential significant benefit but that this has not translated to the present clinical scenario with current protocols.

There are several possible explanatory reasons why this translation cannot be demonstrated. The first major consideration is that the in vivo studies were all performed in healthy younger animals, while obviously the human studies were in patients with multiple comorbidities. Furthermore, hyperlipidaemia and diabetes may have an attenuating effect on ischaemic preconditioning, both important comorbidities frequently present in vascular patients [25, 26].

Table 2.1 Trials specific to vascular surgery

Author	Numbers	Stimulus	Blinding	Propofol	Outcomes
Ali et al. [9]	82 AAA	Iliac clamping	Yes	Yes	Reduced biomarkers
Walsh et al. [10]	40 AAA	Iliac clamping	Yes	Yes	No difference
Murphy et al. [11]	62 AAA	Arm cuff	Yes	Yes	No difference
Li et al. [12]	62 AAA	Arm cuff	Yes	Yes	Reduced inflammatory response lung and intestines
Walsh et al. [13]	70 CEA	Leg cuff	No	Yes	No difference
Walsh et al. [14]	40 EVAR	Leg cuff	No	Yes	No difference
Healey et al. [15]	198 AAA open and EVAR, CEA, limb revascularisation	Arm cuff	No	Not known	No difference
Mouton et al. [16]	69 AAA open or EVAR	Arm cuff	Surgeons blinded	Not known	No difference
Garcia et al. [17]	201 AAA open and EVAR, CEA, limb revascularisation	Arm cuff 12–24 h before surgery	Yes	Not known	No difference
Thomas et al. [18]	85 AAA open and EVAR, limb revascularisation	Arm cuff 24 h before and then following anaesthesia	Yes	Yes	No difference
Coverdale et al. [19]	67 AAA, CEA, limb revascularisation, other	Arm cuff during GA before transfer to OR	Yes	Yes	No difference

AAA abdominal aortic aneurysm, *EVAR* endovascular aortic aneurysm repair, *CEA* carotid endarterectomy

Table 2.2 Meta-analyses of evidence for remote ischaemic preconditioning in vascular surgery

Author	Year	Trials included	Number of studies (participants[a])	Type of study	Major findings and (OR, SMD, and 95% CI)	Risk of bias from included studies
Desai et al. [21]	2011	Vascular and endovascular	4 studies (232 [115:117])	RCT	RIPC improved: Myocardial infarction[b]: (OR 0.31 [1.10–0.90] $p = 0.03$)	Low
					No improvement: Mortality: (OR 1.70 [0.91–5.92] $p = 0.39$)	
					Renal failure: (OR 0.74 [0.35–1.54] $P = 0.42$)	
					Hospital stay: (SMD − 0.12 [−2.38–2.13] $p = 0.91$)	

(continued)

Table 2.2 (continued)

Author	Year	Trials included	Number of studies (participants[a])	Type of study	Major findings and (OR, SMD, and 95% CI)	Risk of bias from included studies
Brevoord [22]	2012	Vascular, endovascular, open cardiac surgery, percutaneous cardiac intervention	23 studies (1878 [954:924])	RCT	RIPC improved: Myocardial infarction[b]: (OR 0.50 [0.31–0.82] $p = 0.005$) Peak troponin levels: (SMD – 0.28 [−0.47 to −0.09] $p = 0.003$) No improvement: Mortality: (OR 1.22 [0.48–3.07] $p = 0.68$) Renal failure: (SMD 1.88 [5.10–8.87] $p > 0.05$) Major cardiac events: (OR 0.65 [0.38–1.14] $p = 0.13$) Length of stay: (SMD 0.04 [−0.21–0.29} $p > 0.05$)	Moderate
Li et al. [23]	2013	Vascular, endovascular, open cardiac surgery, percutaneous cardiac intervention	10 studies (924 [464:460])	RCT	No improvement: Mortality: (OR 1.21 [0.49–2.97] $p = 0.68$) Renal failure: (OR 0.73 [0.50–0.64] $p = 0.18$) Length of stay: (SMD 0.07 [−0.50–0.64} $p = 0.81$)	Moderate
Takagi and Umemoto [24]	2011	Vascular and open cardiac	9 studies (488 unclear)	RCT	RIPC improved: Peak troponin levels: (SMD −0.74 [−0.97 to −0.52] $p < 0.00001$) No improvement Myocardial infarction[b]: (OR −0.02 [−0.06–0.02] $p = 0.28$) Mortality: (OR 0.01 [−0.03–0.05] $p = 0.65$)	Moderate

RCT randomised controlled trial, *RIPC* remote ischaemic preconditioning, *SMD* standardised mean difference
Ref. [20] (Twine CP, Ferguson S, Boyle JR. Review: benefits of remote ischaemic preconditioning in vascular surgery. Eur J Vasc Endovasc Surg. 2014; 48(2):215–9)
[a]Preconditioned—non-preconditioned.
[b]Defined predominantly by troponin levels

As previously discussed, the anaesthetic protocols were heterogeneous throughout these clinical trials and importantly with particular regard to the attenuating effect of propofol. Future clinical trials of remote ischaemic preconditioning in vascular surgery must include clear anaesthetic protocols designed to either exclude or assess the effects of this anaesthetic agent.

The method of remote ischaemic preconditioning has also been variable, with a confounding mixture of the predominantly upper limb and then lower limb together with less commonly intraoperative preconditioning by clamping of major vessels. Of interest there is one trial of remote ischaemic preconditioning in vascular surgery where there was an improvement in biomarkers with cross clamping of the iliac artery but which also caused four episodes of significant damage to the iliac artery [9].

This raises the hypothesis that the extent or mass of rendered tissue ischaemia may be of importance. Compared to cuffed ischaemia of an upper or lower limb, clamping of a common iliac artery will result in activation of the ischaemic reperfusion cascade throughout a much greater mass of tissue. Various authors have further postulated that cuff-based preconditioning may have an effect which is overwhelmed by the attenuation from all of the clinical factors described above. However without exception, all recent authors conclude that there should be further better defined trials of remote ischaemic preconditioning given the overwhelmingly positive evidence in the animal trials and the safety of cuffed-based ischaemic protocols. In the meantime however there is no basis to recommend the routine use of remote ischaemic preconditioning in vascular surgery outside of clinical trials.

References

1. Ovize M, Mewton N. Interventional cardiology: ischaemic POSTconditioning–a long harvest for a little corn. Nat Rev Cardiol. 2014;11:8–10.
2. Przyklenk K, Bauer B, Ovize M, Kloner RA, Whittaker P. Regional ischaemic "preconditioning" protects remote virgin myocardium from subsequent sustained coronary occlusion. Circulation. 1993;87:893–9.
3. Menting TP, Wever KE, Ozdemir-van Brunschot DM, Van der Vliet DJ, Rovers MM, Warle MC. Ischaemic preconditioning for the reduction of renal ischaemia reperfusion injury. Cochrane Database Syst Rev. 2017;3:CD010777. https://doi.org/10.1002/14651858.CD010777.pub2.
4. Kharbanda RK, Nielsen TT, Redington AN. Translation of remote ischaemic preconditioning into clinical practice. Lancet. 2009;374:1557–65.
5. Xing D, Zhang R, Li S, Huang P, Luo C, Hei Z, Xia Z, Gan X. Pivotal role of mast cell carboxypeptidase A in mediating protection against small intestinal ischemia-reperfusion injury in rats after ischemic preconditioning. J Surg Res. 2014;192:177–86.
6. Gi YY, Wang ZD, Wang SF, Wang WT, Yang ZA, Zhou XR, Lei NN, Yue WN. Ischemic preconditioning ameliorates intestinal injury induced by ischemia-reperfusion in rats. World J Gastro Enterol. 2015;21:8081–8.
7. Sardar P, Chatterjee S, Kundu A, et al. Remote ischemic preconditioning in patients undergoing cardiovascular surgery: evidence from a metanalysis of randomised controlled trial. Int J Cardiol. 2016;221:34–41.
8. Kottenberg E, Thielmann M, Bergmann L, et al. Protection by remote ischemic preconditioning during coronary artery bypass graft surgery with isoflurane but not propofol–a clinical trial. Acta Anaesthesiol Scand. 2012;56(1):30–8.
9. Ali ZA, Callaghan CJ, Lim E, et al. Remote ischemic preconditioning reduces myocardial and renal injury after elective abdominal aortic aneurysm repair: a randomized controlled trial. Circulation. 2007;116(11 suppl):I98–I105.
10. Walsh SR, Sadat U, Boyle JR, et al. Remote ischemic preconditioning for renal protection during elective open infrarenal abdominal aortic aneurysm repair: randomized controlled trial. Vasc Endovasc Surg. 2010;44(5):334–40.
11. Murphy N, Vijayan A, Frohlich S, et al. Remote ischemic preconditioning does not affect the incidence of acute kidney injury after elective abdominal aortic aneurysm repair. J Cardiothorac Vasc Anesth. 2014;28(5):1285–92.
12. Li C, Li YS, Xu M, et al. Limb remote ischemic preconditioning for intestinal and pulmonary protection during elective open infrarenal abdominal aortic aneurysm repair: a randomized controlled trial. Anesthesiology. 2013;118(4):842–52.
13. Walsh SR, Nouraei SA, Tang TY, Sadat U, Carpenter RH, Gaunt ME. Remote ischemic preconditioning for cerebral and cardiac protection during carotid endarterectomy: results from a pilot randomized clinical trial. Vasc Endovasc Surg. 2010;44(6):434–9.
14. Walsh SR, Boyle JR, Tang TY, et al. Remote ischemic preconditioning for renal and cardiac protection during endovascular aneurysm repair: a randomized controlled trial. J Endovasc Ther. 2009;16(6):680–9.
15. Healy DA, Boyle E, McCartan D, et al. A multi center pilot randomized controlled trial of remote ischemic preconditioning in major vascular surgery. Vasc Endovasc Surg. 2015;49(8):220–7.
16. Mouton R, Pollock J, Soar J, Mitchell DC, Rogers CA. Remote ischaemic preconditioning versus sham procedure for abdominal aortic aneurysm repair: an external feasibility randomized controlled trial. Trials. 2015;16:377.
17. Garcia S, Rector TS, Zakharova M, et al. Cardiac remote ischemic preconditioning prior to elective vascular surgery (CRIPES): a prospective, randomized, sham-controlled phase II clinical trial. J Am Heart Assoc. 2016;5(10):e003916.
18. Thomas KN, Cotter JD, Williams MJ, van Rij AM. Repeated episodes of remote ischemic precondi-

tioning for the prevention of myocardial injury in vascular surgery. Vasc Endovasc Surg. 2016;50(3):140–6.

19. Coverdale NS, Hamilton A, Petsikas D, McClure RS, Malik P, Milne B, Saha T, Zelt D, Brown P, Payne DM. Remote ischaemic preconditioning in high risk cardiovascular surgery patients: a randomised controlled trial. Semin Thorac Cardiovasc Surg. 2017;30(1):26–33.
20. Twine CP, Ferguson S, Boyle JR. Review: benefits of remote ischaemic preconditioning in vascular surgery. Eur J Vasc Endovasc Surg. 2014;48(2):215–9. https://doi.org/10.1016/j.ejvs.2014.05.008.
21. Desai M, Gurusamy KS, Ghanbari H, Hamilton G, Seifalian AM. Remote ischaemic preconditioning versus no remote ischaemic preconditioning for vascular and endovascular surgical procedures. Cochrane Database Syst Rev. 2011;12:CD008472.
22. Brevoord D, Kranke P, Kuijpers M, Weber N, Hollmann M, Preckel B. Remote ischemic conditioning to protect against ischemia-reperfusion injury: a systematic review and metanalysis. PLoS One. 2012;7:e42179.
23. Li L, Li G, Yu C, Li Y. The role of remote ischemic preconditioning on postoperative kidney injury in patients undergoing cardiac and vascular interventions: a meta-analysis. J Cardiothorac Surg. 2013;8:43.
24. Takagi H, Umemoto T. Remote ischemic preconditioning for cardiovascular surgery: an updated meta-analysis of randomized trials. Vasc Endovasc Surg. 2011;45:511e3.
25. Ungi I, Ungi T, Ruzsa Z, et al. Hypercholesterolaemia attenuates the anti-ischaemic effect of preconditioning during coronary angioplasty. Chest. 2005;128:1623–8.
26. Ishihara M, Inoue I, Kawagoe T, et al. Diabetes mellitus prevents ischaemic preconditioning in patients with a first acute anterior wall myocardial infarction. J Am Coll Cardiol. 2001;38:1007–11.

Part II

Abdominal Aorta

Open Repair of Pararenal Aneurysms: Renal Vessel Surgical Management

3

Daniele Mascia, Alessandro Grandi, Luca Porcellato, Luca Bertoglio, Andrea Kahlberg, Domenico Baccellieri, Germano Melissano, and Roberto Chiesa

3.1 Proximal Abdominal Aortic Aneurysms (P-AAA)

The proximal abdominal aorta constitutes a particular location for the dilative process of the aneurysms because the splanchnic vessels or the renal artery ostium may be involved. As a result, we can make a more specific classification of this type of aneurysms:

- Juxtarenal infrarenal abdominal aortic aneurysms (JR-AAA): The proximal extension of the aneurysms starts adjacent or at the lower margin of the renal artery origins, without involving them in the dilative process.
- Pararenal infrarenal abdominal aortic aneurysms (PR-AAA): One or both renal arteries are involved in the dilative process.
- Suprarenal abdominal aortic aneurysms (SR-AAA): The splanchnic arteries and the renal artery origins are involved in the dilative process.

D. Mascia (✉) · A. Grandi · L. Porcellato
L. Bertoglio · A. Kahlberg · G. Melissano
Vascular Surgery Unit, IRCCS San Raffaele Scientific Institute, Milan, Italy
e-mail: mascia.daniele@hsr.it

D. Baccellieri
Unit of Vascular Surgery, San Raffaele Scientific Institute, Milan, Italy

R. Chiesa
Unit of Vascular Surgery, San Raffaele Scientific Institute, Vita-Salute University, Milan, Italy

3.2 Epidemiology

3.2.1 Incidence

The involvement of the proximal abdominal aorta takes place in 5–15% of all AAAs [1, 2]. AAAs mostly affect the population above 50 years of age; they are two to six times more frequent in men than women and two to three times more common in people of Caucasian descent than in other populations [3–5]. Screening studies have provided us with important information on the incidence and prevalence of this disease: for men above 50 years of age, an incidence of 3.5 for 1000 people/year [6] was shown, while new-onset AAAs were discovered in only 2% of patients at a second examination performed after a mean time of 5.5 years, after a negative result upon first examination. Overall, the incidence by age of ruptured and symptomatic P-AAAs, and the mortality rate of P-AAAs, is six times greater in men than in women. A significant increase in the incidence of asymptomatic AAAs has been observed over the last two decades [7, 8], which may be due to increased diagnostic detection. However, there is emerging proof of a plateau reached by hospitalization numbers for aortic aneurysm repair, perhaps owing to health policies which are finalized to reduce the morbidity and mortality of cardiovascular diseases.

© Springer Nature Switzerland AG 2019
Y. Tshomba et al. (eds.), *Visceral Vessels and Aortic Repair*,
https://doi.org/10.1007/978-3-319-94761-7_3

3.2.2 Prevalence

The asymptomatic prevalence estimate of TAAA (probability of being an AAA carrier) is more accurate compared to the incidence estimate (probability of developing AAA), now that duplex ultrasound screenings are performed on numerous populations. The duplex ultrasound screening studies on the population offer the most accurate information for the prevalence of AAA (>3 cm). Those studies have been conducted both as epidemiologic screening studies (Tromso and Rotterdam) and as randomized studies to evaluate the benefits of the screening itself [Multicentric Aneurysm Screening Study (MASS), Chichester, Viborg, Western Australia]. In Veteran Affairs, a screening study of more than 73,000 patients between 50 and 79 years of age was carried out. The AAA ≥3 cm prevalence was 4.6%, and the AAA ≥4 cm prevalence was 1.4% [9]. The reported prevalence varies according to age and gender. The highest AAA ≥3 cm prevalence was 5.9% that was found in a subpopulation of white males with smoking habits between 50 and 79 years of age [10].

3.3 Preoperative Analysis

3.3.1 Clinical Presentation and Indication for Surgery

AAA is generally a pathology found by chance, as the majority of cases are found to be asymptomatic. Any symptoms related to a locoregional compression by the aneurysm are rare, as there are no structures and organs that suffer the aneurysmal dilation. Ischemic symptoms related to embolization for the crushing of the thrombus near the walls of the aneurysm are even rarer. A typical clinical sign is the appreciation of a pulsating mass in the epi-mesogastrium synchronous with the cardiac cycle, particularly in aneurysms of a certain size and in people of slim build. From a semiotic perspective, the suspicion of a pararenal aneurysm must be present when, during the physical examination, the upper pole of the aneurysmal dilation is not palpable at the arch rib (DeBakey maneuver). In the case of AAAs, the indication for elective surgery arises for aneurysms with a diameter >55 mm, even if intervention must be taken into account for smaller diameters in case of rapid growth and morphological aspects indicating a high risk of ruptures, such as highly eccentric thrombotic material, protrusions (blisters), or even parietal fissures. Currently, the diameter of the aorta is the best criteria for predicting the risk of aortic rupture [11]. According to a study by Juvonen et al., each increase of 1 cm in the diameter of abdominal aortic aneurysms is related to a 1.9-fold increase of the relative risk of rupture [12]. Lo et al. showed that the risk of aortic rupture is precisely calculated, by taking the area of the patient's body surface area (BSA) [13] into account.

3.3.2 Diagnostic Imaging

The use of imaging techniques is crucial in the assessment of AAAs, both to confirm the clinical diagnostic suspicion and to precisely define the critical morphological characteristics indicating surgery.

3.3.2.1 Duplex Ultrasound

The transabdominal ultrasonography is the least invasive examination and more frequently applied, in particular for screening and follow-up. Vessel diameter is measured by ultrasonography, allowing for an inter-operator variability of around 5 mm in 84% of studies, and is more accurate in assessing the anteroposterior than the transverse [14] diameter. The display of the suprarenal aorta and the iliac arteries may be impeded by anatomical characteristics, particularly in obese patients. In such cases, the ultrasound cannot accurately determine the presence of rupture [15] and is often not able to precisely determine the proximal extension of AAA [16]. Ultrasound typically underestimates the anteroposterior diameter of an AAA by 2–4 mm [17–20]. In general, ultrasound is used to diagnose and monitor the AAA until the aneurysm nears a typically operable diameter size. At this point, secondary examinations are required.

3.3.2.2 CT Angiography

The abdominal aorta CT angiography must be performed with an acquisition thickness of 1.25 mm or less, depending on the available CT technology (Fig. 3.1). The overlap (in particular sections, the interval is half of the actual thickness) is recommended to increase the quality of multiplanar images (MPR) and 3D visualization. This phase, without contrast medium, allows for the evaluation of potential wall calcification or the presence of prosthetic aortic grafts in already operated patients. Aneurysms of 3–4.5 cm in diameter require 12-month follow-up with CT scan. This intervention is highly recommended when the diameter increases by 5 mm or more within 6 months or in cases of diameters larger than 55 mm. The CT angiography has become essential for surgical planning [21]. The executive protocol of a CT with contrast enhancement at our center involves the intravenous injection of a high concentration of iodized agent (370–400 mg/mL) at a high flow rate (4–5 mL/s) to obtain a prolonged opacification of the vessels [22]. The interpretation of the CT findings is based on the analysis of a combination of axial images and reformatted images. For some years now, several software applications are available (freeware, OsiriX MD, Pixmeo; paid, TeraRecon, TeraRecon, Inc.) to view and analyze DICOM (Digital Imaging and Communications in Medicine) files, which is the most common format used in medical imaging. This software allows you to automatically download files from any DICOM CD-ROM, regardless of the hospital or the country of origin and rescale. If the acquired images are of sufficient quality, these studies allow a proper assessment, avoiding replication of the CT. The vascular surgeon, who will perform the endovascular or surgical procedure, is personally involved in the assessment of the aortic images and in planning/sizing the case. For the pre-procedural assessment, in addition to morphological information, such as diameter and extension of the aneurysm, angiography provides other fundamental anatomical information such as:

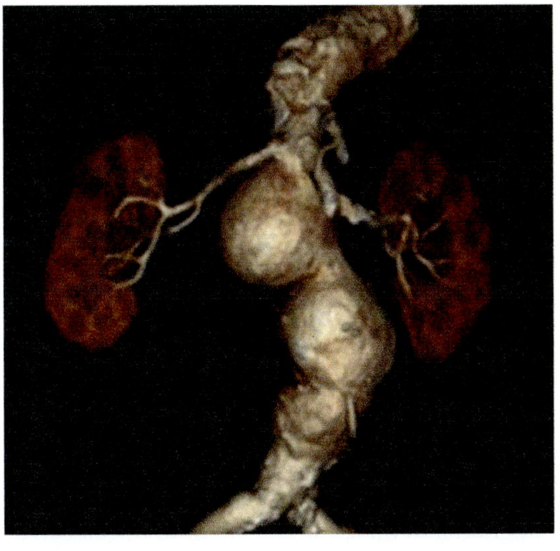

Fig. 3.1 3D reconstruction of a juxtarenal infrarenal abdominal aortic aneurysm

- The quality of the aortic wall
- The involvement of visceral vessels and iliac arteries
- Clamping locations
- Left renal vein (anterior, posterior, or double)
- Visceral vessel-associated diseases (stenosis, occlusion, anatomical abnormalities, such as the "double cluster," hypoplasia)
- Extravascular-associated diseases (pelvic kidney and horseshoe kidney)

The images acquired from CT angiography are equally essential for a thorough follow-up, to recognize quickly and subsequently treat potential complications.

3.3.2.3 MRI

The absence of exposure to ionizing radiation makes the use of magnetic resonance imaging (MRI) for diagnosis and subsequent controls of P-AAAs an apparently advantageous choice compared to CT. Magnetic resonance angiography is comparable to the CT angiography in many aspects but has some shortcomings: the lack of visualization of calcified plaques—it typically owns half of the spatial resolution; it has longer acquisition times and creates more problems for claustrophobic patients, but it can be useful in cases of allergy to iodinated contrast. However, its high cost and limited diffusion do not make it the first choice.

3.3.3 Preoperative Risk Stratification and Patient Optimization

Surgical repair of a proximal abdominal aortic aneurysm is considered a high-risk intervention. Clamping the aorta carries significant hemodynamic stress, which is the reason careful assessment of cardiac, lung, and kidney function is required to determine the eligibility of patients for intervention. Often patients with abdominal aortic aneurysm have comorbidities, such as ischemic heart disease (16–30%), respiratory problems, and kidney failure [23].

3.3.3.1 Heart Function

The European Society of Cardiology (ESC) has recently developed guidelines aimed at helping the choice for a more efficient approach to preoperative evaluation [24]. Vascular interventions are of particular interest because they will involve a significant risk of cardiac complications. These guidelines propose an algorithm to identify patients with a significant risk of cardiac complications during elective surgery. The gradual approach advocated by the ESC has more than one step. The first one is the identification of active heart disease: unstable angina pectoris, recent myocardial infarction (within 30 days), residual myocardial ischemia, acute heart failure, symptomatic valvular disease, and significant cardiac arrhythmias. The second step is the evaluation of functional capacity, which is measured in metabolic equivalents (MET). The third step is the evaluation of the specific risk for surgical procedures. Aortic surgery is considered at high risk (rate of cardiac events at 30 days >5) [25]. It is also important to assess the risk factors in patients with low functional capacity. If there are up to two risk factors, patients can proceed to the intervention, providing a treatment with statins and beta-blockers (including ACE inhibitors in the presence of left ventricular systolic dysfunction are needed). The fourth step is the execution of a noninvasive stress test in patients with a low functional capacity and more than two risk factors, which are scheduled for surgery.

The transthoracic echocardiography is an important noninvasive screening test that assesses the valve function. Coronary CT angiography is becoming the alternative less-invasive method for the visualization of the anatomy of the coronary arteries. The new multi-detector of CT angiography, built to reduce radiation, uses the acquisition of related ECG images allowing us to obtain images of specific phases of the cardiac cycle. In patients with asymptomatic disease, a severe occlusive disease of the coronary arteries can be treated with percutaneous transluminal angioplasty before proceeding to repair the aneurysm.

3.3.3.2 Renal Function

The renal function is traditionally calculated by measuring levels of creatinine, serum electrolytes, and blood urea nitrogen (BUN). These indices are quite sensitive, especially in patients with intermediate and moderate degrees of renal dysfunction. The National Kidney Foundation recommends the use of estimated glomerular filtration rate (GFR) to evaluate kidney function and avoid misclassification based on only one level of serum creatinine [26]. Based on the assessment of GFR, chronic kidney disease has proven to be a strong predictor factor of death after the surgical treatment of abdominal aortic aneurysms, even in patients without clinical evidence of preoperative renal disease. CT angiography, MRI, and ultrasound determine the kidneys' size and renal anatomy. The classification KDOQI has identified five levels of kidney function, based on GFR values. There is also evidence that low levels of GFR and high levels of albuminuria independently correlated with mortality, cardiovascular events, and the probability of progression to kidney failure. This is the reason the latest guidelines suggest the integration of the GFR and albuminuria study for a more accurate assessment of renal function. Of great interest are the data in a meta-analysis conducted by the Chronic Kidney Disease Prognosis Consortium, in which the independent and combined association of the GFR and albuminuria on cardiovascular mortality and on all-cause of death in the general population were evaluated. Compared with a GFR of 95 mL/min, the relative risk of death from all causes was increased by 18% for GFR of 60 mL/min and 57% for GFR of 45 mL/min and was more than tripled for GFR of 15 mL/min. Similarly, the risk-related albuminuria followed linear growth, no threshold effect, and it was already significant at low values of albuminuria or in the presence of traces of proteinuria. Similar results were also found for mortality from all causes. In conclusion, GFR and albuminuria are independent predictors and risk multipliers of mortality in the general population, with no evidence of interactions [27].

3.3.3.3 Respiratory Function

Potential risk factors for respiratory failure are age, gender, aneurysm size, preoperative lung function calculated through the forced expiratory volume in 1 s (FEV1), forced vital capacity (FVC), the relationship between these two units (FEV1/FVC), comorbidities and operative parameters (such as when an extended incision is requested, when there is a left hemi-diaphragm paralysis, or when there is the necessity for a high number of transfusions), timing of aortic clamping operators, and postoperative complications (in addition to the lung, even kidney, failure, bleeding, and infection of surgical wounds). Pre-, intra-, and postoperative blood tests (creatinine, BUN, lactic dehydrogenase, pH) are also important. A standard chest X-ray reveals unexpected abnormalities in approximately 5% of patients between 40 and 60 years and in 6–30% of patients over 60 years. The abnormalities include tracheal deviation, deviation of the left main bronchus, lung or mediastinal masses, lung bubbles, pulmonary edema, pneumonia, atelectasis, fractures of the vertebrae or ribs, cardiomegaly, and dextrocardia. The evaluation of lung function with spirometry and arterial blood gas test is used in all patients who undergo open surgery. The reduction in FEV1 or other spirometric indicators of pulmonary function not within the limits, in addition to arterial blood gas analysis abnormalities, such as hypoxemia or hypercapnia, suggests that the patient is at high risk for the development of postoperative pulmonary complications.

3.4 Surgical Technique

Open surgery for P-AAA is a major vascular procedure with significant mortality and morbidity rates, mostly with regard to renal function. A radial arterial pressure line is always inserted in order to guarantee continuous intraoperative arterial blood pressure monitoring. A central venous catheter (jugular or subclavian) is inserted to rapidly administer medications and fluids and to monitor central venous pressure.

Temperature is monitored by means of a bladder or nasopharyngeal sensor and is used to guide hypothermia when the hypothermic perfusion of renal arteries is required or where long-lasting procedural time or large bleeding may be expected.

Intraoperative transesophageal echocardiography (TEE) enables the dynamic monitoring of hemodynamic status assessing the systolic and diastolic function, ejection fraction, wall motion, dyssynchrony, and valvular function in patients with increased cardiac risk or who develop unexpected nonreversible intraoperative hypotension.

3.4.1 Transperitoneal Access

The patient is usually in a supine position. A median laparotomy from the xiphoid to the symphysis pubis is routinely performed; in patients with specific concerns such as previous median laparotomies, severe obesity, or other technical issues, bilateral subcostal laparotomy may be the alternative (Fig. 3.2). With this access, however, the distal control of iliac arteries is more challenging, and it should be avoided in cases of associated iliac aneurysms. In cases of very large aneurysms, transperitoneal medial

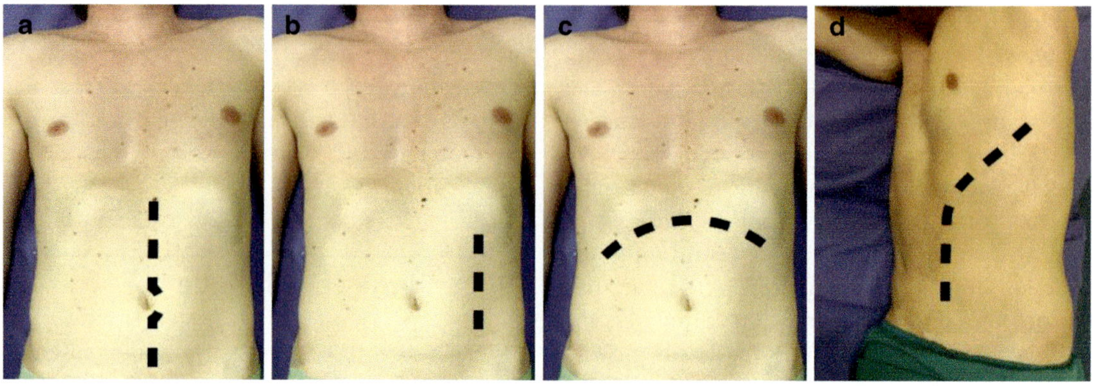

Fig. 3.2 (**a**) Xipho-pubic laparotomic access, (**b**) pararectal laparotomy, (**c**) bilateral subcostal laparotomy access, and (**d**) thoraco-phreno-laparotomy access

visceral rotation is helpful to obtain adequate exposure and proximal aortic control.

3.4.2 Retroperitoneal Access

The patient is positioned in partial right lateral decubitus. The left shoulder is fixed vertically, the pelvis is rotated toward the horizontal plane, and the table broken. The incision usually extends from the lateral border of the left rectus muscle anteriorly to the erector spinae in the eighth intercostal space to the area of the umbilicus. The level and the extent of the incision depend on the patient's anatomy and required exposure. In extensive pathology, a thoraco-phreno-laparotomy may be performed.

3.4.3 Aortic Clamping and Reconstruction

In the preparation of the pararenal aorta, correct management of the left renal vein is mandatory. Usually collocated anteriorly to the aorta, the left renal vein can be mobilized to obtain a greater proximal exposition of the aorta, dividing the gonadic, surrenali, and lumbar ramifications (Fig. 3.3). Alternatively, the left renal vein can be sectioned close to the inferior vena cava; unfortunately, this type of approach increases the postoperative renal insufficiency (Fig. 3.4).

The proximal aortic cross-clamping site is, along with aortic reconstruction technique, the most important issue in the surgical treatment of P-AAA. Suprarenal and supra-celiac clamping (Fig. 3.5) are possibilities. The correct choice depends on the proximal extension of the aneurysm, its morphology, and on the ease of exposing the suprarenal aorta. Sometimes, supra-celiac clamping, especially in inflammatory aneurysm, re-treatment, and emergency treatment can be technically manageable compared to suprarenal one. The need for supra-celiac clamping must be brought forward as much as possible, based on the preoperative imaging, and the presence of extensive calcifications or thrombotic material in pararenal aorta highlighted.

Systemic heparinization is administered before aortic cross-clamping in order to achieve activated clotting time (ACT) of >200 s. Thromboembolism from pararenal aorta to renal arteries is a well-known complication and can be prevented by renal artery cross-clamping before aortic manipulation and clamping. Common iliac arteries and aorta are then cross-clamped. The aneurysm is entered, thrombus is removed, and back-bleeding from lumbar arteries is quickly controlled by the ligation of the ostia (2/0 polypropylene suture reinforced by Teflon pledgets). If the inferior mesenteric artery is patent, it is temporarily clamped with a bulldog clamp, as previously described.

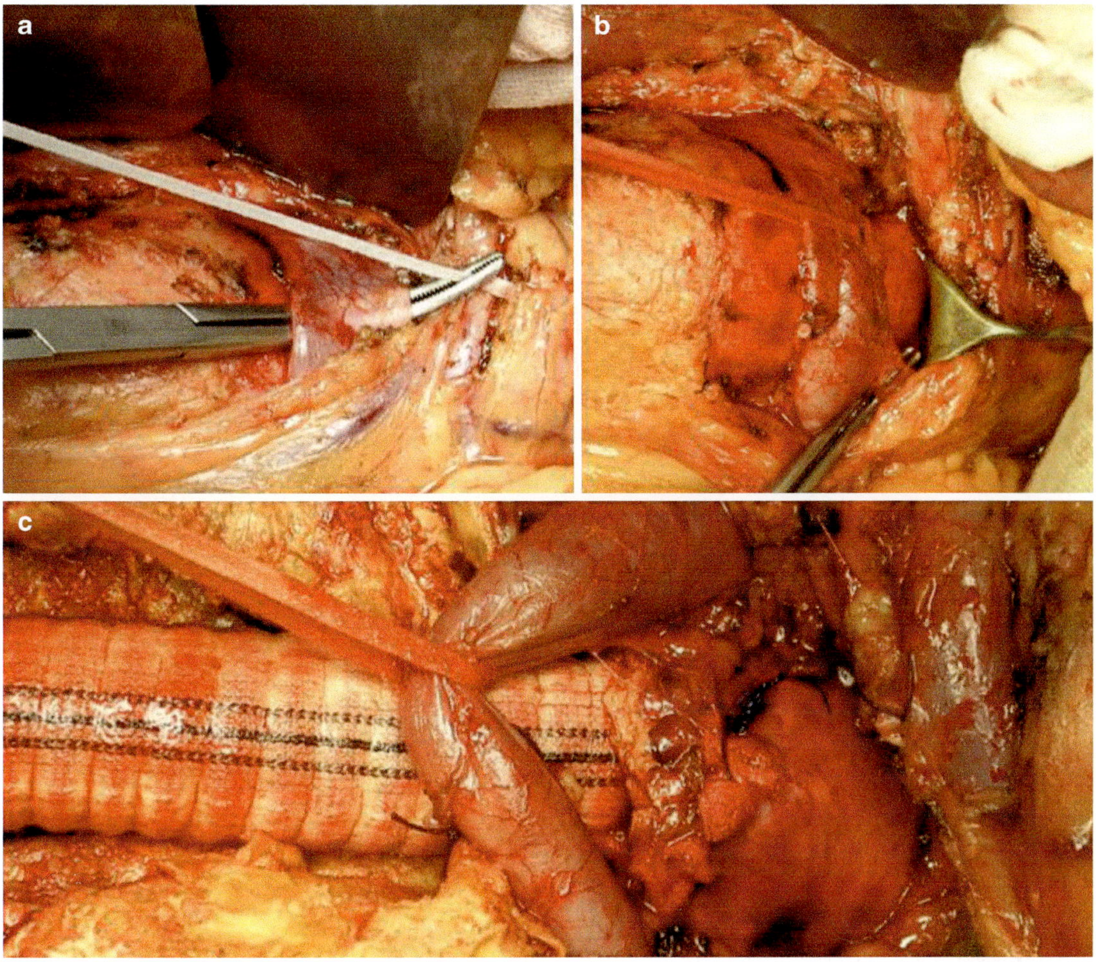

Fig. 3.3 Intraoperative photographs showing the correct steps to mobilize the left renal vein without damaging it

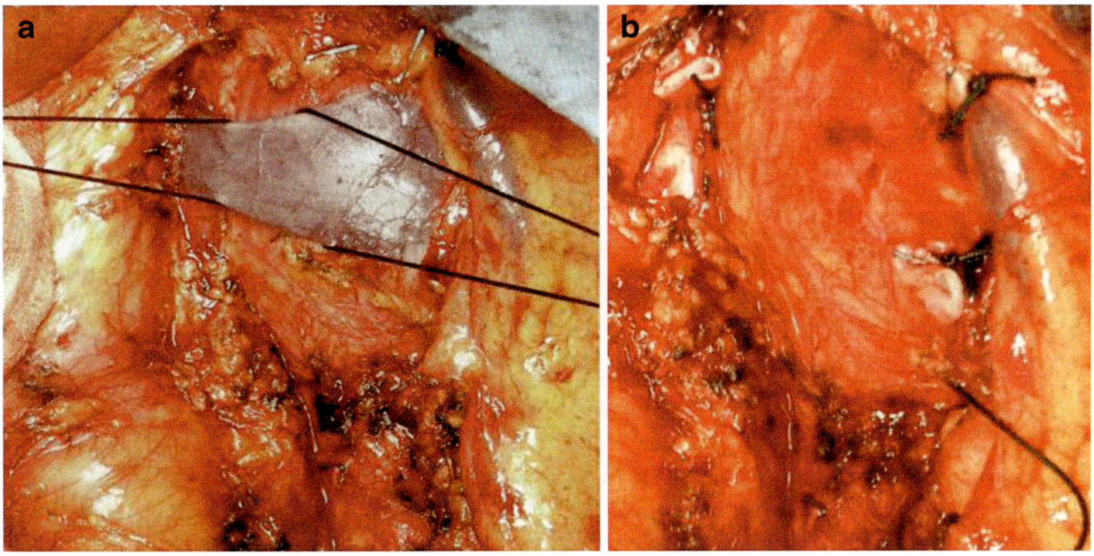

Fig. 3.4 Intraoperative photographs showing the correct steps to section the left renal vein

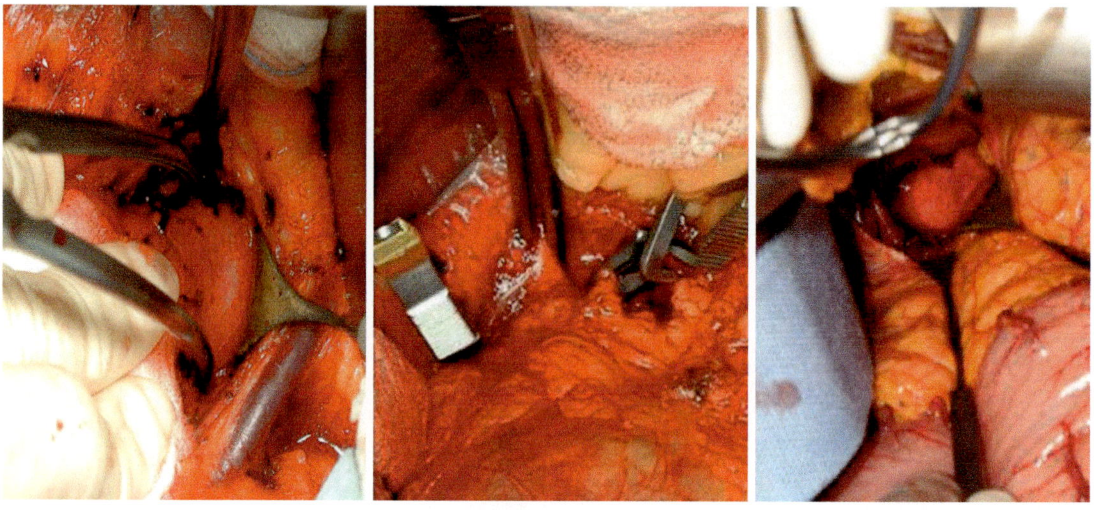

Fig. 3.5 Different clamping sites. From left to right: infrarenal, suprarenal, supra-celiac

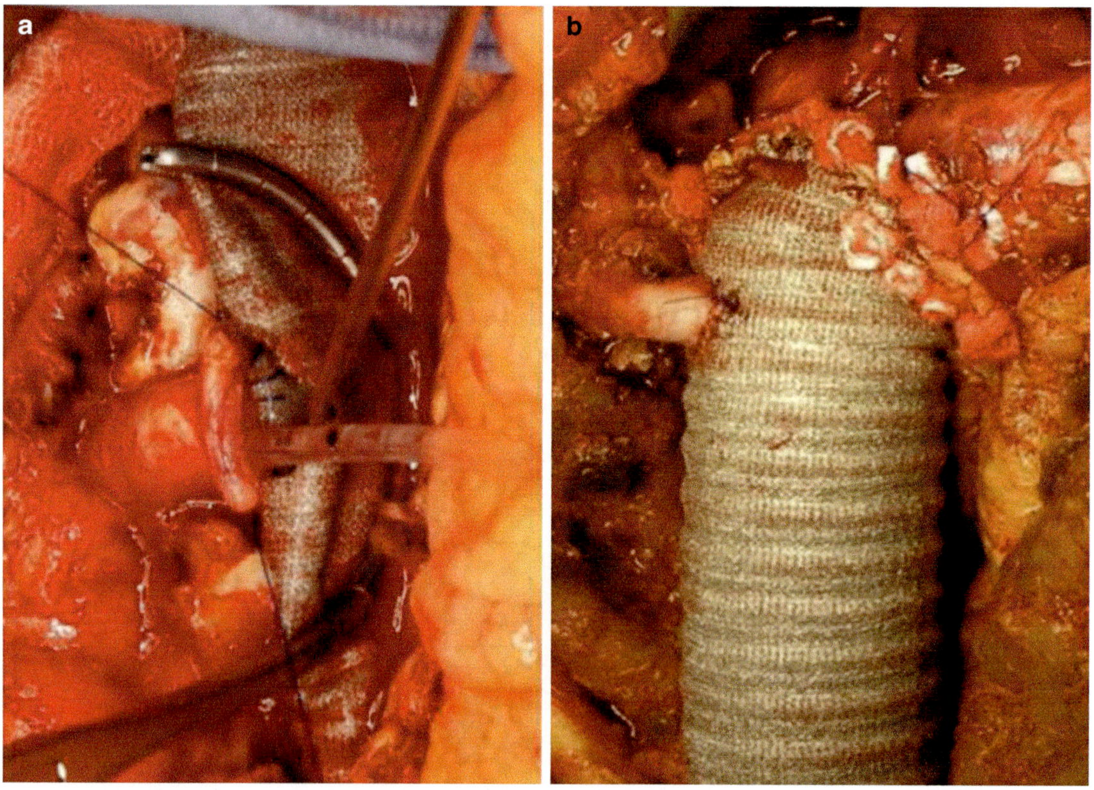

Fig. 3.6 Intraoperative pictures showing (**a**) the right renal artery being perfused while the anastomosis to the aortic graft is completed and (**b**) the final result of a direct renal artery reattachment to the aortic graft

In the case of renal artery involvement with no option of infrarenal aortic reconstruction, we put various strategies in place:

- Aorto-aortic repair with proximal end-to-end anastomosis and direct renal reattachment to the aortic graft (Fig. 3.6)

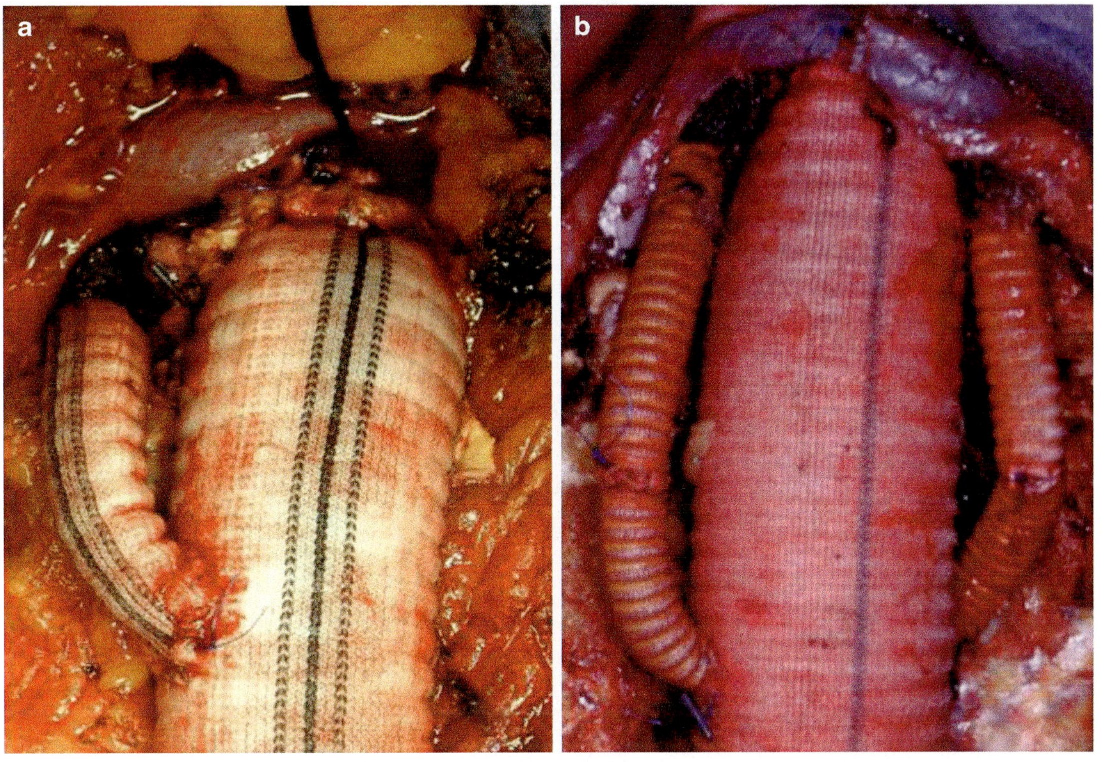

Fig. 3.7 Intraoperative pictures showing aorto-aortic repair with proximal end-to-end anastomosis and (**a**) uni- or (**b**) bilateral aorto-renal bypass grafting

- Aorto-aortic repair with proximal end-to-end anastomosis and uni- or bilateral aorto-renal bypass grafting (Fig. 3.7)
- Aorto-aortic repair with proximal end-to-end anastomosis and uni- or bilateral aorto-renal bypass grafting using a Gore Hybrid graft, inserting the stent in the side into the renal artery, deploying it, and then reinforcing it with four single sutures (Figs. 3.8 and 3.9)
- A proximal beveled anastomosis that includes renal arteries
- Carrel's patch including visceral vessels (celiac trunk, superior mesenteric, and renal arteries) that may be performed by means of a thoraco-phreno-laparotomy or through bilateral subcostal laparotomy with medial visceral rotation

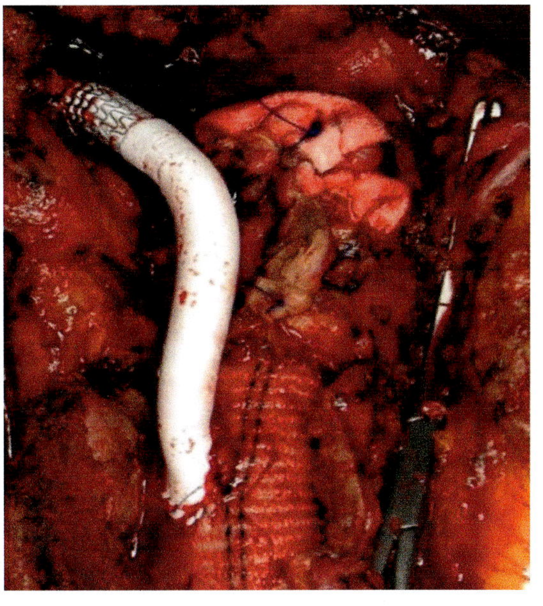

Fig. 3.8 Aorto-aortic repair with proximal end-to-end anastomosis and aorto-renal bypass grafting using a Gore Hybrid graft, inserting the stent in the side into the renal artery, deploying it, and then reinforcing it with four single sutures

3.5 Complications

The perioperative complications are not rare events in the surgical repair of the P-AAAs. It is clear that the perioperative management is crucial

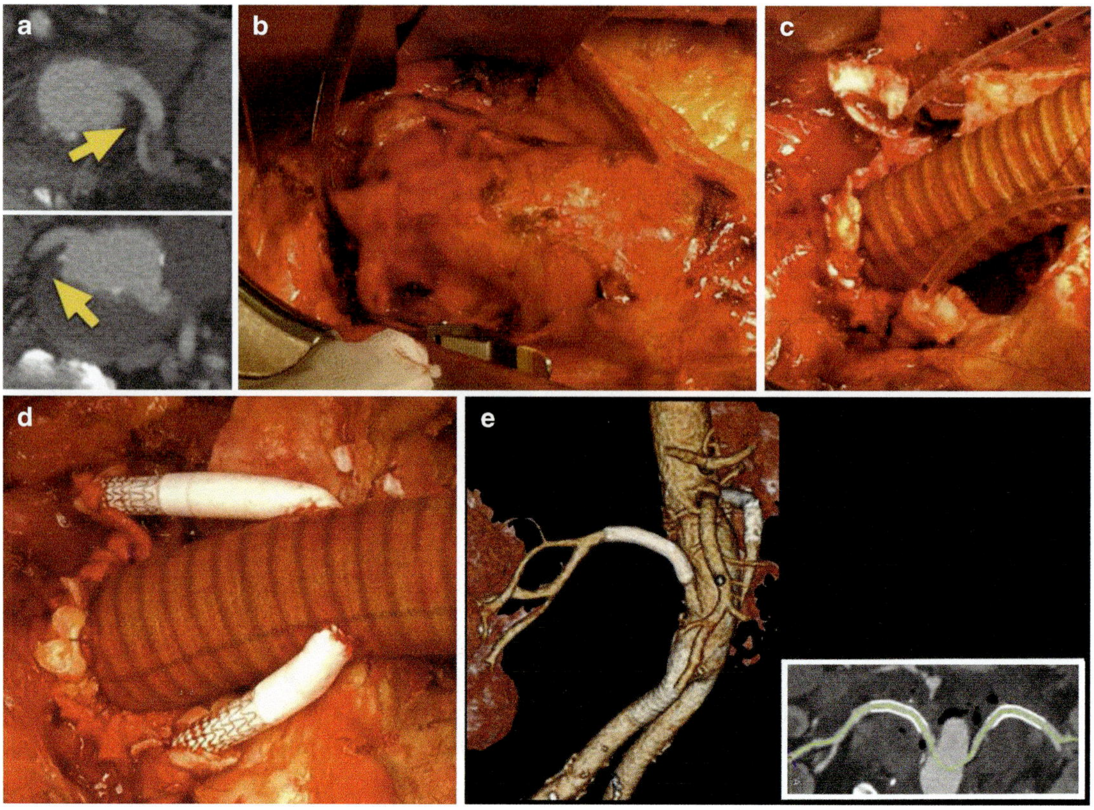

Fig. 3.9 (**a**) Preoperative CT scan showing thrombus close to the ostium of the renal arteries and a dissection of the right renal artery, (**b**) intraoperative picture showing the juxtarenal aortic aneurysm, (**c**) intraoperative picture showing the end-to-end proximal anastomosis and the two renal arteries being selectively perfused, (**d**) intraoperative picture showing renal artery reconstruction with a Gore Hybrid bypass graft, (**e**) postoperative CT scan showing the renal arteries reimplanted on the graft using the Gore Hybrid bypass graft

in reducing postoperative complications. A team of professionals is needed with experience in this type of work, not only from a strictly surgical point of view but also anesthetic and nursing [28, 29].

3.5.1 Bleeding

Because of the type of aneurysmectomy P-AAAs, patients are subject to increased risk of bleeding in the perioperative period. Meticulous attention to hemostasis is essential to minimize the risk of postoperative bleeding, and the surgeon must pay close attention to the fact that there is no active bleeding before closing the retroperitoneum or abdomen. All anastomoses must be checked and all surfaces thoroughly examined. The therapy with blood components should be used to correct the coagulopathy that inevitably occurs. Similarly, topical hemostatic agents can be of great value in treating bleeding of the anastomosis. Despite all, postoperative bleeding can still occur.

The causes of bleeding can be:

- Bleeding from the anastomosis
- Dripping from the wall
- Bleeding from retrograde lumbar branches inadequately controlled
- Insult spleen, often secondary to the use of retractors

3.5.2 Cardiac ischemia

As described above, aortic clamping causes significant hemodynamic disturbances and creates an increase in cardiac workload. Preoperative screening, risk stratification, and appropriate patient selection may help to reduce this. The use of beta-blockers, in the perioperative period, in patients undergoing non-high-risk cardiac surgery, has been shown to reduce cardiovascular events and mortality at 30 days [30–32]. The administration of beta-blockers is associated with a significant reduction in peri- and postoperative mortality [33].

3.5.3 Kidney Failure

Patients undergoing surgical repair of P-AAA have a significant risk of developing kidney complications (Figs. 3.10 and 3.11). The percentage of postoperative renal failure in Medicare rises to 10% study, although with only 0.5% needing renal replacement therapy [34]. A meta-analysis of patients undergoing elective surgery for aortic pararenal aneurysmectomy showed the presence of postoperative renal failure in 15–20% of patients, of which only 3.5% require dialysis [35]. The acute tubular necrosis secondary to renal hypoperfusion is the leading cause of acute renal failure in these patients and occurs because of the important hemodynamic changes that the aortic clamping causes to the renal blood flow, as well as hypovolemia and perioperative hypotension. Particular attention should be paid to blood volume and to the use of crystalloid and colloid during the perioperative period as they are essential in the prevention of recurrent episodes of renal ischemia and for tackling the negative effects of aortic clamping. Despite the evidence that few patients need continuous renal replacement

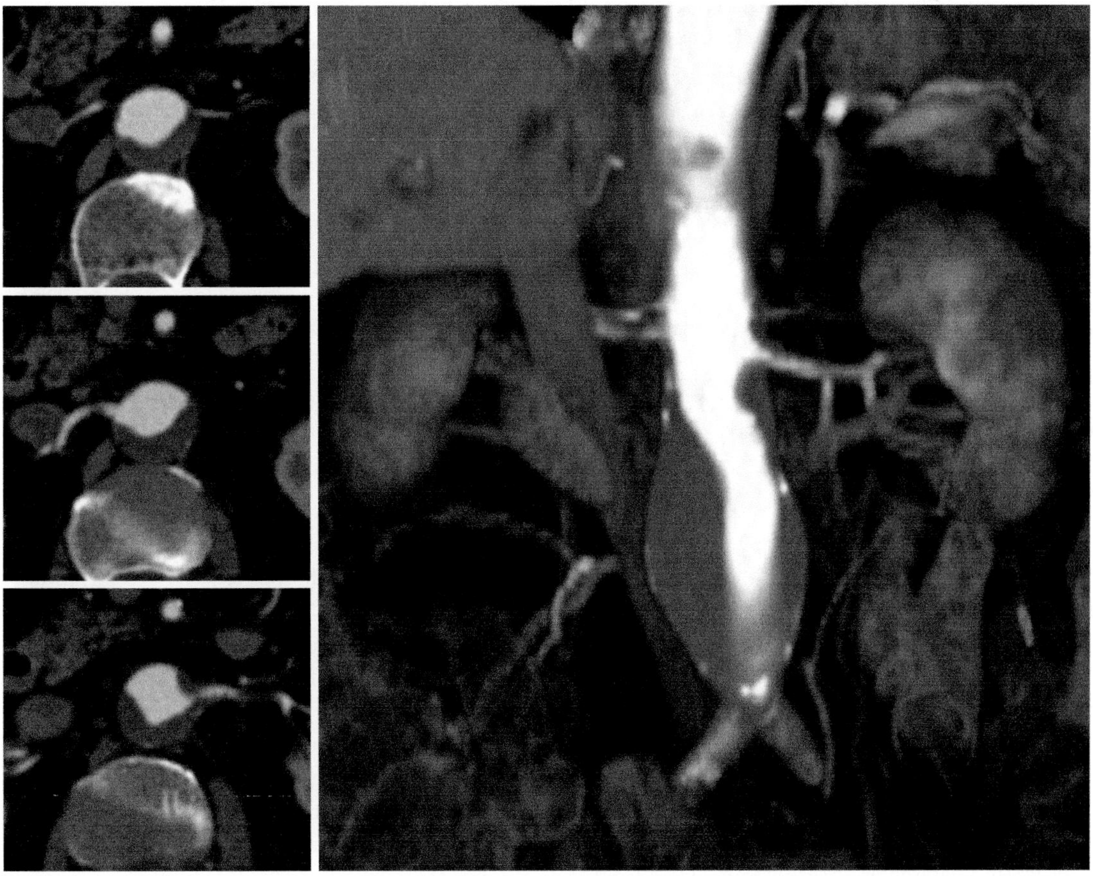

Fig. 3.10 Preoperative CT scan showing parietal thrombus close to the origin of the renal arteries

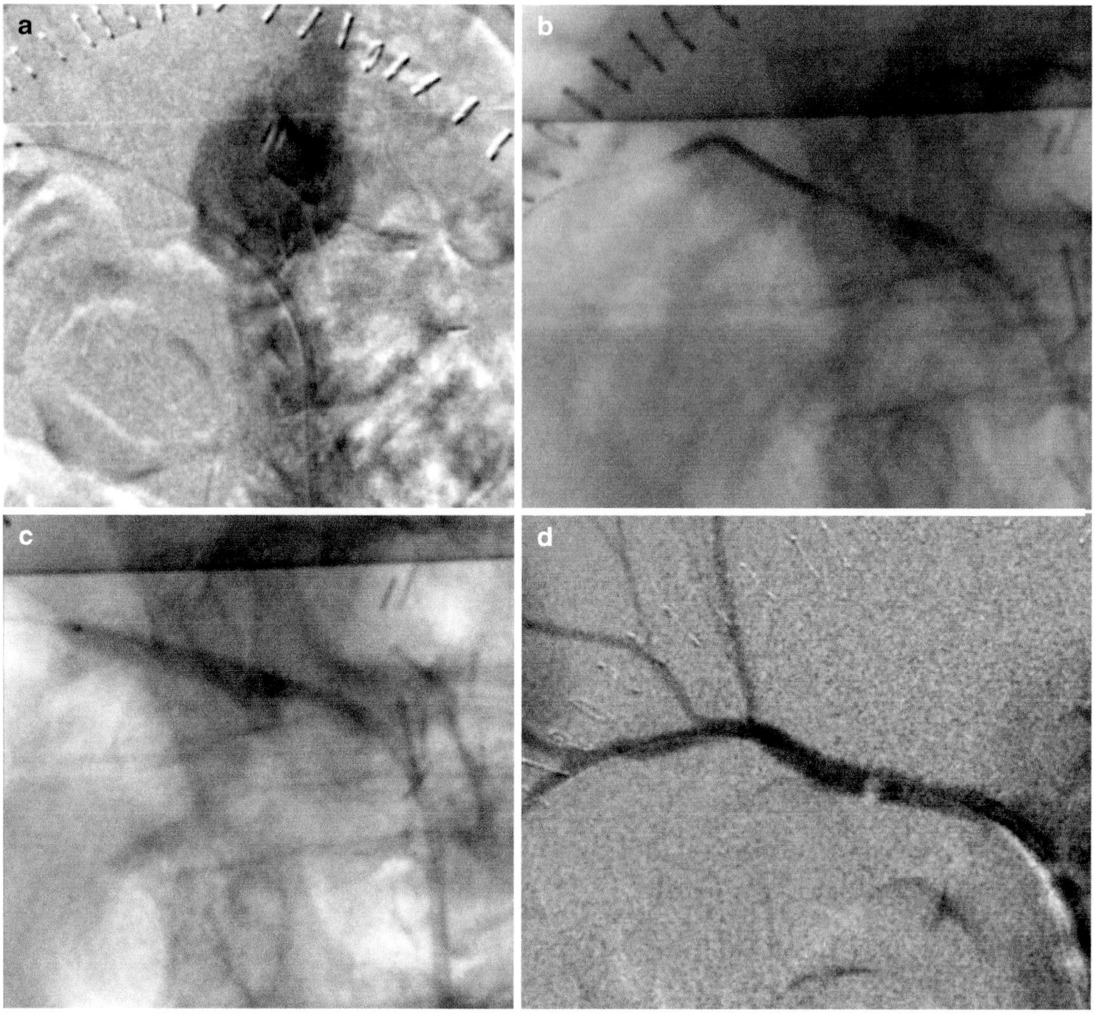

Fig. 3.11 Intraoperative angiography showing (**a**) complete occlusion of both right and left renal arteries, (**b**) catheterization of the right renal artery with a BERN catheter, (**c**) ballooning of the vessels, and (**d**) complete angiography which shows restoration of the blood flow to the right kidney

therapy, it has been shown that even subtle changes in the glomerular filtration rate can have profound long-term effects. The postoperative renal failure, in fact, has been shown to adversely affect the short- and long-term survival after this kind of surgery [36, 37].

3.5.3.1 Classification and Staging of Acute Kidney Injury (AKI)

The KDIGO (Kidney Disease Improving Global Outcomes) guidelines were released in 2012; they associated with the RIFLE (Risk, Injury, Failure, Loss, End-Stage Kidney Disease) and AKIN (Acute Kidney Injury Network) criteria. The KDIGO guidelines introduced a new definition of AKI and a new kidney injury staging system: AKI was defined as an increase in serum creatinine of 0.3 mg/dL or more within 48 h of surgery, or an increase of at least 1.5 times compared to the preoperative value in the last 7 days, or a lower hourly diuresis of 0.5 mL/kg for more than 6 h [38].

3.5.4 Intestinal Ischemia

Intestinal ischemia is a feared complication in the surgical repair of abdominal aortic aneurysm. Binding of the AMI, failure of the hypogastric artery revascularization, iliofemoral occlusive disease, stenosis of the SMA, athero-embolism, injuries from retractor, and previous resection of the colon may contribute to intestinal ischemia, which has a clinical incidence from 0.2% to 6% following surgical repair of AAA [17, 39, 40]. Upon diagnosis, intestinal ischemia requires early and aggressive treatment because it has a generally unfavorable outcome. In some large series, the intestinal ischemia is associated with mortality rates ranging from 25% to 50% [40, 41]. Consequently, all patients should be treated aggressively with intravenously broad-spectrum antibiotics, targeting the bacteria of the intestinal flora. Patients with full-thickness ischemia require emergency treatment with exploratory laparotomy and bowel resection [42].

3.5.5 Long-Term Complications

There is clear evidence from many sources that the proximal aorta continues to reshape over time, regardless of the type of repair [18]. Although the anastomosis with continuous suture allows a robust surgical fixation of the aortic graft, a possible long-term complication is represented by anastomotic pseudoaneurysms. Large cohorts with a significant follow-up pose the incidence of anastomotic pseudoaneurysms to <1% in 6 years, from 1% to 10% at 10 years, and 20% at 15 years, depending on the study [19, 20, 43, 44]. One of these studies, the Mayo Clinic, is significant because it followed 307 patients undergoing AAA repair surgery for an average of 5.8 cases by years [20]. The anastomotic pseudoaneurysm is the most common late complication, with a median of 6 years of onset period; other complications are occlusion (2%), aorto-enteric fistula (1.6%), and the prosthesis infection (1.3%). Taken together, these data show that the result of a correct surgical repair of abdominal aortic aneurysm is excellent, but not perfect. Although the surgery definitively repairs the aneurysmal segment, the underlying aortic disease remains, and this leads to dilation of the proximal and distal portion. This can cause the formation of metachronous aneurysms and pseudoaneurysms, as well as increase the likelihood of rupture of the anastomosis. For these reasons, all patients who underwent surgical repair of abdominal aortic aneurysm require at least a permanent ultrasound monitoring.

References

1. Chaikof EL, Blankensteijn JD, Harris PL, et al. Reporting standards for endovascular aortic aneurysm repair. J Vasc Surg. 2002;35(5):1048–60. https://doi.org/10.1067/mva.2002.123763.
2. Back MR, Bandyk M, Bradner M, et al. Critical analysis of outcome determinants affecting repair of intact aneurysms involving the visceral aorta. Ann Vasc Surg. 2005;19(5):648–56. https://doi.org/10.1007/s10016-005-6843-3.
3. Gillum RF. Epidemiology of aortic aneurysm in the United States. J Clin Epidemiol. 1995;48(11):1289–98. https://doi.org/10.1016/0895-4356(95)00045-3.
4. Katz DJ, Stanley JC, Zelenock GB. Operative mortality rates for intact and ruptured abdominal aortic aneurysms in Michigan: an eleven-year statewide experience. J Vasc Surg. 1994;19(5):804–17. https://doi.org/10.1016/S0741-5214(94)70005-2.
5. LaMorte WW, Scott TE, Menzoian JO. Racial differences in the incidence of femoral bypass and abdominal aortic aneurysmectomy in Massachusetts: relationship to cardiovascular risk factors. J Vasc Surg. 1995;21(3):422–31. https://doi.org/10.1016/S0741-5214(95)70284-9.
6. Wilmink ABM, Hubbard CS, Day NE, Quick CRG. The incidence of small abdominal aortic aneurysms and the change in normal infrarenal aortic diameter: implications for screening. Eur J Vasc Endovasc Surg. 2001;21(2):165–70. https://doi.org/10.1053/ejvs.2000.1285.
7. Melton LJ, Bickerstaff LK, Hollier LH, et al. Changing incidence of abdominal aortic aneurysms: a population-based study. Am J Epidemiol. 1984;120(3):379–86. https://doi.org/10.1093/oxfordjournals.aje.a113902.
8. Wilmink ABM, Quick CRG. Epidemiology and potential for prevention of abdominal aortic aneurysm. Br J Surg. 1998;85(2):155–62. https://doi.org/10.1046/j.1365-2168.1998.00714.x.
9. Lederle FA, Johnson GR, Wilson SE, et al. Prevalence and associations of abdominal aortic aneurysm detected through screening. Aneurysm detection and management (ADAM) veterans affairs cooperative

study group. Ann Intern Med. 1997;126(6):441–9. https://doi.org/10.1056/NEJM200212053472325.
10. Moll F, Powell J, Fraedrich G, et al. Management of abdominal aortic aneurysms clinical practice guidelines of the European society for vascular surgery. Eur J Vasc Endovasc Surg. 2011;41(S1):S1–S58. https://doi.org/10.1016/j.ejvs.2010.09.011.
11. Juvonen T, Ergin MA, Galla JD, et al. Risk factors for rupture of chronic type B dissections. J Thorac Cardiovasc Surg. 1999;117(4):776–86. https://doi.org/10.1016/S0022-5223(99)70299-0.
12. Juvonen T, Ergin MA, Galla JD, et al. Prospective study of the natural history of thoracic aortic aneurysms. Ann Thorac Surg. 1997;63(6):1533–45. https://doi.org/10.1016/S0003-4975(97)00414-1.
13. Lo RC, Lu B, Fokkema MTM, et al. Relative importance of aneurysm diameter and body size for predicting abdominal aortic aneurysm rupture in men and women. J Vasc Surg. 2014;59(5):1209–16. https://doi.org/10.1016/j.jvs.2013.10.104.
14. Beales L, Wolstenhulme S, Evans JA, West R, Scott DJA. Reproducibility of ultrasound measurement of the abdominal aorta. Br J Surg. 2011;98(11):1517–25. https://doi.org/10.1002/bjs.7628.
15. Shuman W, Hastrup W, Kohler T, et al. Suspected leaking abdominal aortic aneurysm: use of sonography in the emergency room. Radiol Clin N Am. 1988;168(1):117–9. https://doi.org/10.1148/radiology.168.1.3289085.
16. Pavone P, Di Cesare E, Di Renzi P, et al. Abdominal aortic aneurysm evaluation: comparison of US, CT, MRI, and angiography. Magn Reson Imaging. 1990;8(3):199–204. https://doi.org/10.1016/0730-725X(90)90089-K.
17. Becquemin J-P, Majewski M, Fermani N, et al. Colon ischemia following abdominal aortic aneurysm repair in the era of endovascular abdominal aortic repair. J Vasc Surg. 2008;47(2):258–63; discussion 263. https://doi.org/10.1016/j.jvs.2007.10.001.
18. Cao P, De Rango P, Parlani G, Verzini F. Fate of proximal aorta following open Infrarenal aneurysm repair. Semin Vasc Surg. 2009;22(2):93–8. https://doi.org/10.1053/j.semvascsurg.2009.04.005.
19. Edwards JM, Teefey SA, Zierler RE, Kohler TR. Intraabdominal paraanastomotic aneurysms after aortic bypass grafting. J Vasc Surg. 1992;15(2):344–53. https://doi.org/10.1016/0741-5214(92)90256-8.
20. Hallett J, Marshall DM, Petterson TM, et al. Graft-related complications after abdominal aortic aneurysm repair: reassurance from a 36-year population-based experience. J Vasc Surg. 1997;25(2):277–86. https://doi.org/10.1016/S0741-5214(97)70349-5.
21. Sun ZH. Abdominal aortic aneurysm: treatment options, image visualizations and follow-up procedures. J Geriatr Cardiol. 2012;9(1):49–60. https://doi.org/10.3724/SP.J.1263.2012.00049.
22. Squillaci E, Fanucci E, Masala S, Nisini A, Tomassini M, Simonetti G. A comparison between two different concentration of contrast media with multidetector CT for the study of abdominal vascular system. Radiol Med. 2002;104(4):341–50.
23. Van Kuijk JP, Flu WJ, Dunckelgrun M, Bax JJ, Poldermans D. Coronary artery disease in patients with abdominal aortic aneurysm: a review article. J Cardiovasc Surg. 2009;50(1):93–107.
24. Poldermans D, Bax JJ, Boersma E, et al. Guidelines for pre-operative cardiac risk assessment and perioperative cardiac management in non-cardiac surgery. Eur Heart J. 2009;30(22):2769–812. https://doi.org/10.1093/eurheartj/ehp337.
25. Thomas D, Anderson D, Hulten E, et al. Open versus endovascular repair of abdominal aortic aneurysm: incidence of cardiovascular events in 632 patients in a department of defense cohort over 6-year follow-up. Vascular. 2014;0(0):1–6. https://doi.org/10.1177/1708538114546207.
26. Inker LA, Astor BC, Fox CH, et al. KDOQI US commentary on the 2012 KDIGO clinical practice guideline for the evaluation and management of CKD. Am J Kidney Dis. 2014;63(5):713–35. https://doi.org/10.1053/j.ajkd.2014.01.416.
27. Cirillo M, Lombardi C, Mele AA, Marcarelli F, Bilancio G. A population-based approach for the definition of chronic kidney disease: the CKD prognosis consortium. J Nephrol. 2012;25(1):7–12. https://doi.org/10.5301/jn.5000045.
28. Pronovost P, Jenckes M, Dorman T, Garrett E. Organizational characteristics of intensive care units related to outcomes of abdominal aortic surgery. JAMA. 1999;281(14):1310–7. https://doi.org/10.1001/jama.281.14.1310.
29. Pronovost PJ, Dang D, Dorman T, et al. Intensive care unit nurse staffing and the risk for complications after abdominal aortic surgery. Eff Clin Pract. 2001;4(5):199–206. http://www.ncbi.nlm.nih.gov/pubmed/11685977
30. Lindenauer PK, Pekow P, Wang K, Mamidi DK, Gutierrez B, Benjamin EM. Perioperative beta-blocker therapy and mortality after major noncardiac surgery. N Engl J Med. 2005;353(4):349–61. https://doi.org/10.1056/NEJMoa041895.
31. Poldermans D, Boersma E, Bax JJ, et al. The effect of bisoprolol on perioperative mortality and myocardial infarction in high-risk patients undergoing vascular surgery. Dutch echocardiographic cardiac risk evaluation applying stress echocardiography study group. N Engl J Med. 1999;341(24):1789–94. https://doi.org/10.1056/NEJM199912093412402.
32. Mangano DT, Layug EL, Wallace A, Tateo I. Effect of atenolol on mortality and cardiovascular morbidity after noncardiac surgery. Multicenter study of perioperative ischemia research group. N Engl J Med. 1996;335(23):1713–20. https://doi.org/10.1056/NEJM199612053352301.
33. Kurzencwyg D, Filion KB, Pilote L, et al. Cardiac medical therapy among patients undergoing abdominal aortic aneurysm repair. Ann Vasc Surg. 2006;20(5):569–76. https://doi.org/10.1007/s10016-006-9078-z.

34. Schermerhorn ML, O'Malley AJ, Jhaveri A, Cotterill P, Pomposelli F, Landon BE. Endovascular vs. open repair of abdominal aortic aneurysms in the Medicare population. N Engl J Med. 2008;358(5):464–74. https://doi.org/10.1056/NEJMoa0707348.
35. Tallarita T, Sobreira ML, Oderich GS. Results of open pararenal abdominal aortic aneurysm repair: tabular review of the literature. Ann Vasc Surg. 2011;25(1):143–9. https://doi.org/10.1016/j.avsg.2010.10.005.
36. Nathan DP, Brinster CJ, Woo EY, Carpenter JP, Fairman RM, Jackson BM. Predictors of early and late mortality following open extent IV thoracoabdominal aortic aneurysm repair in a large contemporary single-center experience. J Vasc Surg. 2011;53(2):299–306. https://doi.org/10.1016/j.jvs.2010.08.085.
37. Grant SW, Grayson AD, Grant MJ, Purkayastha D, McCollum CN. What are the risk factors for renal failure following open elective abdominal aortic aneurysm repair? Eur J Vasc Endovasc Surg. 2012;43(2):182–7. https://doi.org/10.1016/j.ejvs.2011.11.018.
38. Mehta RL, Kellum JA, Shah SV, et al. Acute kidney injury network: report of an initiative to improve outcomes in acute kidney injury. Crit Care. 2007;11(2):R31. https://doi.org/10.1186/cc5713.
39. Bjorck M, Troeng T, Bergqvist D. Risk factors for intestinal ischaemia after aortoiliac surgery: a combined cohort and case-control study of 2824 operations. Eur J Vasc Endovasc Surg. 1997;13(6):531–9. https://doi.org/10.1016/S1078-5884(97)80061-5.
40. Brewster DC, Franklin DP, Cambria RP, et al. Intestinal ischemia complicating abdominal aortic surgery. Surgery. 1991;109(4):447–54. http://www.ncbi.nlm.nih.gov/pubmed/1844392
41. Longo WE, Lee TC, Barnett MG, et al. Ischemic colitis complicating abdominal aortic aneurysm surgery in the U.S. veteran. J Surg Res. 1996;60(2):351–4. https://doi.org/10.1006/jsre.1996.0056.
42. Menegaux F, Trésallet C, Kieffer E, Bodin L, Thabut D, Rouby J-J. Aggressive management of nonocclusive ischemic colitis following aortic reconstruction. Arch Surg. 2006;141(7):678–82. https://doi.org/10.1016/S0749-4041(08)70719-X.
43. Hertzer NR, Mascha EJ, Karafa MT, O'Hara PJ, Krajewski LP, Beven EG. Open infrarenal abdominal aortic aneurysm repair: the Cleveland Clinic experience from 1989 to 1998. J Vasc Surg. 2002;35(6):1145–54. https://doi.org/10.1067/mva.2002.123686.
44. Kalman PG, Rappaport DC, Merchant N, Clarke K, Johnston KW. The value of late computed tomographic scanning in identification of vascular abnormalities after abdominal aortic aneurysm repair. J Vasc Surg. 1999;29(3):442–50. https://doi.org/10.1016/S0741-5214(99)70272-7.

4 Aortic "Coral Reef" with Visceral Artery Involvement: Treatment Options

Enrico Rinaldi, Andrea Kahlberg, Daniele Mascia, Germano Melissano, and Roberto Chiesa

4.1 Introduction

Atherosclerotic occlusive disease of the aorta usually affects its distal portions, and calcifications and obstructions involving the suprarenal aorta are rare and mostly described in case reports [1, 2]. Coral reef aorta (CRA) is an uncommon syndrome caused by a distribution of rock-hard calcifications in the visceral part of the aorta [3]. These heavily calcified plaques that grow into the lumen can cause significant stenoses, which may develop into visceral ischemia, renovascular hypertension, and malperfusion of the lower limbs. Transaortic endarterectomy is accepted as the standard repair, and it is often performed through an extensive thoracoabdominal approach [4]. In the last decade, alternative management of CRA, such as endovascular and laparoscopic approach, has been proposed in order to reduce surgical invasiveness.

Our experience with the operative management of CRA was discussed earlier [5]. In this chapter, we describe the findings, operative procedure, and follow-up of 138 patients treated between 1993 and 2017. We focused on the early outcomes, long-term results, and the frequency of recurrent disease, with special emphasis on the visceral and renal arteries.

E. Rinaldi (✉) · A. Kahlberg · D. Mascia
G. Melissano
Vascular Surgery Unit, IRCCS San Raffaele Scientific Institute, Milan, Italy
e-mail: rinaldi.enrico@hsr.it

R. Chiesa
Unit of Vascular Surgery, San Raffaele Scientific Institute, Vita-Salute University, Milan, Italy

4.2 Materials and Methods

From January 1993 to June 2017, 138 patients (52 men, 86 women, mean age 62.5 years, range 45–86 years) underwent treatment for CRA. Data of patients were recorded and prospectively collected in a database. All patients who presented with the typical signs of CRA in the preoperative ultrasound examination were enrolled. According to our standard practice, patients with severe preoperative renal failure (serum creatinine >2.5 mg/dL) underwent noncontrast computed tomography (NCCT); all the others were studied with contrast computed tomography (CCT) and intra-arterial digital subtraction angiography (DSA). CRA is visualized in the NCCT and in the CCT as white intraluminal blocks in the visceral aorta, with a density comparable with the structure of the bone (Fig. 4.1).

A cloudy formation that narrows the visceral aorta to a very small lumen or total occlusion is the typical morphology of CRA during DSA (Fig. 4.2).

These characteristic signs on preoperative imaging were present in all cases.

© Springer Nature Switzerland AG 2019
Y. Tshomba et al. (eds.), *Visceral Vessels and Aortic Repair*,
https://doi.org/10.1007/978-3-319-94761-7_4

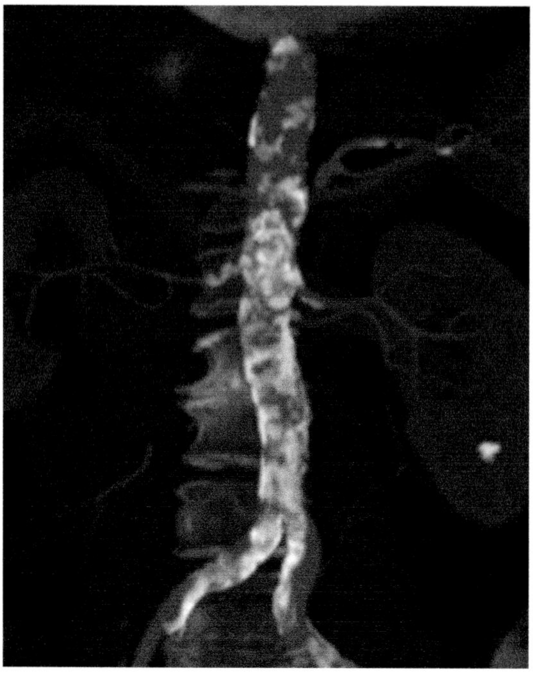

Fig. 4.1 Preoperative CT scan. CRA is visualized as an intraluminal white block in the visceral aorta and at infrarenal level

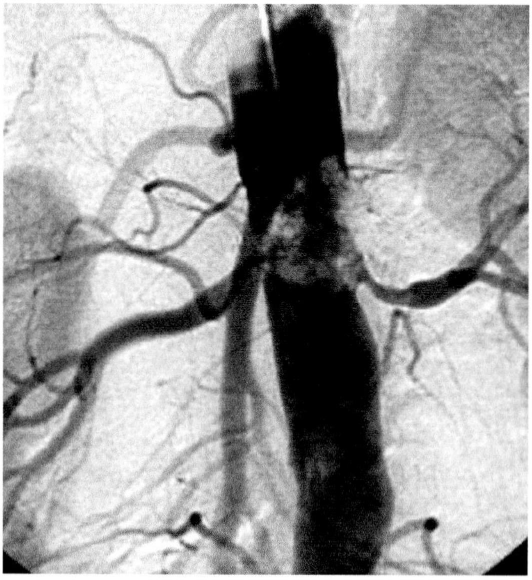

Fig. 4.2 DSA. A typical morphology of CRA involving SMA and renal arteries

Most patients presented with the typical risk factors for arteriosclerosis. Diabetes was found in 23.2% of the patients; heavy smoking (up to 40 cigarettes per day) was found in 70.2% and hypertension with more than two medications in 68.1%. Comorbidities such as tuberculosis, syphilis, or aortitis [6, 7] could not be detected in the study population. All patients underwent a thorough cardiological and neurological examination, including an electrocardiogram, transthoracic echocardiogram, chest X-ray, and Doppler and duplex ultrasound scans of the supra-aortic branches, arms, and limbs. In our experience, CRA is frequently associated with coronary artery disease (CAD) (44 pts., 31.8%); and for this reason, since 2010, all patients with CRA, without severe preoperative renal failure, have been subjected to ECG-gated angio-CT. When significant coronary artery lesions were present, angioplasty of the coronary arteries or coronary bypass surgery was performed before the aortic surgery. After discharge, all surviving patients were introduced in a follow-up protocol with regular clinical and ultrasound evaluation at 1 month, 6 months, and yearly thereafter.

4.2.1 Symptomatology and Findings

Depending on the extent of the disease and the aortic branches involved, three leading symptoms were found, of which the most frequent finding was renovascular arterial hypertension causing headache and vertigo. Ninety-six patients (69.5%) were found to take one (ten patients), two (21 patients), three (40 patients), or more than three (25 patients) medications to control arterial blood pressure. All the patients had developed either severe renal artery stenoses or stenosis of the suprarenal aorta due to protrusion of the coral reef-like calcifications. Intermittent claudication due to peripheral arterial occlusive disease was found in 76 patients (55.0%). The pain-free walking distance was less than 200 m (peripheral arterial occlusive disease Fontaine stage IIb) in 47 patients (34.0%). Forty-three patients (31.1%) presented with chronic visceral ischemia causing diarrhea, weight loss, and abdominal pain. Abdominal angina occurred in 32 of 43 patients (74.4%), and weight loss occurred in 38 of 43 patients (88.3%).

Preoperative examinations showed total occlusion of branches ($n = 38$; celiac trunk $n = 8$, superior mesenteric artery [SMA] $n = 5$, inferior mesenteric artery [IMA] $n = 15$, right renal artery [RRA] $n = 7$, left renal artery [LRA] $n = 3$) and heavily stenotic branches ($n = 94$; celiac trunk $n = 21$, SMA $n = 17$, IMA $n = 27$, RRA $n = 17$, LRA $n = 12$).

4.2.2 Surgical Procedure

One hundred thirty-five (97.8%) of the 138 patients underwent open surgery. Three patients with CRA noneligible for open surgery for severe comorbidities were treated endovascularly. All surgical procedures were performed under general anesthesia. The operative approach was a median laparotomy in 63 patients (46.6%), a bilateral subcostal laparotomy with medial visceral rotation in 29 patients (21.4%), and a left-sided thoracoabdominal approach in 43 patients (31.8%).

After an extensive exposure of the aorta and the visceral and renal vessels (Fig. 4.3), a thromboendarterectomy (TEA) of the aorta was performed in an isolated suprarenal segment in 12 cases (8.8%) and the supra- and infrarenal aorta in 123 cases (91.1%) (Fig. 4.4).

Due to the extension of the plaques into the distal aorta, a TEA of the aortic bifurcation was necessary in 34 patients (25.1%). Distal to the aortic bifurcation, a TEA of the iliac artery (unilateral $n = 4$, bilateral $n = 8$) was performed in 12 cases (8.8%). Blood flow was restored by TEA to the celiac trunk in 25 cases (21 stenosis, 4 total occlusion) (18.5%) and to the SMA in 17 cases (all stenosis) (12.5%).

Whenever possible, visceral vessels were selectively cannulated with occlusion/perfusion Pruitt catheter and perfused with cold crystalloid (Ringer 4 °C).

In three cases of total occlusion, CT was reimplanted with bypass; in one patient with long occlusion of the CT, with a valid collateral network from the SMA, the CT was ligated.

SMA was reimplanted with aortovisceral bypass in five cases of total occlusion.

TEA was performed in 17 cases (12.5%) of stenotic renal artery disease.

In 12 cases (8.8%) with heavily calcified stenosis, the origin of the renal artery was transversely cut and the renal artery reimplanted with a bypass. Renal artery revascularization was not performed in case of occlusion with contract kidney ($n = 10$).

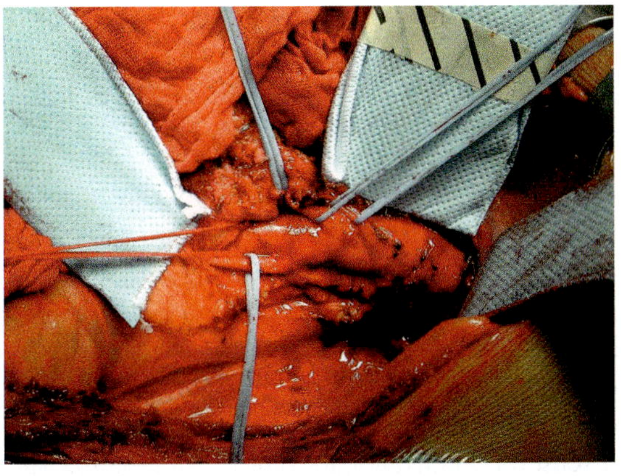

Fig. 4.3 Aortic exposure with visceral and renal artery preparation

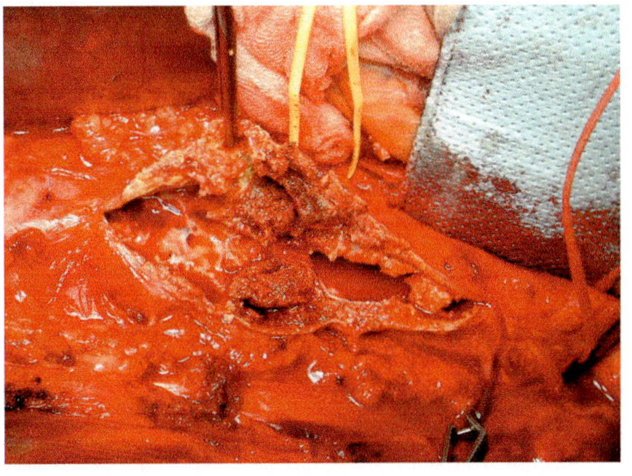

Fig. 4.4 Aortotomy. CRA with supra and infrarenal aortic involvement

Whenever possible, renal arteries were selectively cannulated with occlusion/perfusion Pruitt catheter and perfused. From 1993 to 2010, renal arteries were perfused with cold crystalloid (Ringer 4 °C), but since 2010, following initial encouraging results during thoracoabdominal open repair [8], histidine-tryptophan-ketoglutarate (Custodiol; Dr. Franz-Kohler Chemie GmbH, Bensheim, Germany) was used for renal protection during the procedure (Fig. 4.5).

Aortorenal and aortovisceral bypass were performed using Dacron grafts (n = 9) and polytetrafluoroethylene (PTFE) (n = 7), and after an initial experience during thoracoabdominal open surgery, since 2013 also the Gore Hybrid Vascular Graft (GHVG; W. L. Gore and Associates, Flagstaff, Ariz) has been used for vessel reimplantation (n = 4) [9].

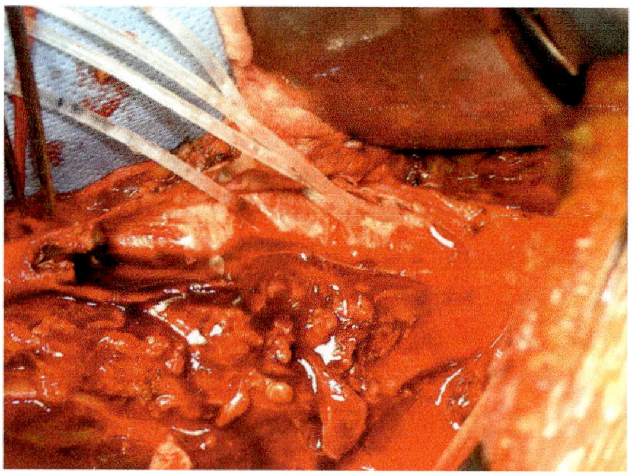

Fig. 4.5 Visceral and renal perfusion. CT and SMA are perfused with Ringer 4 °C; renal arteries are perfused with Custodiol 4 °C

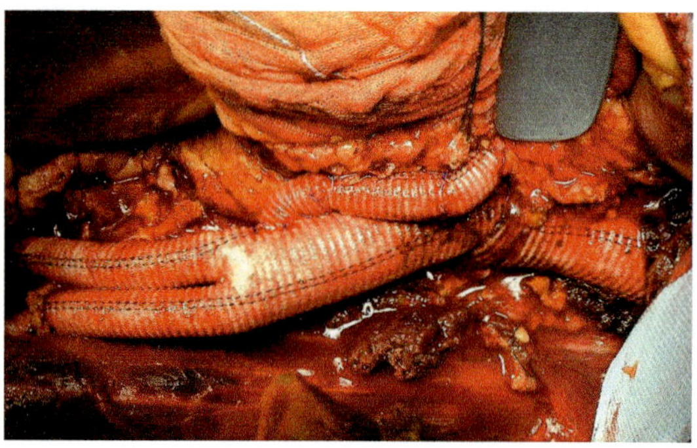

Fig. 4.6 Aortofemoral bypass with Dacron graft with proximal beveled anastomosis on the visceral vessels and right renal artery. Left renal artery is reattached using a bypass

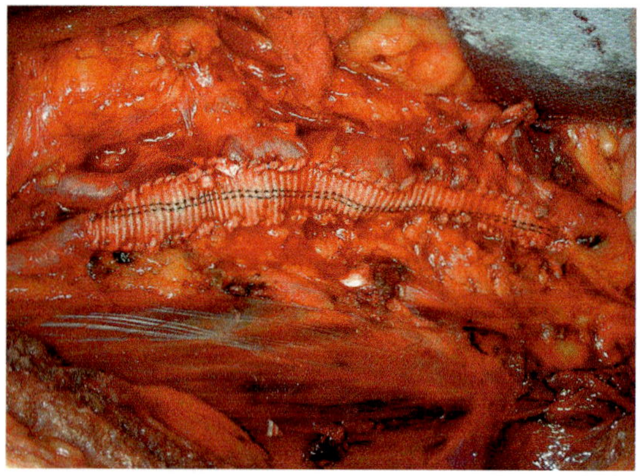

Fig. 4.7 Aortic patch repair

Aortic repair was performed with aortoaortic (n = 27), aortoiliac (n = 31), or aortofemoral (n = 35) bypass with proximal beveled anastomosis on the visceral and renal vessels in the majority of cases (Fig. 4.6); 42 cases were treated instead with aortic patch repair (Fig. 4.7).

Intraoperative angiography at the end of the surgical procedure was performed in 43 cases (31.8%) in order to assess vessel patency in case of extensive TEA or bypass repair of heavily calcified stenosis. In 17 cases, additional simultaneous stenting was performed for persistent stenosis or intraluminal flap (n = 14) or in case of acute angulation of the aortovisceral and aortorenal distal anastomosis (n = 3).

4.3 Results

4.3.1 30-Day Results

Three patients (2.2%) died during or soon after surgery. One patient died from acute cardiac arrest during surgery. One patient died from cardiac arrest (postoperative day 4), and one patient died from multiorgan failure after a prolonged stay in the intensive care unit (postoperative day 22). Postoperative complications that required corrective surgery or additional endovascular procedure occurred in 12 patients (8.8%). The most significant problem was acute ischemia of the lower extremities, which required thrombectomy or femoropopliteal revascularization in five patients. One patient with thoraco-phreno-laparotomy was treated in the intensive care unit with pleural drainage due to prolonged pleural effusion. One patient undergone surgical revision for postoperative bleeding during postoperative day 2. One patient suffered from colon ischemia, which resulted in subtotal colectomy. In one case, acute occlusion after TEA of the aortic bifurcation was treated with aortobifemoral bypass. Three patients required additional endovascular procedures for postoperative complications. Two patients with acute renal failure during postoperative day 2 and 4 with acute renal artery occlusion documented by ultrasound were treated with endovascular recanalization and stenting. In one case, an angiography with additional stenting of CT was performed during postoperative day 2 for acute occlusion.

The overall rate of relevant complications was 25.9% ($n = 35$). Ten patients (7.4%) developed a major adverse cardiac event after surgery requiring coronary artery angioplasty in nine cases and medical treatment in one.

Other relevant complications were temporary renal failure requiring temporary continuous veno-venous hemofiltration in six patients (4.4%), renal failure requiring permanent dialysis in two patients (1.4%), and respiratory failure with necessity of orotracheal reintubation in five patients (3.7%).

4.3.2 Follow-Up

The follow-up examination included medical history, physical examination, and duplex ultrasound scan and was performed after the index procedure at 1 month, 6 months, 1 year, and yearly thereafter. At a mean follow-up of 63 ± 15 months, 18 (13.3%) of the 135 patients died, including the 3 patients who died during the hospital stay post-surgery. One patient died from renal failure, and five patients died from vascular complications (myocardial ($n = 2$) and brain infarction ($n = 3$)).Three patients died from a malignant disease (metastatic lung, pancreatic, and gastric cancer, respectively). In six cases, the cause of death could not be identified.

Late complications leading to secondary surgical or endovascular procedure during follow-up occurred in 12 patients (9.0%) within a time interval of 3–55 months after the first procedure. One patient suffered a thrombotic occlusion of the aortobifemoral prosthesis in one limb, 55 months after surgery, treated with thrombectomy and femoral TEA. Two patients were treated endovascularly with stenting for new-onset limb claudication due to iliac artery stenosis 3 and 21 months after surgery, respectively. One patient was treated endovascularly for iliac anastomotic false aneurysm 32 months after index procedure.

Eight patients with visceral and renal vessel stenosis were treated endovascularly; data regarding visceral and renal vessel patency at follow-up are reported in Table 4.1.

The level of creatinine was comparable with the preoperative period in 122 patients (92.4%), slightly elevated in 6 patients, and elevated in 4 patients.

Among 96 patients suffering from arterial hypertension, 59 patients (61.4%) were still on antihypertensive medication but with reduced medication. In 37 patients with preoperative arterial hypertension, the number of medications was the same as the preoperative period.

Table 4.1 Visceral and renal artery patency at follow-up

At last available follow-up examination						
Vessel	No	Stenosis	Occlusion	Primary patency	Secondary endovascular procedure	Secondary patency
CT	131	2	2	127 (96.4%)	2	129 (98.4%)
SMA	132	1	–	131 (99.2%)	1	132 (100%)
RRA	125	3	4	118 (94.4%)	2	120 (96.0%)
LRA	129	5	6	118 (91.4%)	3	121 (93.7%)
Total	517	11	12	494 (95.5%)	8	502 (97.0%)

All the 43 patients with preoperative chronic visceral ischemia experienced a slow but steady return to normal status after surgical treatment.

Compared with the patients' conditions before surgery, there was significant clinical and diagnostic improvement after surgery in 126 of the 132 follow-up patients (95.4%), and 4 patients remained stable (3.0%). The two patients with renal failure requiring permanent dialysis presented clinical signs of impairment.

4.4 Discussion

Reports on calcification and obstruction of the abdominal aorta were rare before 1984 [10–14], when Qvarfordt et al. described a series of nine patients with a unique disease consisting of isolated stenosis of the suprarenal aorta due to a rock-hard, calcified mass [3]. Since then, many authors have been reporting case series of patients diagnosed with similar lesions.

Schulte et al. reported a series of 21 patients, and the most common symptoms were hypertension, intermittent claudication, abdominal pain, impaired renal function, lower extremity pain at rest, and end-stage renal disease. All patients underwent vascular surgical procedures, including open thromboendarterectomy of suprarenal, infrarenal, or supra- and infrarenal aorta and also thromboendarterectomy of visceral and renal vessels in a high percentage of cases or bypass reconstructions in about one-third of cases [15].

In a series of 70 patients with CRA reported by Grotemeyer et al., the most frequent finding was renovascular hypertension, which caused vertigo, headaches, and visual symptoms in about half of the patients. All patients had developed severe stenosis of the renal artery or suprarenal aorta due to protrusion of the coral reef-like calcifications. Intermittent claudication due to peripheral arterial occlusive disease, with pain-free walking distance less than 200 m, was the second most common symptom. Other symptoms were chronic visceral ischemia that caused diarrhea, weight loss, and abdominal angina. Sixty-nine patients underwent surgery with thromboendarterectomy performed on an isolated suprarenal, infrarenal, or both supra- and infrarenal aorta [4].

CRA is not strictly confined to the suprarenal aortic segment; Sako [10] and Harbison [16] had already described infrarenal disease of the same type. In our experience, 91.1% of patients showed a concomitant supra- and infrarenal presence of typical coral reef atherosclerosis. Additionally, a high percentage of patients also suffered from manifest atherosclerotic disease in other vascular areas, in particular coronary arteries (31.8%). Therefore, CRA cannot be regarded as a disease completely separate from the frequent process of general atherosclerosis but rather denotes one with its own particular manifestations and unusual consequences.

Risk factor analysis in our patients underscored the presence of general risk factors for atherosclerosis but the absence of recognized specific, underlying causes.

The clinical picture in our group is consistent with previous reports and is dominated by the hemodynamic compromise of bowel and kidney and lower limb malperfusion with intermittent claudication.

During preoperative evaluation, duplex scan was used to identify hemodynamic aberrations but was not useful for defining the upper limit of the extent of disease because of the heavy calcification and its position. For this reason, NCCT represents an additional value since it helps in identifying the cranial border of the process and thus in defining the best operative approach, whether abdominal or thoracoabdominal. Moreover, in patients without severe preoperative renal failure, CCT and DSA offer important information about vessel patency and collateral networks.

Additional preoperative work-up includes the coronary and supra-aortic vessels because of the very high incidence of concomitant disease and the perioperative risk of mortality and morbidity from this disease. Due to a not negligible incidence of cardiac postoperative complications in our experience, nowadays all patients with CRA and without a preoperative severe renal function impairment (creatinine serum level

<2.5 mg/dL) underwent ECG-gated angio-CT and are preoperatively treated in case of significant coronary artery disease.

During preoperative evaluation, chest X-rays and an assessment of pulmonary function are useful in view of the pulmonary morbidity of this operative approach in a patient group composed of heavy smokers.

In literature, several surgical accesses have been proposed: from more invasive laparotomy or thoracotomy [3, 4] to lesser invasive lumbotomy [17] and laparoscopy [18]. In our experience, a median laparotomy, a bilateral subcostal laparotomy with medial visceral rotation, and a left-sided thoracoabdominal incision were tailored to any single patient according to disease extension and patient characteristics.

Open TEA of the occluded parts of the aorta and transaortic TEA of the aortic branches are the most widely used surgical procedures for CRA. Flynn [19] was the first to publish results on aortic TEA in 1959. He removed a calcified aortic plug extending from the descending aorta into the renal arteries in a 27-year-old woman suffering from renovascular hypertension. Thromboendarterectomy represents the surgical procedure of choice for this pattern of sclerotic disease [3, 10, 20, 21]. Aortic repair could be performed with prosthetic patch in case of TEA alone. Prosthetic reconstructions can be amended wherever the thickness of the remaining aortic wall after dissection in the adventitial layer or complicated iliac disease renders it inevitable. In case of severe heavily calcified stenosis or occlusion, visceral and renal vessels could be reimplanted using bypass.

Intraoperative angiography offers the possibility to visualize possible residual stenosis or morphological aberrancies after TEA or after bypass reimplantation that could be treated immediately preventing future occlusion of the vessels. In our experience, 43 angiographies were performed after the procedure with 17 additional simultaneous stenting with good angiographic results.

The kidney is one of the major targets of coral reef aortic disease, and a high percentage of patients presented with renal artery stenosis in this series. A large subgroup of these patients suffered from renovascular hypertension, and surgical treatment was effective in ameliorating this symptom with a general reduction of number of medications needed.

If present, abdominal angina produced a severe malnutrition syndrome in our patients. Their deteriorated status should not defer but encourage timely operation, since patients in our group experienced a slow but steady return to normal status after surgical treatment.

Because of the variable extension of aortic plaque, open surgery for CRA is burdened by high mortality and morbidity rates [22]; despite this, transaortic endarterectomy still represents the treatment of choice in such patients in our experience. To reduce surgical invasivity, some authors have reported a successful endovascular treatment by placement of a stent graft [23, 24]. However, the risk for distal embolization and the technical difficulty in the deployment of the stent graft remain important concerns [15], and then this strategy could be addressed only to less severe forms of CRA [17] or in case of patients with severe comorbidities that could not be treated with surgical approach.

4.5 Conclusion

Coral reef aorta is a rare, unique disease of the juxta- and infrarenal aorta that is often associated with severe atherosclerotic disease in other domains. The main symptoms are lower limb claudication, hypertension, deterioration of renal function, and angina abdominalis. Surgical treatment offers good results, and a timely operation is advocated to avoid loss of kidney function, complications of long-standing hypertensive disease, and wasting from intestinal malperfusion.

References

1. Charnsangavej C. Intraluminal calcification and occlusion of the abdominal aorta above the renal arteries. Cardiovasc Intervent Radiol. 1981;4:242–4.

2. Lipchik EO, Rob CG, Schwartzberg S. Obstruction of the abdominal aorta above the level of the renal arteries. Radiology. 1964;82:443–6.
3. Qvarford PG, Reilly LM, Sedwitz MM, Ehrenfeld WK, Stoney RJ. "Coral reef" atherosclerosis of the suprarenal aorta: a unique clinical entity. J Vasc Surg. 1984;1:903–8.
4. Grotemeyer D, Pourhassan S, Rehbein H, Voiculescu A, Reinecke P, Sandmann W. The coral reef aorta–a single centre experience in 70 patients. Int J Angiol. 2007;16:98–105.
5. Chiesa R, Melissano G, Tshombay Y, Moura MRL. Endoarterectomia dell'aorta toraco-addominale nell'ischemia intestinale acuta e cronica. G Ital Chir Vasc. 2000;7:279–90.
6. Axilrod HD. Obstruction of the aortic isthmus by a calcified thrombus. Arch Pathol. 1946;41:63–5.
7. Bialkowski J, Szkutnik M, Bermúdez-Cañete R, Kusa J, Regiec S, Mullins CE. Síndrome de la aorta media causado por enfermedad de Takayasu: Tratamiento con stents y seguimiento a medio plazo. Rev Esp Cardiol. 2002;55:682–5.
8. Tshomba Y, Kahlberg A, Melissano G, Coppi G, Marone E, Ferrari D, et al. Comparison of renal perfusion solutions during thoracoabdominal aortic aneurysm repair. J Vasc Surg. 2014;59(3):623–33.
9. Chiesa R, Kahlberg A, Mascia D, Tshomba Y, Civilini E, Melissano G. Use of a novel hybrid vascular graft for sutureless revascularization of the renal arteries during open thoracoabdominal aortic aneurysm repair. J Vasc Surg. 2014;60(3):622–30.
10. Sako Y. Arteriosclerotic occlusion of the midabdominal aorta. Surgery. 1966;59:709–12.
11. Bercot M, Idatte JM, Piwnica A. Hypertension arterielle sèvère par stènose de l'aorte sous-diaphragmatiqne. Nouv Press Med. 1972;1:2539–42.
12. Borromée L, Frija G, Baglin A, Domart M, Lacombe P, Prinseau J, et al. Pseudo-coarctation due a une masse intra-aortique calcifike. Sem Hop Paris. 1983;59:2827–30.
13. Lipchick E, Rob C, Schwartzberg B. Obstruction of the abdominal aorta above the level of the renal arteries. Radiology. 1964;82:443–5.
14. Cooley D, De Bakey M. Resection of the thoracic aorta with replacement by homograft for aneurysms and constrictive lesions. J Thorac Surg. 1955;29:66–104.
15. Schulte KM, Reiher L, Grabitz L, Sandmann W. Coral reef aorta: a long-term study of 21 patients. Ann Vasc Surg. 2000;14(6):626–33.
16. Harbison S. Arteriosclerotic occlusion of the aorta: a case presenting an unusual location. Surgery. 1957;41:488–90.
17. DeRubertis BG, Jabori SO, Quinones-Baldrich W, Lawrence PF. Retroperitoneal trapdoor endarterectomy for paravisceral "coral reef" aortic plaque. J Vasc Endovasc. 2012;46:487–91.
18. Di Centa I, Coggia M, Javerliat I, Alfonsi P, Maury JM, Kitzis M, et al. Total laparoscopic suprarenal aortic coral reef removal. J Vasc Surg. 2006;44:194–7.
19. Flynn PJ, Kattus AA. Coarctation of the aorta with proximal aortic dilatation and calcific atheromatous degeneration corrected by endarterectomy. J Thorac Cardiovasc Surg. 1959;38:369.
20. Peillon C, Morlet C, Laissy JP, et al. Endoaortic calcific proliferation of the upper abdominal aorta. Ann Vasc Surg. 1989;3:181–6.
21. Patra P, Despins P, Duveau D, et al. Obstructive calcification of the descending thoracic aorta and suprarenal abdominal aorta. Two cases (in French). Presse Med. 1985;14:209–11.
22. Belczak SQ, Sincos IR, Aun R, Costa KV, Araujo EA. Coral reef aorta, emergency surgical: case report and literature review. Einstein (Sao Paulo). 2014;12:237–41.
23. Verma H, Baliga K, George RK, Tripathi RK. Surgical and endovascular treatment of occlusive aortic syndromes. J Cardiovasc Surg. 2013;54:55–69.
24. Holfeld J, Gottardi R, Zimpfer D, Dorfmeister M, Dumfarth J, Funovics M, et al. Treatment of symptomatic coral reef aorta by endovascular stent-graft placement. Ann Thorac Surg. 2008;85:1817–9.

5 Renal Vascular Anatomic Abnormalities During Open Abdominal Aortic Repair

Domenico Baccellieri, Vincenzo Ardita, Gianbattista Tshiombo, Enrico Rinaldi, Yamume Tshomba, and Roberto Chiesa

5.1 Introduction

Renal arteries are defined as a pair of lateral branches from the abdominal aorta. Anatomical dissection studies have revealed that in most cases, each kidney receives one renal artery and one renal vein is deputy to drain blood into the inferior vena cava. The left renal vein also receives left suprarenal and left gonadal veins, in addition to the vein coming out from the kidney.

Variations in number, source, and course of the renal arteries are common, occurring in 60–80% of reported cases [1, 2]. The renal artery may give rise to branches normally derived from other vessels, such as the inferior phrenic, hepatic, suprarenal, gonadal, pancreatic, and lumbar arteries.

The abnormalities in the renal arteries are mainly due to the various developmental positions of the kidney, and the different origin and their variations are explained by the development of mesonephric arteries.

During the development in the pelvis, both kidneys are supplied by common iliac artery branches, but later, during migration into the lumbar region, their arterial supply shifts to the abdominal aorta.

Extrarenal artery may be classified into:

- Aberrant renal artery
- Accessory renal artery

Aberrant renal arteries commonly supply the superior or inferior pole of the kidney.

Accessory renal arteries are a common variant and are present in ~25% (range 20–30%) of the population. They may originate from the abdominal aorta, either above or below the main renal artery or, on rare occasions, from iliac arteries.

Electronic Supplementary Material The online version of this chapter (doi:10.1007/978-3-319-94761-7_5) contains supplementary material, which is available to authorized users.

D. Baccellieri (✉)
Unit of Vascular Surgery, San Raffaele Scientific Institute, Milan, Italy
e-mail: baccellieri.domenico@hsr.it

V. Ardita · E. Rinaldi
Vascular Surgery Unit, IRCCS San Raffaele Scientific Institute, Milan, Italy

G. Tshiombo
Vascular Surgeon, Fondazione Cariplo, Milan, Italy

Y. Tshomba
Unit of Vascular Surgery, Fondazione Policlinico Universitario A. Gemelli IRCCS, Università Cattolica del Sacro Cuore, Rome, Italy

Unit of Vascular Surgery, San Raffaele Scientific Institute, Vita-Salute University, Milan, Italy

R. Chiesa
Unit of Vascular Surgery, San Raffaele Scientific Institute, Vita-Salute University, Milan, Italy

© Springer Nature Switzerland AG 2019
Y. Tshomba et al. (eds.), *Visceral Vessels and Aortic Repair*,
https://doi.org/10.1007/978-3-319-94761-7_5

Accessory renal arteries occur bilaterally in 10–15% of cases:

- Single renal artery arising from the abdominal aorta: 70%
- Double renal arteries ~20% (range 14–23%)
- Triple renal arteries ~2.5% (range 1–4%)
- Quadruple renal arteries <1%

Proper identification is mandatory for surgical planning prior to live donor transplantation, renal artery procedures, and aortic surgery. Techniques proposed for reducing the incidence of renal failure in the presence of aberrant renal arteries and concomitant abdominal aortic aneurysm (AAA) are the aortic patch, single-vessel reattachments through bypass grafts, or direct reattachment (Figs. 5.1 and 5.2 and Movie 5.1).

During aberrant artery reattachment, cold crystalloid perfusion can be used in order to reduce the risk of tubular damage (Movie 5.1).

Renal anomalies are described in the literature and can all be stratified into two categories: the horseshoe kidney and the pelvic kidney.

5.2 Horseshoe Kidney (HSK)

Horseshoe kidney (HSK) is a well-known congenital fusion across the midline of two distinct functioning kidneys found in 0.25% of the general population and is characterized by the medial fusion of the two kidneys anteriorly, or occasionally posteriorly, to the aorta [3–6].

Incidence is between 1:600 and 1:800 and is twice as common in men.

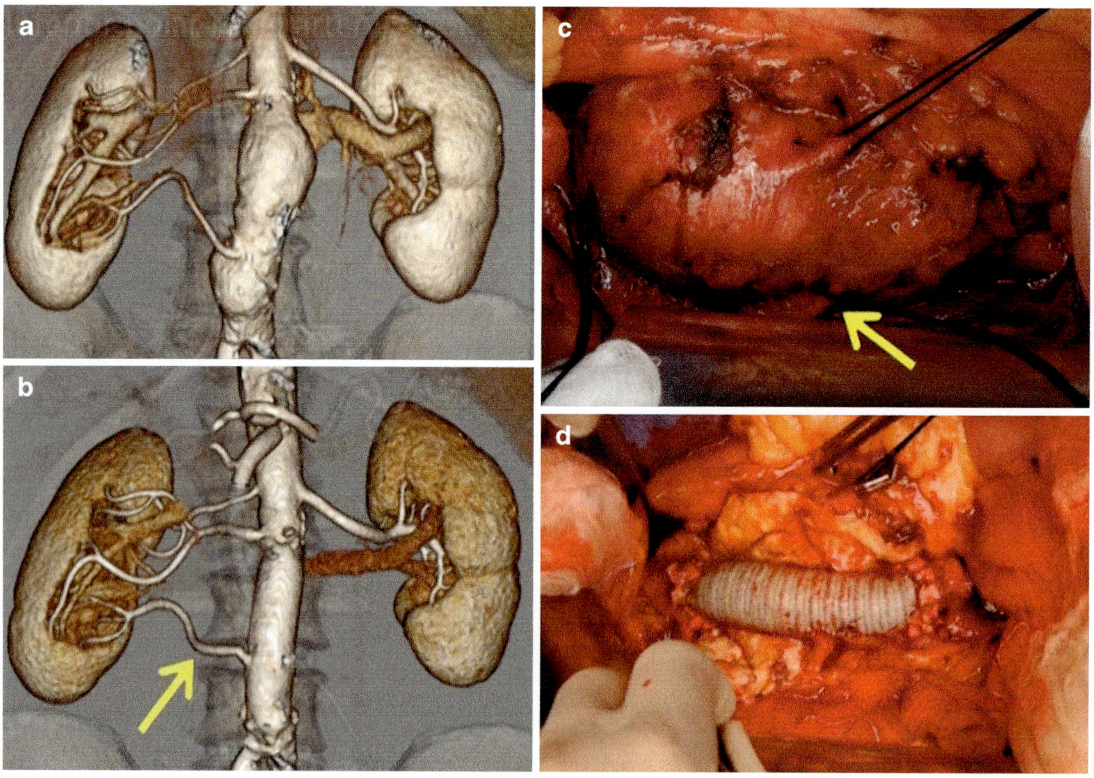

Fig. 5.1 AngioCT showing an infrarenal abdominal aortic aneurysm with an inferior right polar artery requiring reattachment during tube graft repair (**a**) and postoperative angioCT showing the same case after aortic repair and inferior right polar artery reattachment (**b**). The pictures in the operating room show the same case before (**c**) and after repair (**d**). Of note, in (**c**), the arrow indicating inferior right polar renal polar artery and the vessel loop around the inferior mesenteric artery

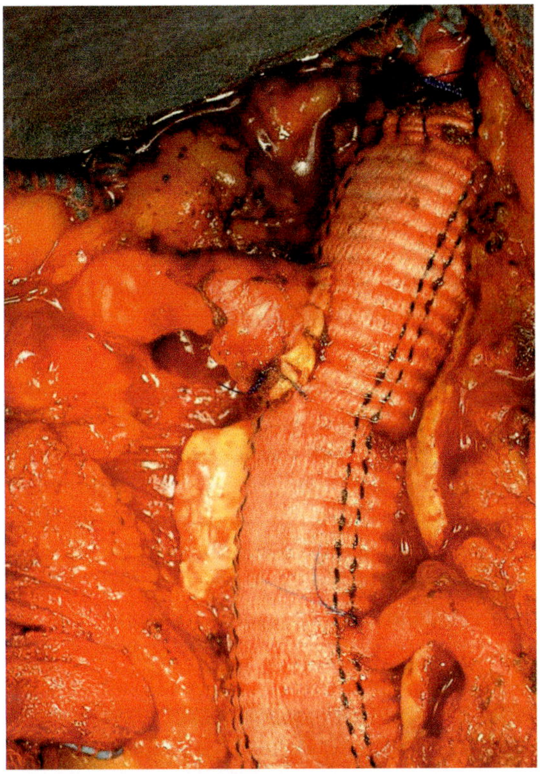

Fig. 5.2 Intraoperative imaging showing direct reattachment of the right renal artery during an AAA tube graft repair with concomitant right aberrant renal artery. Of note, on the right side, the reimplantation of the inferior mesenteric artery as well

The kidneys are connected by an isthmus of either functioning renal parenchyma or fibrous tissue [7]. In the vast majority of cases, the fusion is between the lower poles (90%). The remainder of the superior or both the superior and inferior poles is fused (sigmoid kidney or cake kidney).

As a result of this fusion, the inferior pole of each kidney point medially, ureters leave kidneys and pass anterior to the isthmus, which is typically located immediately below the inferior mesenteric artery. Also, due to the halted ascent, renal vascular anomalies are common: usually, multiple renal arteries arise from the distal aorta or iliac arteries; a wide variety of associated anomalies coexist with HSK, and anomalies for numbers and anatomy are identified in about 80% of the population [8, 9]. Various classifications for the renal blood supply in HSK were proposed, including the commonly used classification of Eisendrath (Table 5.1).

Table 5.1 Eisendrath's classification of renal blood supply in horseshoe kidney (HSK)

Classification	Description
Type I	One renal artery to each side of the kidney
Type II	One renal artery to each side of the kidney and aortic branches to the isthmus
Type III	Two renal arteries to each side of the kidney and one to the isthmus
Type IV	Two renal arteries to each side of the kidney, with one or more from iliac arteries, including isthmus branch
Type V	Multiple renal arteries arising from the aorta, mesenteric, and iliac arteries

Association between HSK and abdominal aortic aneurysm is extremely rare. The combination was first described by Julian in 1956 [10], and since then, more than 200 cases have been described in scientific literature, of which only one case was a cake kidney, a fusion between both poles. Some reports described AAA wrapped with polyester, when most cases were performed with isthmus separation.

Computed tomography (CT) angiography and three-dimensional CT or magnetic resonance (MR) angiography can identify even small branches or accessory renal arteries that may go unnoticed via other diagnostic imaging techniques.

Planning on a workstation is a critical step of the strategy to establish precise measurements of the different anatomic structures considered. In particular, careful attention has to be paid to the urinary excretal structures.

5.2.1 Surgical Techniques

The technical approach to the aorta can be anterior transperitoneal or retroperitoneal, even if the first is the most frequently used [11–14]. However, when arterial disease is limited to the aorta, the retroperitoneal approach avoids problematic dissection of anomalous renal structures [7]. The anterior transabdominal access is preferred in cases of a small isthmus or when the right iliac artery should be reached. This approach assures the best exposure of the kidney, the ureters, the aneurysm, and both iliac vessels; however, the renal isthmus can pose a problem in reimplanting aberrant renal arteries. Therefore, in order to obtain adequate aortic exposure, the isthmus can either be divided or excised. Because of the risks of retroperitoneal urinary leaks, infection, bleeding, and renal ischemia, some surgeons consider it prudent to not divide the isthmus [15]. On the other hand, isthmus division does not provoke complications in cases of vessel sacrifice with diameter <2 mm or in the presence of fibrotic isthmus. Fortunately, it is often enough to mobilize the isthmus anteriorly to place the aortic graft behind it (Fig. 5.3).

The isthmus section is limited to selective cases, especially complex cases or in emergencies (Fig. 5.4 and Movie 5.2).

The retroperitoneal approach could be particularly advantageous when the isthmus is particularly large or in the presence of a rare renal fusion anomaly of the kidneys, widely known as pancake kidney (also known as discoid kidney, disc kidney, lump kidney, fused pelvic kidney, or cake kidney).

Indeed, this approach, with mobilization of the renal mass and its excretory system toward the right, avoids venous and renal anomalies, and the renal arteries can be identified from the inside of the aneurysmal sac. Nowadays, the management of aneurysmal disease of the aorta in the setting of HSK poses several surgical challenges. Endovascular aortic aneurysm repair (EVAR) has been described in several cases of patients unfit to open repair, showing good early and midterm outcomes [16, 17]. The coverage of accessory renal arteries in patients with HSK represents the main drawback of the endovascular approach. As mentioned before, the anomalous renal arteries <2 mm in diameter can be

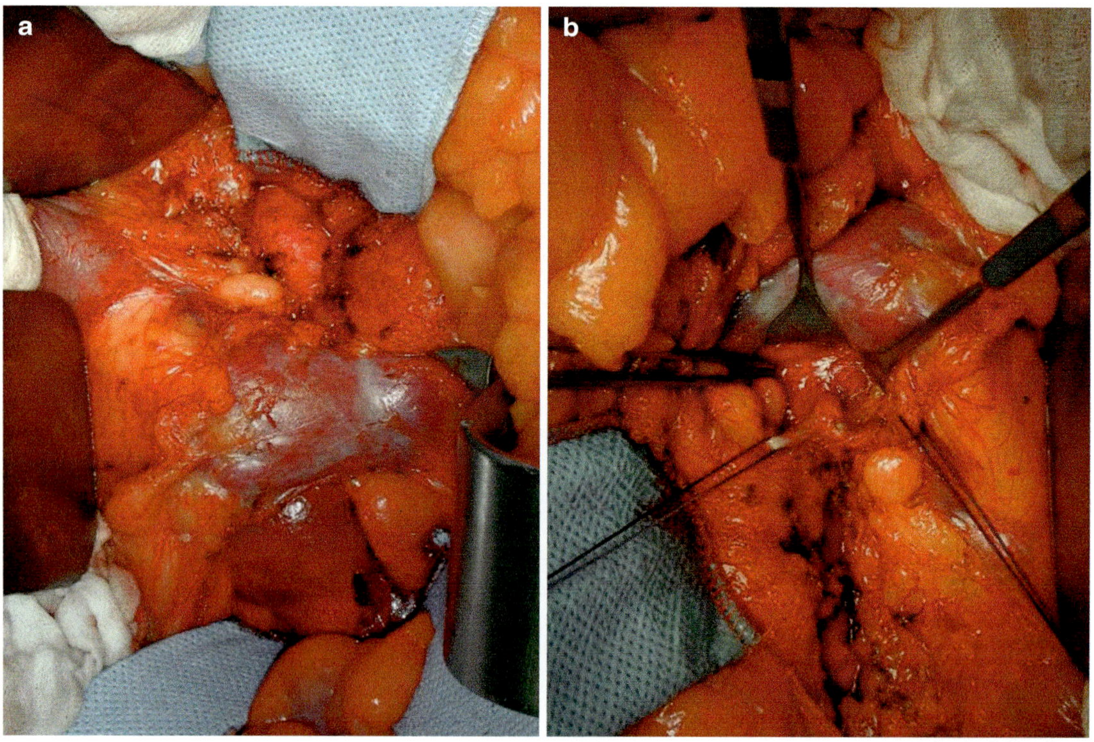

Fig. 5.3 (**a**) Intraoperative image showing the kidney's isthmus exposed above the abdominal aortic aneurysm (AAA) in a patient with concomitant horseshoe kidney. (**b**) Identification of the renal arteries from the horseshoe kidney and mobilization of the kidney isthmus. (**c**) Placing of the aortic graft behind the isthmus of the horseshoe kidney. (**d**) Final imaging of complete end-to-end aorto-aortic Dacron graft bypass reconstruction behind the kidney with renal isthmus and artery preservation

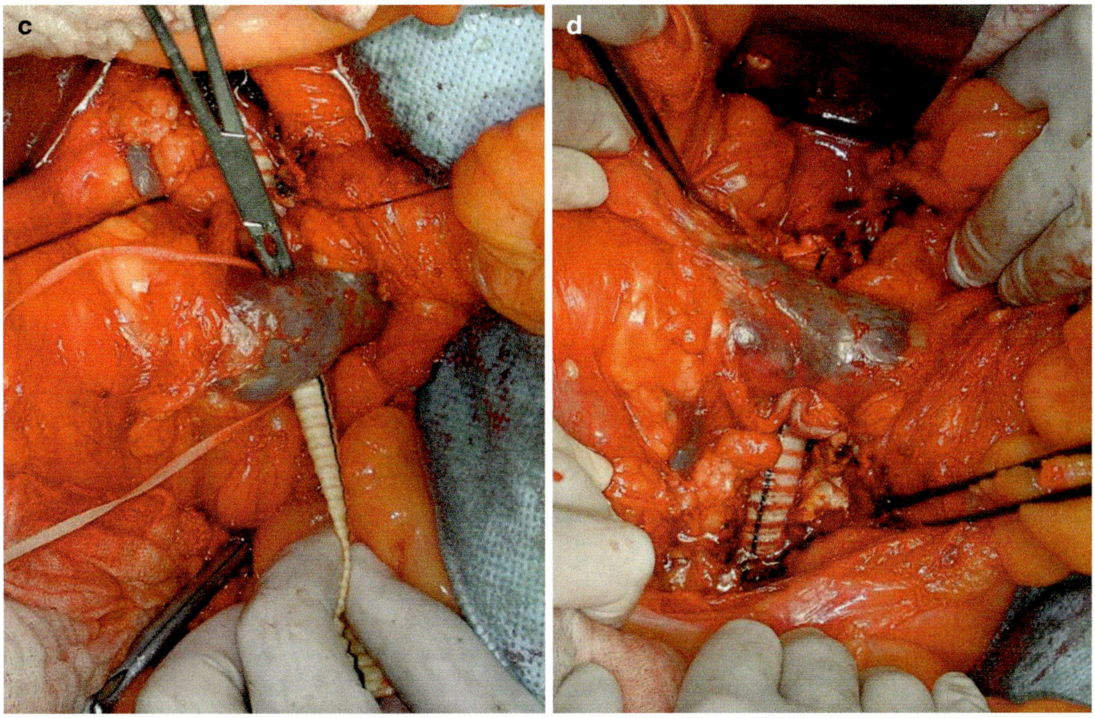

Fig. 5.3 (continued)

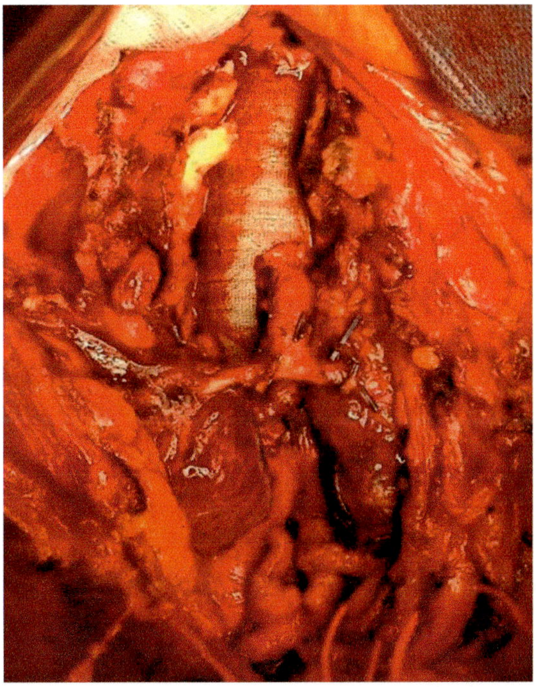

Fig. 5.4 Intraoperative imaging of a ruptured AAA in a patient with concomitant horseshoe kidney. Of note, section and suture of the two stumps at the level of renal isthmus. In Movie 5.1, retroperitoneal hematoma is also shown

sacrificed without a real risk of renal ischemia [15]. However, accessory renal arteries of significant size should be preserved in order to prevent renal infarction. Recently, the use of fenestrated or branched endografts could represent a solution to maintain the accessory renal artery perfusion [18, 19].

5.3 Pelvic Kidney

Ectopic kidney is a less frequent anomaly (0.2–0.03%) with variable locations, as shown in Table 5.2 [20, 21].

Embryologic mechanisms leading to ectopic kidneys remain uncertain, and the combination of congenital pelvic kidney with an aortoiliac aneurysm is extremely rare (Figs. 5.5, 5.6, and 5.7).

A radiological study reported that 0.18% of patients who underwent a major aortic surgery had pelvic kidneys [12]. In 1977, Ezzet et al. [22] documented the first case of a patient with a pelvic kidney associated with AAA. Since then, few cases have been reported in scientific literature.

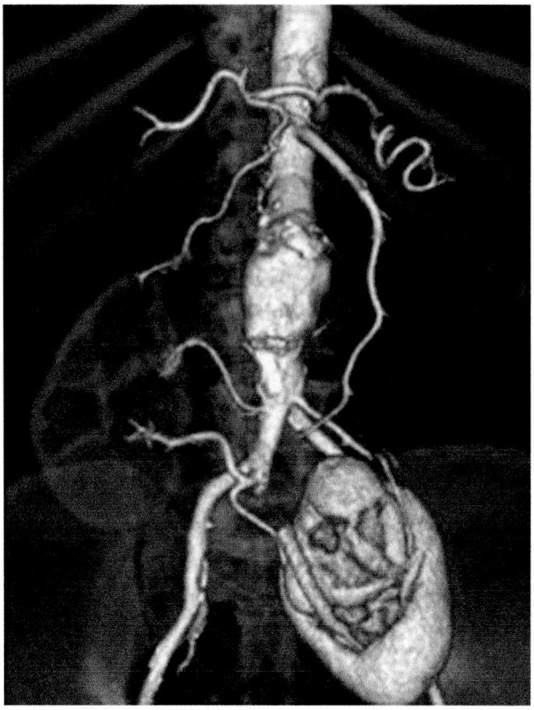

Fig. 5.5 AngioCT showing a case of infrarenal aortic aneurysm associated with ptotic right kidney and left pelvic kidney. Of note, three feeding arteries for the right ptotic kidney originating from the aorta near the superior mesenteric artery, from the origin of the right common iliac artery, and from the right hypogastric artery. Of note, two feeding arteries for the left pelvic kidney originating from the right hypogastric artery and from aortic bifurcation

Table 5.2 Ectopic kidney position

Type	Location
Pelvic	Opposite sacrum, distal to the aortic bifurcation
Lumbar	In the iliac fossa, opposite the sacral promontory
Abdominal	Above the iliac crest, adjacent to the L2 vertebra
Cephalad	Below the diaphragm, near the T10 vertebra
Thoracic	Total or partial location in the chest, above the diaphragm
Crossed ectopia	Ectopic kidney located on the opposite side from its ureteral insertion (1) with fusion, (2) without fusion, (3) solitary crossed ectopia, and (4) bilaterally crossed ectopia

5.3.1 Surgical Approach and Renal Perfusion

The surgical approach is usually the anterior transperitoneal approach, which allows for optimal visualization and control of the ectopic renal arteries usually emerging from the iliac arteries and/or distal abdominal aorta (Fig. 5.6).

The technical challenge is in preserving the function of the pelvic kidney. It is also mandatory to preserve renal perfusion to minimize intraoperative renal ischemia.

A variety of techniques have been described to limit ischemic damage to such abnormal pelvic kidneys [23, 24]. Proximal double clamping of the neck of aneurysm can be used if the aneurysm is entirely limited to the aorta [25, 26]. This technique was reported for the first time in 1986 by Lacombe et al. [27]. The authors affirmed that it does not render the kidney totally ischemic as the kidney is perfused by retrograde flow in the iliac and the lumbar arteries. When the perfusion of the kidney is completely eliminated, then either perfusion of the kidney with cold solution or surrounding it with ice packs reduces its metabolism, thereby minimizing damage. Using this technique, the kidney needs to be reperfused after about 40–45 min of cold ischemia to avoid any damage. However, this technique is limited if the proximal neck of the aneurysm is not long enough to clamp at two sites or if adequate collateral circulation is not established.

Conventional repair with the administration of furosemide and/or mannitol before cross clamping has also been described. These pharmacological agents are thought to induce diuresis before aortic cross clamping, thereby reducing the risk of acute tubular necrosis.

The main drawbacks of these techniques are that it can be a race against time to perfuse the kidney, and the ischemic insult will result in severe impairment to the kidney whose function is previously compromised.

Other options are cold crystalloid perfusion, passive shunts, and extracorporeal circulation [28, 29].

Cold crystalloid perfusion is a safe and easier method compared to extracorporeal circulation

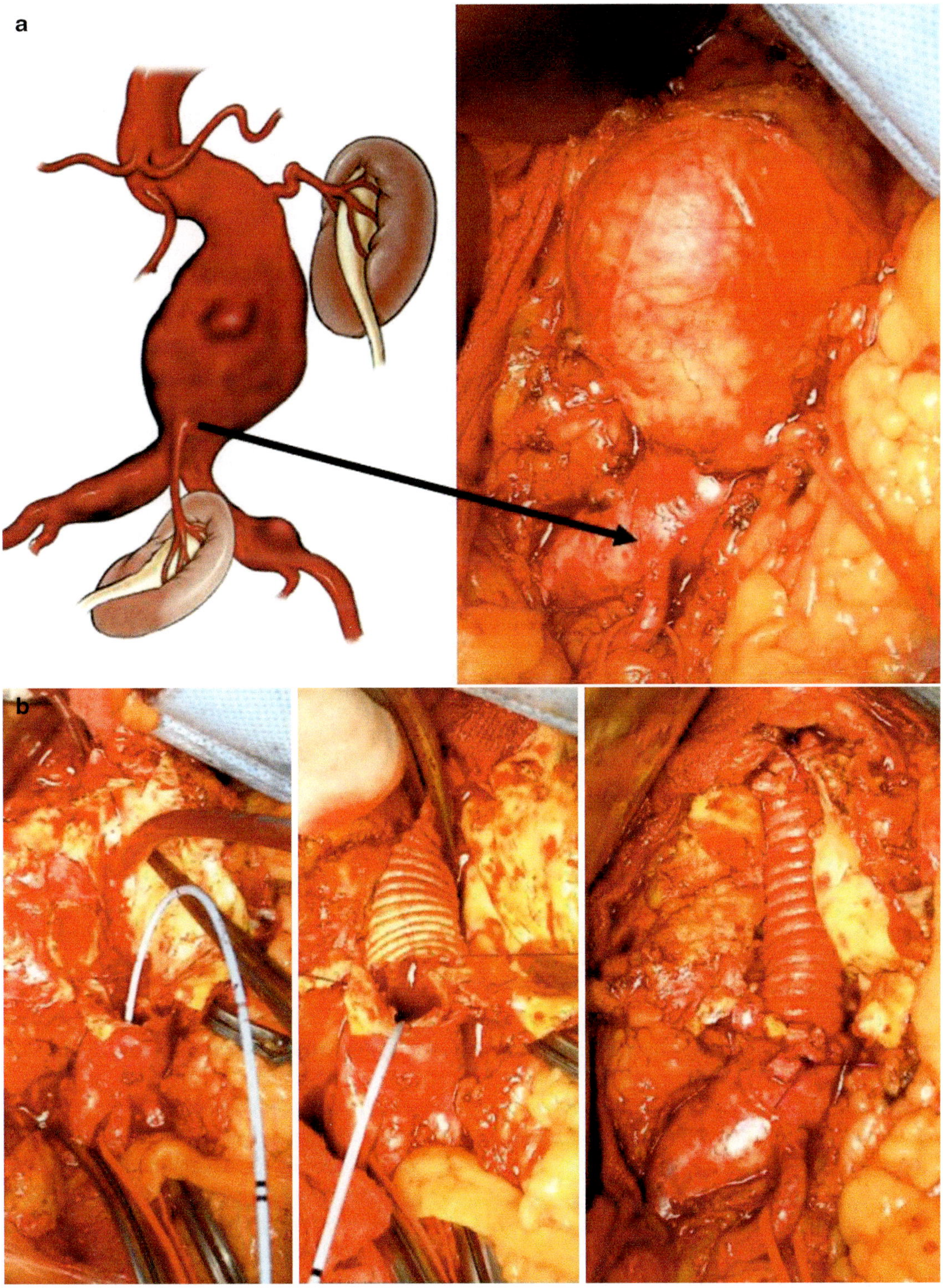

Fig. 5.6 (**a**) A case of infrarenal aortic aneurysm associated with pelvic kidney with the artery originating from the distal aorta. Schematic illustration (left) and intraoperative image (right) showing the abdominal aortic aneurysm and the pelvic kidney feeding artery (arrow). (**b**) Intraoperative images showing perfusion of cold crystalloid into the orifice of the pelvic kidney feeding artery through an occlusion perfusion balloon catheter and end-to-end Dacron aortic bypass with the main pelvic kidney renal artery reimplantation

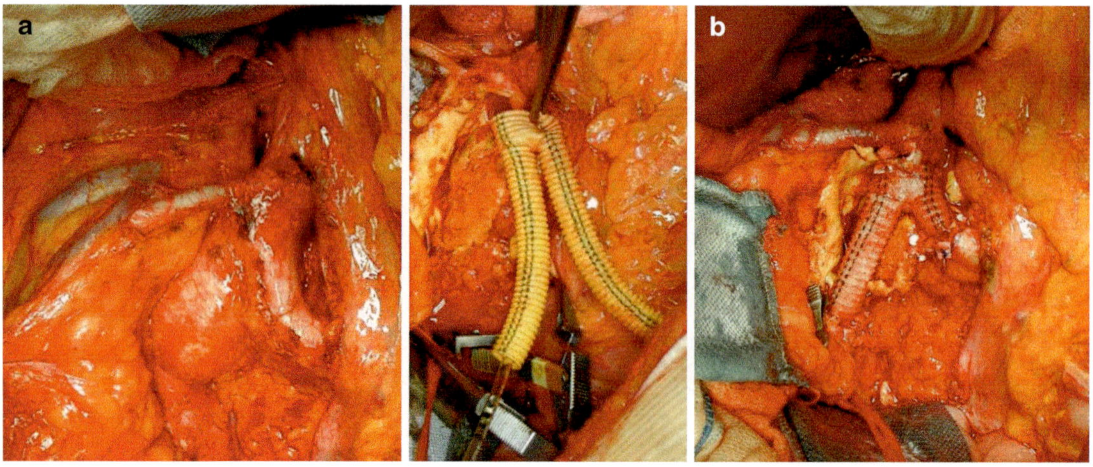

Fig. 5.7 (**a**) A case of right common iliac aneurysm associated with pelvic kidney with a main artery originating from distal aorta immediately above bifurcation. Of note occlusion perfusion balloon catheter inserted into the right limb of the aorto-bi-iliac Dacron graft in order to perfuse with cold crystalloid solution the orifice of the pelvic kidney feeding artery in the distal aorta during proximal anastomosis. (**b**) Intraoperative images showing Dacron aorto-bi-iliac bypass graft with the pelvic kidney feeding artery immediately above the proximal anastomosis

requiring longer renal ischemic time and a pump oxygenator.

As far as the use of a shunt is concerned, embolization and iatrogenic lesions during shunt placement or removal are described [30].

5.3.2 Endovascular Approach

In recent years, developments in endovascular repair of pararenal, juxta-renal, and thoracoabdominal aneurysm (TAAA) have been remarkable, representing, in high-risk patients, a valid alternative to open repair.

However, few cases of aortic aneurysm repair with congenital pelvic kidney have been reported to date.

Morales and Greenberg have described the use of a customized fenestrated graft to repair a TAAA in a patient with a left pelvic kidney supplied by a single left pelvic artery arising from around the aortic bifurcation [31]. In 2012, Spear et al. reported their experience in the treatment of renal artery anomalies and aberrant origins of renal arteries, associated or not with pelvic kidney or horseshoe kidney, using fenestrated and branched endografts. The authors showed satisfactory 6-month outcomes and concluded stating that endovascular treatment with fenestrated and branched endografts should be considered in challenging renal artery anomalies in patients unfit for open repair [32].

However, limitations of fenestrated endografts are the target vessel size <3 mm, and long-term patency rates of these stented arteries may be suboptimal. For these reasons, the use of a customized fenestrated endoluminal graft requires careful preoperative planning and patient selection. This will be an issue to address as fenestrated technology continues to evolve.

5.4 Venous Abnormalities

Congenital venous abnormalities in the retroperitoneal space are relatively infrequent and, under normal circumstances, asymptomatic but have clinical importance in aortoiliac surgery. These anomalies have a low prevalence (5.65%) [33, 34]: type I retroaortic left renal vein (LRV), with an incidence of 0.3–0.9% joining the inferior vena cava (IVC) in orthotopic position [34] (Fig. 5.8); type II LRV that joins the IVC lower, at L4–L5 (0.4–0.9%) [35]; circumaortic renal

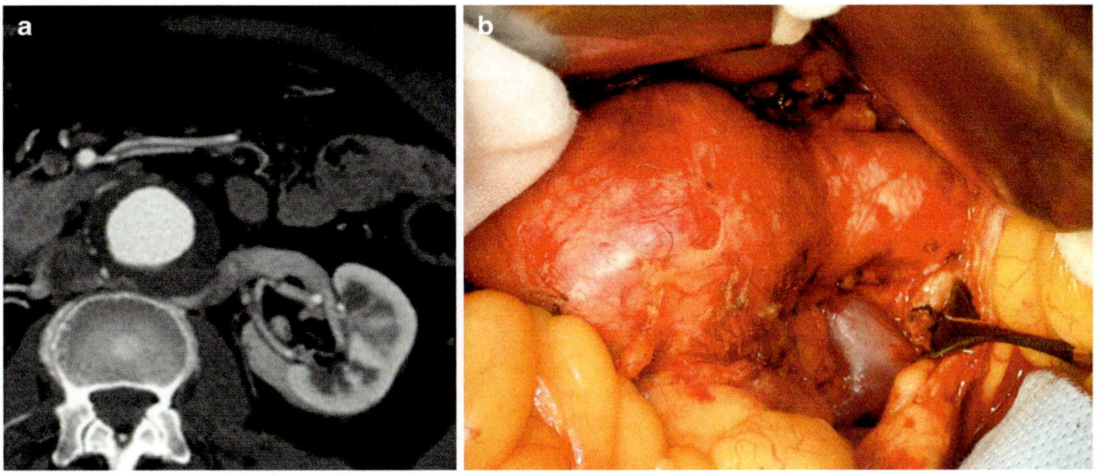

Fig. 5.8 (**a**) AngioCT showing a retroaortic left renal vein in a patient with infrarenal abdominal aortic aneurysm. (**b**) Intraoperative images showing a retroaortic left renal vein in a patient with infrarenal abdominal aortic aneurysm

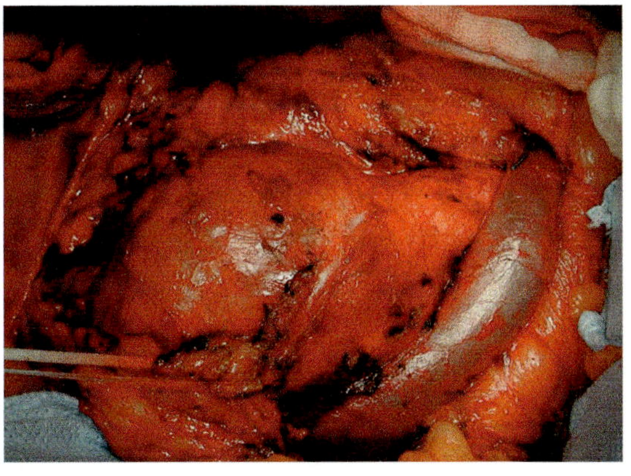

Fig. 5.9 Intraoperative images showing a left-sided inferior vena cava in a patient with infrarenal abdominal aortic aneurysm

collar (0.5–1.4%) [36]; left-sided IVC (Figs. 5.9 and 5.10) and duplication of IVC (0.2–3%) [37] (Fig. 5.10); and the least common anomaly (0.2–0.5%) [33, 35]. The presence of vascular anatomical anomalies can create technical difficulties during aortoiliac surgery, and the patients are most likely to suffer severe bleeding; thus, the surgeon must be alert to detect these anomalies.

There are some variants:

- Retroaortic LRV type I. The ventral preaortic limb of the renal venous collar is obliterated, and the dorsal limb remains on the contrary of the normal evolution, joining the IVC in an orthotopic position, in the neck of the aneurysm.
- Retroaortic LRV type II. The dorsal limb is detected in a lower position, at L4–L5, behind the aneurysm, and joins the IVC, gonadal, or ascending lumbar veins.
- In the circumaortic LRV, both preaortic and retroaortic limbs of the venous collar persist patent.
- Transposition or left-sided IVC develops from the persistence of the left instead of right supracardinal vein, which occurs in the normal evolution. The left-sided infrarenal IVC typically joins the LRV, before it crosses the aorta to form a normal right-sided suprarenal IVC. A complete transposition of the IVC to the left with hemizygous continuation is extremely rare. This case can present itself with or without situs viscerum inversus.
- In the duplication of the IVC, both left and right supracardinal veins persist.
- Preaortic confluence of the iliac veins.
- Although no other anomaly has been encountered behind the left renal vein during this period, communication between the left ascending lumbar vein and the left renal vein is sometimes experienced [38].

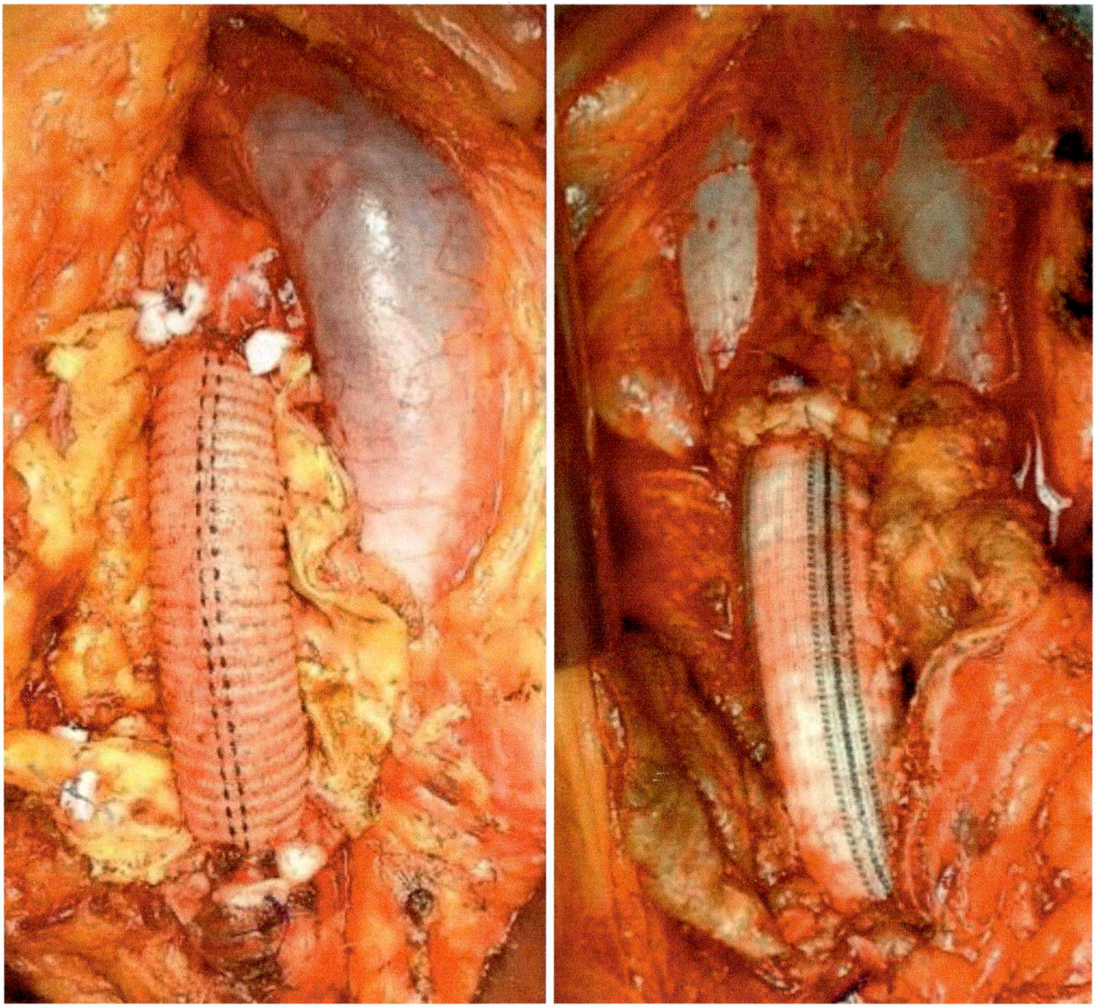

Fig. 5.10 Intraoperative images showing infrarenal aortic tube graft repair in a patient with a left-sided inferior vena cava (left) and a duplication of inferior vena cava (right)

- The superior lumbar veins can be also terminated to the dorsal aspect of the left renal vein [39].

Venous hemorrhage is the most troublesome complication during AAA surgery, occurring particularly during dissection of the proximal infrarenal and lower aorta, the level of CIAs [40].

During elective surgery for AAA, the presence of these rare anomalies can be managed with little additional risk through the use of a long midline incision and transperitoneal route. With a careful blunt dissection, it is possible to gain proximal and distal control mobilizing the "unconventional" caval conformation, which may result strictly adherent to the aorta.

These considerations are valid even in the presence of Kartagener's syndrome.

On the other hand, a large series of aortic interventions showed that the LRV can be readily divided adjacent to the inferior vena cava in order to provide improved exposure during complex aortic reconstruction. Theoretical disadvantages of renal vein ligation such as flank pain or hematuria were not noted in this series [41].

5.5 Conclusion

An in-depth knowledge of variations in the anatomy of the kidneys is mandatory before planning an aortoiliac aneurysm repair. Both arterial and venous vascular anatomies should be carefully evaluated together with possible more complex changes including congenital fusion disorders and ectopia. Accurate preoperative planning with advanced image studies including CT scan or MRN angiography, and, in selected cases, renal artery arteriography and DUS, for complete knowledge of renal vascular anatomy is the key of success in more complex cases. To preserve renal function during open repair, various methods have been reported, but no procedure has still been clearly assessed as the therapeutic gold standard. However, strategies based on reduced renal clamping time, renal branch reattachment/preservation, and renal perfusion with blood or cold crystalloid seem to be effective in minimizing ischemia-reperfusion renal damage.

In selected cases, endovascular repair with fenestrated/branched endografts or CHIMPS may represent an alternative to open repair, even if larger series and longer follow-up are needed.

References

1. Glenn J. Analysis of 51 patients with horseshoe kidney. N Engl J Med. 1959;261:684–7.
2. Sidell PM, Pairolero PC, Payne WS, Bernatz PE, Spittel JA Jr. Horseshoe kidney associated with surgery of the abdominal aorta. Mayo Clin Proc. 1979;54:97–103.
3. Bauer SB, Perlmutter AD, Retik AB. Anomalies of the upper urinary tract. In: Walsh PC, editor. Campbell's urology. 6th ed. Philadelphia: WB Saunders; 1992. p. 1357–44.
4. O'Hara PJ, Hakaim AG, Hertzer NR, Herzer NR, Krajewski LP, Cox GS, et al. Surgical management of aortic aneurysm and coexistent horseshoe kidney: review of a 31 year experience. J Vasc Surg. 1993;17:940–7.
5. Glodny B, Petersen J, Hofmann KJ, Schenk C, Herwig R, Treb T, et al. Kidney fusion anomalies revisited: clinical and radiological analysis of 209 cases of crossed fused ectopia and horseshoe kidney. BJU Int. 2009;103:224–35.
6. Grainger R, Murphy DM, Lane V. Horseshoe kidney-a review of the presentation, associated congenital anomalies and complications in 73 patients. Ir Med J. 1983;76:315–7.
7. Faggioli GL, Freyrie A, Pilato A, Ferri M, Curti T, Paragona O, D'Addato M. Renal anomalies in aortic surgery: contemporary results. Surgery. 2003;133:641–6.
8. Boujnh H, Abid I, Moalla N, Zmerli S. Le rein pelvien. Ann Urol. 1989;23:11–6.
9. Eisendrath DN, Phifer FM, Culver HB. Horseshoe kidney. Ann Surg. 1926;82:735–64.
10. Phelan JT, Bernatz PE, DeWeerd JH. Abdominal aortic aneurysm associated with a horseshoe kidney: report of a case. Mayo Clin Proc. 1957;32:77–81.
11. Bietz DS, Merendno KA. Abdominal aneurysm and horse- shoe kidney: a review. Ann Surg. 1975;181:333–41.
12. Brewster DC, Retana A, Waltman AC, Darling RC. Angiography in the management of aneurysms of the abdominal aorta: its value and safety. N Engl J Med. 1975;292:822–5.
13. Connelly TL, McKinnon W, Smith RB III, Perdue GD. Abdominal aortic surgery and horseshoe kidney: report of six cases and a review. Arch Surg. 1980;115:1459–63.
14. Shortell CK, Welch EL, Ouriel K, et al. Operative management of coexistent aortic disease and horseshoe kidney. Ann Vasc Surg. 1995;9:123–8.
15. Canova G, Masini R, Santoro E, et al. Surgical treatment of abdominal aortic aneurysm in association with horseshoe kidney. Three case reports and a review of technique. Tex Heart Inst J. 1998;25:206–10.
16. Ilic NS, Koncar I, Dragas M, Cvetkovic S, Pejkic S, Kostic D, et al. Technical considerations for transabdominal aortic reconstruction with renal fusion and ectopia: case series. Vascular. 2010;18(5):269–74.
17. Martin MC, Giles KA, Pomposelli FB, Hamdan AD, Wyers MC, Schermerhorn ML. National outcomes after open repair of abdominal aortic aneurysms with visceral or renal bypass. Ann Vasc Surg. 2010;24(1):106–12.
18. Greenberg RK, Lu Q, Roselli EE, et al. Contemporary analysis of descending thoracic and thoracoabdominal aneurysm repair: a comparison of endovascular and open techniques. Circulation. 2008;118:808–17.
19. Chuter TA, Rapp JH, Hiramoto JS, Schneider DB, Howell B, Reilly LM. Endovascular treatment of thoracoabdominal aortic aneurysms. J Vasc Surg. 2008;47:6–16.
20. Faggioli GL, Tarantini S, Stella A, D'Addato M. Aneurisma dell' aorta addominale associato a rene ectopico pelvico e stenosi dell' arteria renale. G It Chir Vasc. 1994;1:47–54.
21. Thompson GJ, Pace JM. Ectopic kidney: a review of 97 cases. Surg Gynecol Obstet. 1937;64:935.
22. Ezzet F, Dorazio R, Herzberg R. Horseshoe and pelvic kidneys associated with abdominal aortic aneurysms. Am J Surg. 1977;134:196–8.

23. O'Hara PJ, Hakaim AG, Hertzer NR, Krajewski LP, Cox GS, Beven EG. Surgical management of aortic aneurysm and coexistent horseshoe kidney: review of 31-year experience. J Vasc Surg. 1993;17:940–7.
24. Eckes D, Lawrence P. Bilateral iliac artery aneurysms and pancake kidney: a case report. J Vasc Surg. 1997;25:927–30.
25. Hollis HW Jr, Rutherford R, Crawford GJ, Cleland BP, Marx WH, Clark JR. Abdominal aortic aneurysm repair in patients with pelvic kidney—technical considerations and literature review. J Vasc Surg. 1989;9:404–9.
26. Schneider JR, Cronenwett JL. Temporary perfusion of congenital pelvic kidney during abdominal aortic aneurysm repair. J Vasc Surg. 1993;17:613–7.
27. Lacombe M. Abdominal aortic aneurysmectomy in renal transplant patients. Ann Surg. 1986;203:62–8.
28. Marone EM, Tshomba Y, Brioschi C, Calliari FM, Chiesa R. Aorto-iliac aneurysm associated with congenital pelvic kidney: a short series of successful open repairs under hypothermic selective renal perfusion. J Vasc Surg. 2008;47:638–44.
29. Campbell DA Jr, Lorber MI, Arneson WA, Kirsh MM, Turcotte JG, Stanley JC. Renal transplant protection during abdominal aortic aneurysmectomy with a pump-oxygenator. Surgery. 1981;90:559–62.
30. Sterioff S, Parks L. Temporary vascular bypass for perfusion of a renal transplant during abdominal aneurysmectomy. Surgery. 1977;82:558–60.
31. Morales JP, Greenberg RK. Customised stent graft for complex thoraco-abdominal aneurysm associated with congenital pelvic kidney. Eur J Vasc Endovasc Surg. 2009;37:557–9.
32. Spear R, Maurel B, Sobocinski J, Perini P, Guillou M, Midulla M, Azzaoui R, Tefera G, Haulon S. Technical note and results in the management of anatomical variants of renal vascularisation during endovascular aneurysm repair. Eur J Vasc Endovasc Surg. 2012;43(4):398–403.
33. Aljabri B, McDonald PS, Satin R, Stein LS, Obrand DI, Steinmetz OK. Incidence of major venous and renal anomalies relevant to aortoiliac surgery as demonstrated by computed tomography. Ann Vasc Surg. 2001;15:615–8.
34. Minniti S, Procacci C. Congenital anomalies of the vena cava: embryological origin, imaging features and report of three new variants. Eur Radiol. 2002;12:2040–55.
35. Bass JE, Redwine MD, Kramer LA, Huynh PT, Harris JH. Spectrum of congenital anomalies of the inferior vena cava: cross-sectional imaging findings. Radiographics. 2000;20:639–52.
36. Giglia JS, Thompson JK. Repair of a thoracoabdominal aortic aneurysm in the presence of a left-sided inferior vena cava. J Vasc Surg. 2004;40:161–3.
37. Karkos CD, Bruce IA, Thomson GJL, Lambert ME. Retroaortic left renal vein and its implications in abdominal aortic surgery. Ann Vasc Surg. 2001;15:703–8.
38. Pilcher JM, Padhani AR. Problem in diagnostic imaging: behind the left renal vein. Clin Anat. 1997;10:349–52.
39. Davis RA, Milloy FJ, Anson BJ. Lumbar, renal, and associated parietal and visceral veins based upon a study of 100 specimens. Surg Gynecol Obstet. 1958;107:1–22.
40. Brener BJ, Darling RC, Frederich PL, Linton RR. Major venous anomalies complicating abdominal aortic surgery. Arch Surg. 1974;108:159–65.
41. Russell H, Samson MD, Michael R, Lepore MD Jr, David P, Showalter MD, Deepak G, Nair MD, Julien B, Lanoue S. Long-term safety of left renal vein division and ligation to expedite complex abdominal aortic surgery. J Vasc Surg. 2009;50:500–4.

Endovascular Aortic Repair: The Renal Side of the Story

6

Mirko Menegolo, Francesco Squizzato, Michele Piazza, Chiara Colacchio, Franco Grego, and Michele Antonello

6.1 Introduction

It is common to find renal function modifications following abdominal aortic aneurysm (AAA) repair, but the precise short-term and long-term effects of open surgical repair (OSR) and endovascular repair (EVAR) on renal function are still unclear. This represents a largely debated topic, especially since the introduction of EVAR in the treatment of infrarenal AAAs with good early and midterm results, even for moderate- to high-risk patients [1, 2]. The advantages of decreased morbidity, mortality, and length of stay [3, 4], in particular, justify the impressive wider use of EVAR in the last two decades; however, a stronger definition of long-term renal effects may help to better select patients for treatment with endovascular techniques.

Renal function impairment may occur after both open and endovascular repairs for several reasons. During open repair (OR), the main factor affecting renal function is the site of aortic cross-clamping, whether infra- or suprarenal, depending on the anatomical characteristics of the aneurysm. Suprarenal clamping is in fact associated with hemodynamic changes that may cause postoperative renal dysfunction in up to 25% of patients [5]. Additionally, embolization into renal arteries or renal artery dissection may occur. On the other hand, EVAR still retains some intrinsic potential adverse effects on renal function due to endoluminal manipulation, which need iodine contrast dye (both for the treatment and the follow-up), and possibly secondary procedures. Moreover, since not all AAAs are amenable to infrarenal endovascular repair, in many cases, where the risky condition of the patient increases the operative mortality of traditional surgery, transrenal fixation (TRF) remains the only option for endovascular treatment [6, 7]. The efficacy of the transrenally placed uncovered stent has been reported, but there are concerns about their effects on renal function. Several reports have indicated an acceptable short-term result of TRF on renal function [8–16]. Other reports seem to demonstrate a decrease of renal function after EVAR, regardless of the fixation level and especially in the long-term period [17–21].

Our experience in this field started more than 10 years ago, when we initially studied the short-term effects of TRF on renal function in a series of patients treated with EVAR. More recently, our aim has been to compare OSR with EVAR

M. Menegolo · F. Squizzato · M. Piazza
C. Colacchio · F. Grego (✉) · M. Antonello
Department of Cardiac, Thoracic and Vascular Sciences, Vascular and Endovascular Surgery, University of Padova, Padova, Italy
e-mail: franco.grego@unipd.it

© Springer Nature Switzerland AG 2019
Y. Tshomba et al. (eds.), *Visceral Vessels and Aortic Repair*,
https://doi.org/10.1007/978-3-319-94761-7_6

(both with TRF and infrarenal fixation (IRF)) regarding long-term effects on renal function in the treatment of infrarenal AAAs.

All of our investigations have been characterized by the use of renal perfusion scintigraphy (RPS) to assess pre- and postoperative renal function. This choice derived from the fact that RPS has a significantly higher sensitivity than conventional serum markers, especially for demonstrating eventual worsening of function limited to a single kidney [22, 23].

6.2 Renal Function Assessment

Overall renal function is traditionally measured as renal clearance. The clearance for a specific compound is defined as the volume of plasma completely cleared of that compound per unit of time ($C_s = U_s \times V/P_s$; C = clearance, U_s = urinary output, P_s = plasma concentration). The clearance depends on all three fundamental renal functions: glomerular filtration, tubular secretion, and tubular reabsorption.

In clinical practice, creatinine clearance (C_{Cr}) is used as an estimate of the GFR (glomerular filtration rate), since creatinine is virtually neither secreted nor reabsorbed by renal tubules. In this situation, GFR results from the following formula: GFR = $C_{Cr} = U_{Cr} \times V/P_{Cr}$. From this concept, it appears that GFR can be estimated from the creatinine plasma concentration and creatinine urinary output in a given period of time, typically requiring 24 h urine collection. An even simpler method to estimate GFR consists in the C_{Cr} calculation based only on P_{Cr} measurement, using the Cockroft-Gault formula (GFR = (140-age) × weight (kg)/(72 × P_{Cr}) with a correction factor of 0.85 to account in part for age-related differences for female patients). An alternative to the Cockroft-Gault formula is the Modification of Diet in Renal Disease (MDRD) study equation, GFR = 175 × $(S_{Cr})^{-1.154}$ × $(\text{Age})^{-0.203}$ × (0.742 if female) × (1.212 if African American), which accounts for a standardized body surface instead of weight.

These methods of GFR estimation based on P_{Cr} (or S_{Cr}, serum creatinine) have the advantage to be simple and readily available in all clinical settings but are limited in that they represent only an estimation of the true GFR that may depend on several other factors such as weight, muscle body mass, sex, age, and comorbidities. Furthermore, P_{Cr} results in a relatively low-sensitive diagnostic tool, since large changes on renal function must occur before a significant increase of P_{Cr}, and, even if CrCl allows a more accurate evaluation of the glomerular filtration rate, this may be overestimated because of a variable tubular secretion of creatinine [23–25]. Another critical point is that C_{Cr} does not allow a renal function determination separately for each kidney, which may be useful, especially in a clinical research scenario.

Thus, a direct measurement of GFR should be advocated to obtain a more precise estimation of renal function. In this regard, RPS represents a more suitable and sensible test, since it evaluates separately the function of the kidneys and it is able to identify subtle renal functional loss [22].

For these reasons, in our studies, renal function has always been evaluated by RPS. This technique is based on the intravenous administration of a radiopharmaceutical and subsequent GFR calculation with the Gates method. For GFR determination, technetium-99m diethylenetriamine pentaacetic acid (DTPA) is typically used, since it is characterized by a negligible protein binding and it is only filtrated by glomerula without being secreted or reabsorbed by tubules. A decrease ≥20% of the GFR was considered clinically relevant. S_{Cr} was anyway tested as well, and Cl_{Cr} was estimated at the same time of S_{Cr}, with the Cockroft and Gault formula. Also in this case, postoperative change ≥20% above the baseline of S_{Cr} and/or Cl_{Cr} was considered significant for renal dysfunction.

As an example of RPS potential, Fig. 6.1 reports the preoperative and follow-up RPS results in a patient treated with EVAR, with a postoperative decrease of GRF in the left kidney, without an overall decrease of S_{Cr}.

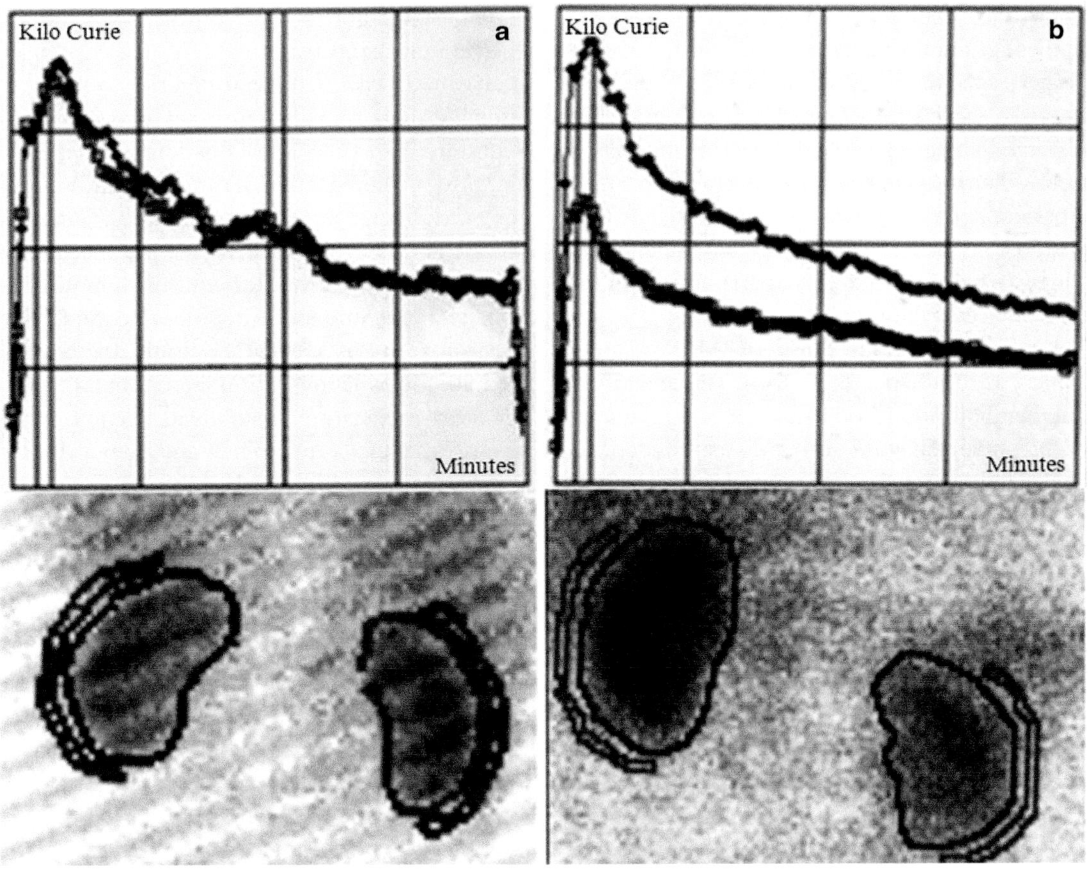

Fig. 6.1 Preoperative renal perfusion scintigraphy (RPS) using ^{99}TC-DTPA (**a**). The postoperative RPS shows a decrease of glomerular filtration rate in the left kidney; in this patient no variation on total serum creatinine levels were observed (**b**)

6.3 Causes of Renal Function Impairment After AAA Repair

6.3.1 Open Surgical Repair

It is common to find a worsening in renal function after OSR of AAAs. This is mostly related to perioperative hypotension leading to acute tubular necrosis, which is more frequent in patients presenting with preoperative renal dysfunction or in patients treated in an urgent/emergent setting. Temporary renal artery occlusion (due to suprarenal aortic clamping), hypovolemic shock, post cross-clamp hypotension, and cardiogenic shock in the perioperative period are the most common causes of acute renal dysfunction in open aortic surgery.

The site of aortic cross-clamping is another crucial factor [5], since suprarenal aortic cross-clamping determines a temporary isolated period of renal ischemia, which can cause postoperative acute renal failure (ARF) in up to 25% of cases. Preoperative chronic renal insufficiency and the duration of cross-clamping are the most important predictors of ARF after suprarenal clamping. For this reason, the overall time of renal ischemia should generally be maintained at less than 40 min, but the period of ischemia may be further prolonged, in particular in pararenal or suprarenal aneurysms requiring renal artery reconstruction. In these cases, a valid alternative consists in temporary renal reperfusion. In fact, in a previous study [24], we demonstrated that the temporary restoration of renal arterial inflow through a Pruitt–Inahara shunt for 3 min after 30 min of cross-clamping ischemia, protected from postoperative renal failure in juxtarenal aortic surgery, is also considered in patients at high risk for acute renal failure.

Another important cause of ARF in aortic surgery is renal atheroembolism. The quantity of microembolization produced during manipulation of the juxtarenal aorta during dissection depends on the embologenic potential of the atheromatous debris and the operative techniques used to prevent such an event. The clinical impact of renal microembolization depends on the quantity of functioning renal units before the procedure and the presence of other causes of ARF. In the absence of other factors favoring ARF and in the presence of normal mass of functioning nephron units, relatively large amounts of atheromatous microemboli can accumulate without immediate impact on renal function. In contrast, in patients with minimal renal reserve, the added insult of even minor microembolizations can lead to decompensation and ARF.

Another issue to consider during aortic OSR is the possible need for left renal vein ligation to gain proper exposure of the aortic neck. This maneuver is generally well tolerated if the operating surgeon takes care to preserve the principal tributaries of the left renal vein (the left gonadal vein, the left ureteral vein, capsular veins, lumbar veins and the ascending lumbar vein from above, and the left middle suprarenal vein and the inferior phrenic vein from below) performing the ligation near the confluence in the cava vein.

6.3.2 Endovascular Repair

Endovascular repair is generally considered a less invasive approach compared to OSR, but the early and long-term effects of EVAR on renal function are usually underestimated, since EVAR may also cause renal impairment through different mechanisms.

The main cause of renal function worsening after EVAR is represented by contrast-induced nephrotoxicity (CIN). This is defined as a 25% increase of the baseline serum creatinine or an absolute increase of at least 0.5 mg/dL (44.2 mmol/L) of serum creatinine, occurring between 24 and 72 h after contrast administration, and not imputable to other factors. The nephrotoxicity is caused by iodinated agents mediating vasoconstriction and tubular damage, and preexisting renal insufficiency, heart failure, diabetes, myeloma, and hypoproteinemia are the major risk factors for CIN. The volume of contrast media, contrast characteristics (including osmolarity, ionicity, molecular structure, and viscosity), and the route of administration (intra-arterial or intravenous) are also relevant. CIN is usually temporary, but in some cases, it may cause persistent renal insufficiency or lead to dialysis. Furthermore, EVAR is characterized by the need for strict follow-up, based on the repeated administration of contrast media for angio-CT scans, with a possible long-term renal function decrease. In this context, endovascular re-intervention performed for midterm and long-term complications (endoleaks, migration, limb occlusion, etc.) may also play a role.

To prevent contrast nephropathy, we administered *N*-acetylcysteine 600 mg orally twice a day for 1 day before and 2 days after EVAR and for any other contrast study during the follow-up period. Furthermore, all patients undergoing angiography or contrast-enhanced computed tomography (CT) receive hydration as guidelines recommend, and all nephrotoxic drugs (angiotensin-converting enzyme inhibitors, angiotensin receptor blockers, nonsteroidal anti-inflammatory drugs, and aminoglycosides) were withdrawn 24 h before contrast exposure [26]. In patients with post-procedural renal dysfunction (GFR < 65 mL/min in men and <60 mL/min in women), the post-EVAR surveillance was usually based on non-contrast-enhanced CT to assess the sac size and the correct device position in duplex ultrasound scanning.

Atheroembolism involving renal arteries may also occur during EVAR, due to manipulation of the juxtarenal aorta with guidewires and catheters. Regarding the clinical consequences of renal atheroembolism, the same considerations already described for OSR are valid.

Another matter to consider is the use of endografts with suprarenal fixation, which has been associated with the concern of short- and long-term renal function worsening due to atheroembolism and renal flow modifications induced by the presence of the free-flow proximal stent through the renal ostia.

An additional issue regards the use of endovascular techniques for the treatment of juxtarenal and pararenal aortic aneurysms, requiring the use of techniques involving the use of renal stents (chimney technique, fenestrated and branched endografts). In these cases, the risk of CIN is increased by the higher dose of contrast needed for the procedure, atheroembolism is increased by the need to cannulate one or both renal arteries, and there is a low but non-negligible risk of stent occlusion during the follow-up.

6.4 The Effect of Transrenal Fixation on Renal Function: Results of a Previous Pilot Study

Our first experience derived from the concern that TRF of abdominal endografts could result in potential renal function impairment due to embolization and flow modifications. Thus, we initially aimed to compare TRF to IRF focusing on the short-term effects on renal function in a cohort of 135 patients treated for infrarenal AAA. Between April 1999 and May 2002, 47 patients (34.8%) had a TRF [25], while 88 had IRF. Indications for TRF included short (1.5 cm, ranging from 0.8 to 1.5 cm) infrarenal proximal neck (28 patients, 59.5%), angulation <120° between the flow axis of the proximal neck and the body of the aneurysm or a pyramidal-shaped proximal neck (11 patients, 23.4%), and the presence of juxtarenal heavy (50% of the circumference) calcification or thrombus (8 patients, 17.1%). The endovascular procedure was always performed in the operating room under general or local anesthesia, and the contrast dye was usually 150 mL (range, 100–160 mL; Omnipaque-350). RPS (99m TC-DTPA) was performed preoperatively on the third postoperative day and repeated at 1 month in patients with worsening of renal function, defined as a decrease of GFR higher than 20%.

The midterm follow-up included routine blood tests (with S_{Cr}) at 3, 6, 12, 18, and 24 months and then yearly and RPS and contrast-enhanced CT scan at 6, 12 months, and yearly thereafter.

In 15 patients (31.9%), a change between the pre- and postoperative RPS was observed; it was permanent in 12 and transient in 3 cases. The permanent changes at RPS were expected in seven patients and unexpected in five. The expected changes were secondary to a segmentary renal infarction (<25% of total renal parenchyma) caused by the planned exclusion of a renal polar artery. Unexpected changes were observed in five patients (10.6%) at the RPS performed postoperatively; three of these patients had a slight preoperative renal insufficiency; and in three of these, a single kidney was involved.

The results of this study strengthened the hypothesis that S_{Cr} is not an accurate index to detect renal impairment since in three (6.3%) patients a significant reduction of GFR (>20%) was observed in the absence of any relevant change of S_{Cr} level. Moreover, the RPS revealed that the impairment of renal function was limited to a single kidney in two patients and bilateral in one. There were no statistical differences in terms of procedural and renal function results between TRF and IRF, but this may be related to the small number of patients (47) in this study.

However, this study showed that some patients are at risk of GFR impairment >20% after EVAR, which can be demonstrated by RPS in 10.6% of cases, and this should be taken into consideration when selecting patients undergoing this procedure, especially in those with preoperative renal insufficiency.

6.5 The Effects on Renal Function of Open and Endovascular Aortic Repair: Long-Term Results

The previous study was limited by the retrospective design, the low number of patients, and the short follow-up limited to early results. However, a comparison of EVAR with OSR would be appropriate in helping to direct patients to the best type of treatment. We then designed a prospective study, conducted from January 2003 to December 2007 [27], to compare OSR with EVAR over a long-term period. The hypotheses of the study were that patients undergoing OSR would demonstrate a lesser decline in renal function over time compared with those undergoing EVAR. In addition, we hypothesized that there would be lower renal function impairment after EVAR with IRF than with TRF. The presence of factors that could affect post-procedural renal function was considered as exclusion criteria: high preoperative renal dysfunction, renal artery stenosis >60%, renal accessory artery planned to be covered by the endograft, a single functioning kidney, hemodialysis and kidney transplant, and pararenal aneurysm requiring suprarenal aortic cross-clamping (Fig. 6.2).

Treatment selection was based on anatomical characteristics and patients' surgical risk. Preoperative angio-CT scan was acquired for all patients.

OSR was offered to patients with unsuitable anatomy, including proximal infrarenal aortic neck of less than 15 mm long or greater than

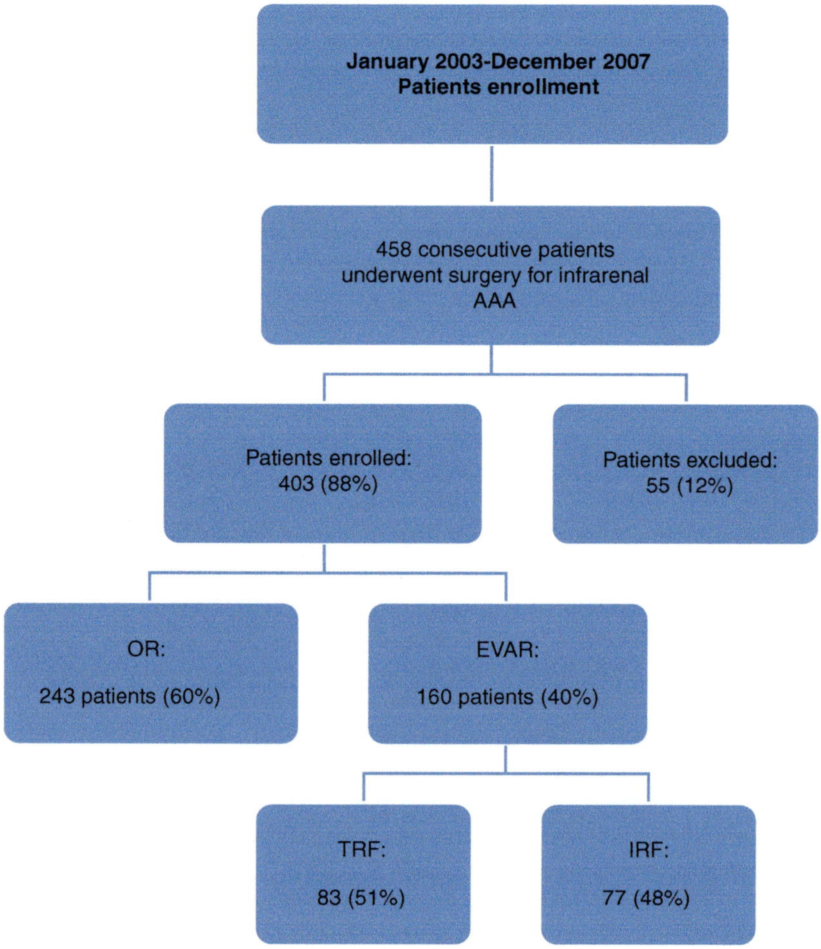

Fig. 6.2 Open surgical (OSR) versus endovascular repair (EVAR) for long-term investigation on renal function. In this study we excluded patients with creatinine clearance <65 mL/min in men and <60 mL/min in women; renal artery stenosis >60%; renal accessory artery planned to be covered by the endograft; single functioning kidney; hemodialysis; kidney transplant; and pararenal aneurysm requiring a suprarenal aortic cross-clamping. Open repair was offered in patients with unsuitable anatomy for EVAR

30 mm in diameter, proximal neck angulation of greater than 60°, extensive neck thrombus, access vessel calcifications (more than 50% circumference involvement) with tortuosity (angulation >60%), common iliac or hypogastric arteries aneurysms of greater than 30 mm in diameter, and associated iliac occlusive disease. OSR was also offered as the first option in patients with long life expectancy, based on age and the absence of significant comorbidities.

The endovascular procedure was always performed in the operating room under general or peridural anesthesia; an intraoperative digital angiography was performed after the device deployment to identify any endoleaks and assess the patency of renal arteries.

Clinical and technical success was defined according to the reporting standards for endovascular repair [28].

RPS was performed preoperatively and postoperatively at 30 days, at 6 and 12 months, and then yearly. Patients that underwent EVAR underwent postoperative contrast-enhanced CT scan at 6 months, 12 months, and annually thereafter; in the OR group, follow-up was based on an annual ultrasound duplex scan.

During the study period, 458 consecutive patients were treated for infrarenal AAA. Fifty-five patients (12.1%) did not meet the inclusion criteria (Fig. 6.2). Among the patients enrolled, 160 (40%) underwent EVAR; 77 had an IRF (Excluder; W.L. Gore & Associates, Flagstaff, Ariz); and 83 had a TRF (Zenith; Cook Inc., Indianapolis, Ind). Of the 243 patients (60%) treated by OSR, 126 (52%) received a bifurcated aortoiliac graft, 98 (40%) received tubular aorto-aortic graft, and the remaining 19 (8%) received bifurcated aortofemoral grafts. The mean infrarenal aortic cross-clamping time was 15.4 ± 5.6 min. No statistical differences were observed between groups for demographics and risk factors, classified according to the Society for Vascular Surgery/International Society for Cardiovascular Surgery reporting standards [27], except for the American Society of Anesthesiologists (ASA) score, coronary artery, and chronic pulmonary occlusive disease which were significantly higher in the EVAR group ($P < 0.0001$ and $P = 0.003$).

In the open repair group, nine (4%) patients died in the early postoperative period, four for myocardial infarction, three after a sigmoid infarction, and two for major arrhythmia.

Endograft deployment was successful in all cases. Two cases (1%) required in the early postoperative period a femoro-femoral crossover for branch occlusion. The angio-CT scan performed after 30 days from the procedure showed the presence of a type II endoleak in 25 cases (15%). No device migration was observed and there were no perioperative deaths.

A significant statistical difference emerged between OR and EVAR for early postoperative death (4% vs 0%, $P = 0.01$). Follow-up ranged from 54 to 126 months (mean, 76 months) for OR and from 54 to 124 months (mean, 74 months) for EVAR (P = NS).

6.5.1 TRF Versus IRF: Effects on Renal Function After EVAR

The mean contrast dye volume per intervention was similar in the two groups (TRF 154 mL ± 11, IRF 148 mL ± 10; $P > 0.05$). No significant changes were observed for mean S_{Cr} between the preoperative and the postoperative periods (fourth day) both in the TRF group (1.1 ± 0.4 to 1.2 ± 0.4) and in the IRF group (1.1 ± 0.2 to 1.0 ± 0.4). Similarly, mean Cl_{Cr} values remained stable in both groups (60.1 ± 13.8 to 59.1 ± 17.1 for TRF and 59.8 ± 12.9 to 61.1 ± 17.6 for IRF).

No statistical differences were observed between the mean GFR measured at the RPS with the Gates method preoperatively and in the 30th postoperative day in both groups (70.5 ± 21.2 to 69.5 ± 23.1 for TRF and 72.3 ± 18.3 to 70.7 ± 20.2 for IRF) (Fig. 6.3). Through analyzing the preoperative and postoperative value of the GFR separately, a significant change (≥20%) emerged in 18 patients (11.2%), 8 (9.6%) from the TRF group and 10 (12.9%) from the IRF group. In seven patients (4.3%, 3 TRF; 4 IRF), a decrease of the GFR was limited to a single kidney; both kidneys were involved in the remaining 11 patients.

6.5.2 OSR Versus EVAR: Long-Term Results

Mean Cl_{Cr} at the RPS did not significantly change between pre- and postoperative (fourth postoperative day) values in both EVAR and OSR groups. Otherwise, analyzing the results separately for each patient, a significantly higher number of patients developed a >20% GFR decrease in the EVAR group (EVAR 14% vs OSR 4%, $P < 0.001$). Interestingly, the GFR impairment was limited to a single kidney in nine patients of the EVAR group.

A deterioration of the GFR was observed in the first 6 postoperative months in both groups, and this effect was more relevant in the EVAR group ($P < 0.001$). In the OSR group, there was no correlation between the type of aortic reconstruction, the time of aortic cross-clamping, and the early decline of renal function. In the EVAR patients, the GFR decreased gradually until 11% over the baseline at 9 years of follow-up (Fig. 6.4). In the OSR group, after the initial postoperative decline (6% with respect to the baseline), there was an almost complete normalization of the GFR at 48 months (decrease of 2%) and a reduction at 9 years of 3% (Fig. 6.4).

6.5.3 Effect of Secondary Procedures on Renal Function in Patients Treated with EVAR

Considering the long-term changes in renal function in patients who underwent EVAR, we aimed to identify who was at increased risk of GFR decrease. Our hypothesis was that patients needing secondary procedures had greater renal function impairment due to the repeated contrast dye administration for endovascular secondary procedures and for CT scans. At least one secondary procedure was performed in 17% of patients undergoing EVAR and in 3% of patients undergoing OR ($P < 0.0001$, Fig. 6.5). During the follow-up, the decline of GFR was remarkably higher in the subgroup needing additional procedures, with a reduction at 9 years of 14% with respect to 7% ($P < 0.005$; Fig. 6.6). In this subgroup of patients, the mean volume of contrast dye used to perform the secondary procedure and the subsequent control angio-CT at 30 days was 223 ± 36 mL.

Furthermore, when comparing the GFR between OR and EVAR patients who did not require a secondary procedure, a significant difference was still present ($P < 0.0005$).

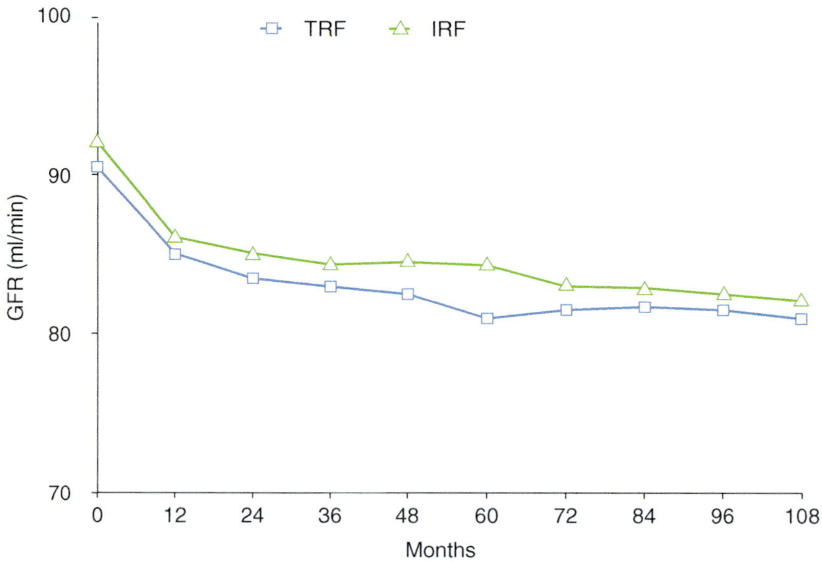

Fig. 6.3 Long-term results on renal function between patient undergoing endovascular aortic repair (EVAR) with transrenal fixation (TRF) and infrarenal fixation (IRF). Glomerular filtration rate (GFR) was estimated using renal perfusion scintigraphy (RPS)

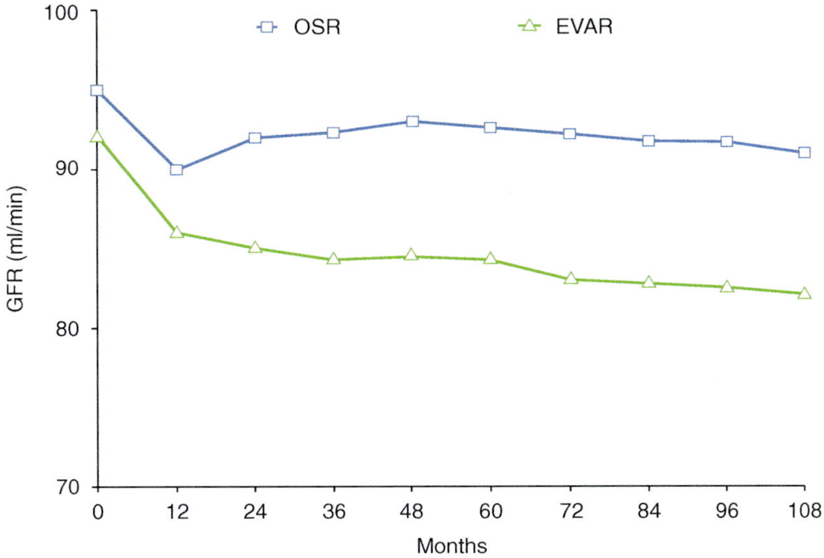

Fig. 6.4 Effects on renal function of open surgical repair (OSR) versus endograft repair (EVAR). Glomerular filtration rate (GFR) was estimated through renal perfusion scintigraphy (RPS). After an initial similar GFR decrease in both groups, a gradual normalization of GFR in the OSR group and a progressive worsening in the EVAR group were observed

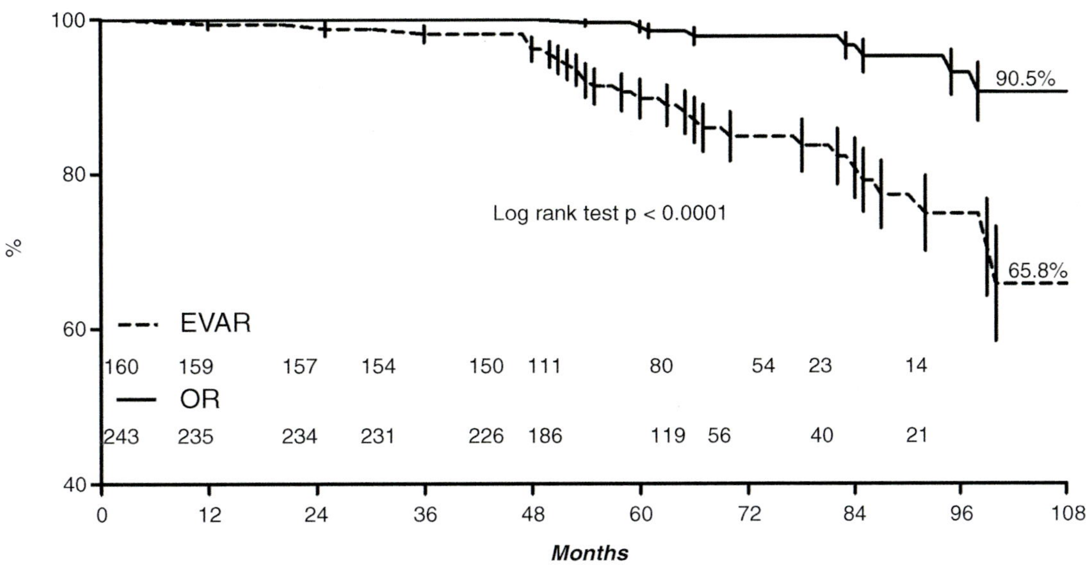

Fig. 6.5 Freedom from secondary procedure after open surgical repair (OSR) and endovascular aneurysm repair (EVAR)

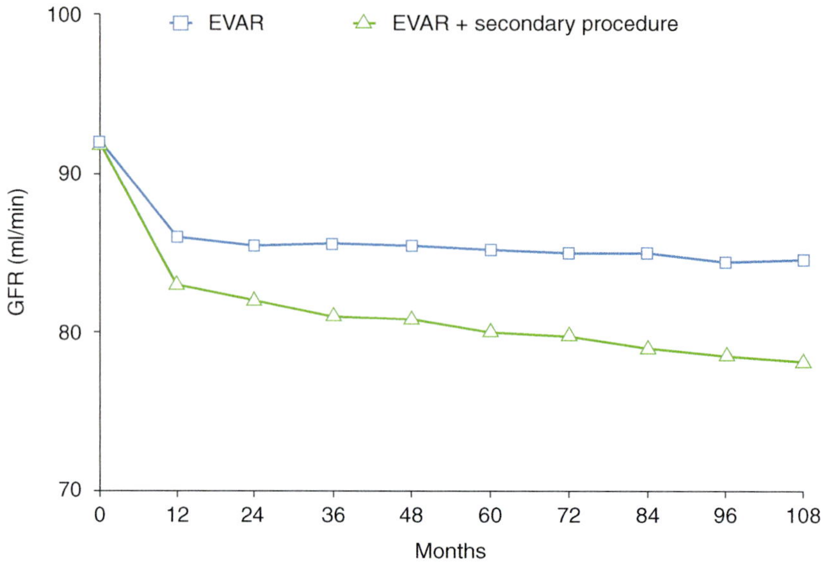

Fig. 6.6 Long-term results on renal function between patients undergoing endovascular aneurysm repair (EVAR) and EVAR with secondary procedure. Glomerular filtration rate (GFR) was estimated through renal perfusion scintigraphy (RPS)

6.6 Discussion

Both endovascular and open repairs of AAAs can be associated with postoperative renal function modifications, but the precise role of these procedures especially on long-term renal outcomes is unclear.

In particular, the effects of EVAR on renal function have been questioned since its introduction, but the question still remains unresolved even if it now represents an accepted method of treatment in appropriate candidates with infrarenal abdominal aortic aneurysm. In this context, the introduction of TRF to improve endograft fixation raised adjunctive concerns regarding its effects on renal function.

The comparison of TRF vs IRF has been largely investigated since flow impairment due to bare stents across the ostia of the renal artery may be a contributing factor in renal function decline [17]. Lau et al. investigated the effect of TRF versus IRF on renal function (assessed by S_{Cr}) and renal artery patency demonstrating that TRF does not lead to significant renal dysfunction or renal artery occlusion [18]. Mehta et al., in a review of their experience with EVAR on 496 patients (111 with IRF, 385 with TRF), found a significant increase of S_{Cr} and a decrease on Cl_{Cr} over the long-term follow-up in both groups [19, 20]. A meta-analysis on this topic provided conflicting results and concluded that the data were insufficient to draw any strong conclusions on the effect of TRF and IRF on renal function [21]. All these studies were based on the use of S_{Cr} and Cl_{Cr} to assess renal function, with the inherent limitations.

On the other hand, our experience is based on RPS to investigate renal function, since it is highly sensitive, can detect even small alterations of GFR, and allows to investigate the two kidneys separately [22, 23]. Moreover, in our studies, we included only patients without severe preoperative renal failure, which represents a known risk factor for renal postoperative renal complications. In a first pilot study in which we analyzed 47 consecutive patients undergoing EVAR with TRF, GFR impairment was documented at RPS in the 10.6% of cases [24], but there was no significant difference in postoperative GFR between IRF and TRF.

Another issue regards the long-term renal outcomes. The analysis of data from the large trials EVAR 1 and EVAR 2 [29] led to the conclusion that the long-term renal function (estimated by the Modification of Diet in Renal Disease calculation) appears to be stable over time with little evidence to suggest any difference attributable to aneurysm management policies. Our experience, however, demonstrated a marked decline over time in renal function in EVAR compared with OR ($P < 0.001$) that started in the early postoperative period (13% vs 4%; $P < 0.001$) and persisted throughout follow-up, with a reduction of the GFR at 9 years of 11% compared with 3% [25]. This may be related to a combination of CIN and renal atheroembolism. It is noteworthy that the RPS revealed a significant reduction (>20%) of the GFR in nine (6%) EVAR patients (four with TRF and five with IRF) that was limited to a single kidney that may be ascribed to microembolism during the endovascular procedure, such as manipulation of the endograft within the aortic neck near the renal ostia and balloon expansion of the proximal stent. This result is in line with findings of punctate renal infarctions on follow-up CT scans that have been described in other studies, suggesting a possible embolic sequela after EVAR [18, 30].

The issue of contrast nephropathy could be particularly relevant in patients who required one or more additional endovascular procedure with the follow-up mainly based on contrast-enhanced CT. The results of our study demonstrated a close relation between adjunctive procedures performed in the long term and the decline in renal function. In fact, in the 24 patients (17%) that required a supplementary endovascular procedure during follow-up, the decline of the GFR at 9 years was remarkably higher ($P < 0.0005$).

In our series, as well as in other reports, type II endoleak was the main cause of secondary procedures; furthermore, these procedures have a low technical success, and up to 40% of patients require additional re-intervention during follow-up [31]. In this scenario, we proposed a modified approach to EVAR consisting in the prevention of type II endoleaks rather than their treatment. This approach, based on aneurysm sac embolization using coil and fibrin glue [31–33], has been demonstrated to reduce type II endoleaks and related re-intervention. Furthermore, we have revised our surveillance protocol in order to reduce contrast dye administration during the follow-up that currently is based on abdominal CT (without contrast dye) and Doppler ultrasound. Contrast-enhanced CT is reserved only in case of aneurysmal sac enlargement, persisting type II endoleak, or signs of endograft migration.

Our study has some limitations that are noteworthy. The small number of patients treated by EVAR (especially if compared with those treated by OR) limits the ability to perform subgroup analysis and to identify statistically significant risk factors for progressive renal function decline. The greater number of ASA IV patients ($P < 0.0001$) in the EVAR groups may influence results on renal function, especially in the long term. However, the greatest advantage of our studies is to have investigated the kidney function by RPS which, in our opinion, overcomes the limitations of the common biochemical markers allowing an accurate assessment of even subtle impairments confined in a single kidney.

Considering all the weaknesses of our experience, it is certainly not possible to draw any strong conclusions about the real nephrological risk of a procedure than another for treatment of AAAs. However, on the basis of our evidence, especially with regard to the GFR impairment after EVAR both with TRF and IRF, it is reasonable to conclude that among the factors that could affect the patient suitability for EVAR, preoperative renal conditions should be taken into account.

6.7 Perspectives

With the technological evolution of endografts, fenestrated and branched endografts are becoming an established type of treatment for juxtarenal, pararenal, and thoracoabdominal aneurysms. These types of endografts require higher volume of contrast dye compared to standard EVAR during the procedure; furthermore, they require renal artery cannulation with guidewires and catheters and stent deployment. These maneuvers, along with contrast media administration during follow-up and the risk of stent compression or occlusion, may have a role, but data are lacking regarding the early and long-term effects of these types of treatment on renal function. On the other hand, open surgery also carries a non-negligible risk of renal function decrease in the treatment of complex AAAs and thoracoabdominal aneurysms, but a direct comparison between the two techniques is needed.

The use of new technologies may limit the dose of contrast dye used for endovascular procedures. The Magellan robotic system (Hansen Medical, Mountain View, CA, USA) has a catheter technology designed to deliver stability and distal tip control of guidewires and catheters and has been demonstrated to reduce the duration of complex endovascular procedures. These advantages could be associated to a decreased need for contrast media and subsequent reduction of renal complications.

Another interesting field is the use of carbon dioxide (CO_2) angiography during endovascular procedures, which is associated to a virtually absent risk of renal impairment. This technology is already used in some centers especially for peripheral procedurals, but large data on feasibility and effectiveness in aortic procedures are needed.

Finally, considering that secondary procedures are strictly associated to renal function worsening during follow-up, improvements in the optimization of patient selection and prevention of complications and secondary endovascular procedures are needed. Considering that type II endoleak represents the most frequent cause of re-intervention after EVAR, in our opinion, the use of type II endoleak-preventing procedures at the time of EVAR could be useful.

References

1. Zarins CK, White RA, Scwarten D, et al. Aneurex stent graft versus open surgical repair of abdominal aortic aneurysms: multicenter prospective clinical trial. J Vasc Surg. 1999;29:292–305.
2. Becquemin JP, Lapie V, JPn F, et al. Mid-term results of a second bifurcated endovascular graft for abdominal aortic aneurysm: the French Vanguard trial. J Vasc Surg. 1999;30:209–18.
3. Ligush J Jr, Pearce JD, Edwards MS, et al. Analysis of medical risk factors and outcomes in patients undergoing open versus endovascular abdominal aortic aneurysm repair. J Vasc Surg. 2002;36:492–9.
4. Veith FJ, Johnston KW. Endovascular treatment of abdominal aortic aneurysms: an innovation in evolution and under evaluation. J Vasc Surg. 2002;35:183.
5. Wartman SM, Woo K, Yaeger A, et al. Outcomes after abdominal aortic aneurysm repair requiring a suprarenal cross-clamp. J Vasc Surg. 2014;60(4):893–9.
6. Sternbergh WC III, Carter G, York JW, et al. Aortic neck angulation predicts adverse outcome with endovascular abdominal aortic aneurysm repair. J Vasc Surg. 2002;35:482–846.
7. Chaikof EL, Fillingar MF, Matsumura JS, et al. Identifying and grading factors that modify the outcome of endovascular aortic aneurysm repair. J Vasc Surg. 2002;35(5):1061–6.
8. Becker GJ, Kovacs M, Mathison MN. Opinion: Transluminal repair of abdominal aortic aneurysm: a call for selective use, careful surveillance, new device design and systematic study of transrenal fixation. J Vasc Surg. 2002;35:611–5.
9. Malina M, Brunkwall J, Ivancev K, et al. Renal artery covered by aortic stents: clinical experience from endovascular grafting of aortic aneurysms. Eur J Vasc Endovasc Surg. 1997;14:109–13.
10. Duda SH, Raygrotzki S, Wiskirchen J, et al. Abdominal aortic aneurysms: treatment with juxtarenal placement of covered stent-grafts. Radiology. 1998;206:195–8.
11. Marin ML, Parsons RE, Hollier LH, et al. Impact of transrenal aortic endograft placement on endovascular graft repair of abdominal aortic aneurysms. J Vasc Surg. 1998;28:638–46.
12. MacIerewicz J, Walker SR, Vincent R, et al. Vascular Surgical Society of Great Britain and Ireland: perioperative renal function following endovascular repair of abdominal aortic aneurysm with suprarenal and infrarenal stents. Br J Surg. 1999;86:696.
13. Bove PG, Long GW, Zelenock GB, et al. Transrenal fixation of aortic stent-grafts for the treatment of infrarenal aortic aneurismal disease. J Vasc Surg. 2000;32:697–703.
14. Lobato AC, Quick RC, Vaugh PL, et al. Transrenal fixation of aortic endografts: intermediate follow-up of a single-center experience. J Endovasc Ther. 2000;7:273–8.
15. Kichikawa K, Uchida H, Maeda M, et al. Aortic stent-grafting with transrenal fixation: use of newly designed spiral Z-stent endograft. J Endovasc Ther. 2000;7:184–91.
16. Izzedine H, Koskas F, Cluzel P, et al. Renal function after aortic stent-grafting including coverage of renal arterial ostia. Am J Kidney Dis. 2002;39:740–36.
17. Birch PC, Start RD, Whitbread T, et al. The effects of crossing porcine renal ostia with various endovascular stents. Eur J Vasc Endovasc Surg. 1999;17:185–90.
18. Lau LL, Hakaim AG, Oldenburg WA, et al. Effect of suprarenal versus infrarenal aortic endograft fixation

on renal function and renal artery patency: a comparative study with intermediate follow-up. J Vasc Surg. 2003;37:1162–8.
19. Cayne NS, Rhee SJ, Veith FJ, et al. Does transrenal fixation of aortic endografts impair renal function? J Vasc Surg. 2003;38(4):639–44.
20. Mehta M, Cayne N, Veith FJ, et al. Relationship of proximal fixation to renal dysfunction in patients undergoing endovascular aneurysm repair. J Cardiovasc Surg. 2004;45(4):367–74.
21. Walsh SR, Boyle JR, Lynch AG, et al. Suprarenal endograft fixation and medium-term renal function: systematic review and meta-analysis. J Vasc Surg. 2008;47:1364–70.
22. Petersen LJ, Petersen JR, Talleruphuus U, et al. Glomerular filtration rate estimated from the uptake phase of ^{99m}Tc-DTPA renography in chronic renal failure. Nephrol Dial Transplant. 1999;14:1673–8.
23. Awad RW, Barham WJ, Taylor DN, et al. The effect of infrarenal aortic reconstruction on glomerular filtration rate and effective renal plasma flow. Eur J Vasc Surg. 1992;6:362–7.
24. Deriu GP, Grego F, Lepidi S. Short-term arterial blood reperfusion of normothermic kidney in renal artery and abdominal aorta reconstructive surgery. Eur J Vasc Endovasc Surg. 2001;21(4):314–9.
25. Grego F, Frigatti P, Antonello M, et al. Suprarenal fixation of endograft in abdominal aortic aneurysm treatment: focus on renal function. Ann Surg. 2004;240(1):169–78.
26. Maeder M, Klein M, Fehr T, et al. Contrast nephropathy: review focusing on prevention. J Am Coll Cardiol. 2004;44(9):1763–71.
27. Antonello M, Menegolo M, Piazza M, et al. Outcomes of endovascular aneurysm repair on renal function compared with open repair. J Vasc Surg. 2013;58(4):886–93. https://doi.org/10.1016/j.jvs.2013.02.249. Epub 2013 May 17.
28. Chaikof EL, Blankensteijn JD, Harris PL, et al. Reporting standard for endovascular aortic aneurysm repair. J Vasc Surg. 2002;35:1048–60.
29. Brown LC, Brown EA, Greenhalgh RM, et al. Renal function and abdominal aortic aneurysm. The impact of different management strategies on long-term renal function in the UK endovascular aneurysm repair (EVAR) trial. Ann Surg. 2010;251:966–75.
30. Kramer SC, Seifarth H, Pamler R, et al. Renal infarction after endovascular aortic aneurysm repair. J Endovasc Ther. 2002;9:98–102.
31. Abularrage CJ, Patel VI, Conrad MF, et al. Improved results using Onyx glue for the treatment of persistent type 2 endoleak after endovascular aneurysm repair. J Vasc Surg. 2012;56:630–6.
32. Zanchetta M, Faresin F, Pedon L, et al. Intraoperative intrasac thrombin injection to prevent type II endoleak after endovascular abdominal aortic aneurysm repair. J Endovasc Ther. 2007;14:176–83.
33. Piazza M, Frigatti P, Scrivere P, et al. Sac embolization during EVAR to prevent type II endoleak: preoperative aneurysm volumetric analysis as predictor of efficacy. J Vasc Surg. 2013;57:934–41.

7 Device Evolution and New Concepts to Preserve Renal Artery Patency in Challenging Infrarenal Aortic Necks

Gianmarco de Donato, Francesco Setacci, Edoardo Pasqui, Mariagnese Mele, Domenico Benevento, Giancarlo Palasciano, and Carlo Setacci

At the beginning of the endovascular aortic repair (EVAR) era, a large number of patients were denied endovascular treatment due to challenging aortoiliac anatomy. In particular, short and angulated neck (so-called complex neck) and narrow access vessels were responsible for EVAR ineligibility in more than 50% of cases [1–5], with women deriving less benefit from EVAR when compared to men [6].

Simultaneously, stent-graft technology has evolved rapidly, limitations of earlier-generation devices have been overtaken, and EVAR eligibility has increased enormously.

Traditional EVAR technology has aimed to both anchor and seal using stents combined with fabric, with neither optimized for their roles and each forced to compete for the same space within their delivery catheters, which inevitably led to larger profile of the delivery system.

The Ovation Prime Abdominal Stent Graft System (TriVascular, Inc., Santa Rosa, CA) is a tri-modular device, designed with the aortic body delivered via a flexible, hydrophilic-coated, ultra-low-profile catheter (14 F outer diameter—OD).

The aortic body is provided with a suprarenal nitinol stent with anchors that provide active fixation, while a network of rings and channels that are inflated with a low-viscosity radiopaque polymer during stent-graft deployment provides effective sealing.

The technical revolution of the Ovation endograft includes the idea of truly uncoupling the stages of stent-graft fixation and seal during the procedure. In the Ovation endograft platform, stent and fabric are not competing for the same space within the delivery system, and an ultra-low-profile delivery can be achieved without compromise. With such a low-profile delivery catheter, approximately 90% of men and 70% of women with AAA have access vessel diameters considered fit for endovascular repair [7, 8].

This chapter focuses on the evolution over the years of endografts in terms of profile and adaptability to challenging infrarenal aortic neck. The final section of the chapter is dedicated to the VENT procedure, a particular EVAR technique that combines the Ovation endograft implantation with open bare-metal stent in the renal arteries and offers a treatment option for patient with unfit challenging neck for traditional endograft.

G. de Donato (✉) · E. Pasqui · M. Mele · D. Benevento · G. Palasciano · C. Setacci (✉)
Vascular Surgery, Department of Medicine, Surgery and Neuroscience, University of Siena, Siena, Italy
e-mail: dedonato@unisi.it; carlo.setacci@unisi.it

F. Setacci
Vascula Surgery, IRCCS Multimedica, Milan, Italy

© Springer Nature Switzerland AG 2019
Y. Tshomba et al. (eds.), *Visceral Vessels and Aortic Repair*,
https://doi.org/10.1007/978-3-319-94761-7_7

7.1 The Evolution of Endograft Delivery Catheter: From 27 to 14 F Profile

More than 25 years ago, Juan Parodi developed a handmade device made of a tube-shaped aorto-aortic graft sutured at each end to a balloon-expandable stent based on the design of radiologist Julio Palmaz. This kind of device was implanted in a human body for the first time on September 7, 1990, in Buenos Aires, Argentina. At that time, the delivery system of this handmade endograft was primitive and extremely rigid, measuring a bulky 27 French (F).

By 1994, the first commercially available devices were launched on the market.

Gradually, they became narrower and much more flexible, allowing for improved access in tortuous vessels, while stent-graft material and design changed in various ways to improve conformability, reduce fracture, and minimize rates of device migration.

The first endograft to enter clinical trials in the United States and the first product to be approved by the FDA in the treatment of abdominal aortic aneurysm was the Ancure Stent Graft (Guidant Corporation). It was made of Dacron, and most of the fixating device was made of Elgiloy, a special alloy produced by CMC of Chicago that was extremely fatigue-resistant. It was a large, bulky, and nonmodular endoprosthesis that required a large (25 F) and complicated delivery system: it was a challenge to implant even in a relatively healthy iliac and femoral anatomy.

Guidant recalled the Ancure endograft due to FDA warnings that this device damaged the already weakened arterial walls and led to complications. The lesson learned was that if it were to reduce endoprosthesis profile, this device would have to be modular.

The AneuRx device (Medtronic AVE, Santa Rosa, CA, USA) was the first endoprosthesis that introduced the concept of "modularity": the flow divider was separated from the contralateral endoleg, therefore reducing the profile to 21 F. The graft consisted of a Dacron mesh, structurally supported by nitinol mesh which was self-expanding upon delivery; moreover AneuRx graft was positioned using radiopaque markers strategically located on the stent graft, combined with orientation indicators on the delivery system.

Soon thereafter, the Talent stent graft (Medtronic AVE, Santa Rosa, CA, USA), which was initially 23 to 24 F, underwent an evolution to a lower-profile device. It consisted in a series of serpentine nitinol stents embedded into woven Dacron fabric. The stents were spaced discontinuously along a full-length nitinol spine. Salient features of talent device included the proximal bare spring (uncovered nitinol stent) and custom manufacturing to fit a wide range of aortoiliac sizes and configurations, as determined preoperatively by CT imaging and angiography.

After these early experiences, a movement began to develop lower-profile devices. The challenge became how to deliver the same amount of fabric and supporting frame in a progressively smaller delivery catheter. This required changes in the design and construction of the device, without compromising the performance and durability of the device. There were two clear ideas on how to accomplish this: either to change the basic design and the materials used or to work with the same materials and reengineer the device.

The first effort to dramatically lower the delivery profile was made by Cordis in 1999 with a AAA device (Cordis Corporation, Bridgewater, NJ) that had a tri-modular design with two 13 F endolegs. It incorporated a polyurethane (Bioseal) sealing gasket in its three-piece design, which was intended to promote a biological seal at the proximal attachment site. Unfortunately, after first clinical development, it was clear that the polyurethane of the sealing gasket was not mechanically robust and did not provide the same effectiveness in a human aorta compared to animal implants. Moreover, the endolegs achieved a lower profile simply by increasing the size of each stent cell (which however became more rigid) and reducing their total number; this led to an increase in the kinkability and torsion of the limbs in tortuous anatomy.

Further efforts to develop a low-profile device involved the planning of new aortic endoprosthesis manufactured with traditional materials and characterized by a new concept of sealing and/or fixation.

Different companies developed their endograft with reduced profile (18–20 F): Zenith Flex LP (Cook Medical Inc., Bloomington, IN), Excluder (Gore & Associates, Flagstaff, AZ), and Endurant (Medtronic Vascular, Inc., Santa Rosa, CA). These new technical solutions consisted in modular low-profile devices which combined a series of barbs or hooks to engage the aortic wall and to provide active fixation, with radial force from self-expanding stent for stability and optimal graft to vessel apposition, and a main body with columnar strength that mimics the natural anatomy of the aorta.

Afterward, a new concept of fixation separated from sealing was expressed for the first time by the low-profile endoprosthesis Powerlink and AFX (Endologix, Inc., Irvine, CA). It combines in a unibody design a highly conformable material (that moves independently from the stent to maximize wall contact, conform to anatomical irregularities, and enhance sealing) with anatomical fixation (that inhibits migration and limb competition). This endograft was delivered through a 17 F introducer sheath (19 F OD).

Further efforts to develop a low-profile device were based on the concept of changing the basic design and the materials used and planning an endoprosthesis without the traditional metallic stent frames to support the fabric. TriVascular (TriVascular Inc., Santa Rosa, CA) developed the first generation of endograft, called eNovus, which was a nonmodular device, presenting a delivery profile of 16 F OD. The device was made of a unique PTFE sleeve with channels for a biocompatible fill polymer as the endoframe for the device and used nitinol stents only for suprarenal and distal endoleg attachments. Unfortunately, the clinical trials revealed some cases of fracture of the suprarenal stent. It was seen that the load created by anatomical flexing was concentrated across a small number of points, leading to a higher potential for fatigue. This problem was rapidly solved with a new design of more uniform strut width that achieves the goal of spreading stress-strain loads more evenly across the stent, thereby significantly improving the resistance to fatigue.

With these design improvements, TriVascular was able to launch the first generation of a new endograft, the Ovation, preserving the unique sealing mechanism of the inflatable sealing rings. Moreover, the other significant improvement in stent design made by TriVascular was that a three-piece modular design with two nitinol endolegs was adopted with a further reduction of profile from 16 F OD to 14 F OD.

Incorporating traditional materials and a three-piece design, the Cordis INCRAFT (Cordis Corporation, a Johnson & Johnson company; Warren, NJ) has recently proposed an ultra-low-profile endograft (14 F). The INCRAFT includes the technologies and designs Cordis acquired from the TERAMed AAA device (also known as Forton) in the design of its endolegs, although the bifurcated component is entirely new. It is made of a low-porosity polyester graft with segmented nitinol stents and a suprarenal fixation: the number of crowns in the suprarenal stent was reduced to a minimum, and instead stent hooks are designed to be fracture-resistant while still affording excellent anchoring with high pullout forces. Moreover, to reduce the profile and increase the durability of the fabric, the attachment of the stent rings to the fabric was modified, minimizing the wear force of attachments and reducing the metal fabric interaction.

The INCRAFT System is approved for investigational device use only, and it is not for sale anywhere in the world. It was initially tested in a phase I-type European study (INNOVATION) with favorable early patient outcomes. The pivotal multicenter US INSPIRATION clinical trial is under way.

7.2 Technical Notes of Endograft Design to Reach Ultra-Low Profile

One of the most frequent reasons for EVAR ineligibility is connected to access. With its ultra-low profile of 14 F OD, the Ovation stent graft allows access in 90% of men and 70% of women with AAA, based on data from the Characterization of Human Aortic Anatomy. In contrast, needing a minimum iliac diameter of 6 mm, many other stent grafts accommodate access in only 70% of men and 40% of women.

From a technical point of view, how can a stent-graft aortic body be packaged in a delivery system with a profile of only 4.66 mm (14 F OD)?

The answer has to be found in a substantial shift in EVAR technology, based on a suggestive change in the conceptual process of two important steps of procedure: the fixation and the sealing.

Actually, the technical revolution of the Ovation endograft includes the idea to truly uncouple the stages of stent-graft fixation and seal during the procedure. This EVAR solution dictated the use of a corresponding segmentation by function, location, and time for the system architecture and its elements. According to this new EVAR technology, a seal is created that must only seal and not be burdened with the additional task of fixation, and a deployed anchor must only hold the implant securely in place and not be asked to do anything more. Additionally, because these components can preferentially engage separate locations within the anatomy, they are not superimposed within the delivery catheter, and their constituents are not all delivered simultaneously.

As a result, in the Ovation endograft platform, stent and fabric do not compete for the same space within the delivery system, and an ultra-low-profile delivery can be achieved without compromise.

The previous EVAR technology has aimed to both anchor and seal using stents combined with fabric, with neither optimized for their roles and each forced to compete for the same space within their delivery catheters, which inevitably led to larger profile of the delivery system.

With the Ovation stent graft, the fixation is acquired by a quite long suprarenal nitinol stent (35 mm), which uses integrally formed anchors. The proximal stent and the anchors are delivered in a staged way, allowing precise placement that is particularly important in short-neck anatomies.

Once the endograft fixation phase is complete, the sealing phase begins. The aortic body is provided with a network of inflatable channels and sealing rings that are filled with a low-viscosity, nonembolic, radiopaque fill polymer. This polymer-filled ring network conforms to the patient's aortic neck, creating an uninterrupted concentric seal reminiscent of O-ring or gasket-like seals that have long been considered the gold standard in other sealing applications. Providing a simple, precise, and reliable seal in a variety of applications and function by introducing a calculated mechanical stress between the O-ring itself and the surface that the ring is in contact with, this kind of design is typically used to prevent the passing of air or fluid between two surfaces.

Being casted in situ to form a custom-molded O-ring seal at the margin of the aneurysm, the polymer guarantees a very high seal conformability of the Ovation to irregular surfaces, such as in the presence of calcium or thrombus.

The polymer-filled O-rings do not apply the kind of chronic outward force on the aorta, which is typically seen with other endografts that employ oversized, self-expanding stents to achieve seal in proximal aortic necks.

Furthermore, the delivery system profile is not affected by the amount of polymer required, since the material is injected in in a liquid state and subsequently solidifies in 20 min.

All these technical details explain how it was possible to package this endograft in a delivery catheter of only 4.66 mm.

7.3 Endograft Design and Aortic Neck Dilatation

At the beginning, very little was known about the role of device design on early procedural success and long-term durability. The idea was just to create endograft simulating those used for open surgical repair, replacing the aortic suture line with stents to achieve fixation.

But how could the device stay in place and guarantee to seal off the aneurysm for years? Of course, a radial force applied by a stent at the proximal aortic neck is needed.

Unfortunately, already in the late 1990s, it was clear that the wall of the aortic neck is never a completely healthy arterial segment, but rather it has to be considered a delicate and weaken area. A significant dilatation of the proximal aortic neck may be experienced in up to one-third of patients following open repair, questioning the efficacy of EVAR over time [1, 2] when a chronic outward force is applied on the proximal neck.

In 2000, Wever et al. reported a 15.5% rate of dilatation of the proximal neck after EVAR [3], which was not correlated with the graft diameter or amount of graft oversizing. At that time, this major concern was confirmed by the failure of the EVT/Ancure graft (formerly Guidant Corporation straight tube graft), which revealed that aortic growth may occur after EVAR leading to failure of aortic seal that occurred in the distal aortic seal zone [4]. This failure of endovascular aorto-aortic tube grafts led to the suggestion of preferential use of bifurcated grafts, abandoning the idea of sealing in the distal infrarenal aorta and moving to the concept of creating healthy seal zones, proximal in the aorta next to the renal arteries and distal in a normal iliac artery.

The following trials performed in the first years of the twenty-first century proved successful with EVAR, with excellent outcome [5, 9–12], although neck dilatation was still reported in single-center studies as being related to excessive device oversizing and chronic outward force applied by the self-expanding stents at the level of the proximal neck [13–17].

Contrary to self-expanding stents, balloon-expandable stents do not place continued outward force on the aortic wall. Studies reporting results on the only two endografts with balloon-expandable stents to generate fixation and sealing in EVAR (the MEGS device—Montefiore endovascular graft system—and the LifePath device, Edwards Lifesciences Corporation, Irvine, CA) revealed an extremely low aptitude to cause aortic neck dilatation. Malas et al. [18] described the complete lack of aortic neck dilatation noted in those patients who underwent AAA repair with the MEGS device. Dalainas et al. [19], studying a cohort of 200 and 42 patients after EVAR, reported a 27.5% rate of aortic neck dilatation in those treated with self-expanding stent grafts versus 7.1% in those treated with balloon-expandable stent grafts.

As well as the balloon-expandable stents, the sealing rings of the Ovation Prime device do not place chronic outward force on the aorta. Up to today, 4-year data from the premarket approval application for the Ovation device have revealed stability of the seal zone without aortic neck dilatation, migration, or proximal endoleak evolution in 100% of cases [20].

7.3.1 Device Evolution and Challenging Infrarenal Aortic Necks

Traditional self-expanding stent grafts (SESG) require an infrarenal non-aneurysmal aortic neck to adequately seal the aneurysmal sac from chronic circulatory pressures. Sealing is then procured by oversizing the stent graft (from 10 to 30%) at that level, prospecting that the chronic radial force exerted longitudinally against the aortic wall will circumferentially avert any leakage. Since the first EVAR experiences, this sealing concept has restricted the application of stent grafts [1]. Typically, the feasibility of EVAR for infrarenal AAA has mainly been related to aortic morphology, with the majority of IFU manufacturers originally requiring an adequate non-aneurysmal proximal neck of 10–15 mm, an aortic diameter <30 mm, and an infrarenal angulation <60°.

In patients with complex aortic necks, proximal graft sealing remains a challenge with traditional SESG [21–24]. As expected, applications outside of anatomically specific IFU variables have an incremental negative effect on late results [25, 26]. In a systematic review and meta-analysis of the literature, Spanos et al. [27] identified patients with large AAA and short necks as those at highest risk of graft migration after EVAR after implantation of an old-generation stent graft. Of note, neck diameter and neck angulation did not have any important influence on stent-graft migration.

With the availability of new-generation devices, an increasing number of EVARs have been performed outside IFU [28]. Violations of IFU are particularly focused on unfavorable proximal aortic neck anatomy. Out of a total of 10,228 patients from the MS2 database undergoing EVAR, only 42% of patients had anatomy that met the most conservative definition of IFU, while 69% met the most liberal definition of IFU [29].

A systematic review and meta-analysis of outcomes following EVAR in patients with hostile neck anatomy (as defined by the presence of a neck length <15 mm, neck diameter >28 mm, or angulation >60° alone or in combination) revealed a significant increase in 30-day type I endoleaks (OR 2.92) and late type I endoleaks (OR 1.71), in comparison with patients with favorable neck anatomy [21].

There are two main consequences of an inadequate choice of the right landing zone: inappropriate fixation with high risk of stent-graft migration and failure of complete aneurysm exclusion with the presence of endoleaks that represent the most important cause of aneurysm progression and rupture.

The so-called hostile neck is typically defined as the presence of any or all of the following features [23]:

- Length <10 mm
- Angle >60°
- Diameter >28 mm
- ≥50% circumferential thrombus
- ≥50% circumferential calcified neck
- Reverse taper morphology

The "chimney" technique has been proposed to manage visceral vessel during endovascular repair of hostile neck or aortic juxtarenal aneurysms (Ch-Evar). It consists in a parallel stent-graft positioning that provides the perfusion to the branch via a stent graft between the aortic wall and aortic graft. In doing so, the sealing zone can be moved proximally, maintaining the perfusion of visceral artery originating from the part of the aorta that will be covered by the body of the aortic graft. It is called "chimney," because the stent protrudes above the aortic endograft; the chimney graft could be also named "snorkel" when the proximal part is extended proximally or "reverse chimney" or "periscope" when stents are extended caudally. Initially, the chimney technique was used when the aortic endograft was positioned across the renal artery, either intentionally or inadvertently. Depending on the percentage of the covered ostium, the stent had to extend proximally, resulting in this peculiar appearance.

The first successes of this technique, as a bail-out procedure, encouraged surgeons to use it during planned intervention for unusual or complex cases, also widening the indications for iliac internal artery, aortic arch, etc.

The complexity of this technique requires a large endovascular experience; the final outcome may vary depending on appropriate selection of patient, planning, and execution.

In order to overcome the difficulties caused by challenging anatomies of the proximal neck of abdominal aortic aneurysms, new devices have been studied and designed. In parallel, innovative endovascular techniques have been created.

The following section describes a new technique as alternative to traditional chimney EVAR to treat challenging short-neck or juxtarenal aneurysm in patients with small iliac access vessels.

7.3.2 VENT Technique

In simple terms, VENT consists of the implantation of the Ovation stent graft [Endologix™, Santa Rosa, CA] with a modified technique that includes synchronous placement of renal bare-metal stents.

To understand how the technique works, it is crucial to remark some of the peculiarities of the Ovation design. The three-modular graft provides a suprarenal fixation by a 35-mm-long nitinol stent, enriched by several hooks. This fundamental part sticks to the aortic wall in the suprarenal part, maintaining renal perfusion and assuring the stability of the entire device. The remaining part is made by a low- profile PTFE (polytetrafluoroethylene) and a network of rings, without any metallic structures. The network of inflatable rings is typically filled with a liquid polymer that solidifies during the deployment procedure.

The filling polymer consists of three different components that are mixed before the injection. Upon mixing and injection into the graft, the components form a radiopaque polymer that fills the proximal sealing rings in the wall of the aortic body graft and the ribs in the aortic body graft legs. The polymer radiopacity dissipates over time and may not be visible on fluoroscopy, X-ray, or CT beyond 1–2 months post-implant.

The low-density polymer is deployed, thanks to an auto-injector system; the "O-rings" are filled both proximally and distally, assuring the right stability to the entire system and reducing endoleak rate.

This new kind of sealing system has been proposed to overcome complex proximal neck issue: non-cylindrical necks, with parietal thrombus and/or calcification. The sealing procedure is gradual, and there are two reasons for this: better adaptability to the aortic wall and to redistribute pressures along the entire stent graft [30].

The Ovation endograft, with its new concept of sealing by non-expansive circumferential apposition of polymer-filled rings to the aortic wall, generates no chronic outward power at the infrarenal aortic level. In August 2010, the Ovation endograft received CE Mark approval and was commercially accessible in Europe. At that time, the device-specific instructions for use (IFU) facilitated the treatment of aneurysms with a proximal aortic neck of only 7 mm, being the first device ever approved for neck shorter than 10 mm.

Currently, the sealing secured with the Ovation endograft is not longitudinal but circumferential, based on the apposition of the polymer-filled ring to the aortic wall, and, theoretically, allows the treatment of a range of aortic neck diameters independent of their length. As a result, a number of patients have been treated even in the presence of an aortic neck length <7 mm, provided that the aortic neck diameter was compatible with the endograft ring sizes.

Lately, in April 2014, the FDA approved changes to the indication statement for the Ovation Abdominal Stent Graft, and since then, it has been the only FDA-approved EVAR stent graft that is not restricted by the conventional measurement of aortic neck length in its labeling [31]. Actually, the expanded indication for use statement eliminates the minimum aortic neck length requirement. Neck length is only considered in assessing angulation: patients with a proximal neck length of less than 10 mm are indicated with an aortic angle of less than or equal to 45°; otherwise, angles up to 60° are indicated.

Instructions for use (IFU) make the Ovation Abdominal Stent Graft usable in abdominal aortic aneurysm with adequate iliac/femoral access with:

- Proximal landing zone with an inner wall diameter of no less than 16 mm and no greater than 30 mm at 13 mm below the inferior renal artery and with an aortic angle of ≤60° if proximal neck is ≥10 mm and ≤45° if proximal neck is <10 mm
- Distal iliac landing zone: With length of at least 10 mm and with an inner wall diameter of no less than 8 mm and no greater than 25 mm

The VENT technique consists of the deployment of the sealing ring of the Ovation stent graft at between 1 and 3 mm below the lowermost renal artery rather than 13 mm as suggested by IFU (Fig. 7.1), with the proximal edge of the fabric lying above the orifice of the renal artery. Short bare-metal stent deployed simultaneously in the renal orifice (Fig. 7.2) and protruding few millimeters into the aorta allows renal patency preservation by moving the proxi-

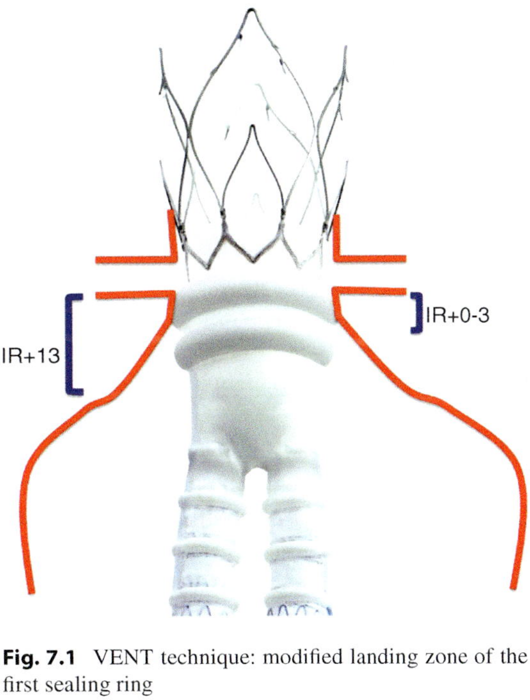

Fig. 7.1 VENT technique: modified landing zone of the first sealing ring

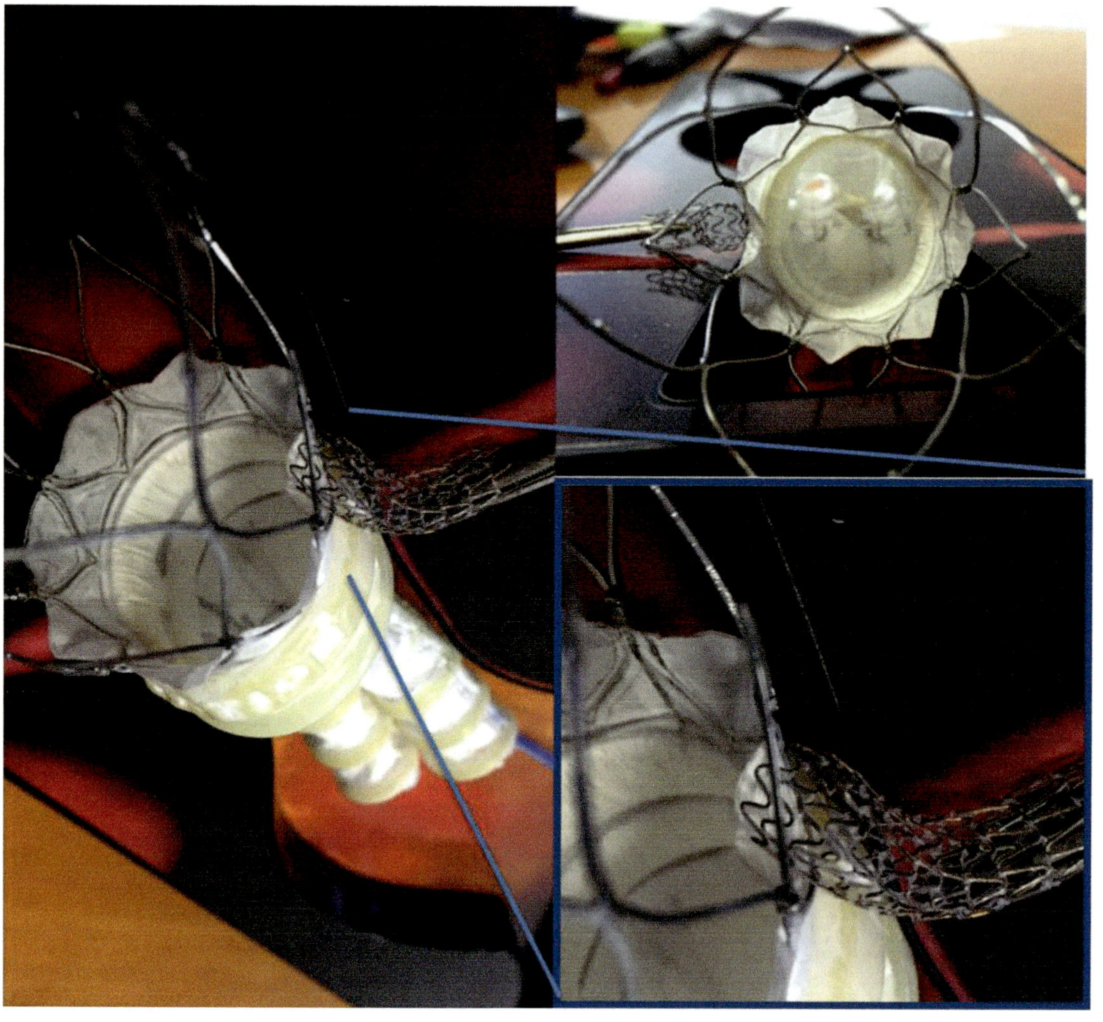

Fig. 7.2 VENT technique at bench test

mal edge of the fabric present just above the first ring (so-called collar zone).

In cases of challenging infrarenal aortic necks or juxtarenal aortic aneurysms, EVAR usually involves the use of custom-made fenestrated stent grafts, which typically require large-diameter access vessels, higher cost, and several weeks between graft planning and delivery.

These limitations with the practice of vascular surgery have been partially addressed with chimney EVAR, whose role is still controversial, largely due to concerns over gutter endoleaks. The proposed VENT technique is an alternative to traditional chimney EVAR that addresses the same limitation in treating short challenging neck/juxtarenal aneurysm in patients, in particular in patients with small iliac access vessels.

Of note, unlike the chimney technique, bare-metal stents positioned during the VENT technique do not compete with the main graft, avoiding the appearance of the so-called gutters. Principal differences between VENT and chimney techniques are summarized in Table 7.1.

Figure 7.3 shows a typical case of a short proximal aortic neck (5 mm) treated by the VENT technique.

Landing with the sealing ring just a couple of millimeters below the lowest renal artery is planned (Fig. 7.4).

Table 7.1 Comparison between Chimney and VENT technique

Chimney	VENT
Renal covered stents (6-8 Fr)	Bare metal stents (5F)
10-15 mm protrusion outside renal arteries	2-4 mm protrusion into the aorta
Chimney & enograft competing for the same room (gutters)	Renal stents & endograft ring are not competing for the same room

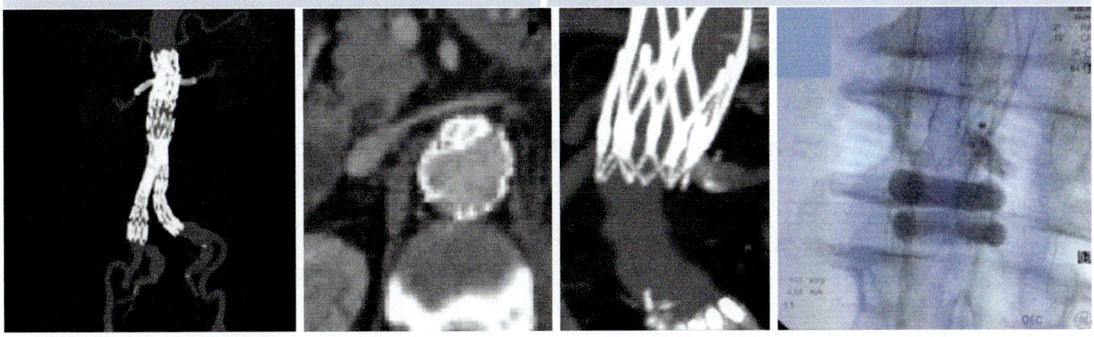

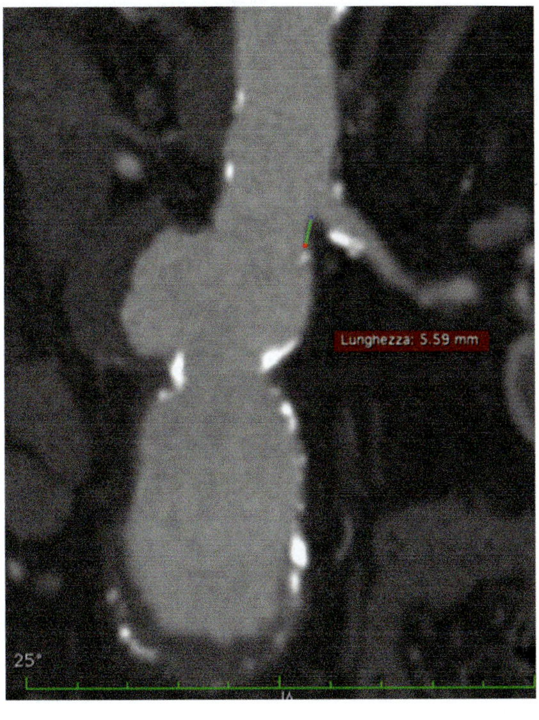

Fig. 7.3 Typical case of a short proximal aortic neck (5 mm) suitable for treatment by the VENT technique

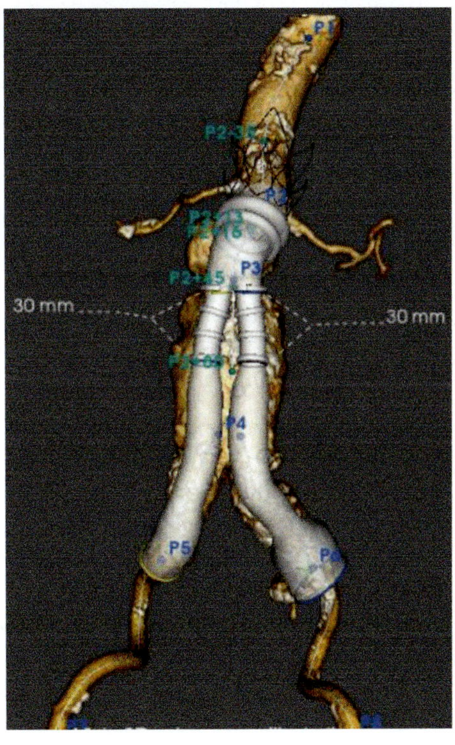

Fig. 7.4 Planning for Ovation implantation with VENT technique

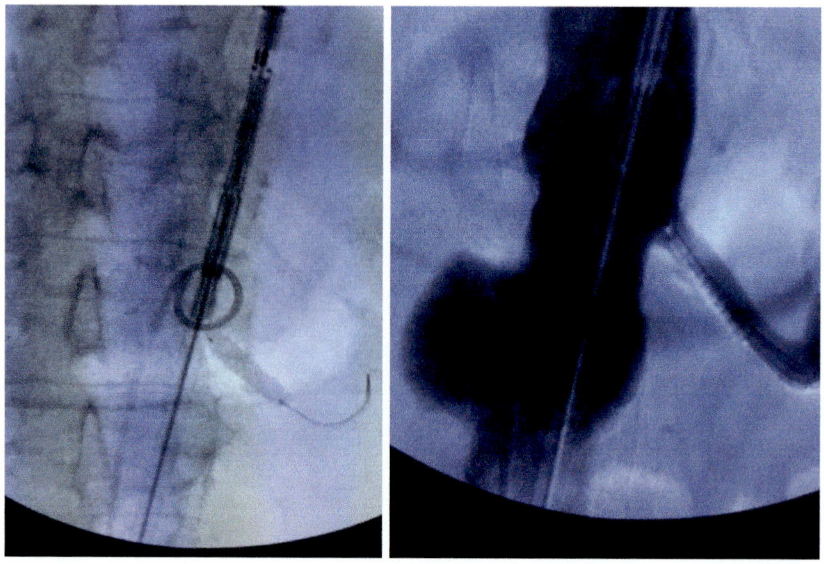

Fig. 7.5 VENT technique: bare-metal stent is advanced at the level of the renal ostium from the brachial access; the main body of an Ovation endograft is advanced at the same level from the femoral access

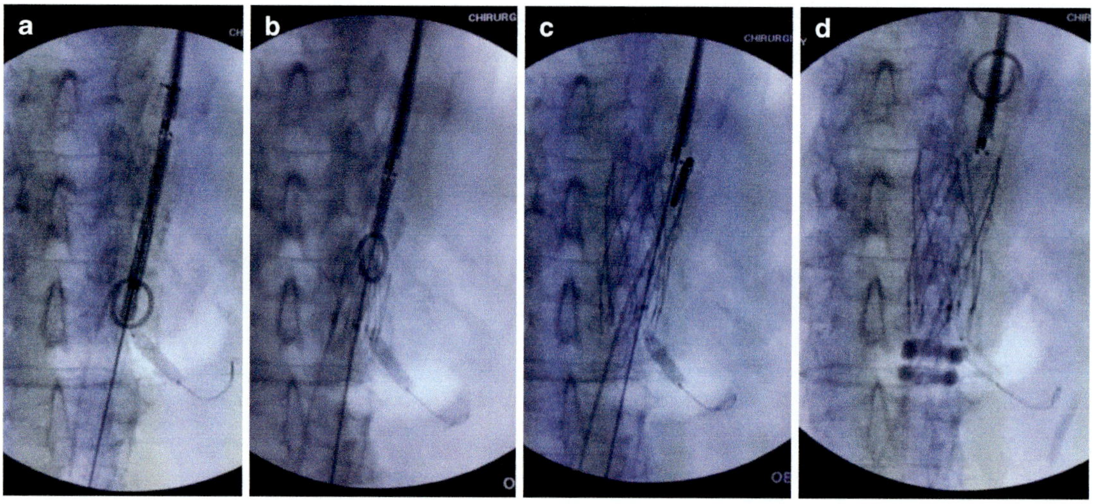

Fig. 7.6 Simultaneous renal stent and main body endograft deployment: (**a**) renal stent deployment; (**b**) first step of the Ovation main body deployment; (**c**) complete deployment of the Ovation main body deployment; (**d**) injection of polymer

With a percutaneous brachial access and a long 5 F introducer sheath, the bare-metal stent is positioned at the level of the renal ostium, while the main body of an Ovation endograft is advanced at the same level from the femoral access (Fig. 7.5).

Simultaneous renal stent and main body endograft deployment is shown in Fig. 7.6. The Ovation is released with the sealing ring landing exactly at the level of the short infrarenal neck. The synchronized release of the short renal bare-metal stent (6/18 mm), which protrudes just a couple of millimeters into the aortic lumen, allows the "ventilation" of the left renal artery by moving the thin fabric of the collar zone.

Complete sac exclusion and left renal artery patency are demonstrated at final angiography. Of note, the renal stent and the first ring of the Ovation endograft are strictly in contact but do not compete for the same room. The ring is

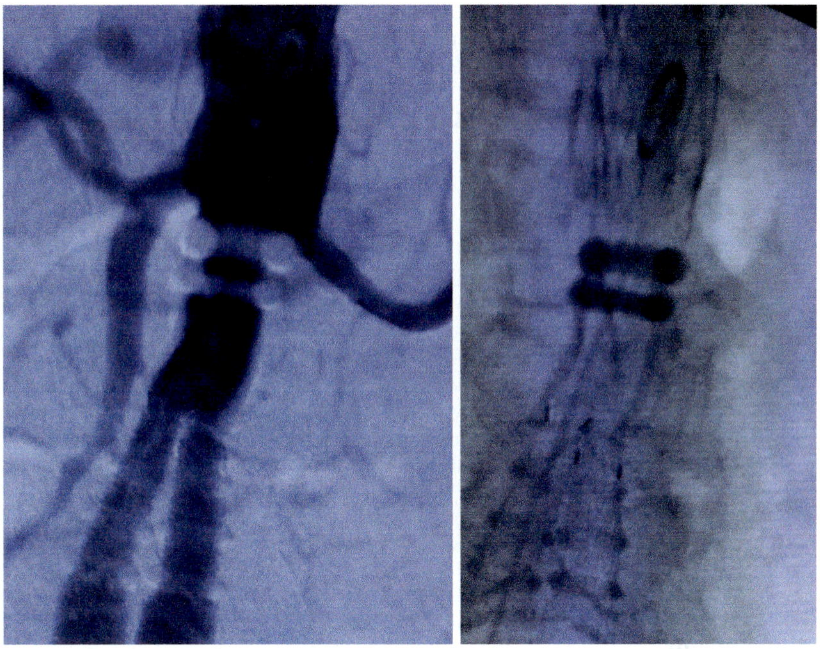

Fig. 7.7 Final angiography: the renal stent and the first ring of the Ovation endograft are strictly in contact but do not compete for the same room. The renal stent is preserving the renal perfusion by moving the thin and flexible fabric of the collar zone

responsible for the circumferential sealing at the level of the short neck (1–3 mm below the left renal artery), while the renal stent is preserving the renal perfusion by moving the thin and flexible fabric of the collar zone (Fig. 7.7).

References

1. Hallett JW Jr, Marshall DM, Petterson TM, et al. Graft-related complications after abdominal aortic aneurysm repair: reassurance from a 36-year population-based experience. J Vasc Surg. 1997;25:277–84; discussion 285-276.
2. Illig KA, Green RM, Ouriel K, et al. Fate of the proximal aortic cuff: implications for endovascular aneurysm repair. J Vasc Surg. 1997;26:492–9; discussion 499-501.
3. Wever JJ, de Nie AJ, Blankensteijn JD, et al. Dilatation of the proximal neck of infrarenal aortic aneurysms after endovascular AAA repair. Eur J Vasc Endovasc Surg. 2000;19:197–201.
4. Faries PL, Briggs VL, Rhee JY, et al. Failure of endovascular aortoaortic tube grafts: a plea for preferential use of bifurcated grafts. J Vasc Surg. 2002;35:868–73.
5. Zarins CK. The US AneuRx Clinical Trial: 6-year clinical update 2002. J Vasc Surg. 2003;37:904–8.
6. Mehta M, Byrne WJ, Robinson H, et al. Women derive less benefit from elective endovascular aneurysm repair than men. J Vasc Surg. 2012;55:906–13.
7. Sweet MP, Fillinger MF, Morrison TM, Abel D. The influence of gender and aortic aneurysm size on eligibility for endovascular abdominal aortic aneurysm repair. J Vasc Surg. 2011;54:931–7.
8. Mehta M, Valdes FE, Nolte T, et al. One-year outcomes from an international study of the Ovation abdominal stent graft system for endovascular aneurysm repair. J Vasc Surg. 2014;59:65.
9. Greenberg RK, Chuter TA, Cambria RP, et al. Zenith abdominal aortic aneurysm endovascular graft. J Vasc Surg. 2008;48:1–9.
10. Carpenter JP. The Powerlink bifurcated system for endovascular aortic aneurysm repair: four-year results of the US multicenter trial. J Cardiovasc Surg. 2006;47:239–43.
11. Peterson BG, Matsumura JS, Brewster DC, Makaroun MS. Five-year report of a multicenter controlled clinical trial of open versus endovascular treatment of abdominal aortic aneurysms. J Vasc Surg. 2007;45:885–90.
12. Turnbull IC, Criado FJ, Sanchez L, et al. Five-year results for the talent enhanced low profile system abdominal stent graft pivotal trial including early and long-term safety and efficacy. J Vasc Surg. 2010;51:537–44; 544, e531-532.
13. Cao P, Verzini F, Parlani G, et al. Predictive factors and clinical consequences of proximal aortic neck dilatation in 230 patients undergoing abdominal aorta aneurysm repair with self-expandable stent-grafts. J Vasc Surg. 2003;37:1200–5.
14. Sternbergh WC 3rd, Money SR, Greenberg RK, Chuter TA. Influence of endograft oversizing on

device migration, endoleak, aneurysm shrinkage, and aortic neck dilation: results from the Zenith multicenter trial. J Vasc Surg. 2004;39:20–6.
15. Tonnessen BH, Sternbergh WC 3rd, Money SR. Late problems at the proximal aortic neck: migration and dilation. Semin Vasc Surg. 2004;17:288–93.
16. Sampaio SM, Panneton JM, Mozes G, et al. Aortic neck dilation after endovascular abdominal aortic aneurysm repair: should oversizing be blamed? Ann Vasc Surg. 2006;20:338–45.
17. Conners MS 3rd, Sternbergh WC 3rd, Carter G, et al. Endograft migration one to four years after endovascular abdominal aortic aneurysm repair with the AneuRx device: a cautionary note. J Vasc Surg. 2002;36:476–84.
18. Malas MB, Ohki T, Veith FJ, et al. Absence of proximal neck dilatation and graft migration after endovascular aneurysm repair with balloon-expandable stent-based endografts. J Vasc Surg. 2005;42:639–44.
19. Dalainas I, Nano G, Bianchi P, et al. Aortic neck dilatation and endograft migration are correlated with selfexpanding endografts. J Endovasc Ther. 2007;14:318–23.
20. de Donato G, Setacci F, Bresadola L, TriVascular Ovation Italian Study, et al. Aortic neck evolution after endovascular repair with TriVascular Ovation stent graft. J Vasc Surg. 2016;63(1):8–15. https://doi.org/10.1016/j.jvs.2015.07.099. Epub 2015 Sep 26.
21. Stather PW, Wild JB, Sayers RD, et al. Endovascular aortic aneurysm repair in patients with hostile neck anatomy. J Endovasc Ther. 2013;20(5):623–37. https://doi.org/10.1583/13-4320MR.1.
22. Jordan WD Jr, Ouriel K, Mehta M, Aneurysm Treatment using the Heli-FX Aortic Securement System Global Registry ANCHOR, et al. Outcome-based anatomic criteria for defining the hostile aortic neck. J Vasc Surg. 2015;61(6):1383–90.
23. Aburahma AF, Campbell JE, Mousa AY, et al. Clinical outcomes for hostile versus favorable aortic neck anatomy in endovascular aortic aneurysm repair using modular devices. J Vasc Surg. 2011;54(1):13–21.
24. Stather PW, Sayers RD, Cheah A, et al. Outcomes of endovascular aneurysm repair in patients with hostile neck anatomy. Eur J Vasc Endovasc Surg. 2012;44(6):556–61.
25. Abbruzzese TA, Kwolek CJ, Brewster DC, et al. Outcomes following endovascular abdominal aortic aneurysm repair (EVAR): an anatomic and device-specific analysis. J Vasc Surg. 2008;48(1):19–28. https://doi.org/10.1016/j.jvs.2008.02.003. Epub 2008 Apr 28.
26. Hobo R, Kievit J, Leurs LJ, et al. Influence of severe infrarenal aortic neck angulation on complications at the proximal neck following endovascular AAA repair: a EUROSTAR study. J Endovasc Ther. 2007;14:1–11.
27. Spanos K, Karathanos C, Saleptsis V, et al. Systematic review and meta-analysis of migration after endovascular abdominal aortic aneurysm repair. Vascular. 2015;24(3):323–36.
28. Antoniou GA, Georgiadis GS, Antoniou SA, et al. A meta-analysis of outcomes of endovascular abdominal aortic aneurysm repair in patients with hostile and friendly neck anatomy. J Vasc Surg. 2013;57:527–38.
29. Schanzer A, Greenberg RK, Hevelone N, et al. Predictors of abdominal aortic aneurysm sac enlargement after endovascular repair. Circulation. 2011;123(24):2848–55.
30. Georgakarakos E, Ioannou CV, Georgiadis GS, Storck M, Trellopoulos G, Koutsias S, et al. The Ovation abdominal stent graft for the treatment of abdominal aortic aneurysms: current evidence and future perspectives. Expert Rev Med Devices. 2016;13:253–62.
31. Mehta M. Rethink the neck. How the Ovation prime system is revolutionizing the way we approach EVAR. Endovascular Today. 2014. p. 3–6.

8 Hypogastric Artery Management During Open and Endovascular Aortoiliac Repair

Aaron Fargion, Carlo Pratesi, Fabrizio Masciello, Walter Dorigo, and Giovanni Pratesi

8.1 Demographic, Pathogenesis, and Natural History

While iliac artery aneurysms (IAAs) are frequently associated with abdominal aortic aneurysms (AAAs) [1, 2], isolated IAAs are rare, with a frequency between 0.5% and 2% of all arterial aneurysms [3] and an incidence among general population of about 0.03% [4].

IAAs are defined as an increase in iliac artery diameter of at least 100% [2]; and considering that a normal common iliac artery has an approximate diameter of 1.2 cm, 2.5 cm is considered the threshold limit for the definition of IAAs [5]. As far as general demographic data are concerned, IAAs are more frequent in men, with a 5:1 ratio with women, and in patients aged 70 or older [2]. More than 70% of IAAs involve the common iliac artery (CIA), between 20 and 25% involve the hypogastric artery (HA), and isolated external iliac artery (EIA) aneurysms are quite rare, probably due to its different embryogenesis [6]. Frequently an aneurysmatic lesion is detected in more than one iliac artery, and it is bilateral in almost one third of the patients (Fig. 8.1).

A. Fargion · C. Pratesi (✉) · F. Masciello · W. Dorigo
Department of Vascular Surgery,
University of Florence, Florence, Italy
e-mail: carlo.pratesi@unifi.it

G. Pratesi
Department of Vascular Surgery, University of Rome
Tor Vergata, Rome, Italy

It has been suggested that IAAs share the same multifactorial pathogenetic pathway promoting the development of AAAs. More than 90% of the lesions has an atherosclerotic cause; among other causes, collagenopathies (Marfan's syndrome, Ehlers-Danlos' syndrome) and inflammatory arterial diseases (Takayasu's disease, Behçet's disease, and polyarteritis nodosa) have to be considered. Infective aneurysms are quite rare and often anecdotally reported.

As AAAs, their natural history contemplates a constant lesion growth, progressively increasing risk of aneurysmal rupture. In the largest published study reporting the fate of untreated IAAs, Santilli

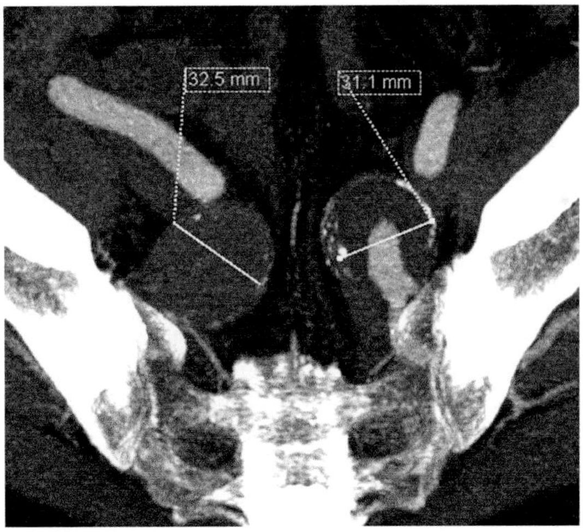

Fig. 8.1 MIP reconstruction of bilateral internal iliac aneurysms

© Springer Nature Switzerland AG 2019
Y. Tshomba et al. (eds.), *Visceral Vessels and Aortic Repair*,
https://doi.org/10.1007/978-3-319-94761-7_8

et al. [7] followed over 300 people with iliac aneurysms of <3 cm in diameter over a 4-year period and found a slow average expansion rate of 1 mm/year. In this study growth rate accelerated to 2.6 mm/year when iliac diameter exceeded 3 cm. Furthermore, expansion rates of isolated iliac aneurysms were similar regardless of laterality, presentation site, and association with an AAA. Differently, other studies suggest for IIA expansion comparable to AAAs [8]. Unfortunately, despite general growth rates, current literature on rupture risk by aneurysmal size is scarce. Currently available information is based on a series of large, symptomatic iliac aneurysms or autoptic findings on the diameters of ruptured IAAs (mean diameter ~5.5 cm) [1, 2]. Considering the rupture rate of untreated IAAs with a maximum diameter of >3 cm ranging between 14 and 70% and that perioperative risk in elective and urgent conditions varies from 3–5% [3] to 30%, current guidelines recommend this threshold as an indication for surgical repair [9, 10]. However, a recent survey involving more than 500 members of the Vascular Societies of Great Britain and Ireland showed that most physicians would wait until an IAA reached 4 cm in diameter before considering intervention [11]. Obviously, in the presence of symptoms and/or of lesions with a 5.5 cm diameter, a prompt or urgent intervention is required.

8.2 Clinical and Instrumental Diagnosis

8.2.1 Clinical Diagnosis

IAAs are usually asymptomatic, and diagnosis is made by the patient, who reports a pulsatile mass in the abdomen, and by the physician during a clinical examination or during instrumental examinations performed for unrelated causes. The presence of an IAA must be suspected in the evidence of a pulsatile mass in the lower abdominal regions; in patients with distal CIAAs or HAs, such a finding cannot be appreciated but sometimes can be found during rectal examination.

However, differently from what usually happens in patients with AAAs, such lesions are more prone to cause compression to adjacent structures, which can be found in up to 30% of cases. The compression of the ureter can lead to hydronephrosis associated with urinary infections or hematuria, whereas the rectal compression can cause pain and tenesmus. Pelvic nerves can also be compressed, causing hypoesthesia of the lower limb, while radicular compression can cause sciatic pain. When rupture occurs, it is usually contained in the retroperitoneal space, causing typical lumbar and flank pain, often referred also to the groin and to the gluteal region. Contained rupture can cause long-lasting symptoms (days or weeks) due to the inflammation and distension of the retroperitoneum. Usually, the classical triad of lumbar pain, hypotension, and pulsatile mass in the iliac region is a strong index of suspicion for a contained rupture of an IAA. Open rupture with massive bleeding is rare at first presentation but represents the final event of an undiagnosed contained rupture. Rarely a contained rupture can occur in adjacent structures, such as iliac veins, causing acute congestive right heart failure, or rectum and ureter, causing acute or chronic bleeding.

Thrombosis or embolism of the aneurysm may cause other possible complications. Aneurysmal thrombosis can cause acute limb ischemia or, more frequently, gluteal or thigh claudication with impotence. Peripheral embolism is usually referred to microembolic events, causing a "blue toe syndrome," but patients may also present an acute/subacute limb ischemia due to macro-embolization.

8.2.2 Instrumental Diagnosis

The first-level diagnostic tool is the duplex ultrasound (DUS), which can identify the presence of the IAA with high accuracy and reproducibility and low costs [12]. Even with all the limits related to the patient conformation [13], DUS is reliable in detecting these aneurysms and assessing their diameters. Moreover, it can help in the diagnosis of impending rupture, if modifications of intraluminal thrombus, sudden enlargement, or presence of periarterial fluid or thickening are found. Angio-computed tomography (CT) scan, even if more expensive and not applicable to all patients, is the gold standard in the evaluation of the morphological presentation of the lesion and in the evaluation of its proximal and distal extension. Its use is especially suggested in patients addressed to surgical repair, particularly when an endovascular procedure has to be planned, thanks to the possibility of 3D reconstructions with dedicated software. It is also mandatory in stable patients with suspected rupture, to assess endovascular feasibility and to accurately depict the status of other abdominal vessels. Angio-magnetic resonance (MR) scan, even if it provides similar accuracy to angio-CT in anatomical evaluation of IAAs, is more expensive, and high-resolution machines (>1.5 T) are usually less accessible. It may be useful in patients with contraindications to iodine contrast medium, and it represents an alternative to angio-CT scan in selected patients but does not allow to properly assess vessel calcifications. Digital subtraction angiography (DSA) is no longer used as a diagnostic tool due to its invasiveness and to the related local and general risks.

8.2.3 Prevention and Medical Treatment

Due to the lack of knowledge concerning the pathophysiology of IAA and of aneurysmal disease in general, a real prevention strategy still does not exist. Congenital factors associated with the development of IAAs are not yet possible to detect and correct. For this reason, strict control of commonly acquired risk factors for atherosclerosis is crucial in controlling lesion growth, rather than their appearance, so as to avoid the end-stage rupture. Smoking has been shown to be associated with an increased aneurysmal growth; for this reason, smoking cessation is mandatory. Several drug treatments, used to control cardiovascular risk factors, have been proposed to reduce aneurysmal growth rate during surveillance; however, no strategy has been demonstrated to be beneficial [14]. ACE inhibitors and statins seem to determine a slowing increase of AAAs, and this could also be suggested in patients with IAAs [15]. For other drugs (β-blockers, doxycycline, roxithromycin), the benefit is uncertain, and their routine use is not recommended. Future developments could come from micromolecular techniques (proteomics, genomics, microRNA), possibly allowing to create drugs selective for the arterial wall, preventing its susceptibility to aneurysmal degeneration.

Since no formal recommendations for the surveillance of iliac aneurysms exist, most clinicians have adapted schedules used for small AAAs, monitoring them more frequently with increasing size. Even if the documented slow expansion rate of iliac aneurysms <3 cm in diameter would support a policy of annual monitoring [16], many opt to multiply controls when they reached 2.6–3 cm. New research into surveillance intervals for AAAs, however, has suggested that current schedules remain overcautious and could be significantly longer without increasing rupture rate [17].

8.2.4 Surgical Treatment

The aim of invasive treatment of IAAs is to surgically replace affected iliac segments or to exclude lesions from the blood flow reducing arterial wall stress, to prevent further dilatation and rupture.

As previously reported [7, 9, 10, 18], current guidelines suggest treating asymptomatic lesions with a diameter exceeding 3 cm and symptomatic ones independently from the diameter. Smaller and asymptomatic lesions should be followed up with DUS evaluation following the schedule previously described. Current treatment options include open surgery and endovascular repair. The choice for one of the two options derives from the careful evaluation of patients' general operative risk and lesion morphology [19].

8.2.4.1 Open Surgery

Conventional open surgical repair represented the only option for patients with AAAs and IAAs for nearly 50 years, and it is still widely used in clinical practice. It consists in aneurysmal resection with graft substitution (aneurysmectomy and graft interposition). The intervention is usually performed under general anesthesia, with a urinary catheter, a nasogastric tube, a central venous line, and an arterial line preliminary placed. In recent years, a fast-track strategy has increasingly been used, to reduce intra- and postoperative patient stress by minimizing the gastrointestinal injuries, using locoregional anesthesiological techniques, and promoting an early postoperative nutrition [20].

Access to the iliac vessels is achieved with two different approaches: median transperitoneal and retroperitoneal. The former is commonly used in patients with bilateral lesions or with a concomitant AAA, while the latter is preferred in patients with unilateral iliac involvement. During aneurysmal dissection (Fig. 8.2), attention must be paid to avoid injuries to adjacent structures, mainly iliac veins, which lie in a deeper plane and can cause severe bleeding, ureters, which lie above and laterally the iliac axis, and nerves (pelvic plexus).

Before the proximal and distal vessels are clamped, systemic heparinization is performed, usually at the dose of 30 IU/kg; longitudinal incision of the sac is then performed, and the intraluminal thrombus is evacuated. The following step is the reconstitution of the arterial continuity.

In the presence of saccular aneurysms or limited blisters or blebs of the arterial wall, aneurysmal resection with primary closure of the arteriotomy can be safely performed. In most cases, however, a prosthetic graft interposition is required, whose extension and morphology depend on the aneurysm extension and on number of involved vessels.

In patients with IAA of the CIA, if adequate proximal and distal neck are available, a tube graft can be used to replace the affected artery in an "end-to-end" fashion; if the iliac bifurcation is involved, the ostium of the HA should be included in the anastomosis cuff. If this is not possible, the distal anastomosis should be performed on the EIA or the HA and the other vessel reimplanted on the graft.

A similar strategy should be used also in case of concomitant aneurysms of the CIA and HA or isolated lesions of the HA, especially when bilateral. Even if several authors suggested in the past years that bilateral ligation of hypogastric arteries was relatively safe and advocated selective IMA reimplantation to prevent pelvic ischemic complication (stump pressure cutoff value <0.6 compared to radial pressure) [21], the vast majority of the surgeons agree to preserve at least one side, paying particular attention to the IIA status (extent of dilation and patency of outflow branches). If the aneurysm is limited to the proximal segment of the artery, a direct revascularization with a short graft starting either from native CIA or from a tube graft between CIA and EIA ("T" fashion reconstruction) is the ideal strategy; if the aneurysm involves the anterior and posterior branches of the vessel, an aneurysmorrhaphy with inside ligature of the branches is suggested. Unfortunately, depending on the size of the aneurysmal sac, surgical dissection down into the pelvis to isolate iliac branches may be extremely difficult and exposes the patient to an increased risk of bleeding and damage of adjacent structures. Recently a hybrid device made of an expanded PTFE prosthesis with a nitinol-reinforced self-expanding section at one end has been

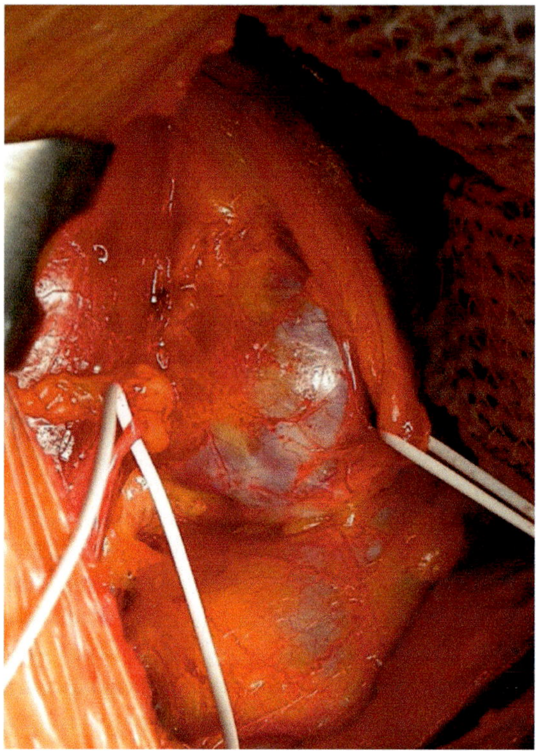

Fig. 8.2 Laparotomic isolation of an isolated iliac aneurysm

used to address this issue. This device, originally developed for hemodialysis accesses, was already implanted during complex aortic procedures for arch or visceral debranching allowing a sutureless revascularization of target vessels and decreasing overall clamping time [22]. The nitinol end is inserted on a 0.035″ guidewire inside the target artery directly through the ostium (direct cannulation) or with a small incision on the side wall avoiding extensive surgical dissection. After the self-expanding portion is released distally and post-dilated, it is ensured with three 5-0 or 6-0 polypropylene stitches to avoid possible migrations. The standard PTFE side is then anastomosed end to side on a graft or native artery. This technique was originally proposed to treat complex thoracoabdominal aneurysms using standard self-expanding covered stents as bridges for visceral arteries to be sewn to the aortic tube graft or native iliacs, as in hybrid procedures, and was defined as "VORTEC" technique [23–25]. Finally, in patients with unilateral or bilateral iliac aneurysms associated with AAA, the surgical strategy usually adopted consists in a bifurcated graft distally brought to the EIAs or HAs with concomitant reimplantation or bypass of the remaining vessels (Fig. 8.3).

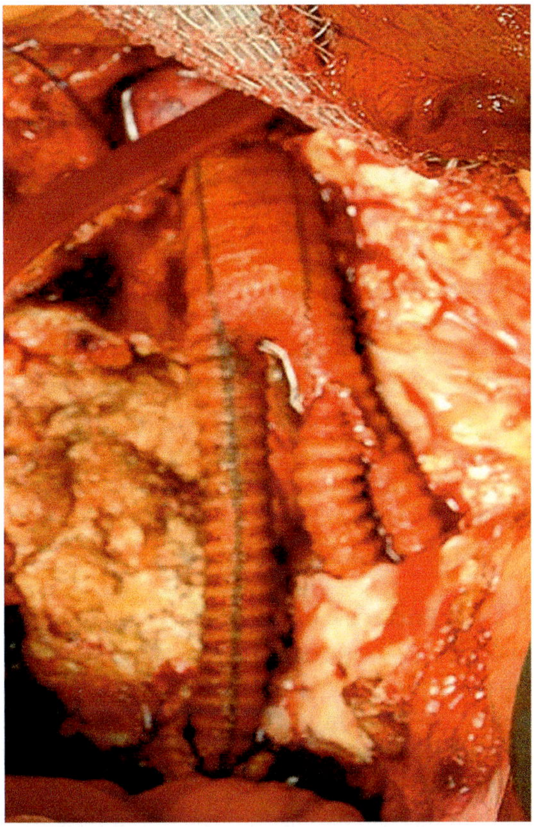

Fig. 8.3 Aorto-bi-iliac graft and end-to-side bypass to the internal iliac

Open surgical treatment of IAAs in an elective setting is, nowadays, a safe procedure. Due to improvements in anesthesiological techniques and postoperative medical protocols, perioperative mortality rates have progressively decreased over the past years, and in most recent series, it does not exceed 2% [26]. As expected, in urgent conditions, mortality rises to 7–10%. The rate of nonfatal perioperative complications is however not negligible, ranging from 5% [2] up to 15% [26]. Complications could be systemic or local. Among the former, the most common are cardiac (acute myocardial infarction, congestive heart failure), respiratory (pneumonia, acute respiratory insufficiency), and renal. Among local complications, the most frequent is the early postoperative bleeding, sometimes requiring surgical revision. Thrombosis of the graft leading to limb ischemia is rare but requires surgical revascularization; the most feared complications are related to pelvic and intestinal ischemia, due to both hemodynamic (prolonged hypotension, acute bleeding) and surgical factors (lack of preservation of hypogastric flow, hypogastric diffuse microembolization). Other minor complications include wound infection, reported in up to 10% of cases, and wound dehiscence, for which the reported frequency is lower than 1%.

The risk of late intervention-related complications is low, rarely exceeding 5% at 5 years, and the long-term survival of the operated patients, once the perioperative risk is overcome, is similar to a matched population for age and sex, without IAAs [27]. Among graft-related complications, anastomotic aneurysms (dilation of the arterial wall sutured to the graft), graft thrombosis, and infection have to be cited. More frequently, patients may develop new aneurysms proximally or distally to the intervention site during follow-up. Particularly, the most studied issue is the possible aneurysmatic evolution of the abdominal aorta years after treatment of an isolated IAA. Regarding this, there is no clear evidence in the literature concerning replacement of an ectatic abdominal aorta in patients with IAAs (maximum diameter lower than 3 cm). Some authors suggest that the risk of AAA development in patients with mild dilatation of the aorta is substantial, and for this reason, it should be treated along with the IAA [28]. More recent studies showed, on the contrary, that a 5 mm increase in the diameter of the abdominal aorta after 5 years occurs only in 15% of patients operated on for IAA, suggesting the possibility of effectively following those patients up over time, leaving the ectatic abdominal aorta at the time of the first operation [29, 30].

8.2.4.2 Endovascular Repair

Endovascular aneurysm repair of abdominal aortic aneurysms (EVAR), conceived and realized by N. Volodos in the Soviet Union and by J. Parodi in Argentina and the United States [31], represented a real revolution in the management of aortoiliac aneurysmal disease. Initially, it was reserved for elderly patients in poor general condition at high risk for open surgery, but nowadays it is increasingly used also in patients at intermediate risk, providing excellent results, mainly in the perioperative period. The use of endovascular techniques in the iliac vessels took its origin as a consequence of the frequent involvement of the iliac arteries in patients with AAA, and it was later applied to patients with isolated IAAs, considering that anatomical and technical issues are quite similar in those subgroups of patients. In fact, the involvement of iliac arteries significantly increases the complexity of the endovascular repair, negatively affecting early outcomes and late graft-related complications [32].

The main issue during endovascular management of IAAs is related to the lack of adequate distal neck in the CIA resulting in the need to find a suitable landing zone in the EIA. In the first experience, the only possible solution was to land with the endograft iliac limb down into the EIA and overstenting the HA ostium. This technique usually required a concomitant embolization of the HA, to prevent the risk of type II endoleak development. The embolization can be performed before or during endograft implantation, placing coils or plugs in the HA main trunk or in division branches (Fig. 8.4).

This procedure is associated with several complications addressed to the development of pelvic ischemia. In several different series, up to 30% of the patients undergoing HA emboli-

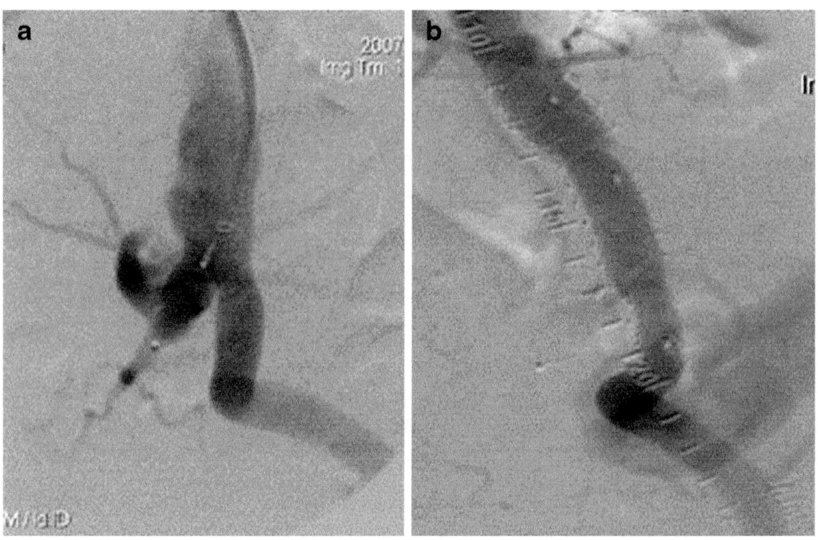

Fig. 8.4 (**a**) IIA embolization and (**b**) overstenting of the IIA ostium

zation reported a combination of bowel, spinal cord, or nerve ischemia, sexual impotence, buttock or thigh claudication, and buttock necrosis [33–37]. A systematic review [33] of 18 studies, including 643 patients with unilateral or bilateral HA embolization, reported 31% vs 35% of buttock claudication and 17% vs 24% of impotence, respectively. There are few data in the literature concerning risk factors for the developing symptoms of pelvic ischemia when an HA occlusion is performed; among them, presence of diabetes, multilevel occlusive disease, and differences in patients' age have been largely examined.

Buttock claudication has a higher presentation rate in younger patients with an active lifestyle and in elderly patients with reduced inflow due to cardiac disease. Moreover, in patients with concomitant occlusive disease of the contralateral HA and/or of the ipsilateral common femoral artery, symptoms are frequent due to lack of collateral flow to the embolized vessel [38]. In these subgroups of patients, antegrade flow in the HA should be preserved to avoid pelvic ischemia. This issue can be achieved with different techniques during open surgical repair (see description above) or hybrid procedures [39] (Fig. 8.5a). Several possible endovascular options have been used: the bell-bottom technique, the multilayer stent technology, the chimney or sandwich technique, the iliac branch device, and, more recently, the endovascular aneurysm sealing.

The *bell-bottom technique*, proposed by Karch et al. [40] in 2001, consists of an off-label use of an aortic proximal cuff to achieve sealing in ectatic CIAs with diameter between 14 and 18 mm. Although designed for the proximal aortic neck, the extension cuffs were implanted into the distal portion of the iliac limb. The result was a flared iliac limb in a bell-bottom configuration, which achieved adequate hemostatic seal in the enlarged or aneurysmal iliac segments (Fig. 8.6). For many years, large-diameter iliac limbs have been commercially available on the European market. Even if long-term results are favorable [41], flared limb size limits such technique to iliacs of up to 24 mm in diameter in the seal zone.

A *multilayer stent* is made of a three-dimensional matrix of nitinol wires derived from neuroradiological concept of flow diverter stents. The theory behind the function of this technology is the action on blood flow: reducing turbulence inside the aneurysmal sac and maintaining laminar flow into the main artery and its collaterals. Even if the aneurysmal sac is not immediately excluded from the blood flow after its placement, the progressive reduction of flow velocity potentially favors intra-sac thrombus formation with aneurysmal exclusion, while main collaterals tend to remain patent (Fig. 8.5b). While there are several published series

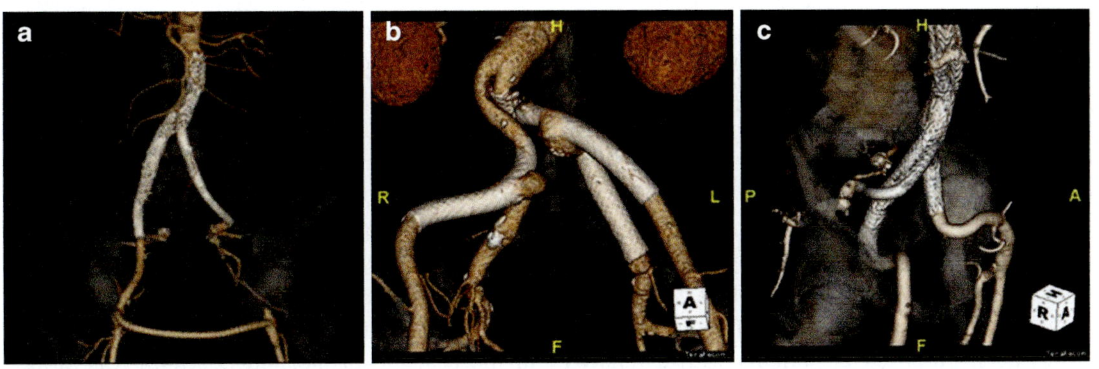

Fig. 8.5 (**a**) Complex hybrid treatment of bilateral iliac aneurysm with EIA occlusion, (**b**) multilayer stent technique, and (**c**) sandwich or double-barrel technique

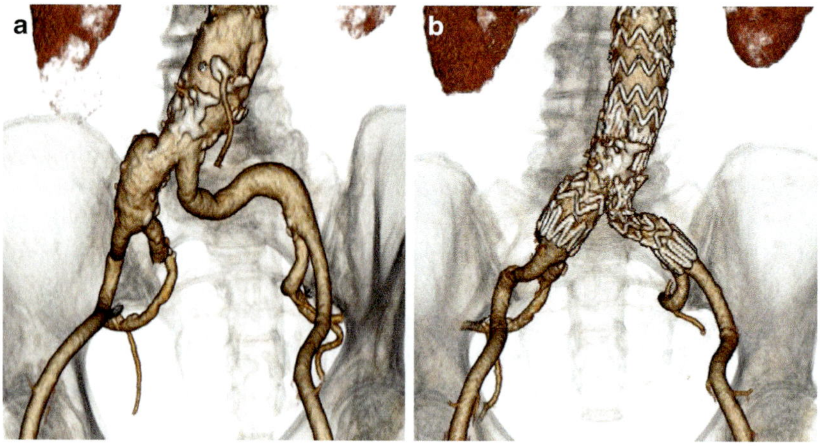

Fig. 8.6 (a, b) Hypogastric preservation with a bell-bottom iliac limb

concerning the use of such device in the treatment of visceral and peripheral aneurysms [42, 43], there are still few data concerning its application in the aortoiliac vessels [44], and its effectiveness has still to be determined.

The *chimney technique* was initially used as a bailout to restore the patency of inadvertently covered vessels (usually renal arteries) during aortic endografting [45]. It consists in the cannulation of target collateral vessels, originating from the covered part of the aorta, parallel to the released graft and stent placement (usually covered or bare metal balloon-expandable stents) to restore antegrade blood flow. The use of this technique has been recently proposed in patients with complex aneurysms, involving visceral and iliac vessels (Fig. 8.5c) [46, 47]. However, with the introduction and technical improvements of fenestrated and branched endografts, the role of the chimney technique remains limited to the treatment of unexpected intraoperative complications or in urgent setting, as custom-made endografts are associated with a not negligible crafting time and off-the-shelf devices may not be available.

When the stents used to preserve flow in the collaterals are released proximally inside an iliac limb or a tube graft, it is called "sandwich technique" (or double-barrel technique) [48, 49]. It has been proposed in patients with extensive thoracoabdominal or aortoiliac aneurysms to achieve proximal seal using a graft as a safe landing zone when a native one is not present. The early- and midterm results are promising; however, the technique is complex and technically demanding, often requiring a brachial access to engage HAs and is often associated with the early phase of the follow-up with the presence of the so-called small-gutter endoleaks. These are technique-specific type III endoleaks related to the mutual disposition of graft materials and generally disappear after a period up to 6 months postoperatively and may require a reintervention (filling the space between the grafts with glue or coils) if this does not happen.

The most widespread technique to treat iliac aneurysms and to prevent early and late complications related to the coverage or embolization of the HA is *the iliac branch device (IBD)*. This technology was born by adapting a small bifurcated body of a standard endograft to fit in a CIA, using a covered stent as bridge between the contralateral gate and a suitable distal neck inside the main trunk of the HA to preserve blood flow to the pelvis while providing a safer distal landing zone in the EIA (Fig. 8.7) [37, 50]. Iliac branch devices (IBDs) are one of the most popular options when anatomically feasible [3] (Fig. 8.8). Instructions for use (IFU) for IBDs recommend complete aortic repair with a proximal bifurcated aortic endograft. However, in the case of an isolated common iliac artery aneurysm, a stand-alone IBD implant has been proposed when an adequate landing zone is found

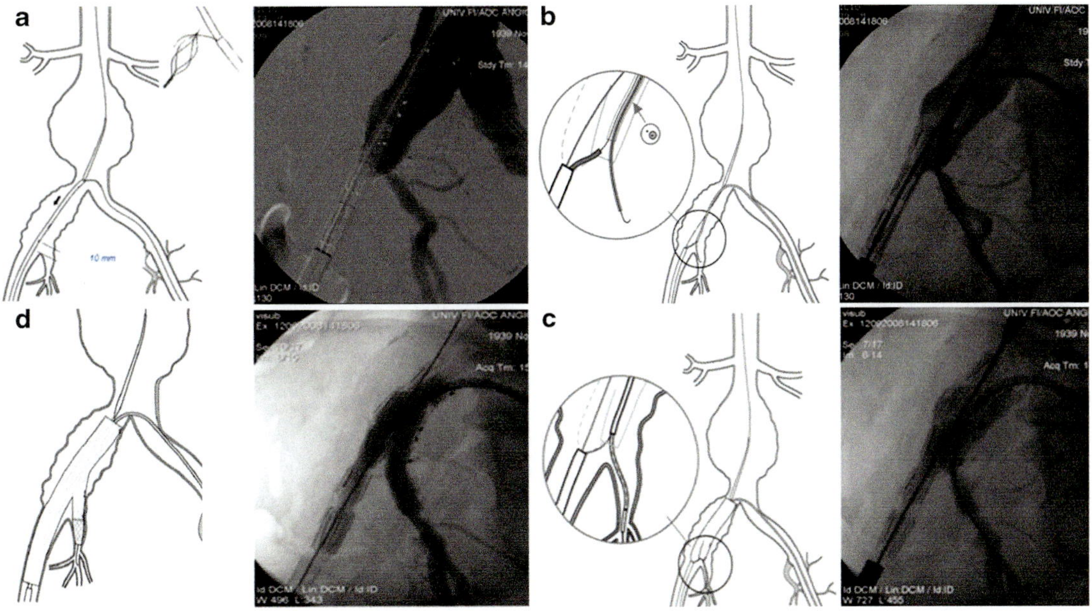

Fig. 8.7 (**a**–**d**) Steps of IBD deployment

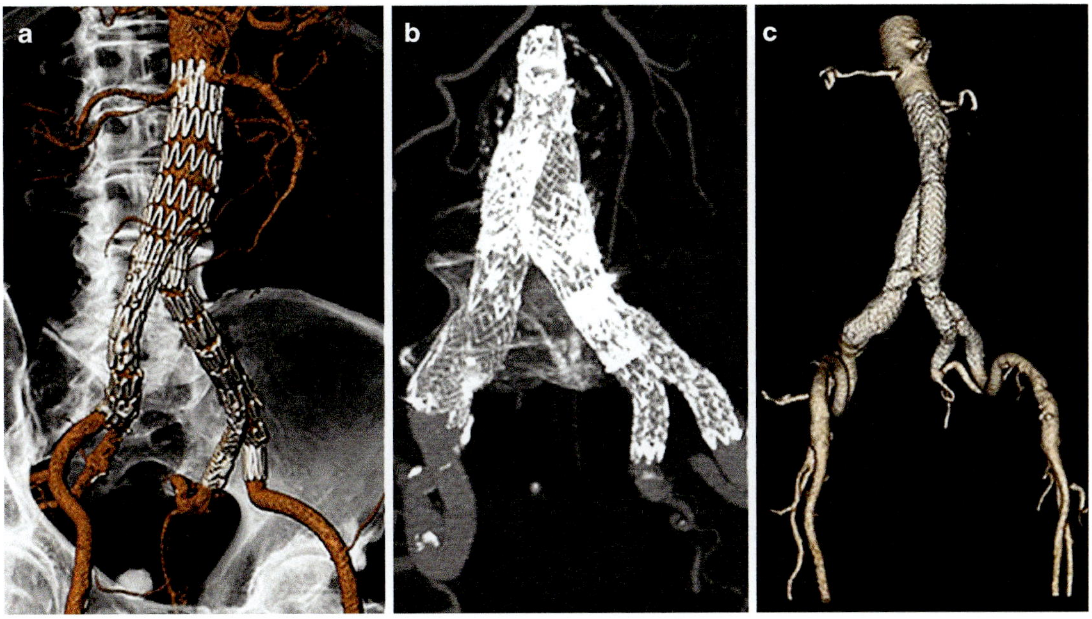

Fig. 8.8 (**a**) Endovascular exclusion with ZBIS IBD and (**b**, **c**) IBE device

in the proximal CIA (Figs. 8.9 and 8.10). The main limitation is related to several anatomical criteria needed to assess the feasibility: a length of CIA >50 mm, a diameter of the iliac bifurcation >16 mm, the presence of iliac and femoral access adequate to the dimensions of the devices, a landing zone on the EIA of 20 mm length with a diameter between 8 and 11 mm, and a landing zone on the HA of 10 mm length with a diameter adequate for an optimal sealing [51]. Among

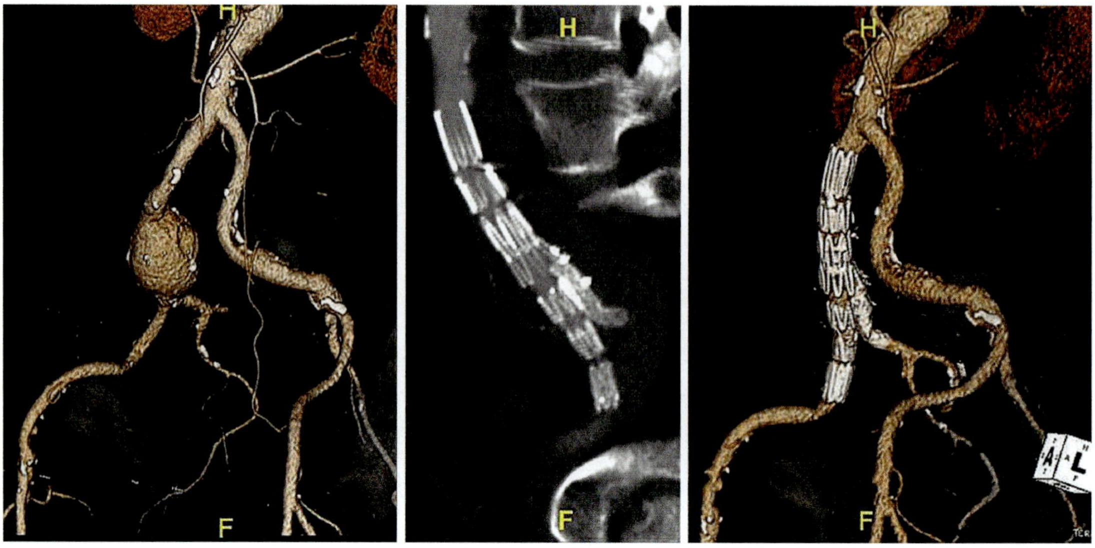

Fig. 8.9 Endovascular exclusion of an IIA with ZBIS IBD

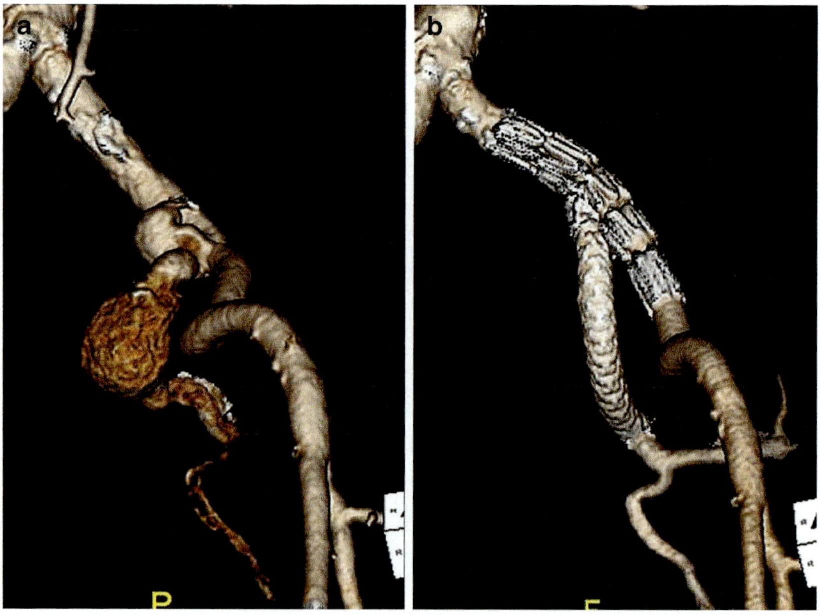

Fig. 8.10 (**a**) Isolated hypogastric aneurysm and (**b**) ZBIS IBD landing into distal main trunk

contraindications, severe tortuosity and calcifications of the iliac axis, severe kinking of the iliac bifurcation, and an extensive aneurysmal involvement of the HA are the most commonly encountered (Fig. 8.11). For this reason, a proper case selection along with an accurate planning is mandatory, and a detailed preoperative imaging is crucial. It can usually be obtained with a spiral angio-CT scan with 1 mm axial slices and high-resolution multiplane reconstructions. Fortunately, the fast evolution of materials has brought about new generation devices that are able to treat even complex anatomies with severe angulations in the origin of the EIA and HA and to reduce potential risk of kinking, dislocation, and migration. Good experience in both aortic

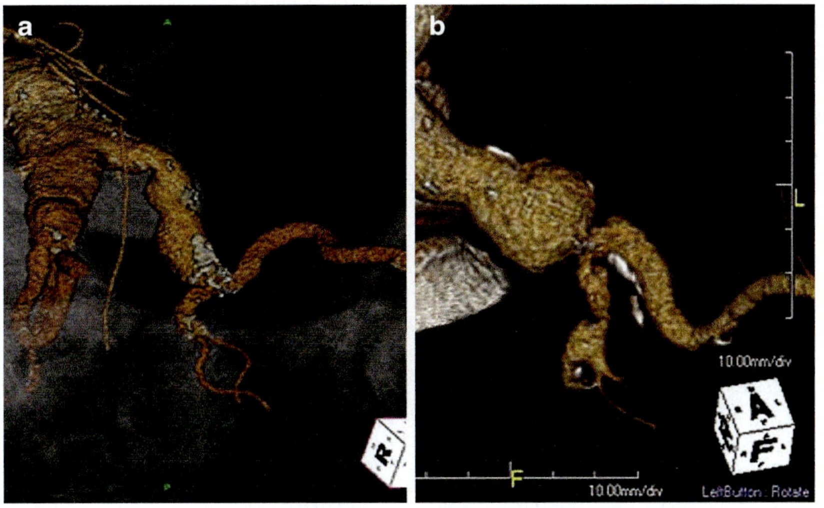

Fig. 8.11 (**a**) Wide hypogastric takeoff angle and (**b**) tight iliac bifurcation

and visceral endovascular interventions together with sufficient advanced endovascular techniques is required to perform an IBD treatment; thus, an adequate learning curve due to the relative complexity of the procedure must be considered.

Several studies have demonstrated that the use of IBD is associated with a reduction in the risk of developing buttock claudication and pelvic ischemia in comparison with alternative techniques [37, 52–54]. Furthermore, a recent retrospective study evaluating the long-term results of IBDs in a series of 575 patients and 650 implants performed in 6 high-volume European centers reported satisfying rates of estimated 8-year freedom from IBD and target HA occlusion (87% and 95.1%, respectively) and freedom from reintervention due to occlusion and/or type I endoleak (85.7%) [55]. These results (especially in the mid and long term) allowed the IBD to be considered as the first-choice treatment in young patients with active lifestyles, who may suffer from a significant impact of ischemic pelvic complications in their everyday activities. Technical success rates approach 97%, and the risk of long-term graft-related complications is negligible [52]. Moreover, its use is suggested in patients with previous or concomitant treatment of multilevel complex aortic disease (Fig. 8.12) that can benefit from hypogastric flow preservation in terms of prevention of spinal cord ischemia.

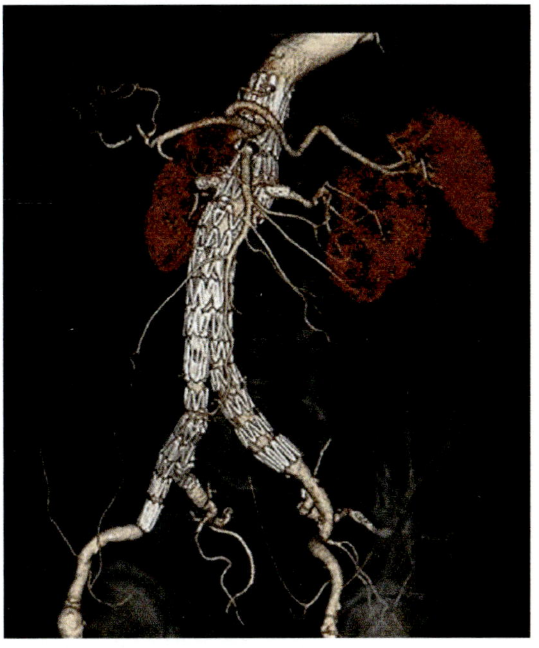

Fig. 8.12 Hypogastric preservation during complex aortic procedures

Recently, the *endovascular aneurysm sealing* (EVAS), proposed as an alternative method to EVAR for AAA treatment, has been extended also to the visceral and iliac segments. This technique consists of a balloon-expandable stent graft with surrounding polyurethane endobag. Once the stent grafts are deployed, a polymer solution is injected into the endobags to fill the blood lumen outside the stents, thereby sealing the aneurysm. These stents have been used also in a "chimney technique" fashion in combination with covered or bare metal stents inside visceral or iliac arteries achieving sealing of the aneurysmal sacs with the bags and leaving blood flow to collaterals. Early results (usually with a mean follow-up less than 12 months) in the literature are also promising in patients with IAAs, but long-term studies are mandatory to assess efficacy and possible complications [56].

References

1. McCready RA, Pairolero PC, Gilmore JC, et al. Isolated iliac artery aneurysms. Surgery. 1983;93:688–93.
2. Richardson JW, Greenfield LJ. Natural history and management of iliac aneurysms. J Vasc Surg. 1988;8:165–71.
3. Sandhu RS, Pipinos II. Isolated iliac artery aneurysm. Semin Vasc Surg. 2005;18:209–15.
4. Brunkwall J, Hauksson H, Bengtsson H, et al. Solitary aneurysms of the iliac arterial system: an estimate of their frequency of occurrence. J Vasc Surg. 1989;10:381–4.
5. Williams SK, Earnshaw JJ. Intervention criteria for iliac aneurysms. In: Greenhalgh RM, editor. Vascular and endovascular controversies update. London: BIBA; 2012.
6. Giordano J. Embryology of the vascular system. Philadelphia: W. B. Saunders; 2000.
7. Santilli SM, Wernsing SE, Lee ES. Expansion rates and outcomes for iliac artery aneurysms. J Vasc Surg. 2000;31:114–21.
8. Rutherford RB. Management of abdominal aortic aneurysms: which risk factors play a role in decision-making? Semin Vasc Surg. 2008;21:124–31.
9. Chaikof EL, Brewster DC, Dalman RL, et al. The care of patients with an abdominal aortic aneurysm: the Society for Vascular Surgery practice guidelines. J Vasc Surg. 2009;50(4 Suppl):2–49.
10. Pratesi C, Alberti V, Apostolou D, et al. Patologia aneurismatica dell'aorta infrarenale, aneurismi viscerali ed aneurismi periferici. Ital J Vasc Endovasc Surg. 2016;23(Suppl 1):1–54.
11. Williams SK, Campbell WB, Earnshaw JJ. Survey of management of common iliac artery aneurysms by members of the Vascular Society of Great Britain and Ireland. Ann R Coll Surg Engl. 2014;96:116–20.
12. Antignani PL, Benedetti-Valentini F, Aluigi L, et al. Diagnosis of vascular diseases. Ultrasound investigations - guidelines of the Italian Society for Vascular Investigation. Int Angiol. 2012;31(5 Suppl 1):1–7.
13. Wilmink AB, Forshaw M, Quick CR, et al. Accuracy of serial screening for abdominal aortic aneurysms by ultrasound. J Med Screen. 2002;9:125–7.
14. Golledge J, Powell JT. Medical management of abdominal aortic aneurysm. Eur J Vasc Endovasc Surg. 2007;34:267–73.
15. Schouten O, van Laanen JH, Boersma E, et al. Statins are associated with a reduced infrarenal abdominal aortic aneurysm growth. Eur J Vasc Endovasc Surg. 2006;32:21–6.
16. Buckley CJ, Buckley SD. Technical tips for endovascular repair of common iliac artery aneurysms. Semin Vasc Surg. 2008;21:31–4.
17. Thompson SG, Brown LC, Sweeting MJ, et al. Systematic review and meta-analysis of the growth and rupture rates of small abdominal aortic aneurysms: implications for surveillance intervals and their cost-effectiveness. Health Technol Assess. 2013;17:1–118.
18. Krupski W. Iliac artery aneurysms. Philadelphia: W. B. Saunders; 2001.
19. Katsargyris A, Oikonomou K, Klonaris C, et al. Common iliac and hypogastric aneurysms: open and endovascular repair. J Cardiovasc Surg. 2015;56:249–55.
20. Muehling BM, Ortlieb L, Oberhuber A, et al. Fast track management reduces the systemic inflammatory response and organ failure following elective infrarenal aortic aneurysm repair. Interact Cardiovasc Thorac Surg. 2011;12:784–8.
21. Bacharach JM, Slovut DP. State of the art: management of iliac artery aneurysmal disease. Catheter Cardiovasc Interv. 2008;71:708–14.
22. Levack MM, Bavaria JE, Gorman RC, et al. Rapid aortic arch debranching using the Gore hybrid vascular graft. Ann Thorac Surg. 2013;95(6):163–5.
23. Lachat M, Mayer D, Criado FJ, et al. New technique to facilitate renal revascularization with use of telescoping self-expanding stent grafts: VORTEC. Vascular. 2008;16(2):69–72.
24. Chiesa R, Kahlberg A, Mascia D, et al. Use of a novel hybrid vascular graft for sutureless revascularization of the renal arteries during open thoracoabdominal aortic aneurysm repair. J Vasc Surg. 2014;60(3):622–30.
25. Tyagi S, Pineda D, Zheng H, et al. A novel method for the treatment of bilateral hypogastric aneurysms using hybrid polytetrafluoroethylene graft. Vasc Endovasc Surg. 2017;51(4):199–202.
26. Buck DB, Bensley RP, Darling J, et al. The effect of endovascular treatment on isolated iliac artery aneurysm treatment and mortality. J Vasc Surg. 2015;62:331–5.
27. Hallett JW Jr, Marshall DM, Petterson TM, et al. Graft-related complications after abdominal aortic aneurysm repair: reassurance from a 36-year population-based experience. J Vasc Surg. 1997;25:277–84.
28. Kasirajan V, Hertzer NR, Beven EG, et al. Management of isolated common iliac artery aneurysms. Cardiovasc Surg. 1998;6:171–7.

29. Dorigo W, Pulli R, Troisi N, et al. The treatment of isolated iliac artery aneurysm in patients with non-aneurysmal aorta. Eur J Vasc Endovasc Surg. 2008;35:585–9.
30. Troisi N, Dorigo W, Marek J, et al. Treatment for isolated iliac aneurysms. In: Setacci C, Gasparini D, Reimers B, Cremonesi A, Rossi P, editors. Aortic surgery: new developments and perspectives. Turin: Edizioni Minerva Medica; 2009. p. 429–3.
31. Parodi JC, Palmaz JC, Barone HD. Transfemoral intraluminal graft implantation for abdominal aortic aneurysms. Ann Vasc Surg. 1991;5:491–9.
32. Greenhalgh RM, Powell JT. Endovascular repair of abdominal aortic aneurysms. N Engl J Med. 2008;398:454–501.
33. Rayt HS, Bown MJ, Lambert KV, et al. Buttock claudication and erectile dysfunction after internal iliac artery embolization in patients prior to endovascular aortic aneurysm repair. Cardiovasc Intervent Radiol. 2008;31:728–34.
34. Bratby MJ, Munneke GM, Belli AM, et al. How safe is bilateral internal iliac artery embolization prior to EVAR? Cardiovasc Interv Radiol. 2008;31:246–53.
35. Vandy F, Criado E, Upchurch GR Jr, et al. Transluminal hypogastric artery occlusion with an Amplatzer vascular plug during endovascular aortic aneurysm repair. J Vasc Surg. 2008;45:1121–4.
36. Wyers MC, Schermerhorn ML, Fillinger MF, et al. Internal iliac occlusion without coil embolization during endovascular abdominal aortic aneurism repair. J Vasc Surg. 2002;36:1138–45.
37. Verzini F, Parlani G, Romano L, et al. Endovascular treatment of iliac aneurysm: concurrent comparison of side branch endograft versus hypogastric exclusion. J Vasc Surg. 2009;49:1154–61.
38. Yano OJ, Morrissey N, Eisen L, et al. Intentional internal iliac artery occlusion to facilitate endovascular repair of aortoliac aneurysms. J Vasc Surg. 2001;34:204–11.
39. Pratesi G, Pulli R, Fargion A, et al. Alternative hybrid reconstruction for bilateral common and internal iliac artery aneurysms associated with external iliac artery occlusion. J Endovasc Ther. 2009;16:638–41.
40. Karch LA, Hodgson KJ, Mattos MA, et al. Management of ectatic, nonaneurysmal iliac arteries during endoluminal aortic aneurysm repair. Management of ectatic, nonaneurysmal iliac arteries during endoluminal aortic aneurysm repair. J Vasc Surg. 2001;33:33–8.
41. Torsello G, Schönefeld E, Osada N, et al. Endovascular treatment of common iliac artery aneurysms using the bell-bottom technique: long-term results. J Endovasc Ther. 2010;17:504–9.
42. Ruffino M, Rabbia C, Italian Cardiatis Registry Investigators Group. Endovascular treatment of visceral artery aneurysms with Cardiatis multilayer flow modulator: preliminary results at six-month follow-up. J Cardiovasc Surg. 2011;52:311–21.
43. Sfyroeras GS, Dalainas I, Giannakopoulos TG, et al. Flow-diverting stents for the treatment of arterial aneurysms. J Vasc Surg. 2012;56:839–46.
44. Natrella M, Castagnola M, Navarretta F, et al. Treatment of juxtarenal aortic aneurysm with the Multilayer stent. J Endovasc Ther. 2012;19:121–4.
45. Greenberg RK, Clair D, Srivastava S, et al. Should patients with challenging anatomy be offered endovascular aneurysm repair? J Vasc Surg. 2003;38: 990–6.
46. Moulakakis KG, Mylonas SN, Avgerinos E, et al. The chimney graft technique for preserving visceral vessels during endovascular treatment of aortic pathologies. J Vasc Surg. 2012;55:1497–503.
47. Mosquera Arochena N, Rodríguez Feijoo G, Carballo Fernandez C, et al. Use of modified sandwich-graft technique to preserve hypogastric artery in EVAR treatment of complex aortic aneurysm anatomy. J Cardiovasc Surg. 2011;52:643–9.
48. Lobato AC, Camacho-Lobato L. The sandwich technique to treat complex aortoiliac or isolated iliac aneurysms: results of midterm follow-up. J Vasc Surg. 2013;57:26–34.
49. Lim CS, Naji Y, Hussain ST, et al. Modified sandwich-graft technique employing Aorfix and Viabahn stent-grafts to preserve hypogastric flow in cases of complex aortoiliac and isolated common iliac artery aneurysms including the internal iliac artery ostium. Eur J Vasc Endovasc Surg. 2016;51:364–70.
50. Fernández-Alonso L, Fernández-Alonso S, Grijalba FU, et al. Endovascular treatment of abdominal aortic aneurysms involving iliac bifurcation: role of iliac branch graft device in prevention of buttock claudication. Ann Vasc Surg. 2013;27:851–5.
51. Delay C, Deglise S, Lejay A, et al. Zenith bifurcated iliac side branch device: mid-term results and assessment of risk factors for intraoperative thrombosis. Ann Vasc Surg. 2017;41:141–50.
52. Loth AG, Rouhani G, Gafoor SA, et al. Treatment of iliac artery bifurcation aneurysms with the second-generation straight iliac bifurcated device. J Vasc Surg. 2015;62:1168–75.
53. Pratesi G, Fargion A, Pulli R, et al. Endovascular treatment of aorto-iliac aneurysms: four-year results of iliac branch endograft. Eur J Vasc Endovasc Surg. 2013;45:607–9.
54. Simonte G, Parlani G, Farchioti L, et al. Lesson learned with the use of iliac branch devices: single centre 10 year experience in 157 consecutive procedures. Eur J Vasc Endovasc Surg. 2017;54(1):95–103.
55. Donas KP, Inchingolo M, Cao P, et al. Secondary procedures following iliac branch device treatment of aneurysms involving the iliac bifurcation: the pELVIS registry. J Endovasc Ther. 2017;24(3):405–10.
56. Youssef M, Nurzai Z, Zerwes S, et al. Initial experience in the treatment of extensive iliac artery aneurysms with the Nellix aneurysm sealing system. J Endovasc Ther. 2016;23:290–6.

9 Operative Management of Type II Endoleaks After Aortic Endovascular Repair

Anna Maria Ierardi, Filippo Pesapane, Francesca Patella, Enrico Maria Fumarola, Salvatore Alessio Angileri, Mario Petrillo, Matteo Crippa, and Gianpaolo Carrafiello

9.1 Introduction

Endoleaks (ELs) are the most common complications after endovascular aneurysm repair (EVAR), with an incidence that varies between 10% and 50% [1–4]. They are defined as persistent flow within the excluded aneurysm sac and the graft [1–4]. Endoleaks are classified according to the underlying etiology and localization [5, 6]. The risk of rupture of the aneurysmatic sac depends on the type and persistency of endoleaks. The type II endoleak (T2EL) is the most common form and occurs in about 20–30% of patients after treatment, persisting in 10–15% of patients after 6 months [3]. T2EL occurs when a retrograde flow of blood supplies the aneurysm sac through branch vessels such as lumbar arteries or a patent inferior mesenteric artery (IMA) [4]. T2EL usually has a complex architecture because it should be featured by more than one inflow and outflow vessel, which communicates through a channel [5]. For this reason, a further differentiation of T2EL was proposed: type IIA, when it is related to only one patent branch, and type IIB, when it is complex with two or more patent branches and creating a flow-through situation [4].

Fifty percent of type II ELs resolve spontaneously, 10–15% are persistent on long-term follow-up, and recurrent T2EL develop in 5–10% [2, 4, 7, 8].

A conservative approach with regular follow-up is accepted for stable T2EL [9, 10], whereas treatment of T2EL is normally required when the aneurysm sac diameter increases more than 5 mm between sequential Computed Tomography (CT) follow-up examinations, because this is indicative of high sac pressure [3].

In the past, T2EL were usually treated surgically, both with graft explantation and with retroperitoneal ligation of collateral feeding vessels [5]. These invasive methods require hospital admission and they increase morbidity of surgery [11]. For this reason, over the years, new less invasive techniques for the treatment of T2EL have made their way through. Nowadays, the most common treatment for patients with T2EL is transarterial embolization (TAE), with the aim of occluding the feeding arteries and/or the EL nidus [12]. In order to achieve successful embolization, the inflow vessels and the channel(s) need to be embolized [5]. A critical step of the procedure is

A. M. Ierardi · S. A. Angileri · M. Petrillo
G. Carrafiello (✉)
Department of Health Sciences, Diagnostic and Interventional Radiology, San Paolo Hospital, University of Milan, Milan, Italy
e-mail: gianpaolo.carrafiello@unimi.it

F. Pesapane · F. Patella · E. M. Fumarola
Postgraduation School in Radiodiagnostics, Università degli Studi di Milano, Milan, Italy

M. Crippa
Surgery Department, San Paolo Hospital, University of Milan, Milan, Italy

© Springer Nature Switzerland AG 2019
Y. Tshomba et al. (eds.), *Visceral Vessels and Aortic Repair*,
https://doi.org/10.1007/978-3-319-94761-7_9

the identification of the artery feeding the sac, which allows reaching the nidus of the endoleak and delivering embolic agents for complete occlusion. Failure is primarily due to the inability to reach the nidus or to coil the aneurysmatic sac [13].

Angiographic identification of the feeding artery may be time-consuming, because sequential angiographic image acquisitions are usually necessary. Moreover, determination of the specific artery responsible for the EL is difficult when the arterial vasculature has a complex branching pattern [13, 14]. Several studies presented the value of intraprocedural Cone-Beam CT (CBCT) and Advanced Vessel Detection (AVD) software as problem-solving tool to aid in safe catheterization of offending vessels during TAE of gastrointestinal [15, 16] and visceral arterial bleedings [4, 17, 18] while decreasing total procedure time, contrast dose, and radiation exposure [15, 19]; recently the same technology was used to detect the feeders of the ELs [15, 16]. When TAE is not feasible (e.g., there are no arterial routes) or unsuccessful, direct percutaneous sac injection (DPSI) and transcaval embolization (TCE) are alternative endovascular methods validated for the treatment of T2EL [5, 20–23].

Actually, no treatment is considered the gold standard for T2EL management, and consequently, a tailored treatment should be preferred [1, 23, 24].

A variety of embolic agents have been used either in isolation or in combination for treatment of T2EL [5]. Liquid embolic agents and coils are the main embolic agents used [12], but there are no guidelines for the choice of embolic material, and the final decision is often made on the basis of the operator experience and confidence [5].

Patient preparation and management is the same as for any standard endovascular procedure. Prophylactic antibiotics for secondary interventions are advisable, although there is no convincing evidence of benefit for the prevention of infection in the literature [4].

9.2 Endovascular Embolization

Percutaneous TAE is the most common intervention for T2EL [12]. This procedure involves a percutaneous transfemoral or transbrachial approach, with the aim of catheterizing the nidus of the endoleak via its collaterals.

Treatment of T2EL is feasible when IMA is supplied via the arch of Riolano through the collaterals of the SMA. Another possible approach is from the internal iliac arteries when the endoleak arises from lumbar arteries (LA), through collaterals of the iliolumbar arteries [25].

Briefly, for transarterial embolization of an IMA T2EL, catheterization of the middle colic artery (MCA) through the SMA, a microcatheter must be advanced via the arch of Riolano until the catheterization of the IMA [26] (Fig. 9.1). With regard to the embolization of a LA T2EL, a short sheath is

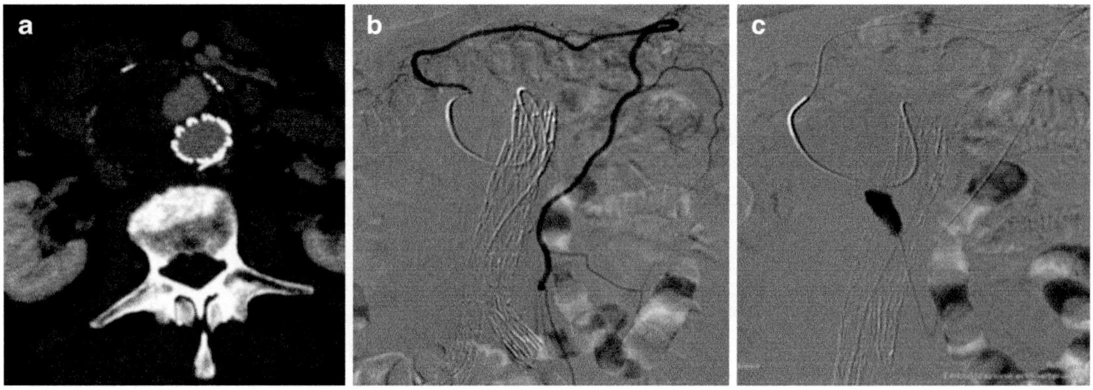

Fig. 9.1 CT Angiography revealed T2EL supplied from IMA (**a**); a microcatheter has to be advanced via the arch of Riolano until the catheterization of the IMA (**b**) and to reach the nidus (**c**)

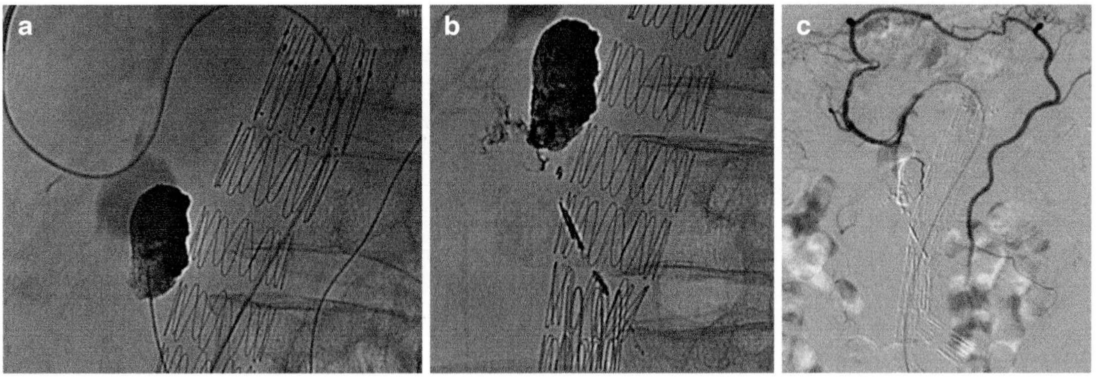

Fig. 9.2 Endoleak nidus was reached and the embolic agent was injected to fill the nidus and the feeding vessel (**a**, **b**); final angiogram confirmed complete embolization of the EL (**c**)

placed into the ipsilateral femoral artery, and the internal iliac artery is catheterized. As the majority of lumbar T2EL communicate with the iliolumbar artery, it is generally necessary to catheterize the iliolumbar artery with a microcatheter and an angled microwire, a passage which can be extremely challenging [26].

In both cases, when the EL's nidus is reached, it is possible to inject or deploy the embolic agent until the nidus and the feeding vessels are occluded [12] (Fig. 9.2).

This procedure may be difficult, time-consuming, and not possible in all patients because of anatomic limitations [27]; as literature data has demonstrated, embolization of a single feeding or draining artery may be ineffective in most cases, because additional flow is often recruited from other adjacent branches [14]; it is highly suggested to try to achieve a permanent cessation of flow occluding the entire nidus, in order to interrupt the communication to all patent communicating aortic side branches, including the inflow and outflow vessels [28].

The final goal is to definitively stop the blood flow in these collateral arteries with appropriate embolic agents which should cause thrombosis and cessation of the EL [29].

EL embolization can be performed with many different embolic agents. Glue (*n*-butyl cyanoacrylate (NBCA)), coils, thrombin, and polymers (ethylene-vinyl alcohol copolymer (EVOH)) are the most commonly used ones [30].

Among these agents, polymer Onyx (Liquid Embolic System; ev3 Neurovascular, Irvine, California) is particularly suitable for EL embolization. EVOH is dissolved in dimethyl sulfoxide (DMSO). When Onyx comes into contact with blood, it precipitates and forms a cast, with a harder outer layer and a semiliquid central core. These proprieties can be helpful especially in cases with tortuous and small feeding vessels, when microcatheter positioning into the nidus is unachievable. In these situations, Onyx can be injected from a more distant catheter position through the network of collateral vessels and pushed into the nidus, thanks to its unique proprieties [31].

However, a recently-published retrospective study, despite an encouraging post-procedural high success rate (88.9%), after a mean follow-up period of 32.8 months, 44.4% of patients required a second intervention for EL recurrence or delayed clinical failure [32].

So, despite some encouraging results on Onyx and other liquid agents, there are no conclusive data on the advantages or disadvantages of the different embolic materials [26].

A large and recent review that considered seven different studies which reported outcomes for transarterial procedures, for a total of 120 interventions, showed an overall clinical success rate of 62.5%, defined as no evidence of recurrent T2EL during follow-up. In this cohort of patients, 22.5% required further intervention for failed embolization

[33]: development of new type II ELs, persistent blood flow through the coils of the treated EL, and growth of anastomoses around the coiled vessel are all reasons suggested as being correlated to clinical failure [2].

As already pointed out, the critical step in the procedure is to identify the feeding sac artery, which then allows to reach the nidus and deliver embolic agents for complete occlusion. Failure occurs primarily due to an inability to reach the nidus or to embolize the aneurysmatic sac [13].

Technology is moving fast and new tools are available and can help to spare time and to improve outcomes. In particular, C-arm CBCT is considered the most impactful breakthrough in the last decade [34].

CBCT and AVD software may be a useful option in case of angiographically occult T2EL or complex vasculature, permitting to identify safely and quickly the feeding artery [15].

9.3 Percutaneous Sac Puncture

Percutaneous sac puncture (PSP) is an interventional procedure consisting in the direct injection of an embolizing agent into the aneurysmatic sac through a percutaneous access [20].

It has been proposed as an alternative option for treatment of T2EL in case of unsuccessful TAE [4, 35] or whether endovascular approach is not feasible [20].

PSP can be performed with two different techniques: with a transabdominal or a translumbar approach (Fig. 9.3). The first method should be preferred if the EL is located or extended anteriorly, while the second one should be selected whether the EL is visualized in the posterior portion of the sac or when bowel or other important structures are interposed [25, 36]. Indeed, the most important advantage of the translumbar approach is that it does not imply the passage into cavities or organs [35, 37]. However, this method imposes an uncomfortable position of the patient, who is supposed to stay in a prone position [36].

Conversely, the principal advantage of the transabdominal technique is that the patient can be placed in a supine position; moreover a simultaneous transarterial angiography should be performed if needed. The risk of organ injury during the transabdominal approach can be minimized, using real-time US guidance [36].

In both cases, in order to confirm the T2EL and to assess its origin (lumbar and/or mesenteric), PSP requires a pre-interventional imaging evaluation, that can be provided either by CEUS [5] or CT angiography or MRI angiography [36] or CT/MRI and CEUS.

The procedure can be performed under local anesthesia [20].

Briefly, PSP technique involves the percutaneous puncture under US or CT/fluoroscopic guidance of the aneurysmatic sac, generally using a 21G needle [36]. Once blood flashback is obtained, a wire is advanced into the sac, to allow the positioning of a larger introducer sheath and the subsequent introduction of a 4 or 5 F angiographic catheter [25]. Then, after an angiogram of the aneurysmatic sac to assess the features of the EL and to identify the inflow and

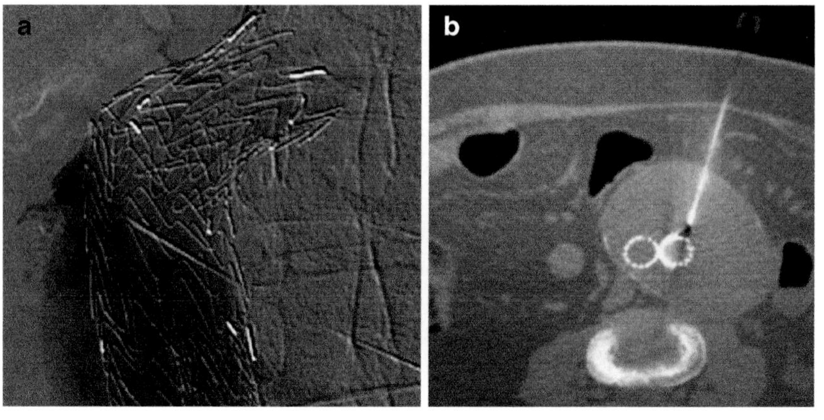

Fig. 9.3 PSP can be performed with translumbar (**a**) or transabdominal (**b**) approach

outflow vessels, the embolization of the sac and of the feeding vessels can be performed [25, 36].

As above reported, there are no guidelines for the choice of the embolic material; a variety of embolic agents either combined or alone can be used for the treatment of T2EL. However, permanent agents such as coils, NBCA, thrombin, and EVOH are advisable [5]. In addition, the selection of a liquid embolic agent allows to completely fulfilling the aneurysmatic sac, including all in- and outflow vessels, creating a solid cast which results in an uncompressible structure that impedes recanalization, providing a hypothetic more durable repair than coils. Specifically, EVOH has a lava-like flow pattern within blood vessels without any fragmentation during the injection. It is also associated with a lower inflammatory reaction and the absence of polymerization heat compared with NBCA [38].

Featured by almost 100% of technical success rate and 70% of secondary clinical success rate, percutaneous and endovascular treatments have overlapping outcomes [25], but PSP is usually a faster procedure, able to reduce consistently the ionizing radiation dose, especially if US-guidance is used.

Complications are rare and include nontarget embolization, puncture site hematomas, and perforation of vessels or bowel during the passage of the needle [25].

However, treatment results must be checked by a strict imaging follow-up, generally provided by CT angiography or Contrast-Enhanced UltraSound (CEUS) at 30 days, at 6 months, and at 12 months postoperatively and annually thereafter [5].

In conclusion, PSP can be a helpful minimally invasive therapeutic option for treatment of T2EL, allowing the sac obliteration, as well as a significantly shorter procedure and fluoroscopy time compared to endovascular approach.

9.4 Transcaval Embolization

TCE has been proposed instead of the direct translumbar approach as the initial treatment of T2EL and in cases where transarterial embolization failed. The indications for treatment are the same as those reported in the introduction of this chapter [24].

Compared with TAE, TCE is less time-consuming and can be also performed in T2EL with no direct lumbar collateral vessels. Another advantage of TCE is the utilization of supine positioning, which facilitates patient comfort and concomitant arterial access allowing the confirmation of the EL, verification of EL obliteration and, if necessary, concurrent TAE. If the T2EL originates from lumbar or middle sacral vessel, we directly access the aorta via either a translumbar or TCE, with the approach dictated by the localization of the T2EL and the aorta relative to the inferior vena cava (IVC) and lumbar spine [39]. Furthermore, with TCE, the IVC is punctured through one wall instead of both, as required when the right translumbar approach is performed, and lower risk of retroperitoneal hemorrhage or inadvertent bowel injury may be anticipated [24, 39].

The TCE is viable in almost all patients; however, direct puncture should be difficult when the aneurysmatic sac diameter is small and is associated with an increased risk of stent graft puncture.

Preoperative planning allows identification of radiographic markers (e.g., stent graft, graft bifurcation, device overlap points, or aortic wall calcifications) that may guide transcaval puncture facilitating the access to the T2EL [39]. In order to optimize needle orientation into the aneurysm sac, an intraoperative CT or CBCT can be performed [15, 19]. After confirmation of successful embolization, the puncture system may be removed, and an imaging examination should be performed to determine if there is any evidence of aortocaval fistula or contrast extravasation. Usually the patient is admitted overnight and undergoes noncontrast CT at 24 h to evaluate the immediate success of embolization and to identify any complications related to the procedure [24, 39]. Potential complications include the thrombophlebitis at the site of femoral percutaneous venous access, inadvertent intracaval embolization of coils, retroperitoneal hematoma, and caval-aortic fistulas [24, 39]. However, TCE requires a thin needle cannula and a 5 F catheter, which is quite small in caliber and only causes small holes in the caval walls. The caval hole is expected to close immediately after the removal of the 5 F catheter [21, 24].

To the best of our knowledge, the cumulative combined reported success of transarterial and translumbar procedures is ≤70%, and this is comparable to the early results of TCE [39].

Follow-up CT should be performed following the same protocol described above [24].

In conclusion, TCE seems to be a safe and technically feasible management option for T2EL which require treatment; nevertheless, further studies are needed to confirm its role as a complementary technique to existing methods of T2EL management.

9.5 Conclusions

The described techniques permit to treat T2EL and to avoid surgery, with the main advantages of mini-invasivity and less morbidity and mortality.

More studies with longer follow-up will allow for more information about embolic agents and tools to reach the nidus (CBCT and AVD software).

Compliance with Ethical Standards

Conflict of interest: The authors declare that they have no conflict of interest.

References

1. Veith FJ, Baum RA, Ohki T, et al. Nature and significance of endoleaks and endotension: summary of opinions expressed at an international conference. J Vasc Surg. 2002;35(5):1029–35.
2. Solis MM, Ayerdi J, Babcock GA, et al. Mechanism of failure in the treatment of type II endoleak with percutaneous coil embolization. J Vasc Surg. 2002;36(3):485–91.
3. Bryce Y, Rogoff P, Romanelli D, Reichle R. Endovascular repair of abdominal aortic aneurysms: vascular anatomy, device selection, procedure, and procedure-specific complications. Radiographics. 2015;35(2):593–615.
4. Rand T, Uberoi R, Cil B, Munneke G, Tsetis D. Quality improvement guidelines for imaging detection and treatment of endoleaks following endovascular aneurysm repair (EVAR). Cardiovasc Intervent Radiol. 2013;36(1):35–45.
5. Ierardi AM, Micieli C, Angileri SA, et al. Ethylene-vinyl alcohol copolymer as embolic agent for treatment of type II endoleak: our experience. Radiol Med. 2017;122(2):154–9.
6. Gelfand DV, White GH, Wilson SE. Clinical significance of type II endoleak after endovascular repair of abdominal aortic aneurysm. Ann Vasc Surg. 2006;20(1):69–74.
7. Harris PL, Dimitri S. Predicting failure of endovascular aneurysm repair. Eur J Vasc Endovasc Surg. 1999;17(1):1–2.
8. Baum RA, Carpenter JP, Golden MA, et al. Treatment of type 2 endoleaks after endovascular repair of abdominal aortic aneurysms: comparison of transarterial and translumbar techniques. J Vasc Surg. 2002;35(1):23–9.
9. Moll FL, Powell JT, Fraedrich G, et al. Management of abdominal aortic aneurysms clinical practice guidelines of the European society for vascular surgery. Eur J Vasc Endovasc Surg. 2011;41(Suppl 1):S1–S58.
10. EVAR Trial Participants. Endovascular aneurysm repair and outcome in patients unfit for open repair of abdominal aortic aneurysm (EVAR trial 2): randomised controlled trial. Lancet. 2005;365(9478):2187–92.
11. Wisselink W, Cuesta MA, Berends FJ, van den Berg FG, Rauwerda JA. Retroperitoneal endoscopic ligation of lumbar and inferior mesenteric arteries as a treatment of persistent endoleak after endoluminal aortic aneurysm repair. J Vasc Surg. 2000;31(6):1240–4.
12. Avgerinos ED, Chaer RA, Makaroun MS. Type II endoleaks. J Vasc Surg. 2014;60(5):1386–91.
13. Kasirajan K, Matteson B, Marek JM, Langsfeld M. Technique and results of transfemoral superselective coil embolization of type II lumbar endoleak. J Vasc Surg. 2003;38(1):61–6.
14. Nevala T, Biancari F, Manninen H, et al. Type II endoleak after endovascular repair of abdominal aortic aneurysm: effectiveness of embolization. Cardiovasc Intervent Radiol. 2010;33(2):278–84.
15. Ierardi AM, Pesapane F, Rivolta N, et al. Type 2 endoleaks in endovascular aortic repair: cone beam CT and automatic vessel detection to guide the embolization. Acta Radiol. 2018;59(6):681–7.
16. Patil VV, Fischman AM, Patel RS, et al. GI hemorrhage arising from splenic artery: intraprocedure cone-beam CT as problem-solving tool to aide in safe catheterization of offending vessel. Clin Imaging. 2015;39(5):928–30.
17. Miyayama S, Yamashiro M, Okuda M, et al. Usefulness of cone-beam computed tomography during ultraselective transcatheter arterial chemoembolization for small hepatocellular carcinomas that cannot be demonstrated on angiography. Cardiovasc Intervent Radiol. 2009;32(2):255–64.
18. Ronot M, Abdel-Rehim M, Hakime A, et al. Cone-beam CT angiography for determination of tumor-feeding vessels during chemoembolization of liver Tumors: comparison of conventional and dedicated-software analysis. J Vasc Interv Radiol. 2016;27(1):32–8.

19. Carrafiello G, Ierardi AM, Duka E, et al. Usefulness of cone-beam computed tomography and automatic vessel detection software in emergency transarterial embolization. Cardiovasc Intervent Radiol. 2016;39(4):530–7.
20. Park YS, Do YS, Park HS, Park KB, Kim DI. Experience of direct percutaneous sac injection in type II endoleak using cone beam computed tomography. Ann Surg Treat Res. 2015;88(4):232–5.
21. Stavropoulos SW, Carpenter JP, Fairman RM, Golden MA, Baum RA. Inferior vena cava traversal for translumbar endoleak embolization after endovascular abdominal aortic aneurysm repair. J Vasc Interv Radiol. 2003;14(9 Pt 1):1191–4.
22. Ellis PK, Kennedy PT, Collins AJ, Blair PH. The use of direct thrombin injection to treat a type II endoleak following endovascular repair of abdominal aortic aneurysm. Cardiovasc Intervent Radiol. 2003;26(5):482–4.
23. Baum RA, Carpenter JP, Cope C, et al. Aneurysm sac pressure measurements after endovascular repair of abdominal aortic aneurysms. J Vasc Surg. 2001;33(1):32–41.
24. Mansueto G, Cenzi D, Scuro A, et al. Treatment of type II endoleak with a transcatheter transcaval approach: results at 1-year follow-up. J Vasc Surg. 2007;45(6):1120–7.
25. Yang RY, Tan KT, Beecroft JR, Rajan DK, Jaskolka JD. Direct sac puncture versus transarterial embolization of type II endoleaks: an evaluation and comparison of outcomes. Vascular. 2017;25(3):227–33.
26. Chung R, Morgan RA. Type 2 endoleaks post-EVAR: current evidence for rupture risk, intervention and outcomes of treatment. Cardiovasc Intervent Radiol. 2015;38(3):507–22.
27. Baum RA, Stavropoulos SW, Fairman RM, Carpenter JP. Endoleaks after endovascular repair of abdominal aortic aneurysms. J Vasc Interv Radiol. 2003;14(9 Pt 1):1111–7.
28. Stavropoulos SW, Park J, Fairman R, Carpenter J. Type 2 endoleak embolization comparison: translumbar embolization versus modified transarterial embolization. J Vasc Interv Radiol. 2009;20(10):1299–302.
29. Kuziez MS, Sanchez LA, Zayed MA. Abdominal aortic aneurysm type II endoleaks. J Cardiovasc Dis Diagn. 2016;4(5):255.
30. Golzarian J, Maes EB, Sun S. Endoleak: treatment options. Tech Vasc Interv Radiol. 2005;8(1):41–9.
31. Muller-Wille R, Wohlgemuth WA, Heiss P, et al. Transarterial embolization of type II endoleaks after EVAR: the role of ethylene vinyl alcohol copolymer (Onyx). Cardiovasc Intervent Radiol. 2013;36(5):1288–95.
32. Khaja MS, Park AW, Swee W, et al. Treatment of type II endoleak using Onyx with long-term imaging follow-up. Cardiovasc Intervent Radiol. 2014;37(3):613–22.
33. Sidloff DA, Stather PW, Choke E, Bown MJ, Sayers RD. Type II endoleak after endovascular aneurysm repair. Br J Surg. 2013;100(10):1262–70.
34. Angle JF. Cone-beam CT: vascular applications. Tech Vasc Interv Radiol. 2013;16(3):144–9.
35. Binkert CA, Alencar H, Singh J, Baum RA. Translumbar type II endoleak repair using angiographic CT. J Vasc Interv Radiol. 2006;17(8):1349–53.
36. Choi SY, Won JY, Lee DY, et al. Percutaneous transabdominal approach for the treatment of endoleaks after endovascular repair of infrarenal abdominal aortic aneurysm. Korean J Radiol. 2010;11(1):107–14.
37. Rial R, Serrano Fj F, Vega M, et al. Treatment of type II endoleaks after endovascular repair of abdominal aortic aneurysms: translumbar puncture and injection of thrombin into the aneurysm sac. Eur J Vasc Endovasc Surg. 2004;27(3):333–5.
38. Molyneux AJ, Coley SC. Embolization of spinal cord arteriovenous malformations with an ethylene vinyl alcohol copolymer dissolved in dimethyl sulfoxide (Onyx liquid embolic system). Report of two cases. J Neurosurg. 2000;93(2 Suppl):304–8.
39. Scali ST, Vlada A, Chang CK, Beck AW. Transcaval embolization as an alternative technique for the treatment of type II endoleak after endovascular aortic aneurysm repair. J Vasc Surg. 2013;57(3):869–74.

10 Vascular Reconstructions in Kidney Transplantation

Massimiliano Veroux, Alessia Giaquinta, Giuseppe D'Arrigo, Alberto Davì, Angelo Sanfiorenzo, and Pierfrancesco Veroux

10.1 Introduction

Kidney transplantation is the preferred treatment for patients in end-stage renal disease, since it improves the overall quality of life and patient survival [1].

The original surgical technique of kidney transplantation was described in 1951 and has only evolved slightly over 60 years [2]. The gold standard surgical procedure is still open and still in either the right or left iliac fossa, with an end-to-side anastomosis with the external iliac vessels [1, 2]. Although the surgical technique has not significantly evolved over the last decades, many improvements have been made in the graft conservation solutions and in the procurement of the aortic cuff and extension of the right renal vein using the inferior vena cava [1, 3–5]. Particularly, the extension of the right renal vein using the inferior vena cava (*cava conduit*) significantly decreases the rate of renal vein thrombosis and graft loss [3]. Moreover, the use of older donors to increase the donor pool and to face the increasing demand for kidney transplantation has prompted the use of vascular reconstructions to manage the atherosclerotic aortic and renal arteries. Moreover, kidneys with multiple arteries often require a surgical reconstruction to reduce the number of anastomoses and the cold ischemia time.

Vascular surgery may also be required to manage immediate and late complications of kidney transplantation, mainly the pseudoaneurysm of the renal artery, which is a life-threatening condition, occurring mainly as a consequence of a graft infection.

In this chapter we will describe the main vascular reconstructions adopted in renal transplant surgery.

10.2 Kidney Transplantation with Multiple Arteries

The use of grafts with multiple renal arteries (MRA) is a potential risk factor that could impair the outcome of kidney transplantations. Autopsy studies have reported an incidence of 17–35% MRA grafts, depending on the donor's ethnic origin [6, 7]. The incidence of multiple arteries in deceased donors is variable: a study among 400 deceased donors reported double arteries in 23%, triple arteries in 4%, and quadruple arteries in 1% of donors [6–10]. Contradictory results have been reported in literature, and while many studies examining the use of kidneys with multiple renal arteries for renal transplantation did not find that graft survival and function were

M. Veroux (✉) · A. Giaquinta · G. D'Arrigo · A. Davì · A. Sanfiorenzo · P. Veroux
Vascular Surgery and Organ Transplant Unit, Department of Surgery, University Hospital of Catania, Catania, Italy
e-mail: veroux@unict.it; pveroux@unict.it

© Springer Nature Switzerland AG 2019
Y. Tshomba et al. (eds.), *Visceral Vessels and Aortic Repair*,
https://doi.org/10.1007/978-3-319-94761-7_10

adversely affected by multiple arteries and that vascular reconstructions did not influence recipient creatinine levels or ureteral complication rates [10], many other studies reported an increased incidence of vascular complications, delayed graft function (DGF), and increased warm ischemia time in graft from MRA [3, 6–10].

A recent meta-analysis by Zorgdrager et al. [6] showed that kidney grafts from any type of donor with MRA were associated with a lower 1-year graft survival, a higher complication rate, and an increased frequency of DGF compared to SRA grafts. Both vascular (10.8%) and urological complications (5.5%) are more frequent in MRA grafts. However, no significant differences were observed in the 5-year graft survival and 1- and 5-year patient survival rates. Furthermore, there was a trend toward a longer WIT and higher 1- and 5-year creatinine levels in MRA grafts.

The technique of vascular reconstruction may differ significantly when using graft from deceased or living donor. Although ligation of polar arteries supplying <5–10% of renal parenchyma may be frequently encountered with an increase in urological complication [11], the presence of MRA often requires vascular reconstruction on bench surgery.

Multiple arteries from kidney grafts from deceased donors may be spatulated together to provide a common outflow or anastomosed end-to-side to the main renal artery, even in the case of arterial injury during organ retrieval (Fig. 10.1). Alternatively, in case of >3 arteries, a vein patch could be used. These techniques have been also used successfully in dual kidney transplantations (DKT) [12, 13]. In an interesting study, Veroux et al. [13] reported the results of grafts with multiple arteries in 12 patients who underwent monolateral dual kidney transplantation. In six patients, the accessory arteries were anastomosed end-to-side or side-to-side on the aortic patch. In six patients, with three or more accessory arteries, vascular reconstruction with an inferior vena cava patch was performed, before implanting the kidney (Fig. 10.2). There were no intraoperative complications in the entire series, and there were no immediate vascular complications.

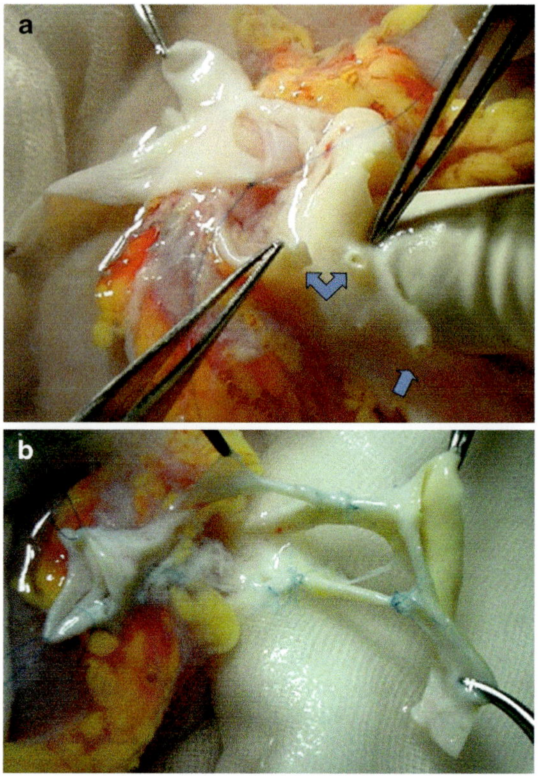

Fig. 10.1 (**a**) Arterial injury. The renal artery and an accessory renal artery were completely transected from its origin on the aortic patch, during organ retrieval (arrow); (**b**) the arteries were sutured at bench surgery through an end-to-end anastomosis between the injured renal artery and the aortic patch

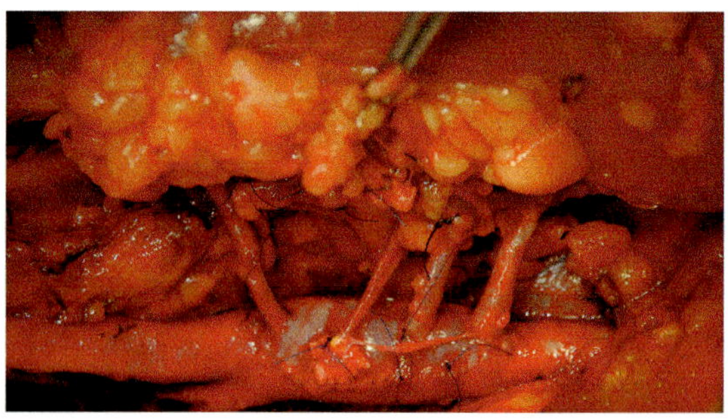

Fig. 10.2 Intraoperative view of reconstructed renal artery on an inferior vena cava patch during a dual kidney transplantation. Four branches are clearly visible

Usually, when feasible, a single anastomosis is preferable to reduce the anastomotic time in the recipient, which has a known wrong effect on graft function.

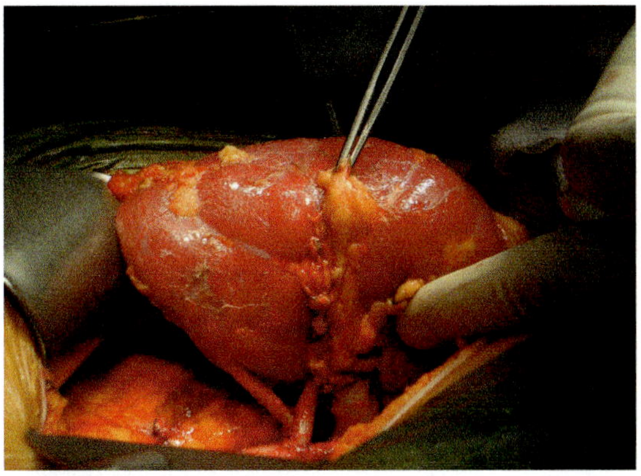

Fig. 10.3 End-to-side anastomosis between an accessory artery and the main renal artery in a living donor kidney transplantation. The kidney was correctly perfused with no signs of parenchymal ischemia

With the increasing demand for organ transplantation due to the increasing number of patients on the waiting list, a growing experience on the use of living donor kidney graft with multiple arteries has accumulated recently, with similar graft and patient outcomes.

Multiple renal artery reconstruction follows the same principles of deceased donor grafts (Fig. 10.3), but recent studies reported excellent outcomes with arterial reconstruction with recipient's own internal iliac artery [14].

10.3 Vascular Reconstruction in Dual Kidney Transplantation

Dual kidney transplantation (DKT) of marginal kidneys could offer transplant candidates very satisfactory kidney transplantation in terms of renal function. However, DKT might be considered a major surgical procedure and, in older recipients, has a potentially greater risk of surgical complications compared with single kidney transplantation [12, 13, 15–17].

While different surgical techniques have been described, including the positioning of one kidney for each side extraperitoneally and the positioning of both kidneys intaperitoneally, most transplant centers, to reduce the intraoperative time and the rate of surgical complications, positioned both grafts on the same side [12, 15, 16].

Ekser et al. [15] analyzed the results of 100 unilateral dual kidney transplantations performed at a single center. When compared with a cohort of single kidney transplantations, surgical complications were similar between the two groups.

A recent review [16] compared the three techniques of bilateral placement, unilateral placement with separate anastomoses, and unilateral placement with patch anastomoses, in dual kidney transplantation, and they reported a similar graft and patient survival among the three groups.

However, in order to reduce the number of anastomoses and the operative time, some transplant centers tried to develop new surgical techniques in dual kidney transplantation. By employing techniques used to conjoin organ vasculature ex vivo, the number of in situ anastomoses is reduced, thereby minimizing operative ischemic time and potential for complications associated with extensive vascular dissection [13, 16, 18–20]. Moreover, these techniques could be used even in those patients with a moderate-to-severe atherosclerosis of the iliac vessels, which is usually a contraindication for dual kidney transplantation [18].

Nghiem [19] proposed a novel technique of transplanting both kidneys en bloc using a single arterial and single venous anastomosis by implanting the renal vein end-to-side alternatively to the left renal vein or on the vena cava. Veroux et al. [18] proposed a new technique of monolateral dual kidney transplantation by joining the two renal veins and the two arteries in one single anastomosis. The technique included a running suture between the posterior margin of the vein of the left kidney and the anterior margin of the right renal vein while the two aortic patches were sutured together (Fig. 10.4).

More recently, Tran et al. [20] described an alternative technique of dual kidney transplantation in 22 patients by using the donor's common iliac artery with its internal and external branches for performing an interposition Y-graft to join the left and the right renal artery of the graft. The suprarenal vena cava was oversewn in a running

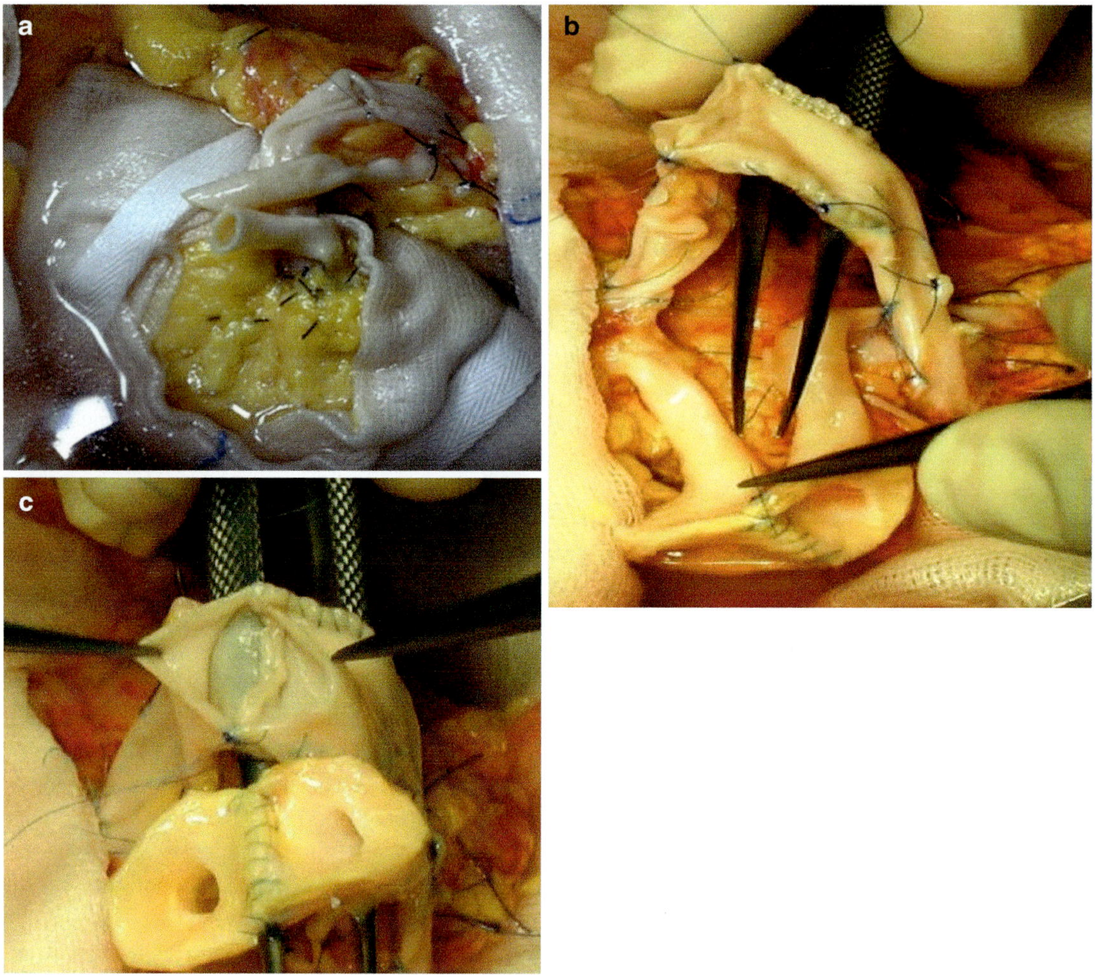

Fig. 10.4 Technique of cojoining renal vessels in dual kidney transplantation. After elongation of the right renal vein with the vena cava, (**a**) the two renal veins were sutured together, joining the posterior margin of the vein of the left kidney with the anterior margin of the right renal vein. Then (**b**) the two aortic patches were sutured together. (**c**) Final result with the joined arteries and veins

fashion, and the distal part of the inferior vena cava was used for anastomosis.

10.4 Renal Aneurysm and Pseudoaneurysm

Renal artery aneurysms (RAAs) are defined as dilation of all three layers of the arterial wall >1 cm in diameter [21–23]. Renal artery aneurysms (RAAs) are very uncommon, with a widely accepted incidence of 0.1% in the general population [21, 22]. Approximately 75% of true RAAs are saccular in shape, and 25% are found to be fusiform. RAAs most commonly affect the main bifurcation but can be located anywhere in the arterial tree [21].

In a kidney transplant setting, the evidence of an aneurysm of the main renal artery or one of its branches is an uncommon finding but usually requires surgical repair to allow for its use for kidney transplantation. The most frequently adopted technique is similar to the ex vivo technique adopted in patients with an aneurysm of native kidneys, and the technique involves a resection of the renal artery aneurysm and a suture of the arterial wall [23].

Renal pseudoaneurysm (RPA) forms as a consequence of arterial wall injury: the kidney tissue surrounding the site of injury exerts a compressive force to slow or completely stop the bleeding, so that a hematoma forms around the arteriotomy [24]. The subsequent clot retraction and the reactive fibrosis form a structure resembling an aneurysmal sac, which can be eventually connected with the intraluminal space, leading to expansion of the pseudoaneurysmal sac and pain or rupture.

Renal pseudoaneurysm is a life-threatening condition because it involves an arterial injury that is occluded solely by hematoma and connective tissue. The degree of bleeding depends on the delicate balance between the tamponade effect of the surrounding hematoma and connective tissue and the intraluminal hydrostatic pressure changes [24]. Anastomotic pseudoaneurysm of renal allograft is a rare and life-threatening vascular complication after kidney transplantation, occurring in <1% of cases. Intrarenal pseudoaneurysms are more common and usually resolve spontaneously. In contrast, extrarenal pseudoaneurysms are related to a mycotic infection at the site of anastomosis and usually occur in the early weeks after transplantation as a result of anastomotic defects, such as suture rupture, anastomotic leakage, vessel wall ischemia, or arterial dehiscence caused by local infection. In the case of infection, the risk of pseudoaneurysm rupture and graft loss is high. Fungal infection may originate from the donor or, more likely, from exogenous sources leading to contamination during graft handling and implantation [23].

Pseudoaneurysms of the transplant renal artery are usually asymptomatic, and the diagnosis is mainly incidental, during follow-up outpatient visits. Although rare, these complications may have a high risk of anastomotic leakage or arterial wall rupture, resulting in hemorrhagic shock and graft loss [23].

Surgical repair of transplant renal artery pseudoaneurysm is challenging and often requires specialized treatment, due to the inflammatory tissue surrounding the renal artery, and, in most cases, transplant nephrectomy may ultimately be required: in the series of six patients with anastomotic pseudoaneurysm of the renal transplant artery reported by Bracale et al. [25], a transplant nephrectomy was needed in all but one patient.

However, in a recent report, Ardita et al. [26] reported a successful pseudoaneurysm repair with in situ bypass (Fig. 10.5) between the internal iliac artery and the renal artery, while the common iliac artery was revascularized through an autologous vein bypass between the proximal external iliac artery and the common femoral artery.

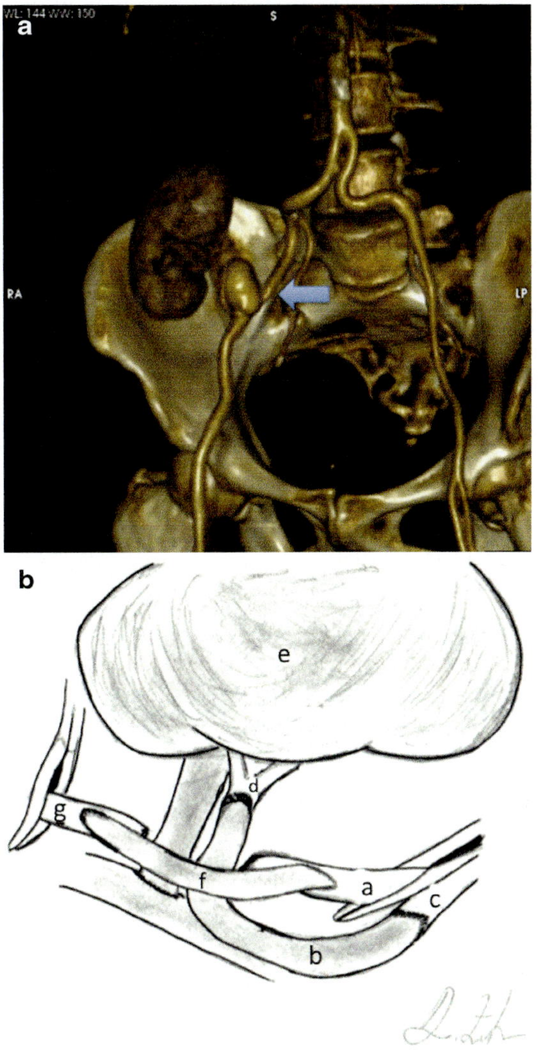

Fig. 10.5 Anastomotic pseudoaneurysm of the renal transplant artery. (**a**) Computed tomography angiography demonstrated a 3-cm anastomotic pseudoaneurysm of the graft. (**b**) Scheme of surgical procedure after resection of the anastomotic pseudoaneurysm. The external iliac artery (*a*) was dissected, and a bypass (*c*) was performed between the internal iliac artery (*b*) and the renal artery (*d*) of kidney transplantation (*e*). External iliac artery was revascularized through a bypass between proximal external iliac artery and common femoral artery (*f*)

10.5 Summary and Conclusions

Vascular reconstructions are often required in the kidney transplant setting.

Multiple arteries are frequently encountered and usually require a surgical reconstruction to minimize the number of vascular anastomoses. Renal artery aneurysm and pseudoaneurysms are rare but potentially life-threatening and require a challenging surgical repair. Vascular reconstruction techniques may also be used in dual kidney transplantation to reduce the operative ischemic time and potential for complications associated with extensive vascular dissection.

References

1. Veroux M, Corona D, Veroux P. Kidney transplantation: future challenges. Minerva Chir. 2009;64(1):75–100.
2. Kuss R, Teinturier J, Milliez P. Some attempts at kidney transplantation in man. Mem Acad Chir (Paris). 1951;77:755.
3. Bessede T, Droupy S, Hammoudi Y, et al. Surgical prevention and management of vascular complications of kidney transplantation. Transpl Int. 2012;25:994–1001.
4. Benoit G, Jaber N, Moukarzel M, et al. Incidence of vascular complications in kidney transplantation: is there any interference with the nature of the perfusion solution? Clin Transpl. 1994;8:485.
5. Fung LC, McLorie GA, Khoury AE, Churchill BM. Donor aortic cuff reduces the rate of anastomotic arterial stenosis in pediatric renal transplantation. J Urol. 1995;154:909.
6. Zorgdrager M, Krikke C, Hofker SH, et al. Multiple renal arteries in kidney transplantation: a systematic review and meta-analysis. Ann Transplant. 2016;21:469–78.
7. Khamanarong K, Prachaney P, Utraravichien A, et al. Anatomy of renal arterial supply. Clin Anat. 2004;17:334–6.
8. Bessede T, Droupsy S, Hammoudi Y, et al. Surgical prevention and management of vascular complications of kidney transplantation. Transpl Int. 2012;25:994–1001.
9. Osman Y, Skokeir A, Ali-el-Dein B, et al. Vascular complications after live donor renal transplantation: study of risk factors and effect on graft and patient survival. J Urol. 2003;169:859–62.
10. Hellegering J, Visser J, Kloke HJ, et al. Deleterious influence of prolonged warm ischemia in living donor kidney transplantation. Transplant Proc. 2012;44:1222–6.
11. Kok NF, Dols LF, Hunink MG, et al. Complex vascular anatomy in live kidney donation: imaging and consequences for clinical outcome. Transplantation. 2008;85:1760–5.
12. Veroux M, Corona D, Gagliano M, et al. Monolateral dual kidney transplantation from marginal donors. Transplant Proc. 2007;39(6):1800–2.
13. Veroux M, Giuffrida G, Ekser B, et al. Vascular reconstruction in monolateral dual kidney transplantation with multiple arteries. Clin Transpl. 2012;26(3):443–6.
14. Hiramitsu T, Futamura K, Okada M, et al. Impact of arterial reconstruction with recipient's own internal iliac artery for multiple graft arteries on living donor kidney transplantation: strobe study. Medicine (Baltimore). 2015;94(43):e1811.
15. Ekser B, Furian L, Broggiato A, et al. Technical aspects of unilateral dual kidney transplantation from expanded criteria donors: experience of 100 patients. Am J Transplant. 2010;10(9):2000–7.
16. Cocco A, Shahrestani S, Cocco N, et al. Dual kidney transplant techniques: a systematic review. Clin Transpl. 2017;31(8):28544075.
17. Renaud S, Tinsit MO, Rabant M, et al. Dual kidney transplantation: is it worth it? Transplantation. 2017;101:488–97.
18. Veroux P, Giuffrida G, Cappellani A, et al. Two-as-one monolateral dual kidney transplantation. Urology. 2011;77:227–30.
19. Nghiem DD. Simultaneuos double adult kidney transplantation using single arterial and venous anastomoses. Urology. 2006;67:1076–8.
20. Tran KC, Li D, Taqi A, et al. Dual en bloc technique for adult renal transplantation. Clin Transpl. 2017;31(8):28523715.
21. Orion KC, Abularrage CJ. Renal artery aneurysms: movement toward endovascular repair. Semin Vasc Surg. 2013;26:226–32.
22. Colemna DM, Stanley JC. Renal artery aneurysms. J Vasc Surg. 2015;62:779–85.
23. Veroux P, Giaquinta A, Zerbo D, De Marco E, Sanzone A, Veroux M. Surgery for the renal arteries. In: Chiesa R, Setacci C, Castelli PM, editors. Tip and tricks in open vascular surgery. Torino: Edizioni Minerva Medica; 2017. p. 93–100. ISBN: 978-88-7711-885-1.
24. Ngo TC, Lee J, Gonzalgo ML. Renal pseudoaneurysm: an overview. Nat Rev Urol. 2010;7:619–25.
25. Bracale UM, Santangelo M, Carbone F, et al. Anastomotic pseudoaneurysm complicating renal transplantation: treatment options. Eur J Vasc Endovasc Surg. 2010;39:565–8.
26. Ardita V, Veroux M, Zerbo D, et al. Non-mycotic anastomotic pseudoaneurysm of renal allograft artery. Case report. Ann Ital Chir. 2016;87:27319817.

11 Renal Transplantation and Aortic Disease: Operative Management

Gabriele Piffaretti, Matteo Tozzi, Marco Franchin, and Patrizio Castelli

11.1 Introduction

In the last decade, we recognized three main facts that dramatically changed the perspective on kidney transplant. Firstly, progress in surgical technique and the development of new immunosuppressant protocols have lengthened graft survival; secondly, population affected by end-stage kidney disease (ESKD) has become even older; and finally, renal transplant has increased the longevity of graft recipients. As a result, kidney transplant recipients (KTRs) are more and more exposed to chronic degenerative pathologies, such as atherosclerosis. Additionally, it is necessary to emphasize the relationship existing between ESKD, long-term hemodialysis, and accelerated atherosclerosis [1]. Subsequently, an increase in the prevalence of aortic atherosclerotic disease, either occlusive or dilatative, in KTR must be expected.

It is remarkable how Brekke et al. in 1993 reported a prevalence of both aneurysmal and occlusive diseases in only 1.86% of patients waiting for kidney transplant. Accordingly, in a literature review published in 1994, Panneton et al. described the concomitance of aortic aneurysm and kidney transplant as a very rare event and reported only 51 cases of aortic reconstruction performed in organ recipients in the previous 30 years [2]. Nowadays, according to the Michigan Transplant Centre Registry, prevalence of aortic aneurysm between KTRs has increased to 4% [3].

In a review by Droupy et al. on 1110 kidney transplants, a severe occlusive disease affecting iliac arteries was documented in 9.6% of KTR. Among them 3.4% required endarterectomy at the time of the transplant. In analyzing follow-up data, they concluded that overall graft survival was significantly lower if compared to patients without iliac atheroma [4–6].

It means that in the future, a new challenge for vascular and transplant surgeons will be represented by the aortoiliac reconstruction in KTR.

The management of many problems associated to aortic surgery needs to be solved in prospective, preoperative evaluation and screening, risk stratification and surgical planning, graft protection from ischemia and reperfusion injury during aortic surgery, and follow-up.

11.2 Consideration on Open Surgery in Kidney Transplant Recipients and Graft Protection Techniques

Sehti et al. in 1976 were the first to report a case of thoracic aorta repair in a KTR for a ruptured type B dissecting aneurysm [6]. Soon after, Shons

G. Piffaretti · M. Tozzi · M. Franchin (✉) · P. Castelli
Vascular Surgery, Department of Medicine and Surgery, Circolo University Teaching Hospital, University of Insubria School of Medicine, Varese, Italy

© Springer Nature Switzerland AG 2019
Y. Tshomba et al. (eds.), *Visceral Vessels and Aortic Repair*,
https://doi.org/10.1007/978-3-319-94761-7_11

et al. and Sterioff et al. reported two cases of abdominal aortic aneurysm repair in KTR [7, 8]. Unfortunately, the three patients died after intervention, and the first to report a successful abdominal aortic aneurysm repair with a femoro-femoral partial extracorporeal circulation was Campbell in 1981 [9].

Open surgery for the management of aortic aneurysms in KTR presents various problems. The first and most relevant is that renal graft derives blood supply from the iliac artery below the aneurysm. Consequently, aortic repair can be responsible for transient or permanent ischemic injuries and even graft loss. Second, the previous kidney transplant can be associated with perivascular fibrosis and consequently difficulty in dissecting vessels and higher risk of graft parenchyma and ureter damage.

Graft protection technique continues to be the main and open question in literature. The options commonly adopted by surgeons for graft protection are:

- No protection
- Topical cooling with sterile ice
- In situ graft cold perfusion (static or dynamic perfusion technique)
- Ex situ graft cold storage (static storage or dynamic perfusion technique)
- Distal aortic perfusion with a shunt or bypass
- General hypothermia

The technical choice should be influenced by many factors including:

- Graft fitness
- Complexity of aortic repair
- Estimated duration of kidney ischemia
- Confidence with a specific preservation technique

Adjunctive renal protection measures must be taken into account in case of difficult surgical anatomies including arterial graft anastomosis on large iliac aneurysms and impaired graft function (creatinine serial level >250 μmol/L).

Unfortunately, literature mainly reports case reports or small series concerning personal author experience. The analysis of these results does not demonstrate the superiority of a particular technique. A "clamp and go" technique without graft protection and short cross-clamp time can be considered a safe alternative in an experienced hand. Otherwise, the protective technique can prolong operative time and can be prone to graft damage, thrombosis, or sometimes ischemic injury if not done correctly.

11.2.1 None Graft Protection

During the 1970s, when this surgery was first developed, it was postulated that aortic clamping would be responsible for total graft warm ischemia [7, 8]. Otherwise, with experiences conducted between 1973 and 2005, Lacombe demonstrated that during the aortic clamp, the graft continued to be perfused by the retrograde flow from the lumbar, inferior mesenteric, and both iliac arteries. Lacombe proved that during aortic clamp the back pressure through the collateral pathway is always >35 mmHg [10], while Morris et al. showed experimentally that the minimum pressure needed for kidney viability is 25 mmHg [11]. Accordingly, total graft ischemia would occur only during renal artery reattachment when necessary. However, it has been demonstrated that the kidney can tolerate periods of total artery occlusion of up to 50 min, more than the time required for anastomosis [12]. Lacombe reported a successful experience conducted on 18 KTRs without the aid of vascular shunts. When the surgeon does not adopt a preservation method, Lacombe suggested to apply small but substantial modifications to the standard surgical technique. Particularly, he recommended to make a suprarenal transverse section of the aorta between two clamps followed by an end-to-end anastomosis of the prosthesis to the aorta. The second step is represented by the revascularization of the kidney by the prosthetic graft anastomosis on the iliac axis proximal to the transplant artery or by the renal artery reattachment on the prosthetic graft. The third step is the management of the aneurysmal sac and the opposite limb revascularization [10].

11.2.2 In Situ Cold Perfusion and Ex Situ Preservation

Many authors suggested that in situ static cold perfusion with Ringer's lactate (4 °C) through the common iliac artery combined with topical cooling may be the faster and easiest alternative for graft preservation [13]. More recently, Tshomba et al. showed better results in terms of perioperative renal function after aortic clamp with Custodiol over Ringer's lactate [14]. Alternatively, our experience suggests that ex situ static cold storage with a standard preservation solution (Celsior or University of Wisconsin solution) and the subsequent re-transplantation of the organ on the prosthetic graft represent a safe, effective, and viable alternative. The main advantages offered by this technique are comfort and the possibility of extending the surgical time without substantial risk of compromising residual renal function. Possible complication is represented by the risk of renal artery dissection during cannulation and perfusion, especially in case of marginal graft. Additionally, we must remember possible complications related to cold injury and reperfusion (see Chap. XXX).

11.2.3 Distal Aortic Perfusion with Shunt or Bypass

A wide range of techniques have been described in literature. Mostly, we can group them between axillo-femoral and aortofemoral shunts.

Shons et al. first reported the use of axillo-femoral permanent bypass with an 8 mm woven Dacron graft. The aorta was ligated distally to the renal artery and common iliac artery and proximally to the origin of hypogastric. Graft anastomoses were performed on the external iliac vessels [7]. Temporary axillo-femoral shunts were described by Gibbons et al. and Roach et al. with satisfactory results in five patients. They admitted an increase in operating time, but deterioration in renal function was not seen in any case [15, 16].

More frequently, temporary aortofemoral bypass with Gott shunt has been described [17, 19]. Other authors have adopted polyvinyl tubes as the shunt with optimal perfusion pressure (only 15 mmHg less than systemic pressure) maintained for long cross-clamp times [8, 18]. Finally, successful results have been obtained with modified techniques, adopting an inline shunt instead of separate aortic cannulation [19].

11.3 Endovascular Aortic Reconstruction

A safe and effective alternative to open surgery is represented by endovascular reconstruction for both aneurysm and aortic occlusive diseases. This surgery was proposed for the first time in 2000 by Sawhney et al. in the treatment of abdominal aortic aneurysms with aorto-uni-iliac right graft and femoro-femoral crossover bypass to perfuse a left-sided renal transplant and homolateral lower limb [20]. In 2001, Forbes described the first treatment of a large aneurysm with an endovascular approach bifurcated graft [21]. Endovascular aortic repair (EVAR) demonstrated two main potential advantages if compared to open conventional surgery. Firstly, aorta and iliac cross clamping is not required, minimizing ischemic risk. Additionally, in cases of abdominal aortic aneurysms, it is not necessary to take into account the limitations associated with proximal neck morphology and length (pararenal and juxta-renal aneurysms) because of the possibility of proximal extension [22]. Actually, tube graft use is limited to those cases that are characterized by severe, not crossable, atherosclerosis of the common iliac artery. Bifurcated devices are largely used. The main body must be introduced through the contralateral iliac artery, while the lower profile limb is delivered from the donor iliac artery. It is not actually clear if the newer lower profile prosthesis has better results in terms of complications over conventional grafts. In fact, potential risks associated to endovascular procedures may be renal graft or vessel iatrogenic lesions. In a recent review of 17,213 cases of EVAR for abdominal aneurysm from the Vascular Quality Initiative dataset, Bostock et al. did not find any difference in technical outcomes between KTR and conventional patients (KTRs were 0.2% of all patients). Endoleak occurred in 20% of KTR ($p = 0.46$), while no graft migration and infection were seen [23]. According to everyday experience, limitations to endovascular aortic procedures remain femoro-iliac atheromasia and obstinate stenosis that can obstacle the sheath progress. Additionally, large delivery systems can produce vascular lesions, plaque dissections, or renal graft artery damage. For that reason, the manipulation of catheters and wires should be kept at a minimum. Large-bore delivery systems and sheaths must be placed downstream of the orifice of renal graft artery, and they should be removed as soon as possible to avoid unintentional artery occlusion or damage. Surprisingly, Bostock et al. reported a very low incidence of arterial injuries requiring open repair with no statistical difference between the two cohorts ($p = 0.62$). In every case, surgical correction was not related to kidney dysfunction. Finally, in their large review, they did not describe any event of kidney graft damage or renal artery lesions.

Another possible complication related to endovascular aorta reconstruction in KTRs is contrast-induced nephropathy. According to literature, transplanted kidneys and autogenous kidneys are prone to contrast-induced nephropathy in the same way [24, 25]. Once again, Bostock et al. seem to contradict what was previously reported in literature. In fact, they showed that renal dysfunction defined as acute kidney injury (elevation of serum creatinine 0.5 mg/dL) or necessity of postoperative hemodialysis was three times more frequent in KTRs over conventional patients ($p = 0.02$). They saw a significant prevalence of renal dysfunction in patients with lower glomerular filtration rate before EVAR [27]. Patient hydration, diuresis stimulation, and antioxidant agents as *N*-acetylcysteine have been largely recommended [25–27]. Additionally, it is suggested to reduce the contrast dose to a minimum. Comprehensive procedure planning and correct C-arm angulation help to minimize the contrast amount [27]. Other advanced imaging modalities, such as image fusion technology, have been described as alternatives to standard fluoroscopy [28, 29]. Bostock et al. did not find any difference in terms of absolute iodinate contrast dose in KTRs that developed postoperative nephropathy and not. However, KTR with renal dysfunction received a significantly higher dose of contrast in relation to the preoperative glomerular filtration ratio (iodine/GFR ratio 0.78 vs 0.39, $p = 0.02$) [22]. This remark should be taken into account when considering aortic repair in KTRs.

11.4 Final Remarks: Aortoiliac Reconstruction Prior, Concomitant, or After Transplant

Galazka et al. described an experience of over 1553 patients where 201 (13%) required intervention for aortoiliac atherosclerosis. Surgery consisted in iliac endarterectomy and anastomosis of the renal graft to the hypogastric artery when patent. They also described the use of Y-shaped ilio-iliac vascular graft for iliac revascularization and kidney anastomosis [4]. Tsivian et al. reported that in their series of 1554 transplants, aortoiliac surgery was necessary in 2% of cases, and among them 80% of lesions were discovered intraoperatively [30]. Many other papers have been published on the same topics, and we can argue that intervention schedule is not usually the result of careful planning but rather the consequence of casual intraoperative findings. Piquet and Gouny investigated the correct timing for aortoiliac reconstruction in KTRs. They concluded that concomitant procedure, sometimes involving prosthetic grafts, had higher risks of infections. Consequently, they suggested delaying renal transplantation to at least 6–12 weeks after vascular reconstruction [31–32]. On the contrary, Coosemans et al. in a prospective trial compared different interventional timing, concluding that transplant concomitant to reconstruction is safe and effective, is cheaper, and has fewer difficulties and risks of graft injuries [33]. Tsivian et al. confirmed that concomitant reconstruction and transplant is safe, even if it would be preferable to

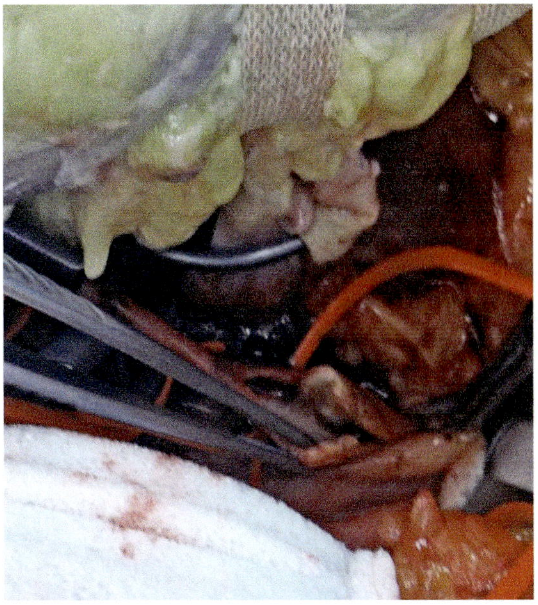

Fig. 11.1 Aortic and common iliac artery endarterectomy before kidney transplant

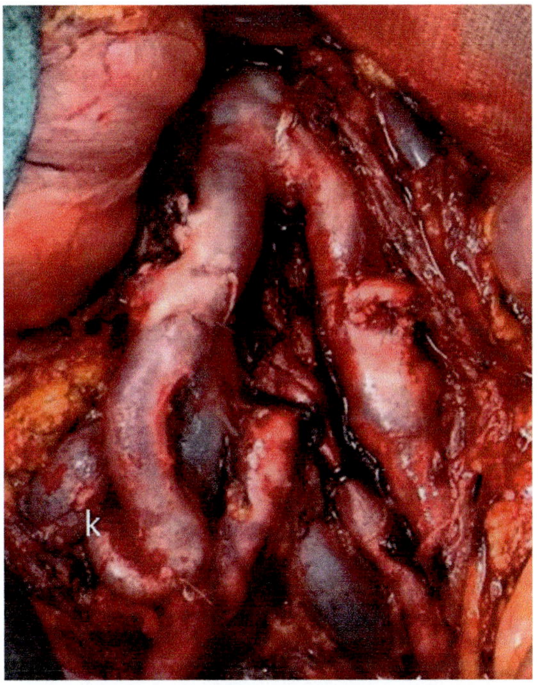

Fig. 11.2 Aorto-bisiliac composite cadaveric homograft bypass and concomitant kidney graft (k) transplant

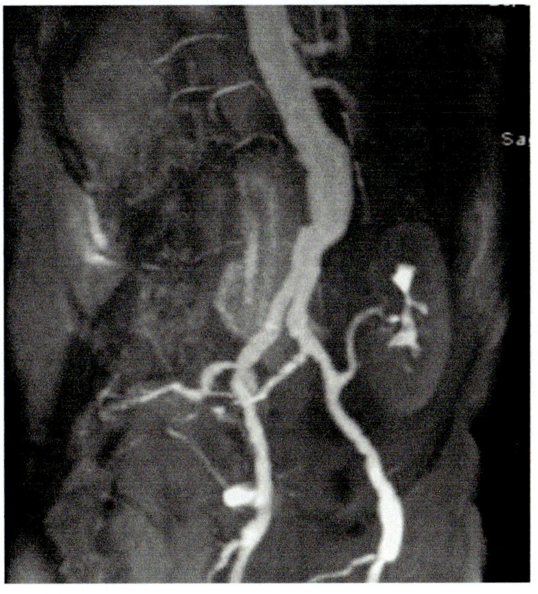

Fig. 11.3 Magnetic resonance imaging of aorto-bisiliac bypass and graft

anticipate the aortoiliac surgery [30] (Fig. 11.1). Possible benefit could be obtained using autologous grafts instead of synthetic prosthesis, and consequently, the single-stage surgery is preferable (Figs. 11.2 and 11.3). Additionally, endovascular treatment had better results in terms of infection in comparison to prosthetic grafts.

Gill et al. suggested that proper planning cannot be separated from a correct diagnostic study. They recommended Doppler ultrasound screening in patients at high risk for atherosclerosis disease. When physical examination or Doppler is suggestive of a disease, completion angiography should be performed [34]. Tozzi et al. recommended performing CT angiography scan in all patients on the waiting list for kidney transplant with risk factors for atherosclerosis. They suggested aortoiliac stenosis can be treated simultaneously with kidney transplant. It is important to be mindful of the risk that atherosclerosis lesions could increase, therefore worsening both graft and limb vascularizations (Fig. 11.4). On the contrary, both symptomatic stenosis and aortic aneurysm (especially >5 cm in diameter) should be treated before transplant, in order to reduce complications while on the waiting list. In particular, endovascular repair before transplant does not compromise retroperitoneal tissue and vascular integrity [35].

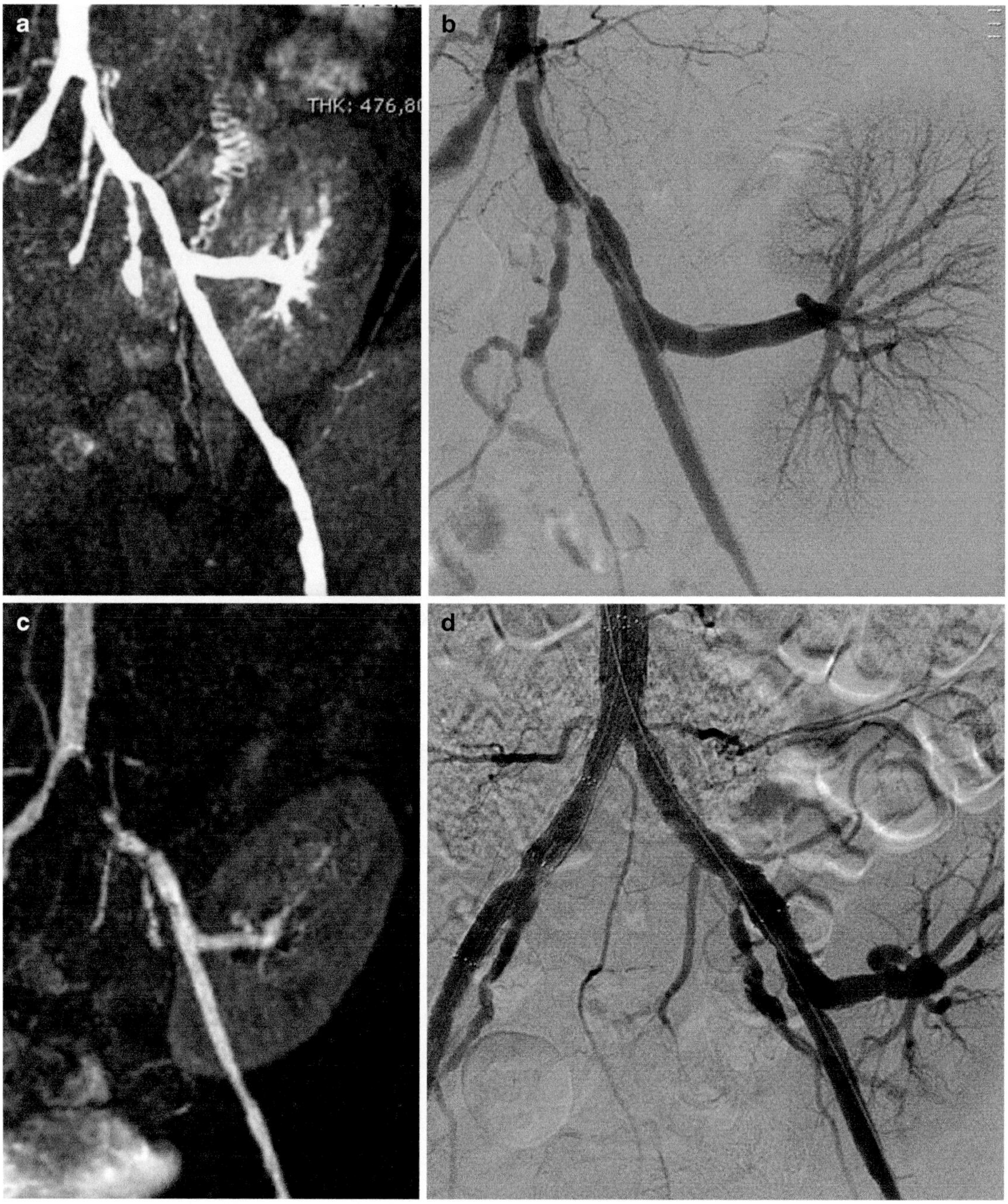

Fig. 11.4 (**a**) A 68-year-old female patient was referred to our center for bilateral claudication, 3 years after kidney transplant. (**b**) The patient was treated with bilateral angioplasty. (**c**) After 6 months, bilateral claudication and moderate increase in creatinine serial levels were present. (**d**) The patient was treated with kissing stent. Complete resolution of claudication and restoration of kidney function. Seven years follow-up

References

1. Lindner A, et al. Accelerated atherosclerosis in prolonged maintenance hemodialysis. N Engl J Med. 1974;290:697–701.
2. Panneton JM, et al. Aortic reconstruction in kidney transplant recipients. Ann Vasc Surg. 1996;10(2):97–108.
3. Cron DC, et al. Aneurysms in abdominal organ transplant recipients. J Vasc Surg. 2014;59(3):594–8.
4. Galazka Z, et al. Kidney transplant in recipients with atherosclerotic iliac vessels. Ann Transplant. 1999;4:43.
5. Droupy S, Eschwège P, Hammoudi Y, Durrbach A, Charpentier B, Benoit G. Consequences of iliac arterial atheroma on renal transplantation. J Urol. 2006;175(3 Pt 1):1036–9.
6. Sehti GK, et al. Renovascular hypertension and acute aortic dissection in a patient with renal transplant. Am Surg. 1976;132:97–9.
7. Shons AR, et al. Renal transplantation with blood supply by axillofemoral bypass graft. Am J Surg. 1976;132:97–9.
8. Sterioff S, et al. Temporary vascular bypass for perfusion of a renal transplant during abdominal aneurysmectomy. Surgery. 1977;82:558–60.
9. Campbell DA Jr, et al. Renal transplant protection during abdominal aortic aneurysmectomy with a pump-oxygenator. Surgery. 1981;90:559–62.
10. Lacombe M. Surgical treatment of aortoiliac aneurysms in renal transplant patients. J Vasc Surg. 2008;48(2):291–5.
11. Morris GC Jr, et al. The protective effect of subfiltration arterial pressure on the kidney. Surg Forum. 1956;6:623–4.
12. Lacombe M. Non traumatic acute obstructions of the renal artery. J Cardiovasc Surg. 1992;33:163–8.
13. Nghiem DD, et al. In situ hypothermic preservation of a renal allograft during resection of abdominal aortic aneurysm. Am Surg. 1982;48:237–8.
14. Tshomba Y, et al. Comparison of renal perfusion solution during thoracoabdominal aortic repair. J Vasc Surg. 2014;59(3):623–33.
15. Gibbons GW, et al. Aortoiliac reconstruction following renal transplantation. Surgery. 1982;91:435–7.
16. Roach DM, et al. Aortic aneurysm repair with a functioning renal transplant: therapeutic options. ANZ J Surg. 2004;74:65–7.
17. Hughes JD, et al. Renal transplant perfusion during aortoiliac aneurysmectomy. J Vasc Surg. 1985;2:600–2.
18. O'Mara CS, et al. Use of a temporary shunt for renal transplant protection during aortic aneurysm repair. Surgery. 1983;94:512–5.
19. Kashyap VS, et al. Abdominal aortic aneurysm repair in patients with renal allograft. Ann Vasc Surg. 1999;13:199–203.
20. Sawhney R, Chuter TA, Wall SD, Reilly LM, Kerlan RK, Canto CJ, Jean-Claude J, Faruqi RM. Aortic stent-grafts in patients with renal transplants. J Endovasc Ther. 2000;7(4):286–91.
21. Forbes TL, DeRose G, Kribs S, Abraham CZ, Harris KA. Endovascular repair of abdominal aortic aneurysm with coexisting renal allograft: case report and literature review. Ann Vasc Surg. 2001;15(5):586–90.
22. Silverberg D, Yalon T, Halak M. Endovascular repair of abdominal aortic aneurysms in the presence of a transplanted kidney. Cardiovasc Intervent Radiol. 2015;38(4):833–9.
23. Bostock IC, Zarkowsky DS, Hicks CW, Stone DH, Eslami MH, Malas MB, Goodney PP. Outcomes of endovascular aortic aneurysm repair in kidney transplant recipients: results from a National Quality Initiative. Am J Transplant. 2016;16(8):2395–400.
24. Aspelin P, Aubry P, Fransson SG, Strasser R, Willenbrock R. Berg KJ; nephrotoxicity in high-risk patients study of iso-osmolar and low-osmolar nonionic contrast media study investigators. nephrotoxic effects in high-risk patients undergoing angiography. N Engl J Med. 2003;348(6):491–9.
25. Vigneau C, Fulgencio JP, Godier A, Chalem Y, El Metaoua S, Rondeau E, Tuppin P, Bonnet F. The use of contrast media in deceased kidney donors does not affect initial graft function or graft survival. Kidney Int. 2006;70(6):1149–54.
26. Ruiz Fuentes MC, Moreno Ayuso JM, Ruiz Fuentes N, Vargas Palomares JF, Asensio Peinado C, Osuna Ortega A. Treatment with N-acetylcysteine in stable renal transplantation. Transplant Proc. 2008;40(9):2897–9.
27. MacNeill BD, Harding SA, Bazari H, Patton KK, Colon-Hernadez P, DeJoseph D, Jang IK. Prophylaxis of contrast-induced nephropathy in patients undergoing coronary angiography. Catheter Cardiovasc Interv. 2003;60(4):458–61.
28. Maurel B, Hertault A, Sobocinski J, Le Roux M, Gonzalez TM, Azzaoui R, Saeed Kilani M, Midulla M, Haulon S. Techniques to reduce radiation and contrast volume during EVAR. J Cardiovasc Surg. 2014;55(2 Suppl 1):123–31.
29. Carrafiello G, Ierardi AM, Radaelli A, De Marchi G, Floridi C, Piffaretti G, Fontana F. Unenhanced cone beam computed tomography and fusion imaging in direct percutaneous sac injection for treatment of type II endoleak: technical note. Cardiovasc Intervent Radiol. 2016;39(2):323.
30. Tsivian M, et al. Aortoiliac surgery concomitant with kidney transplant: a single centre experience. Clin Transpl. 2009;23:164.
31. Piquet P, et al. Aortoiliac reconstruction and renal transplantation: staged or simultaneous. Ann Vasc Surg. 1989;3:251.
32. Gouny P, et al. Aortoiliac surgery and kidney transplantation. Ann Vasc Surg. 1991;5:26.
33. Coosemans W, et al. Renal transplantation in patients with a vascular aortoiliac prosthesis. Transplant Proc. 1999;31:1925.
34. Gill R, et al. Management of peripheral vascular disease compromising renal allograft placement and function: review of the literature with an illustrative case. Clin Tranplant. 2011;25:337–44.
35. Tozzi M, Franchin M, Soldini G, Ietto G, Chiappa C, Molteni B, Amico F, Carcano G, Dionigi R. Treatment of aortoiliac occlusive or dilatative disease concomitant with kidney transplantation: how and when? Int J Surg. 2013;11(Suppl 1):S115–9.

12

Ex Vivo Open Reconstruction of Hilar Renal Artery Aneurysms: A Single-Center Experience

Mirko Menegolo, Elda Chiara Colacchio, Lucrezia Furian, Paolo Rigotti, Jacopo Taglialavoro, Michele Piazza, Michele Antonello, and Franco Grego

12.1 Epidemiology and Guidelines

The renal artery aneurysms (RAAs) represent 3% of all visceral aneurysms. Their incidence rate is about 0.1% in the general population [1], even if angiographic findings report a little higher incidence (0.3–2.5%) [2] with a modest prevalence in female patients.

RAAS are mainly detected in the sixth–seventh decade, and female patients are associated with an earlier incidence [3]. True RAAs are extra-parenchymal in 90% of cases, while intraparenchymal RAAs represent 10% of cases, and they are often multiple and congenital. RAAs can be saccular in 75% of cases or fusiform. Saccular RAAs usually affect the main renal artery bifurcation, while fusiform aneurysms often involve the main arterial trunk [4].

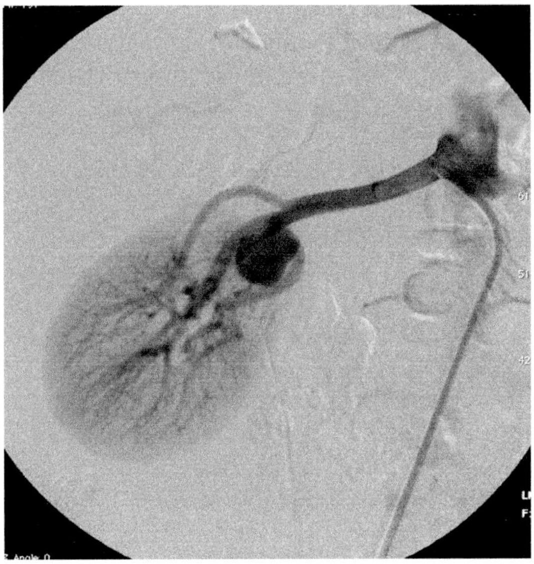

Fig. 12.1 Hilar renal artery aneurysm. The digital subtraction angiography shows the distal location of the renal aneurysm involving the origin of the terminal branches

RAAs can be bilateral (10–20%) or associated with a multiple location. High calcifications are detected in 18–68% of cases [1].

HRAAs represent a rare subgroup of RAAs, located in the distal part of the renal artery, very close to the renal hilum even though they are considered extra-parenchymal (Fig. 12.1).

In addition to "true aneurysms," the main renal arteries and their collaterals can be affected by:

M. Menegolo (✉) · E. C. Colacchio · J. Taglialavoro
M. Piazza · M. Antonello · F. Grego
Department of Cardiac, Thoracic and Vascular Sciences, Vascular and Endovascular Surgery, University of Padova, Padova, Italy
e-mail: mirko.menegolo@unipd.it; michele.antonello.1@unipd.it; franco.grego@unipd.it

L. Furian · P. Rigotti
Department of Surgery, Oncology and Gastroenterology, Surgery and Organ Transplantation Unit, University of Padova, Padova, Italy
e-mail: lucrezia.furian@unipd.it; paolo.rigotti@unipd.it

© Springer Nature Switzerland AG 2019
Y. Tshomba et al. (eds.), *Visceral Vessels and Aortic Repair*,
https://doi.org/10.1007/978-3-319-94761-7_12

- Pseudoaneurysms, which can occur after trauma or invasive procedures, such as renal biopsy, nephrostomy, or selective catheterization of renal arteries.
- Arteriovenous malformations, congenital or posttraumatic, that can evolve in dangerous dilatative diseases.
- Aneurysms following artery dissection.
- Mycotic aneurysms.
- Aneurysms secondary to pathologies, such as panarteritis nodosa, tuberculosis, neurofibromatosis, and Kawasaki disease; they are generally intraparenchymal and lead to nephrectomy.

RAAs have a slow growth rate (0.06–0.6 mm/year) [1] with no difference in terms of aneurysm morphology or calcification. The rupture rate is estimated at 3–5% with a non-gestational mortality <10% [1]. For those reasons, the surgical indications are still controversial. Actually, indications for RAA treatment include diameters of more than 2 cm, aneurysms of any size in females within childbearing age, symptoms such as pain, medical refractory hypertension, thromboembolism, concomitant symptomatic dissection, and rupture [1, 5, 6].

12.2 Clinical Presentation

Most RAAs are asymptomatic, and before the routine use of computed tomography angiography (CTA), their incidence was much lower since they were mainly detected during autopsy.

Currently, RAAs are often discovered during instrumental examinations for other pathologies or during investigation for medically refractory hypertension.

Hypertension seems to be the most common symptom, in approximately 70–100% of patients [1], and it is still unclear whether the presence of the aneurysm causes hypertension. Many theories have been advanced to explain this association:

- Hemodynamic changes from turbulent blood flow within the aneurysm resulting in decreased distal renal artery perfusion [7]
- Distal parenchymal embolization causing microvascular ischemia with a consequent releasing of angiotensin II [8]
- Compression or kinking of renal artery branches [1]
- Coexistent renal artery steno-occlusive disease that has been identified in 7–66% of patients with RAA [1]

Most authors report a significant reduction in arterial blood pressure in the postoperative period, both after surgical and endovascular correction [9].

Other symptoms include acute flank pain and hematuria, especially if the aneurysm is associated with dissection or hydronephrosis, in cases of large intrarenal RAAs [4].

RAAs may manifest with clinical signs of intra-abdominal arterial rupture and therefore must be treated as a vascular surgical emergency.

The highest rupture rate occurs in saccular aneurysms and during pregnancy with a maternal/gestational mortality of 80% [10].

12.3 Diagnosis

The patient's history and the medical examination are generally silent, except for large aneurysms in very lean patients. The diagnosis of RAAs often occurs by chance, especially during investigation for other diseases.

The first-level examination in the diagnosis of a RAA is ultrasound (US). It should be performed by experienced staff, and it gives morphological and flow information that are important both in the preoperative period (to exclude associated steno-occlusive diseases) and in the follow-up, in order to evaluate arterial patency and kidney perfusion.

The US technique has the advantage of being inexpensive and noninvasive. However, it is operator-dependent, and favorable anatomical conditions are needed (lean patient, localization of the aneurysm, poor intestinal meteorism) [11].

Computed tomography angiography (CTA) is a second-level exam, and it is essential both for diagnosis and for postoperative follow-up. It is a

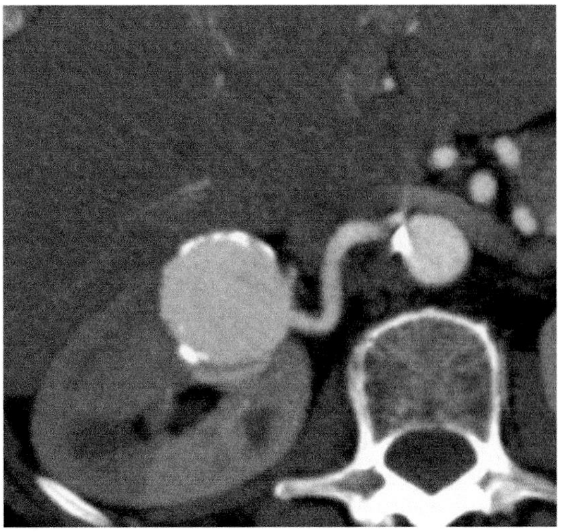

Fig. 12.2 The computed tomography allows in the majority of cases the perfect anatomical definition of renal artery aneurysm even if located closely to the kidney parenchyma

low-invasive technique that accurately identifies RAAs and allows for adequate anatomical definition and precise preoperative planning. CTA is as accurate as conventional angiography, with the advantage of being faster, cheaper, and less invasive. CTA should be the first choice in evaluating an RAA [12] (Fig. 12.2).

Magnetic resonance angiography (MRA) is a diagnostic exam similar to CTA. It provides information about the location of RAA and the vascular anatomy. It is superimposable to angiographic findings in 93% of cases [13].

However, CTA gives a better spatial 3D resolution than MRA. Moreover, MRA does not provide detailed information about the vessel wall [14].

In this regard, while CTA is preferable for preoperative planning, MRA can be used for follow-up avoiding X-ray exposure and nephrotoxicity of contrast medium.

Digital subtraction angiography (DSA) is still the diagnostic tool of choice especially in cases involving renal artery bifurcations or when the morphology of the aneurysm is not easy to analyze with CTA (Fig. 12.3). It provides the most accurate images of arterial flow, precise location of the aneurysm, and vascularization of the organ [14]. However, this examination must be considered not only a diagnostic tool, but it must be aligned with the surgical procedure.

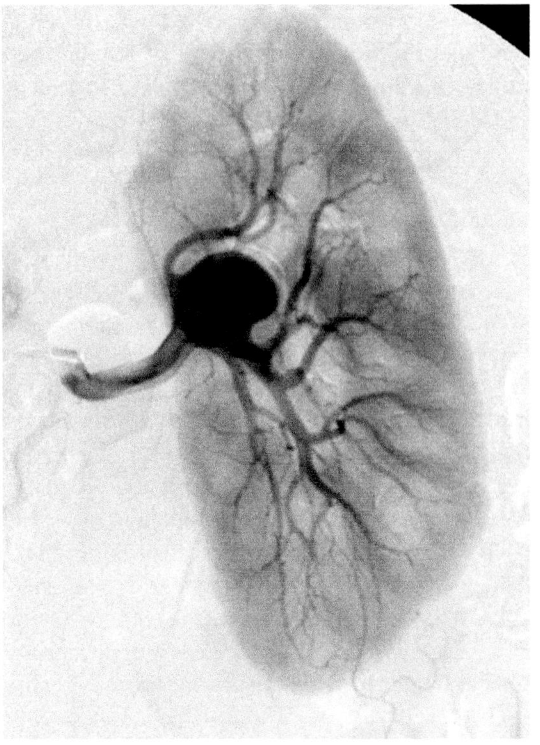

Fig. 12.3 Digital subtraction angiography of a hilar renal artery aneurysm involving collateral branches

Despite its invasiveness, the risk associated with arterial puncture, use of contrast medium, and intra-arterial devices (catheters, guidewires, etc.) is very low [14].

12.4 Treatment

The patient history provides key information on the surgical indication and the best treatment solution. It is important to know the age, sex, fertility (for women), symptoms (e.g., hypertension), and comorbidities that could influence the surgical choice (kidney failure, drug or iodine contrast allergies, heart diseases, coagulation disorders, previous abdominal surgery, or medical therapy).

Treatment of RAAs is still controversial and several techniques have been proposed over the years.

Given the difficulties associated with the treatment and the usual slow growth of RAA, some authors have proposed a conservative treatment and to monitor patients by ultrasonography, reserving surgery only for selected cases [1, 15]. However, in the majority of cases, a treatment solution should be identified.

The best treatment must be decided considering anatomical features, surgeon's ability, and availability of devices and materials.

For several years, open repair (OR) has been the only treatment available, despite the difficulties associated with this very peculiar district.

The endovascular approach has become popular, given its low invasiveness. It includes two main techniques: coil embolization and/or exclusion of the aneurysm by stent positioning [16]. Patients must be selected considering the anatomy of the vessels. However, in expert hands, even cases with a complex renal artery anatomy can be treated if the right devices are available (Fig. 12.4) [17].

HRAAs were classically excluded for both ER and OR and often candidate to nephrectomy, because of their very distal location close to the renal parenchyma. Even nowadays, in the endovascular era, the majority of HRAAs results that are unsuitable for an endo-approach because of the difficulty to be super-selective in small vessels. For the same reasons, the conventional "in vivo" open surgical approach could not be feasible either.

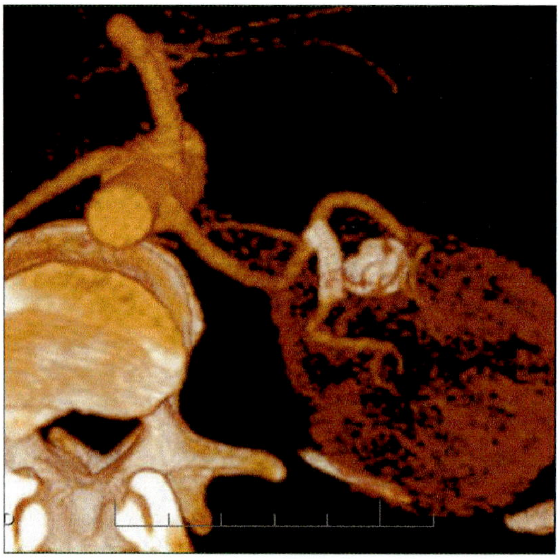

Fig. 12.4 Post-procedural computed tomography of a collateral branch renal artery aneurysm successfully excluded by a covered stent

"Ex vivo" repair with backbench reconstruction and kidney autotransplantation may facilitate the surgical reconstruction despite the high invasiveness of this approach. In this regard, a total laparoscopic nephrectomy can reduce the surgical impact: the subsequent backbench vascular repair provides many advantages both for the surgeon and for the patient. Kidney autotransplantation can finally be carried out through an extraperitoneal approach in the iliac fossa.

This technique, or the hand-assisted laparoscopic approach, has already been described in small series [5, 18].

12.5 Our Experience

From September 2011 to December 2017, we treated five patients affected by hilar RAAs using the "ex vivo technique" via a total or hand-assisted laparoscopic approach and kidney autotransplantation.

Mean age was 60 ± 4 years, and two were male patients. Table 12.1 summarizes clinical and demographic characteristics.

The indication for treatment was the diameter of the aneurysm >2 cm (mean, 2.9 ± 0.74 cm).

Surgical treatment was performed along with general surgeons, who carried out the nephrectomy and subsequent autotransplantation in all cases.

Table 12.1 Patients demographics, aneurysms characteristics, and arterial reconstructions

Variables	*N* (%) or mean ± SD
Sex (males)	2 (40)
Age	60 ± 4
Aneurysm diameter (cm)	2,9 ± 0,74
Aneurysm side (left)	3 (60)
Arterial reconstruction	
Aneurysmectomy + GSV patch	2
Aneurysmorrhaphy	3

SD standard deviation, *GSV* great saphenous vein

12.5.1 Surgical Technique

The patient was placed in a lateral decubitus position, with the hips rotated behind and the arms extended above the head.

This position allowed a rapid surgical conversion with a median laparotomy in case it was needed. The pneumoperitoneum was obtained through a Hasson "open technique" in all cases, with a small paramedian abdominal incision, just above the umbilicus (a "closed technique" with a Veress needle via umbilical access, or left iliac fossa is a superimposable approach).

After the total laparoscopic kidney dissection (releasing it from the adrenal gland and from the peripheral adipose tissue, paying attention to not injure the spleen, the tail of the pancreas, and the adrenal gland), the ureter was cut as far as possible without damaging its vascularization.

Endovenous 5000 IU of heparin and 20 mg of furosemide were administered before cutting the kidney vessels with a laparoscopic stapler (Endo GIA – Covidien).

The kidney was finally extracted by an EndoCatch bag introduced through a Pfannenstiel incision and then perfused with a cold renal preservation Celsior solution [19].

In our series, two patients were treated for a right HRAA, and in these cases, a hand-assisted laparoscopic approach was adopted.

The backbench surgery was performed by vascular surgeons inside a Celsior solution [19].

Aneurysmorrhaphy was performed in three cases, while aneurysm resection with autologous saphenous vein angioplasty was the choice in the other two patients (Fig. 12.5).

At the end of the procedure, the kidney was placed in the right iliac fossa, using a Gibson incision (Fig. 12.6).

Arterial and venous anastomoses were performed in a termino-terminal fashion between the renal artery and the hypogastric artery and between the renal vein and the external iliac vein in all cases. The anastomosis between the ureter and the bladder was performed according to the technique of Lich-Gregoir, which consists in the reimplantation of the ureter on the anterolateral wall of the bladder with an

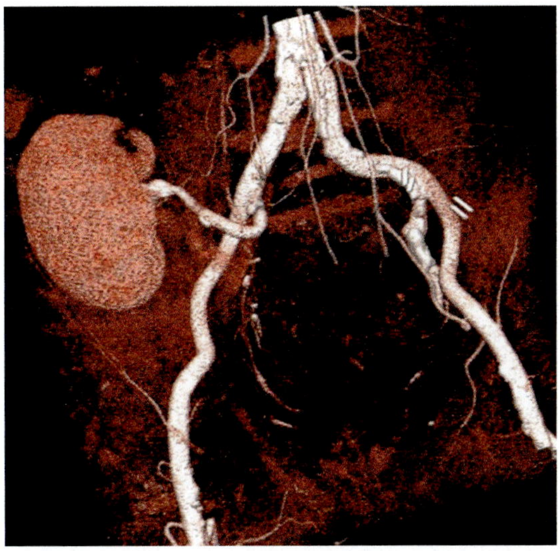

Fig. 12.6 Postoperative computed tomography showing a well-perfused reimplanted kidney in the iliac fossa

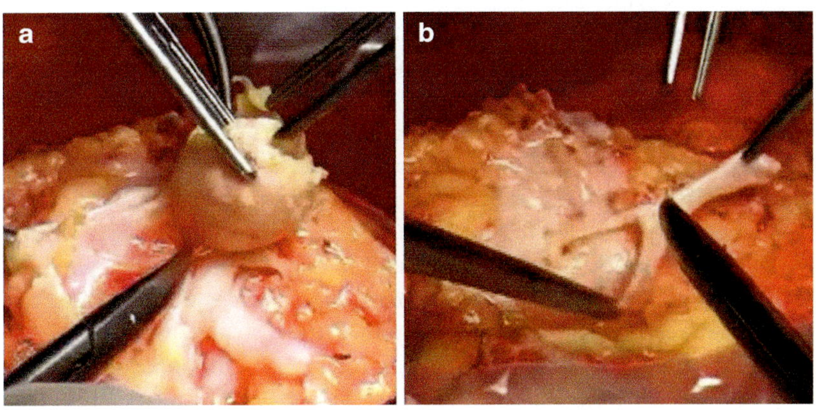

Fig. 12.5 Ex vivo bench surgery of a hilar renal artery aneurysm. The removal of a high calcified aneurismal wall (**a**) allows the reconstruction of the renal artery (**b**)

anti-reflux plastic, after positioning a double-J catheter.

A sequential renal perfusion scintigraphy was performed in all patients postoperatively before discharge from hospital.

The follow-up of all patients was achieved by CTA at 1 month and then by US at 6 and 12 months and then yearly, along with renal function monitoring.

12.5.2 Results

An aneurysm resection with primary closure was performed in three cases and aneurysm resection with patch angioplasty with great saphenous vein in the other two.

Patients were dismissed after performing renal scintigraphy, which documented the correct functioning of the transplanted organ in four cases (80%). Acute renal artery thrombosis occurred only in one case and a nephrectomy was necessary.

All patients were discharged from hospital. The medium follow-up was 9 months (2–36 months). No postoperative deaths were recorded. No postoperative complications occurred in three patients. One patient developed hypertension and it was necessary to introduce medical therapy. There was a doubt regarding a stenosis on the arterial anastomosis, but a CTA excluded it.

12.6 Discussion and Conclusions

RAAs are uncommon and, between them, HRAAs are even rarer.

They pose a technical challenge, and they are often unsuitable both for OR and ER.

The ex vivo technique is a potentially valid treatment option and an alternative to nephrectomy for HRAAs where endovascular repair and in situ open repair are not feasible.

The first step is the nephrectomy, and in our series a total or hand-assisted laparoscopic technique was adopted in order to reduce the invasiveness of this approach. In this regard, since pneumoperitoneum reduces renal blood flow, it is important to keep the patient well-hydrated, and a topical application of papaverine on the renal artery to prevent vasospasm may be considered [20].

Diuresis should always be stimulated with a bolus administration of mannitol, and a high level of hydration must be maintained.

Many authors perform the total laparoscopic nephrectomy only in the left kidney, with a single renal artery. The right renal vein is usually too short, and this could eventually increase the risk of venous thrombosis. Furthermore, a total laparoscopic technique could become more difficult to perform with multiple renal arteries. However, experiences of a total laparoscopic technique with a right kidney and/or multiple renal arteries are described [21]. In our series, we adopted the hand-assisted laparoscopic approach for right diseases.

After the nephrectomy, the following step is backbench surgery, which allows the surgeon to choose the best technical solution for the aneurysm repair.

In this series, both aneurysmorrhaphy and aneurysm resection were performed with autologous saphenous vein angioplasty. The vascular surgeon will make a therapeutic decision based on preoperative imaging but especially on the macroscopic findings. It depends on many factors: the anatomy of the aneurysm, the quality of the arterial wall, and the need to preserve as much of the collateral vessels as possible, with the goal of obtaining a safe, effective, and fast solution. Aneurysmectomy with primary anastomosis between inflow and outflow arteries and replacement of the aneurysmatic tract with autologous veins or prosthetic bypasses are other possible technical options.

During backbench repair, some caution should be exercised in the care of the kidney.

Numerous studies have shown that a warm kidney ischemia time longer than 30 min may cause permanent kidney damage [22–25]. It is also necessary to consider some risk factors related to the patient that can reduce tolerance to ischemia, such as age, diabetes mellitus, and hypertension.

In order to prevent renal ischemic damage, it is mandatory to hydrate the patient during surgery and administer mannitol (25–50 g) via intravenous infusion 5–10 min before renal artery cross-clamping, in order to reduce cellular swelling.

If the ex vivo surgery time exceeds 30 min, in situ kidney hypothermia is recommended in order to minimize the ischemic damage of the organ. Cooling the kidney surface can extend the duration of the ischemia by up to 3 h without any permanent damage.

The optimal temperature is 10–15 °C [18]. The safest method for this purpose is to cool the organ with frozen and shredded saline granules.

In our series, kidneys were perfused with a "Celsior solution," which was first created for cardiac transplantation [19]: it is a high-concentrate solution of Na+, mannitol, lactobionic acid (as in the Wisconsin University solution), and histidine (as in Bretschneider's HTK solution) which prevents cellular edema and removes free radicals.

In conclusion, in the endovascular era, open surgery remains a safe and valid option for treatment of RAAAs even if their location is very distal and proximal to the kidney hilum; in these cases, the ex vivo technique could be considered as an alternative to nephrectomy since the ER and in situ OR are not often feasible.

The total laparoscopic approach for nephrectomy allows this approach to be less invasive, and in this regard, the teamwork (collecting different specialists as vascular surgeons, transplant surgeons/urologists) is mandatory in order to achieve the best results in terms of technical success, patency of renal artery reconstructions, and renal function preservation. However, larger series are needed to assess the real effectiveness of this approach.

References

1. Coleman DM, Stanley JC. Renal artery aneurysms. J Vasc Surg. 2015;62(3):779–85.
2. Henke PK, Cardneau JD, Welling TH 3rd, Upchurch GR Jr, Wakefield TW, Jacobs LA, Proctor SB, Greenfield LJ, Stanley JC. Renal artery aneurysms: a 35-year clinical experience with 252 aneurysms in 168 patients. Ann Surg. 2001;234(4):454–62.
3. Pfeiffer T, Reiher L, Grabitz K, Grunhage B, Hafele S, Voiculescu A, et al. Reconstrucion for renal artery aneurysm: operative techniques and long-term results. J Vasc Surg. 2003;37:293–300.
4. Calligaro KD, Dougherty MJ. Renovascular disease: aneurysms and arteriovenous fistulae. In: Cronenwett JL, Johnston KW, editors. Rutherford's vascular surgery. 8th ed. Philadelphia: Saunders; 2014.
5. Gallagher KA, Phelan MW, Stern T, Bartlett ST. Repair of complex renal artery aneurysms by laparoscopic nephrectomy with ex vivo repair and autotransplantation. J Vasc Surg. 2008;48(6):1408–13.
6. Klausner JQ, Lawrence PF, Harlander-Locke MP, Coleman DM, Stanley JC, Fujimura N, Vascular Low-Frequency Disease Consortium. The contemporary management of renal artery aneurysms. J Vasc Surg. 2015;61(4):978–84.
7. Tham G, Ekelund L, Herrlin K, Lindstedt EL, Olin T, Bergentz SE. Renal artery aneurysms. Natural history and prognosis. Ann Surg. 1983;197:348–52.
8. Hupp T, Allenberg JR, Post K, Roeren T, Meier M, Clorius JH. Renal artery aneurysm: surgical indications and results. Eur J Vasc Surg. 1992;6:477–86.
9. Reiher L, Grabitz K, Sandmann W. Reconstruction for renal artery aneurysm and its effect on hypertension. Eur J Vasc Endovasc Surg. 2000;20:454–6.
10. Stanley JC. Natural history of renal artery stenosis and aneurysms. In: Calligaro KD, Dougherty MJ, Dean RH, editors. Modern management of renovascular hypertension and renal salvage. Baltimore: Williams & Wilkins; 1996. p. 15.
11. Bielsa AA, Rodriguez JP, Castromil RG. Extraparenchymal renal artery aneurysms: is hypertension an indication for revascularization surgery? Ann Vasc Surg. 2002;16:339–44.
12. Dib M, Sedat J, Raffaelli C, Petit I, Robertson WG, Jaeger P. Endovascular treatment of a wide-neck renal artery bifurcation aneurysm. J Vasc Interv Radiol. 2003;14:1461–4.
13. Bui BT, Oliva VL, Leclerc G, Courteau M, Harel C, Plante R, et al. Renal artery aneurysm: treatment with percutaneous placement of a stent-graft. Radiology. 1995;195:181–2.
14. Tateno T, Kubota Y, Sasagawa I, Sawamura T, Nakada T. Successful embolization of a renal artery aneurysm with preservation of renal blood flow. Int Urol Nephrol. 1996;28:283–7.
15. JP MC Jr, Marshall VF, Whitsell JC 2nd. Indications for surgery on renal artery aneurysms. J Urol. 1975;114(2):177–80.
16. Wei X, Sun Y, Wu Y, Li Z, Zhu J, Zhao Z, Feng R, Jing Z. Management of wide-based renal artery aneurysms using noncovered stent-assisted coil embolization. J Vasc Surg. 2017;66(3):850–7.
17. Menegolo M, Frigatti P, Antonello M, Grego F. Stent graft exclusion of a renal artery aneurysm at hilum in a case with complex anatomy. Perspect Vasc Surg Endovasc Ther. 2009;21(4):240–3. Epub 2010 May 20
18. Laser A, Flinn WR, Benjamin ME. Ex vivo repair of renal artery aneurysms. J Vasc Surg. 2015;62(3):606–9.

19. Catena F, Gazzotti F, Amaduzzi A, Fuga G, Montori G, Cucchetti A, Coccolini F, Vallicelli C, Pinna AD. Pulsatile perfusion of kidney allografts with Celsior solution. Transplant Proc. 2010;42(10):3971–2.
20. Sorokin I, Stevens SL, Cadeddu JA. Periarterial papaverine to treat renal artery vasospasm during robot-assisted laparoscopic partial nephrectomy. J Robot Surg. 2017;12(1):189–91.
21. Ham SW, Weaver FA. Ex vivo renal artery reconstruction for complex renal artery disease. J Vasc Surg. 2014;60(1):143–50.
22. Desai MM, Gill IS, Ramani AP, Spaliviero M, Rybicki L, Kaouk JH. The impact of warm ischaemia on renal function after laparoscopic partial nephrectomy. BJU Int. 2005;95(3):377–83.
23. Zargar H, Akca O, Ramirez D, Brandao LF, Laydner H, Krishnan J, Stein RJ, Kaouk JH. The impact of extended warm ischemia time on late renal function after robotic partial nephrectomy. J Endourol. 2015;29(4):444–8.
24. Novick AC. Renal hypothermia: in vivo and ex vivo. Urol Clin North Am. 1983;10:637–44.
25. Ward JP. Determination of the optimum temperature for regional renal hypothermia during temporary renal ischaemia. Br J Urol. 1975;47:17–24.

13 Pulsate Perfusion of Allografts

Matteo Tozzi, Gabriele Piffaretti, Marco Franchin, and Patrizio Castelli

'If one could substitute for the heart a kind of injection of arterial blood, either natural or artificial made, one would succeed easily in maintaining alive indefinitely any part of the body'

Julien Jean Cesar Le Gallois,
French physiologist (1770–1814)

13.1 Introduction

Since the introduction of organ transplantation surgery more than 50 years ago, static cold storage (SCS) has been considered as the gold standard of organ preservation. However, the discussion on optimal composition of preservation solution and duration and methods of preservation (normothermic vs hypothermic, static vs pulsate) is still open.

Studies on continuous organ perfusion appeared in the late nineteenth century. In the 1930s, Carrel et al. refined those studies with the idea that continuous flow could help in eliminating toxic metabolic products providing nutrients [1]. Thirty years later, Starzl's group employed extracorporeal femoro-femoral canine perfusion for sub-normothermic preservation with satisfactory results. Belzer et al. combined the principle of continuous flow with hypothermia, with the aim of reducing cellular metabolic demand [2, 3]. Despite initial encouraging results both on kidney and liver grafts, continuous organ perfusion was abandoned in favour of SCS, mainly for logistic reasons after the commercialization of new and more effective preservation solutions [4]. Finally, in the 1990s, the increased utilization of less than optimal kidneys from expanded criteria donors (ECD) and non-heart-beating donors (NHBD according to Maastricht classification) gave new interest to this technique [5].

Nowadays, dynamic perfusion (DP) machine is largely adopted for the following advantages:

- Providing nutrition to cellular supply
- Washing out toxins
- Triggering a series of protective mechanisms by innate immune responses and adaptive immune responses
- Evaluating organ function with haemodynamic data

13.2 The Machine Perfusion

13.2.1 Dynamic Perfusion Characteristics and Settings

During DP, recirculating perfusate is continuously pumped (roller or centrifugal pump) through the organ vasculature by a machine perfusion (MP). There are two modalities of preser-

M. Tozzi · G. Piffaretti · M. Franchin (✉) · P. Castelli
Vascular Surgery, Department of Medicine and Surgery, University of Insubria School of Medicine, Circolo University Teaching Hospital, Varese, Italy

© Springer Nature Switzerland AG 2019
Y. Tshomba et al. (eds.), *Visceral Vessels and Aortic Repair*,
https://doi.org/10.1007/978-3-319-94761-7_13

vation: in situ (in vivo regional perfusion) and ex situ. During in vivo regional perfusion, a pump sends the perfusate to the graft through the artery, while the vein cannulation guarantees the elimination of the perfusate. In the ex situ modality, after procurement, the graft is placed in an organ chamber and connected to a circuit. In case of liver DP, a separate circulation is sometimes predisposed for the portal vein and hepatic artery through different pumps with different pressure/flow settings.

A heat exchanger regulates temperature from hypothermia (4–10 °C) to sub-normothermia (20–25 °C) and normothermia (35–37 °C).

According to the literature, hypothermic DP should be set by pressure and not by flow velocity, preferring low pressure in avoiding injuries to the graft [6, 7]. Perfusion can be both continuous (CP) and pulsate (PP), and the perfusate can be nonoxygenated or oxygenated. Generally, hypothermic DP employs acellular perfusates that differ from those used for SCS.

It is noticeable that comparative studies on PP and CP did not demonstrate significant outcome benefit in terms of graft survival [8]. Additionally, no difference was seen in terms of renal graft function after transplant [9]. However, continuous flow has been correlated with increased vascular impedance [10] and impaired platelet function [11]. The kidneys are generally treated with PP (25–30 mmHg) [12–15]. Livers are generally treated with continuous low-pressure flow (3–5 mmHg) through the portal vein. The role of hepatic artery perfusion to maintain the peribiliary vascular plexus is still debated [6, 16].

The rationale of oxygen supply under hypothermia with acellular perfusate is debated. Firstly, we must underline how oxygen solubility is moderated at atmospheric pressure conditions also at low temperature. Additionally, increased electric charges due to colloidal agents decrease gas solubility. Consequently, the only possibility is to increase partial pressure of oxygen in the perfusate with the aid of a pressurized oxygenator up to 700 mmHg. Experimental models of liver and kidney transplant showed significant improvement in the outcome. Nevertheless, we have only a little evidence on possible complications, due to hyperoxygenation as substrate for reactive oxygen species (ROS) [5].

With sub-normothermic DP, both cellular and acellular perfusates are adopted. The kidneys are generally treated with pulsate flow (40 mmHg). Livers are generally treated with continuous low-pressure flow (4–8 mmHg) through the portal vein. With normothermic DP, an oxygenated perfusate is always necessary, and an oxygen carrier is mandatory (usually red blood cells) [17, 18]. Near-physiological pressure is used. The kidneys are generally treated with pulsate flow (70–90 mmHg). Livers are generally treated with continuous flow (60–105 mmHg). We have to notice that in case of machine malfunction, hypothermic and sub-normothermic grafts can be rapidly and safely stored with static cold technique. On the contrary, grafts treated with normothermic perfusion will be vulnerable to warm ischemia.

13.2.2 Organ Preservation Solution

Anoxia associated with hypothermia triggers a biological cascade driving apoptosis and toxic metabolite production. Goals for preservation solution are:

- Limit ischemia damage during cold preservation.
- Limit reperfusion damage.
- Maintain electrolyte balance.
- Supply metabolites.

The first experimental application of DP, during the 1960s, showed that one of the most relevant complications associated with continuous flow was interstitial oedema and cell swelling. This phenomenon was mainly associated with high capillary resistance. This problem was solved with the development of a new generation of perfusate solution with higher oncotic properties by the addition of hydroxyethyl starch (HES).

The most commonly used cold preservative solutions are:

- ViaSpan (University of Wisconsin solution): High-potassium low-sodium solution, HES,

adenosine and raffinose. Main disadvantages are high viscosity, tendency for crystallization and risk of hypercalcaemic cardiac arrest.
- Celsior: Low-potassium high-sodium solution, which employs mannitol and lactobionate to decrease cellular oedema.
- Custodiol – histidine-tryptophan-ketoglutarate (HTK): Low-potassium low-viscosity crystalloid not requiring filtering.
- Perfadex: Low-potassium solution lightly buffered dextran-containing, pulmonary-specific preservation solution.

Actually, Belzer solution is the most commonly used in clinical routine DP. Its main characteristic is the presence of a ribose and a zwitterionic organic buffering agent [2-hydroxy-ethylpiperazine-*N*′-2-ethanesulfonic acid (HEPES)].

13.3 Dynamic Perfusion Impact on Graft Physiology

13.3.1 Hypothermia, Sub-normothermia, Adenosine Triphosphate Depletion and Oxygen Free Radical Production

The rationale of hypothermic preservation is to reduce adenosine triphosphate (ATP) depletion to control the cascade of ischaemic injury. Many physiological processes are driven by ATP and mainly electrolyte balance. In fact, sodium/potassium membrane pump is dependent on ATP, and its depletion is responsible for the loss of electrolyte cellular gradient and membrane integrity. With such a result, cellular oedema and increment of intracellular calcium concentration are seen and, subsequently, phospholipase activation leading to inflammation and apoptosis. During normal oxidative metabolism, ATP breakdown is converted to urea by xanthine dehydrogenase. During ischemia, xanthine dehydrogenase is converted to xanthine oxidase. After reperfusion, in the presence of oxygen, xanthine oxidase transforms the accumulated ATP breakdown into xanthine, and superoxide anion is responsible for lipid peroxidation and cell membrane lesion. ATP metabolism is slowed from 1.5 to 2 times for every 10 °C drop in temperature [19].

The rationale of sub-normothermic DP is to maintain the graft at a low temperature, reducing metabolism and oxygen requirements, without the risk of cold-induced injuries.

13.3.2 Dynamic Perfusion, Apoptosis and Inflammation

Isolated graft tissues produce large quantity of oxygen free radicals that, in association with anoxia, results in mitochondrial damage [20]. Additionally, ROS are involved in many signalling pathway activations, triggering the expression of pro-inflammatory mediators such as interleukins 1 and 6 (IL1, IL6) and tumour necrosis factor alpha (TNFα), providing for intracellular calcium overload and apoptosis. Inflammation leads to cell proliferation, extracellular matrix (ECM) remodelling and degradation [21]. Vascular cell adhesion molecule-1 (VCAM-1) and e-selectin produce an increment of immunogenicity and subsequent organ damage after graft reperfusion [5]. Tozzi et al. outlined how PP significantly reduces tissue antigen expression of soluble intracellular adhesion molecule-1 (sICAM-1) and pro-inflammatory cytokine (TNF-α, IL-2 and IL-1β) compared to SCS controls, resulting in the reduction of leucocyte stimulation (particular neutrophils) and a decrease in post-reperfusion activated inflammation-mediated acute-phase proteins that are responsible for ischemia/reperfusion injury (IRI). Many authors have stressed the correlation between IRI, cell apoptosis, delayed graft function (DGF) and chronic renal failure [22, 23]. Apoptosis is a reversible programmed cell death [24]. It is noteworthy that apoptosis is responsible for the loss of renal tubular epithelial cells, chronic tubular atrophy and the loss of podocytes [17, 25–27]. One of the crucial phases of apoptosis is represented by cell membrane degeneration [28]. Many authors focus their attention on ezrin-radixin-moesin (ERM) proteins and plasma membrane-actin cytoskeleton linkers, particularly expressed in epithelial cells [18, 29]. Ezrin-radixin-moesin proteins are considered anti-apoptotic proteins activated by a phosphoinositide 3-kinase signalling pathway (PI3K/AKT/mTOR) [30]. Zhang et al. demonstrated that DP enhances the expression of ERM through PI3K/AKT/mTOR pathway with an anti-apoptotic effect. Another crucial element involved in apoptosis is represented by caspase, a protein family that plays a significant role in apoptosis signalling. Among them, Caspase 3 is a key execution molecule that functions in many ways in the apoptotic signal transduction. A significant reduction in activated Caspase 3 was documented in graft cells treated with DP over SCS [31].

In addition to cell apoptosis, ECM damage affects graft functional recovery. Matrix metalloproteinases (MMPs) are a family of calcium-dependent zinc-containing gelatinase responsible for ECM remodelling. Overexpression of MMP-2 and MMP-9 is commonly observed after large endothelial damage such as tumour invasion, inflammation or IRI [32]. Metalloproteinases show temporal variability. In particular, MMP-2 and MMP-9 reach a peak of concentration 6 h after graft reperfusion, subsequently gradually decrease and finally present another peak 24 h later [33]. Metalloproteinase activation occurs due to ROS and nitric oxide by s-nitrosylation and oxidation [34]. Fu et al. described a lower statistical expression of MMP-9 in PP over SCS [35]. The washout of toxins produced by PP is quite probably responsible for those events.

In contrast to SCS, PP maintains continuous flow with more physiologic haemodynamic forces and promotes microcirculatory perfusion. In fact, fat emboli, lipoprotein aggregation, vasoconstriction and cortical hypoperfusion are responsible for tissue hypoxia and oedema. Furthermore, pulsate perfusion has shown itself to be responsible for microvasculature perfusion improvement and reduction in blood component aggregation [36]. Furthermore, haemodynamic shear stress regulates gene expression of endothelial cells [37, 38], while flow cessation increases pro-thrombotic and inflammatory characteristics of endothelium [39]. In particular, flow stop is associated with the decrease in Kruppel-like factor 2 (KLF-2) expression and with an increase of adhesion molecules. The KLF-2 is a transcription factor that acts as part of the vasoprotective phenotype against thrombosis [40–43].

13.4 Kidney

13.4.1 General Issues and Results of Conventional Grafts

Although the acute rejection rate is not significantly different between grafts treated with PP or SCS, molecular evidence is clear in terms of DGF and primary nonfunction (PNF) risk reduction [4]. Accordingly, Wight et al., in a systemic review of 20 studies, suggested a 20% overall reduction of DGF with PP [44]. The limitation of the paper was the inclusion of small and underpowered studies. Nevertheless, results were confirmed by Moers et al. in a randomized trial including 336 paired kidneys confirming an overall reduced incidence of DGF in PP grafts [45]. Schold et al., in a large register retrospective analysis of 907 paired kidneys treated with concluding for PP superiority. Surprisingly, authors demonstrated that prolonged time of pulsate cold ischemia was associated with better results in terms of DGF risk reduction [46]. Interestingly, Chueh et al. emphasized the benefit of prolonged time of pulsate cold ischemia (>24 h). In fact, due to their remote geographical location, they had the possibility to compare DGF rate and serum creatinine recovery curve of the kidney with an average time of ischemia above 21–23 h. Grafts that received pulsatile perfusion had less delayed graft function (3.6% vs 23.4%, $p = 0.02$) and faster graft recovery ($p < 0.001$) [47].

13.4.2 Expanded Criteria Donors, Non-heart-Beating Donors and the Role of Haemodynamic Data

The utility of PP over SCS is even more evident if we focus our attention on ECD and NHBD. Aged ECD grafts are known to have decreased functional capacities and are more susceptible to ischemia-related damage [48]. Grafts from NHBD are subjected to a significant period of warm ischaemic injury (from 10 to 45 min) between cardiac arrest and perfusion with cold solution [19]. Over 50% of the kidneys from NHBD suffer from an extended period of DGF, requiring continued dialysis until recovery [49].

The retrospective analysis of 6057 kidney transplants from the Organ Procurement and Transplantation Network (OPTN) showed better results in terms of DGF reduction and was found when the donor age was higher than 60 years [50]. Treckmann et al., in an international randomized controlled trial, enrolled 91 consecutive ECD kidneys, obtaining meaningful results in terms of DGF and PNF risk. In addition, 1-year graft survival resulted significantly higher in the machine-perfused kidney compared with the cold-stored kidney [12]. Conversely, the analysis of 170 kidney transplants from donors older than 65 years from Eurotransplant Senior Program found statistical differences in terms of PNF in PP population over SCS (3.5% vs 12.9%, $p = 0.02$). On the contrary, the overall frequency of DGF was similar in the two groups [4].

Preliminary results of PP applied to graft from NHBD were not equally satisfactory. In fact, a UK multicentre randomized controlled trial conducted in 2010 of 91 kidney transplants from NHBD did not show statistically significant differences in GFR rate (53.3% vs 57.8%, $p = 0.8$) and 1-year graft survival (93.3% vs 97.8%, $p = 0.3$) between the cohorts of graft treated with SCS and PP. Notably, this study showed a significant difference in terms of acute rejections (22% vs 7%, $p = 0.06$) [13]. On the contrary, a large review of the National Scientific Registry of Transplant Recipient (SRTR) database of 4923 kidney transplants demonstrated how grafts from NHBD stored with SCS technique had a higher risk of DGF. Data analysis suggested PP was beneficial on DGF over SCS in both ECD and NHBD [51]. In our opinion, the encouraging results obtained with perfusion machine are not only explained by the intrinsic benefit of pumped perfusion, especially in this population. In fact, in addition to therapeutic use, pulsatile perfusion machine allows us to obtain fundamental pre-transplantation haemodynamical information: perfusion flow, pressure and intraparenchymal renovascular resistances (Fig. 13.1). These data were correlated by different authors on post-transplant outcome. In fact, it is well demonstrated how elevated vascular resistance is more likely to show reduced survival 1 year after transplant together with increased risk of DGF or PNF.

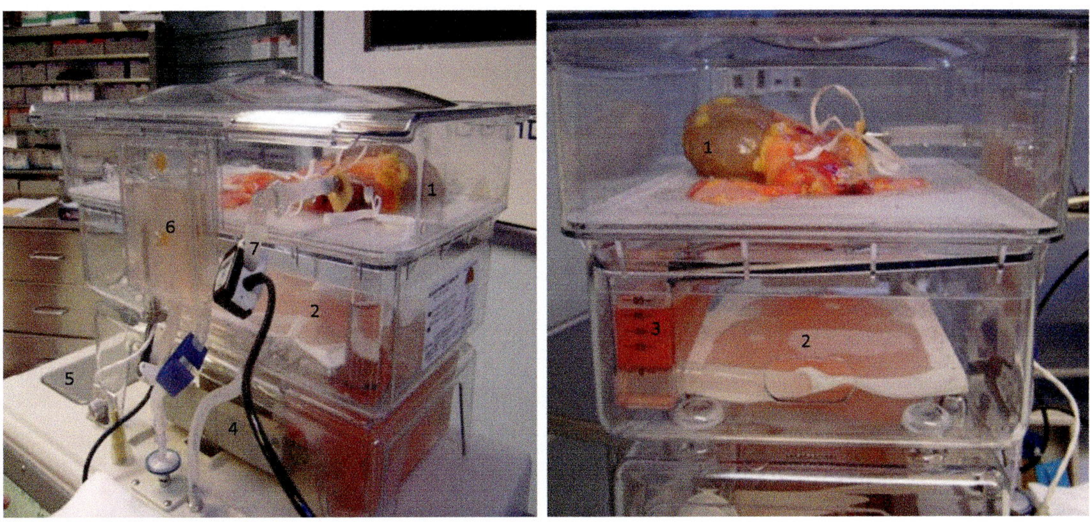

Fig. 13.1 Example of pulsate perfusion machine: (1) kidney graft connected to the circuit, (2) the perfusate excrete through the ureter is filtered by a membrane, (3) the perfusate is collected and (4) sent to the pulsate pump. (5) A cooler is responsible for perfusate temperature control. (6) The perfusate is sent to a bubble evacuator and subsequently to the graft. (7) A flow detector gives haemodynamic indices

13.5 Other Organs

Dynamic perfusion was first developed for kidney and liver grafts. From the beginning, it was clear that the kidneys present characteristics that make this treatment safer and with better results. For that reason, PP treatment on the liver, heart, lung and pancreas had been relegated for a long time to a research and preclinical area. The "rediscovery" of DP occurred as consequence of the increased demand for organs and the resulting need to extend the criteria for graft procurement. As seen before, the marginal graft is more affected by hypothermic preservation injury, and consequently new strategies have been required.

13.5.1 Liver

Because of its unique anatomy and physiology, the liver is a challenge for DP. In particular, the competition between hepatic artery and portal vein inflow and the sensitivity of hepatic endothelial cells to high pressures are the main problems affecting DP [52, 53]. Organs from the elderly, steatosic or NHBD have elevated risk of moderate to severe preservation injury and related biliary complications [54]. Possible complications are represented by PNF and the need for retransplantation in 3–7% [55], early allograft dysfunction, cholestasis and infections [56]. The study of DP on animal models started in 1967 at the first attempt to obtain PP of the hepatic artery alone using hypothermic crystalloid solution in hyperbaric oxygen condition with unsatisfactory results [57]. Starzl group proposed the perfusion of both the hepatic artery and the portal vein in a canine model with a solution of blood and preservation solution with excellent results [58]. Soon after, the same procedure was successfully applied to seven patients [59]. Unexpectedly, this technique was never accepted, and static cold storage was largely adopted.

Only at the beginning of the 1980s, Kamada et al. started novel investigation on dynamic hypothermic perfusion [60]. Further investigation on animal models gave promising results [61]. Guarrera et al. were the first to describe a prospective cohort pilot study in humans. Results confirmed safety and feasibility of liver DP. They did not document any difference in terms of PNF, a small reduction of early allograft dysfunction ($p = 0.08$) and a significant benefit in terms of hospitalization ($p = 0.004$). Further studies comparing DP and SCS are in progress. Many trials are in progress, evaluating both portal vein and combined hepatic artery and portal vein perfusion. Preliminary evidence suggests perfusate oxygenation is necessary to prevent IRI; otherwise, ideal partial oxygen pressure is still unknown [19]. Guarrera et al. reported perfusate oxygen tension >120 mmHg in an open system without active oxygenation [56]. More data from larger trials on both cold and normothermic continuous preservation are expected.

13.5.2 Lung

Steen et al. described first ex vivo lung continuous hypothermic perfusion in clinical use. The most relevant problem researchers found during preclinical phase was pulmonary oedema consequent to endothelial circuit-induced injury and increased vascular resistance. This experience enabled the first pulmonary transplant to be performed with graft from NHBD. The available data does not demonstrate superiority of DP over SCS with conventional grafts [51]; otherwise, Ingermansson and Cypel's experiences proved the advantage of DP for reconditioning of high risk for transplant grafts (pulmonary oedema and/or PaO2: FiO2 < 300) [62, 63]. A portable Organ Care System (OCS) (TransMedics, Andover, MA, US) was commercialized and specifically designed for the reconditioning of marginal lungs. This device is able to perfuse the graft and allows ventilation for continuous alveoli recruitment at the same time. The machine also allows for bronchoscopy during ventilation [64] to be performed. More recently, another ex vivo MP especially designed for marginal lung reconditioning was commercialized by XVIVO Perfusion System (Gothenburg, Sweden).

13.5.3 Heart

The clinical use of DP for the heart has been a particular focus for most researchers. In fact, this technique could represent a fabulous opportunity to extend the type and numbers of heart donors. Additionally, this technique could be used to identify dysfunctional grafts prior to implantation, reducing the risk of death for recipients. Biomarkers of myocardial injury (pH, lactate, troponins) can be measured during perfusion. Additionally, magnetic resonance and coronarography have been proposed for assessment of left ventricular function, anatomy and viability [52, 65]. A multicentre randomized trial on a new device specifically designed for heart graft perfusion was commercialized by TransMedics' OCS which started in the USA and Europe (PROCEEDII) and demonstrated better outcomes after transplantation in terms of recipient survival and PNF [66].

13.6 Assessment of Graft Viability and Limits

Dynamic perfusion offers the attractive feature of providing useful data to assess organ viability before transplant. It may not always be necessary to understand whether the graft was procured under ideal circumstances or from conventional donors. On the contrary, vascular resistance and flow rate can provide useful information on graft quality in case of marginal donors or when particular events occurred during graft harvesting.

The prediction of outcome of the preserved liver is not currently possible, and transplant viability is sought from donor history, organ appearance and microscopical scoring. During DP, the liver does not produce bile. Some authors suggested that perfusate transaminase and lactate dehydrogenase may correlate with transplant outcome, but data are controversial [56, 61]. For the preserved kidneys, we have a different situation, and 'pour perfusion parameters' have been widely advocated as negative prognostic factors for DGF or PNF. In the literature, the definition of 'poor perfusion parameters' is not univocal. For example, according to Mozes et al., it is defined as resistance inferior to 0.40 mmHg/mL/min and superior to 0.60 mmHg/mL/min [67]. Guarrera et al. defined poor perfusion parameter as flow inferior to 80 mL/min/100 g with resistance above 0.40 mmHg/mL/100 g. De Vries et al. stressed the importance of very high resistance (>3 mmHg/mL/min/100 g) as a sensitive negative prognostic factor [68, 69]. Accordingly, poor perfusion parameters detected in grafts from ECD and NHBD could be responsible for a higher incidence of graft refusals. The retrospective analysis of 6057 kidney transplants from the Organ Procurement and Transplantation Network (OPTN) partially downgraded the relevance of haemodynamical data emphasizing the risk of possible underutilization of grafts [50]. Although the literature stressed the role of haemodynamic data as an independent risk factor in multivariate analysis for DGF, the evidence to suggest its predictive capacity as a stand-alone parameter is scarce [70]. Jochmans et al. demonstrated low sensitivity and positive predictive value (respectively, 17% and 40%) and acceptable specificity and negative predictive value (93% and 81%) [14]. In a recent prospective study, Gomez et al. compared vascular resistance detected with perfusion machine with post-transplant kidney resistance calculated on Doppler ultrasound without finding any statistical correlation. Additionally, authors did not find any statistical association between renal resistances and DGF (p = 0.58) [70]. Those unsatisfactory results can perhaps be explained by the multifactorial nature of DGF or PNF such as obesity, high blood pressure, diabetes mellitus or dyslipidaemia [70, 71]. It is noteworthy that Guarrera et al. assumed that poor perfusion parameters in grafts from donors without other risk factors for DGF should not be taken into count for graft discard [72]. Today, authors suggest organ refusal should be a multidisciplinary choice [50, 69]. Haemodynamic data from perfusion machine could be a complementary tool to kidney biopsy scores [71].

References

1. Carrel A, Lindberg CA. The culture of whole organs. Science. 1935;81:621–3.
2. Belzer FO, Ashby BS, Gulyassy PF, Powell M. Successful seventeen-hour preservation and transplantation of human-cadaver kidney. N Engl J Med. 1968;278:608–10.
3. Belzer FO, Southard JH. Principles of solid-organ preservation by cold storage. Transplantation. 1988;45:673–6.
4. Gallinat A, et al. Machine perfusion versus cold storage for the preservation of kidney from donors ≥65 years allocated in the eurotransplant senior programme. Nephrol Dial Transplant. 2012;27:4458–63.
5. Timsit MO, Tullius SG. Hypothermic kidney preservation: a remembrance of the past in the future? Curr Opin Organ Transplant. 2011;16:162–8.
6. Schlegel A, Rougemont O, Graf R, Clavien PA, Dutkowski P. Protective mechanisms of end-ischemic cold machine perfusion in DCD liver grafts. J Hepatol. 2013;58:278–86.
7. Maathuis MH, Manekeller S, van der Plaats A, et al. Improved kidney graft function after preservation using a novel hypothermic machine perfusion device. Ann Surg. 2007;246:982–8.
8. Pegg DE, et al. Renal preservation by hypothermic perfusion. The lack of influence of pulsate flow. Cryobiology. 1976;13:161–7.
9. Gimbrone MA Jr, et al. Endothelial dysfunction, hemodynamic forces, and atherogenesis. Ann N Y Acad Sci. 2000;902:230–9.
10. Travis AR, et al. Vascular pulsatility in patients with a pulsatile- or continuous-flow ventricular assist device. J Thorac Cardiovasc Surg. 2007;133:517–24.
11. Crow S, et al. Comparative analysis of von Willebrand factor profile in pulsatile and continuous left ventricular assist device recipients. ASAIO J. 2010;56:441–5.
12. Treckmann J, Moers C, Smits JM, Gallinat A, Maathuis MH, van Kasterop-Kutz M, Jochmans I, Homan van der Heide JJ, Squifflet JP, van Heurn E, Kirste GR, Rahmel A, Leuvenink HG, Pirenne J, Ploeg RJ, Paul A. Machine perfusion versus cold storage for preservation of kidneys from expanded criteria donors after brain death. Transpl Int. 2011;24(6):548–54.
13. Watson CJE. Cold machine perfusion versus static cold storage of kidney donated after cardiac death: a UK multicentre randomized controlled trial. Am J Transplant. 2010;10:1991–9.
14. Jochmans I, Moers C, Smits JM, et al. The prognostic value of renal resistance during hypothermic machine perfusion of deceased donor kidneys. Am J Transplant. 2011;11:2214–20.
15. Gallinat A, Fox M, Luer B, Efferz P, Paul A, Minor T. Role of pulsatility in hypothermic reconditioning of porcine kidney grafts by machine perfusion after cold storage. Transplantation. 2013;96:538–42.
16. Guarrera JV, Henry SD, Samstein B, et al. Hypothermic machine preservation in human liver transplantation: the first clinical series. Am J Transplant. 2010;10:372–81.
17. Ichii O, Yabuki A, Sasaki N, et al. Pathological correlations between podocyte injuries and renal functions in canine and feline chronic kidney diseases. Histol Histopathol. 2011;26:1243–55.
18. Fiévet B, Louvard D, Arpin M. ERM proteins in epithelial cell organization and functions. Biochim Biophys Acta. 2007;1773:653–60.
19. Luer B, Koetting M, Efferz P, Minor T. Role of oxygen during hypothermic machine perfusion preservation of the liver. Transpl Int. 2010;23:944–50.
20. Mitchell T, Rotaru D, Saba H, Smith RA, Murphy MP, MacMillan-Crow LA. The mitochondria-targeted antioxidant mitoquinone protects against cold storage injury of renal tubular cells and rat kidneys. J Pharmacol Exp Ther. 2011;336:682–92.
21. Barklin A. Systemic inflammation in the brain-dead organ donor. Acta Anaesthesiol Scand. 2009;53:425–35.
22. Yoshida M, Honma S. Regeneration of injured renal tubules. J Pharmacol Sci. 2014;124:117–22.
23. Bonventre JV, Yang L. Cellular pathophysiology of ischemic acute kidney injury. J Clin Invest. 2011;121:4210–21.
24. Toronyi E. Role of apoptosis in the kidney after reperfusion. Orv Hetil. 2008;149:305–15.
25. Andrea H, Steven CB. Apoptosis and acute kidney injury. Kidney Int. 2011;80:29–40.
26. Koçkara A, Kayatas M. Renal cell apoptosis and new treatment options in sepsis-induced acute kidney injury. Ren Fail. 2013;35:291–4.
27. Hartleben B, Wanner N, Huber TB. Autophagy in glomerular health and disease. Semin Nephrol. 2014;34:42–52.
28. Kondo T, Takeuchi K, Doi Y, Yonemura S, Nagata S, Tsukita S. ERM (ezrin/radixin/moesin)-based molecular mechanism of microvillar breakdown at an early stage of apoptosis. J Cell Biol. 1997;139:749–58.
29. Viswanatha R, Bretscher A1, Garbett D. Dynamics of ezrin and EBP50 in regulating microvilli on the apical aspect of epithelial cells. Biochem Soc Trans. 2014;42:189–94.
30. Gautreau A, Poullet P, Louvard D, Arpin M. Ezrin, a plasma membrane-microfilament linker, signals cell survival through the phosphatidylinositol 3-kinase/Akt pathway. Proc Natl Acad Sci U S A. 1999;96:7300–5.
31. Zhang Y, Fu Z, Zhong Z, Wang R, Hu L, Xiong Y, Wang Y, Ye Q. Hypothermic machine perfusion decreases renal cell apoptosis during ischemia/reperfusion injury via the Ezrin/AKT pathway. Artif Organs. 2016;40(2):129–35.
32. Hamada T, Duarte S, Tsuchihashi S, Busuttil RW, Coito AJ. Inducible nitric oxide synthase deficiency impairs matrix metalloproteinase-9 activity and dis-

rupts leukocyte migration in hepatic ischemia/reperfusion injury. Am J Pathol. 2009;174:2265–77.
33. Kunugi S, Shimizu A, Kuwahara N, et al. Inhibition of matrix metalloproteinases reduces ischemia-reperfusion acute kidney injury. Lab Investig. 2011;91:170–80.
34. Gu Z, Kaul M, Yan B, et al. S-nitrosylation of matrix metalloproteinases: signaling pathway to neuronal cell death. Science. 2002;297:1186–90.
35. Fu Z, Ye Q, Zhang Y, Zhong Z, Xiong Y, Wang Y, Hu L, Wang W, Huang W, Ko DS. Hypothermic machine perfusion reduced inflammatory reaction by downregulating the expression of matrix metalloproteinase 9 in a reperfusion model of donation after cardiac death. Artif Organs. 2016;40(6):E102–11.
36. Patal SK, et al. Effect of increased pressure during pulsatile pump perfusion of deceased donor kidney in transplantation. Transplant Proc. 2012;44:2202–6.
37. McCormick SM, et al. DNA microarray reveals changes in gene expression of shear stressed human umbilical vein endothelial cells. Proc Natl Acad Sci U S A. 2001;98:8955–60.
38. Davies PF. Hemodynamic shear stress and endothelium in cardiovascular pathophysiology. Nat Clin Pract Cardiovasc Med. 2009;6:16–26.
39. Garcia-Cardena G, et al. Biochemical activation of vascular endothelium as a determinant of its functional phenotype. Proc Natl Acad Sci U S A. 2001;98:4478–85.
40. Fledderus JO. Prolonged shear stress and KLF2 suppress constitutive proinflammatory transcription through inhibition of ATF2. Blood. 2007;109:4249–57.
41. Dekker RJ, van Thienen JV, Rohlena J, de Jager SC, Elderkamp YW, Seppen J, de Vries CJ, Biessen EA, van Berkel TJ, Pannekoek H, Horrevoets AJ. Endothelial KLF2 links local arterial shear stress levels to the expression of vascular tone-regulating genes. Am J Pathol. 2005;167(2):609–18.
42. Dekker RJ, Boon RA, Rondaij MG, Kragt A, Volger OL, Elderkamp YW, Meijers JC, Voorberg J, Pannekoek H, Horrevoets AJ. KLF2 provokes a gene expression pattern that establishes functional quiescent differentiation of the endothelium. Blood. 2006;107(11):4354–63.
43. van Thienen JV, Fledderus JO, Dekker RJ, Rohlena J, van Ijzendoorn GA, Kootstra NA, Pannekoek H, Horrevoets AJ. Shear stress sustains atheroprotective endothelial KLF2 expression more potently than statins through mRNA stabilization. Cardiovasc Res. 2006;72(2):231–4.
44. Wight JP, Chilcott JB, Holmes MW, Brewer N. Pulsatile machine perfusion vs. cold storage of kidneys for transplantation: a rapid and systematic review. Clin Transpl. 2003;17(4):293–307.
45. Moers C, Smits JM, Maathuis MH, Treckmann J, van Gelder F, Napieralski BP, van Kasterop-Kutz M, van der Heide JJ, Squifflet JP, van Heurn E, Kirste GR, Rahmel A, Leuvenink HG, Paul A, Pirenne J, Ploeg RJ. Machine perfusion or cold storage in deceased-donor kidney transplantation. N Engl J Med. 2009;360(1):7–19.
46. Schold JD, Kaplan B, Howard RJ, Reed AI, Foley DP, Meier-Kriesche HU. Are we frozen in time? Analysis of the utilization and efficacy of pulsatile perfusion in renal transplantation. Am J Transplant. 2005;5(7):1681–8.
47. Chueh S-CJ. The benefit of pulsate machine perfusion of standard criteria deceased donor kidney at a geographically remote transplant center. ASAIO J. 2014;60(1):76–80.
48. Ruggenenti P. Ways to boost kidney transplant viability: a real need for the best use of older donors. Am J Transplant. 2006;6:2543–7.
49. Wells AC. Donor kidney disease and transplant outcome for kidney donated after cardiac death. Br J Surg. 2009;96:299–304.
50. Cantafio AW, et al. Risk stratification of kidney from donation after cardiac death donors and the utility of machine perfusion. Clin Transpl. 2011;25:e530–40.
51. Lodhi SA, Lamb KE, Uddin I, Meier-Kriesche HU. Pulsatile pump decreases risk of delayed graft function in kidneys donated after cardiac death. Am J Transplant. 2012;12(10):2774–80.
52. Balfoussia D, et al. Advances in machine perfusion graft viability assessment in kidney, liver, pancreas, lung, and heart transplant. Exp Clin Transplant. 2012;10:87–100.
53. Op den Dries S, et al. Ex vivo normothermic machine perfusion and viability testing of discarded human donor livers. Am J Transplant. 2013;13:1327–35.
54. Maheshwi A, et al. Biliary complications and outcome of liver transplant from donors after cardiac death. Liver Transpl. 2007;13:1645–53.
55. Plaeg RJ, et al. Risk factors for primary dysfunction after liver transplantation-a multivariate analysis. Transplantation. 1993;55:807–13.
56. Guarrera JV, et al. Hypothermic machine perfusion in human liver transplantation: the first clinical series. Am J Transplant. 2010;10:372–81.
57. Slapak M, et al. Twenty-four hours liver preservation by the use of continuous pulsate perfusion and hyperbaric oxygen. Transplantation. 1967;5(s):1154–8.
58. Brettschneider L, et al. The use of combined preservation technique for extended storage of orthotopic liver homografts. Surg Gynecol Obstet. 1968;126:263.
59. Brettschneider L, et al. Experimental and clinical preservation of orthotopic liver homograft. In: Norman J, editor. Organ perfusion and preservation. New York: Allpeton-Century Crofts; 1968. p. 271–84.
60. Kamada N, et al. Orthotopic rat liver transplantation after long-term preservation by continuous perfusion with fluorocarbon emulsion. Transplantation. 1980;30:43–8.
61. Guarrera JV, et al. Hypothermic machine perfusion of liver graft for transplantation: technical development in human discard and miniature swine models. Transplant Proc. 2005;37:323–5.

62. Ingemansson R, Eyjolfsson A, Mared L, et al. Clinical transplantation of initially rejected donor lungs after reconditioning ex vivo. Ann Thorac Surg. 2009;87:255–60.
63. Cypel M, Yeung JC, Liu M, et al. Normothermic ex vivo lung perfusion in clinical lung transplantation. N Engl J Med. 2011;364:1431–40.
64. Mohite P, Sabashnikov A, Garcia Saez D, et al. Utilization of the organ care system lung for the assessment of lungs form a donor after cardiac death (DCD) before bilateral transplantation. Perfusion. 2014;29:1–4.
65. Ciubotaru A, Haverich A. Ex vivo approach to treat failing organs: expanding the limits. Eur Surg Res. 2015;54:64–74.
66. Koerner MM, Ghodsizad A, Schulz U, et al. Normothermic ex vivo allograft blood perfusion in clinical heart transplantation. Heart Surg Forum. 2014;17:E141–5.
67. Mozes MF, Skolek RB, Korf BC. Use of perfusion parameters in predicting outcomes of machine-preserved kidneys. Transplant Proc. 2005;37:350–1.
68. Jochmans I, Moers C, Smits JM, Leuvenink HG, Treckmann J, Paul A, Rahmel A, Squifflet JP, van Heurn E, Monbaliu D, Ploeg RJ, Pirenne J. Machine perfusion versus cold storage for the preservation of kidneys donated after cardiac death: a multicenter, randomized, controlled trial. Ann Surg. 2010;252(5):756–64.
69. de Vries EE, Hoogland ER, Winkens B, Snoeijs MG, van Heurn LW. Renovascular resistance of machine-perfused DCD kidneys is associated with primary nonfunction. Am J Transplant. 2011;11(12):2685–91.
70. Gómez V, Orosa A, Rivera M, Diez-Nicolás V, Hevia V, Alvarez S, Carracedo D, Ramos E, Burgos FJ. Resistance index determination in the pre and post kidney transplantation time points in graft dysfunction diagnosis. Transplant Proc. 2015;47(1):34–7.
71. Paredes-Zapata D, Ruiz-Arranz A, Rodriguez-Villar C, Roque-Arda R, Peri-Cusi L, Saavedra-Escobar S, Vizcaino-Elias F, Garcia-Rodriguez X, Bohils-Valle M, Rodriguez-Peña S, Quijada-Martorell M, Gonzalez-Rodriguez JJ, Oppenheimer-Salinas F, Alcaraz-Asensio A, Adalia-Bartolome R. Does the pulsatile preservation machine have any impact in the discard rate of kidneys from older donors after brain death? Transplant Proc. 2015;47(8):2324–7.
72. Guarrera JV, Goldstein MJ, Samstein B, et al. When good kidneys pump badly: outcomes of deceased donor renal allografts with poor pulsatile perfusion characteristics. Transpl Int. 2010;23:444–6.
73. Weeder PD, van Rijn R, Porte RJ. Machine perfusion in liver transplantation as a tool to prevent non-anastomotic biliary strictures: rationale, current evidence and future directions. J Hepatol. 2015;63:265–75.
74. Steen S, Sjo¨berg T, Pierre L, Liao Q, Eriksson L, Algotsson L. Transplantation of lungs from a non-heart-beating donor. Lancet. 2001;357:825–9.

Part III

Thoracoabdominal Aorta

14 Physiopathology of Intraoperative Visceral Ischemia and Anesthesiological Management of Supravisceral Aortic Clamping

Fabrizio Monaco, Barucco Gaia, Mattioli Cristina, and De Luca Monica

14.1 Introduction

In patients undergoing aortic surgery, visceral ischemia is the leading cause of visceral dysfunction and injury [1, 2]. In fact, acute kidney injury (AKI), spinal cord ischemia (SPCI), and bowel ischemia are catastrophic complications which may occur during surgical procedures involving the supra- and juxta-renal aorta cross-clamping [2, 3]. Because of the fact that the higher the extent of the surgical aortic repair, the greater the risk of organ dysfunction, thoracoabdominal aortic aneurysm open repair (TAAAr) is more prone to developing visceral ischemia than infrarenal abdominal aortic aneurysm [1, 3]. The application of the aortic clamp, decreasing the blood supply to the organs, is associated with extensive physiological changes which may affect patient outcomes. Therefore, it is important for surgeons and anesthesiologists to understand the pathophysiologic changes occurring during aortic cross-clamping in order to mitigate the deleterious effect of ischemia-reperfusion injuries.

14.2 Physiopathology of Intraoperative Visceral Ischemia

Vascular surgery, in which the aorta is clamped proximally to the celiac artery, is one of the few surgical procedures producing ischemia of the liver, bowel, kidneys, spinal cord, and inferior limbs contemporarily. Aortic cross-clamping produces rapid hemodynamic changes and induces ischemic insults. Following the aortic clamp removal, the reperfusion itself may lead to a sudden drop in blood pressure and cellular damage. Therefore, aortic surgery shows double physiological phenomena named ischemia/reperfusion (I/R) injury which is the major determinant of an extensive systemic inflammatory response and the trigger for postoperative multi-organ dysfunction (MODS) [4, 5]. In particular, after aortic clamping in the district distal to the aortic clamp, visceral tissues suffer a sudden decrease of the blood flow with an acute hypoxic insult, shift from an aerobic to an anaerobic metabolism, production of lactate, and development of acidosis [6]. At the same

Electronic Supplementary Material The online version of this chapter (http://doi.org/10.1007/978-3-319-94761-7_14) contains supplementary material, which is available to authorized users.

F. Monaco (✉) · B. Gaia · M. Cristina · D. L. Monica
Department of Cardiothoracic and Vascular Anesthesia and Intensive Care, IRCCS San Raffaele Scientific Institute, Milan, Italy
e-mail: monaco.fabrizio@hsr.it

© Springer Nature Switzerland AG 2019
Y. Tshomba et al. (eds.), *Visceral Vessels and Aortic Repair*,
https://doi.org/10.1007/978-3-319-94761-7_14

time, cellular membranes increase their permeability, leading to cellular swelling [4, 7, 8]. Following aortic clamp removal, the reperfusion of tissue is responsible for additional injuries on the top of ischemia [4–8]. In some instances, the reperfusion damage may exceed the original ischemic injury; in fact, the restoration of the blood flow account for the activation of several inflammatory pathways and biochemical changes [4]. In the I/R syndrome, polymorphonuclear neutrophils, oxygen radicals (ROS), nitric oxide (NO), complement system, and various cytokines play a pivotal role, showing their effects in both re-perfused tissues and distal organs [9, 10]. The re-oxygenation enhances ROS production, which are associated with lipid peroxidation, complement activation, platelet aggregation, white cell activation, suppression of adenosine triphosphate synthesis, and inactivation of metabolic enzymes [10, 11]. Moreover, the ROS leading to the depletion of antioxidant reserves, disruption of cellular and mitochondrial membrane, derangement of intracellular electrolytes boost the phenomenon of apoptosis [12, 13].

A growing body of literature suggests that polymorphonuclear neutrophils play a central role in the pathophysiology of I/R [10]. In fact, the upregulation of adhesion molecules, chemoattractants, chemokines, and integrins due to I/R stimulates the migration of polymorphonuclear neutrophils from the postcapillary venules to the area of inflammation. Polymorphonuclear neutrophils, then, may disrupt the contiguous tissues by the secretion of proteolytic enzymes, production of free radicals, and microcirculation disarrangement [11]. Of note, the oxidative stress and ROS formation reach their peak during the ischemic attack (15–60 min of clamping), while PMN infiltration is at a maximum during reperfusion [10–12].

Notably, the NO has both cytotoxic and cytoprotective effects. In fact, it is an oxygen-free radical scavenger, maintains normal vascular permeability, inhibits the proliferation of smooth muscle, reduces PMN adherence, and decreases platelet aggregation [13]. However the release of large amounts of NO may account for tissue injury, bacterial translocation, mucosal apoptosis, and pulmonary injury [14–16].

The complement, acting together with ROS, NOS, and PNM, increases vascular permeability and tissue edema [17–20]. It elicits a cascade of pro-inflammatory events with release of high concentration of TNF-α and interleukin (IL)-1 [18, 21]. Finally, the occurrence of edema in the interstitium of the injured organ further decreases the oxygen diffusion gradient from the microcirculation to the cells [9].

14.3 Postoperative Effects of Ischemia/Reperfusion Injury

Interestingly, the I/R injury has an effect on both the organs directly affected by the ischemia and the organs not involved in the ischemic insult, by a systemic release of inflammatory mediators [22]. Therefore, it is not surprising that during aortic surgery, along with the bowel and kidney, even the heart, lungs, and spinal cord may suffer I/R damage [4]. When the damage is extensive, multi-organ failure may occur [22, 23]. Each organ and apparatus has a specific sensitivity to I/R insult and deserves specific considerations.

14.3.1 Bowel

Since labile cells are settled at the tips of the villi and supplied by the end of the distribution of a central arteriole, they are much more vulnerable to the ischemia when compared to cells located within the crypts [24]. The various acute-phase proteins, hydrogen peroxide, hormones, and cytokines produced by intestinal mucosa during I/R injury have deleterious effects onto the intestinal microvasculature and may lead to bowel infarction, short-bowel syndrome, systemic inflammatory response syndrome, acute respiratory distress syndrome, and MOF [25]. Moreover, the impairment of the mucosal barrier allows the release in the systemic circulation of the endotoxin which induces the systemic activation of PMN, complement, and clotting pathways and further increase of the mucosal permeability [26].

14.3.2 Kidney

Acute renal failure (AKI) during aortic surgery is multifactorial and it may occur as a result of I/R damage, hemodynamic changes, bleeding, acute heart failure, and cytotoxic agents [27–36]. The level at which the aortic clamp is applied affects the renal perfusion [37]. In fact, it decreases by 80% in the event of the suprarenal aortic cross-clamping, while it decreases by 45% when the aortic clamp is infrarenal [38]. To counteract the decrease of the renal blood flow, an increase of the renal vascular resistance is mediated by the hormone angiotensin II which redistributes the blood flow away from renal medulla and cortex, significantly decreasing renal perfusion [28, 39]. This effect persists after aortic clamp removal, despite a normal mean perfusion pressure [40]. Similarly, the glomerular filtration rate and renal blood flow may remain impaired for a long period of time after the surgery [31]. Besides this, ROS, complement, IL-1, IL 6, and IL8 released by the damaged mesangial cells increase the local inflammation worsening the renal function [41].

14.3.3 Heart

Aortic surgery is associated with the highest risk of myocardial infarction and cardiovascular complications compared to other noncardiac-related surgeries [42, 43]. The reasons for that include the increase of afterload and preload associated with the aortic cross-clamp, massive bleeding with consequent volume shift, and inflammatory response following I/R injury of abdominal organs [22]. Several authors have proposed that IL-2, IL-1β, IL-6, IFN-γ, and TNF-α may affect the cardiac function [44]. In I/R injury of the heart, the NO is probably involved in the decrease of ventricular compliance [4]. The activation of the NO synthesis leads to higher NO concentration which significantly affects the cardiac adrenergic and cholinergic stimulation [4]. A ventricle with low compliance is "difficult to fill," and it is associated with lower cardiac output and impairment of the coronary blood flow due to a decrease in the aortocoronary pressure gradient. Moreover, the ROS released from the injured myocytes and endothelial cells promotes membrane damage, endothelial injury, and vessel permeability [45, 46]. The treatment of the diastolic dysfunction is challenging: in fact, the administration of exogenous inotropes/vasopressors may further decrease a microcirculation already impaired by the endothelial swelling, exacerbating the ischemic damage [46]. In addition, activation of the coagulation cascade, formation of microthrombi, platelet aggregation stimulated by the use of vasopressors, and accumulation of reactive neutrophils act together impairing the microcirculation and decreasing the myocardial perfusion [47].

14.3.4 Lungs

The respiratory function after aortic surgery is commonly impaired. While in the vast majority of cases, damage is moderate with nonsignificant clinical manifestations; in several circumstances, it may be part of MOF [22]. Since in a physiological state the pulmonary vasculature is a neutrophil reserve, the respiratory system is at the highest risk of developing an inflammatory response during aortic surgery [11]. In fact, it is particularly sensitive to the circulating cytokines released from several organs during the postoperative period [48]. The I/R damage releases "per se" cytokines, which activate the pulmonary endothelium, stimulate the leucocytes migration into the interstitial and alveolar space, and promote inflammation [22]. Similarly, the anaphylatoxins C3a and C5a play a role in increasing the pulmonary vascular tone, favoring capillary leakage, and activating the mast cells which release histamine [49, 50]. The most severe clinical respiratory manifestation of this "vicious circle" is the acute respiratory distress syndrome which is associated with refractory hypoxia and death in a high percentage of patients [51].

14.3.5 Spinal Cord

Spinal cord ischemia is one of the most dreadful complications in aortic surgery [1–3]. The abrupt interruption of the blood flow to the spinal cord leads to ischemic injury [52–56]. Even when the thoracic aorta is not involved (abdominal aorta aneurysm open repair), a profound shock may impair the medulla perfusion pressure causing SCI [53]. The pathogenesis includes oxygen-free radical-induced lipid peroxidation, intracellular calcium overload, leukocyte activation, inflammatory response, and neuronal apoptosis. All these factors acting together cause the disruption of the blood-spinal cord barrier, which in turn exacerbates the spinal cord edema, increases the leukocyte infiltration, and amplifies inflammation and oxidative stress [57].

14.4 Anesthesiological Management of Supravisceral Aortic Clamping

Given the complexity of the physiopathology of the visceral ischemia in procedures involving supravisceral aortic clamping, the aim of the anesthesiological management is to avoid the hemodynamic fluctuations which may induce irreversible damage to organs and apparatus.

14.5 Hemodynamic Response to Cross-Clamping

Generally speaking, the higher the location of the aortic clamp, the greater the increase of the afterload against which the heart has to work [58]. The immediate effect of aortic clamping is a rapid increase of blood pressure due to an increase in systemic vascular resistance (SVR) [58, 59] (Fig. 14.1). Reasons for that are higher impedance to aortic flow, increased venous return (preload) from the viscera, and release of catecholamines and angiotensin [6, 58–62]. In particular, in the event of supraceliac aortic clamping, a rapid decrease of venous capacity in the splanchnic district is associated with a blood volume shift proximal to the clamp site [63]. When the aortic clamp is infra-celiac, the increase of preload is directly related to the splanchnic venous tone: with a lower preload when the venous tone is low and higher preload if the venous tone is higher [38, 63]. The consequence of the increase of afterload and preload is the improvement in contractility [59]. The increase of the left ventricular end-diastolic pressure, following the increase in arterial blood pressure, leads to a transitory subendocardial ischemia which triggers the augmentation of the coronary blood flow toward the endocardia (Anrep effects) [64]. The effect is an increase of contractility and then of cardiac output [65]. On the contrary, patients with low coronary reserve, due to coronary artery disease, fail to respond to the subendocardial ischemia with an increase of the coronary flow leading to subendocardial ischemia and low cardiac output. In this case, vasodilators may improve the Anrep effect, increasing coronary blood flow and reducing, at the same time, pre- and afterload [66]. When a distal perfusion technique is not provided and an aortic clamp is present, the perfusion of the vital tissues distal to the aortic clamp is provided by collateral vessels and depends upon the proximal perfusion pressure [62]. Thus, hypotension should be avoided as much as possible [62, 66, 67].

When the aortic clamp is released, the rapid decrease in vascular resistance produces hypotension. Reperfusion of previous ischemic tissues which are vasodilated for the effect of hypercapnia, acidosis, and high concentration of adenosine and lactate [58] leads to central hypovolemia. Furthermore, the washout into the systemic circulation of myocardial depressant metabolites from ischemic area is associated with further vasodilation and decrease in cardiac output [59] (Fig. 14.2).

Following aortic clamp removal, a transient increase in CO_2 is commonly observed due to both CO_2 washout from the ischemic tissues into the systemic circulation and increased CO_2

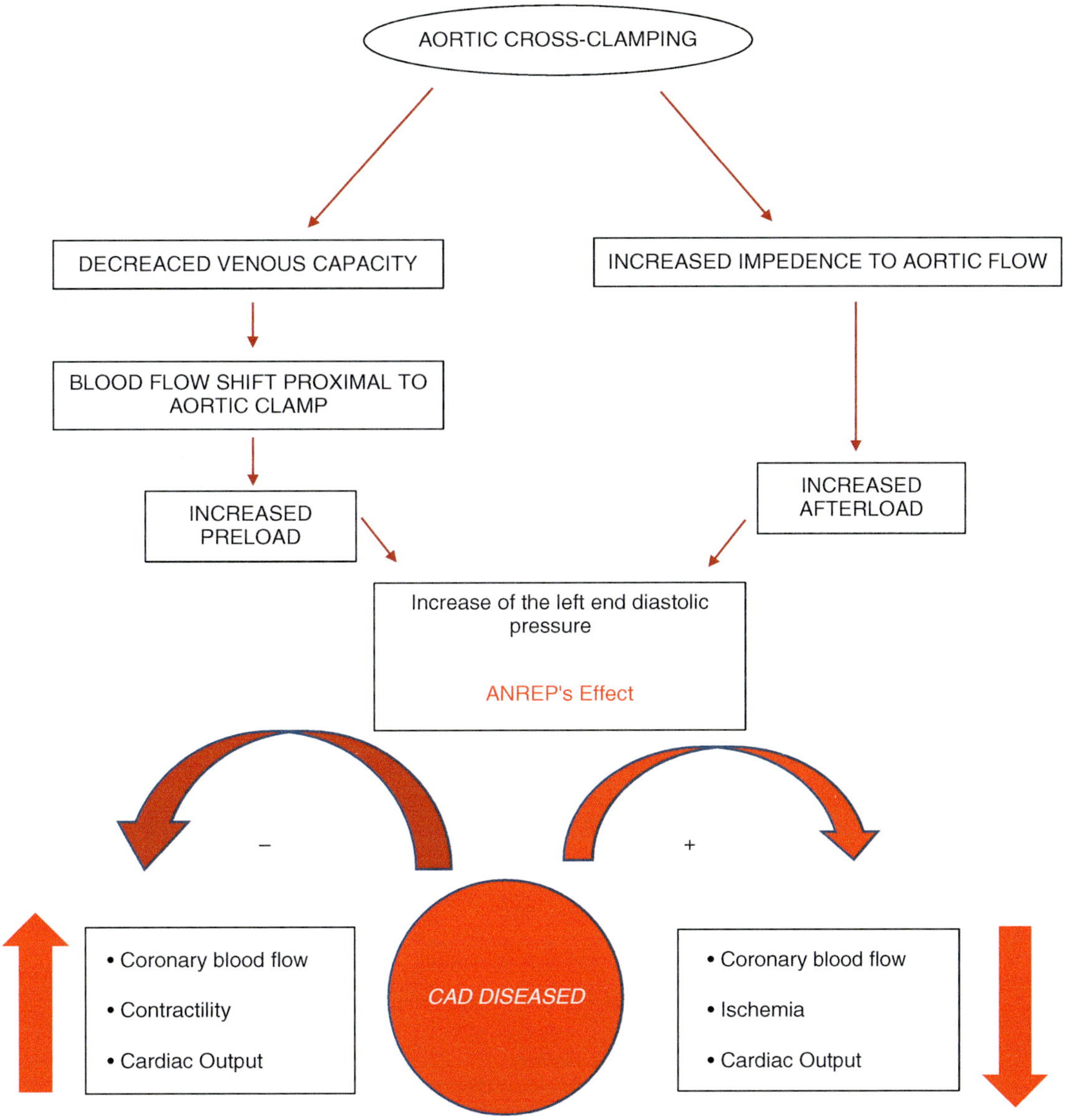

Fig. 14.1 Hemodynamic response to aortic cross-clamping

production secondary to increased oxygen consumption of the re-perfused tissues [58, 59]. Carbon dioxide causes further vasodilation [68].

Hypotension after aortic cross-clamp release can be prevented and treated with volume loading, infusion of vasoactive medications, prompt treatment of metabolic abnormalities, and gradual release of aortic cross-clamp. In this dynamic setting, the anesthesiologist has to continuously assess the patient's global hemodynamic status, integrating cardiac function, intravascular volumes (estimated from transesophageal echocardiography, filling pressures, or both), blood loss, and the total amount of fluid administered [59, 60]. Moreover, adequate tissue perfusion is based on the availability of oxygen delivered. In situations where the blood flow is suboptimal, an arterial oxygen saturation as high as possible and a hemoglobin concentration above 10 g/dL are mandatory [69].

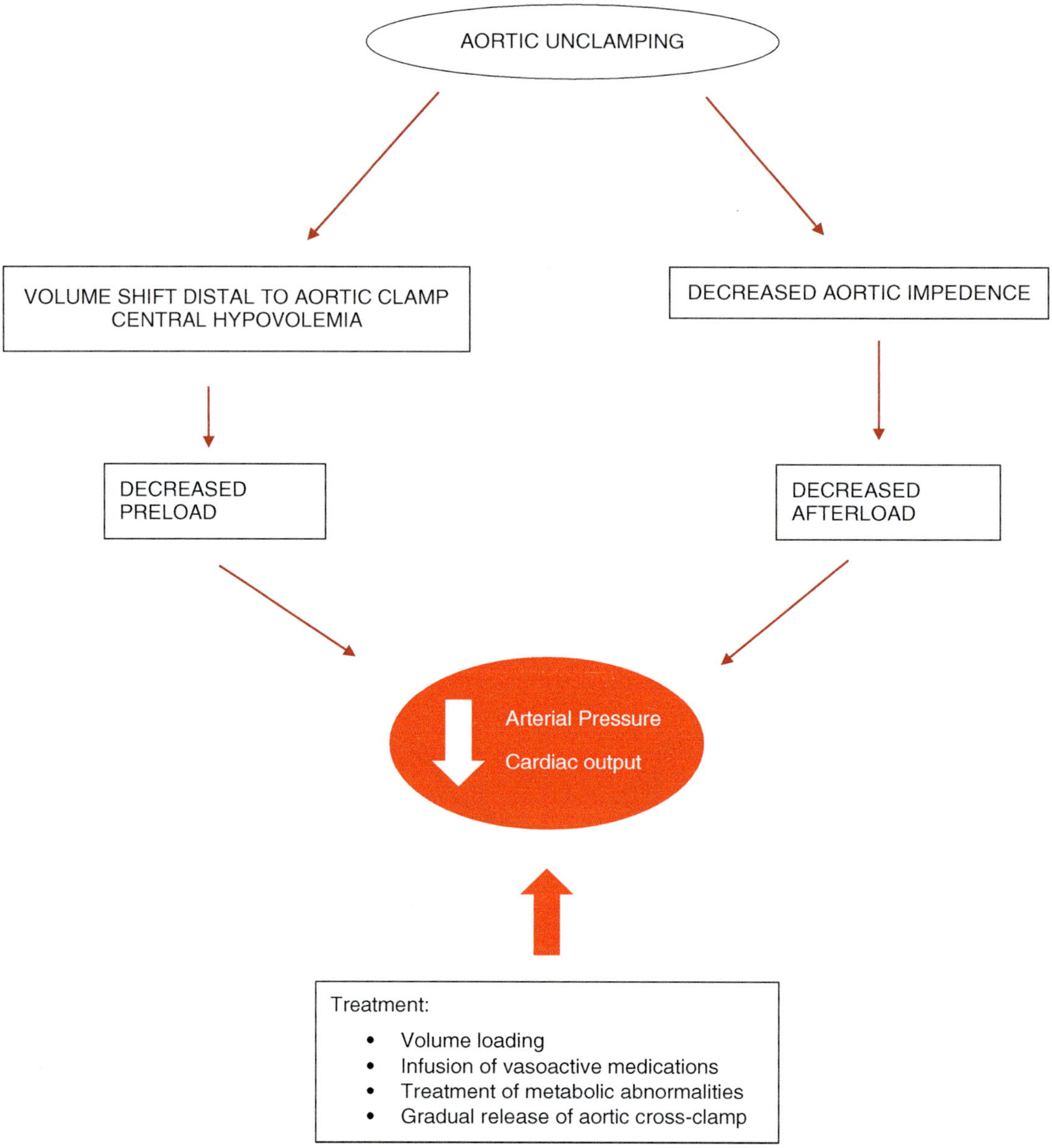

Fig. 14.2 Hemodynamic response to aortic unclamping

14.6 The Distal Perfusion Technique as a Strategy to Prevent Visceral Ischemia

Cross-clamping of the descending thoracic aorta produces visceral, spinal cord, kidney, bowel, and limb ischemia and is also challenging for the heart due to an abrupt increase of the pre- and afterload. In order to prevent and mitigate the consequences of visceral ischemia, several pharmacological and mechanical strategies have been proposed [70]. To date, distal organ perfusion is universally recognized as the best technique to limit ischemic injury in the organs distal to the clamp site, to support the heart, and to control proximal hypertension during thoracoabdominal aneurysm open repair [71, 72]. Distal perfusion may be performed by partial cardiopulmonary bypass (CPBP), left bypass (LBP), or left heart bypass (LHBP). Among these, LHBP is

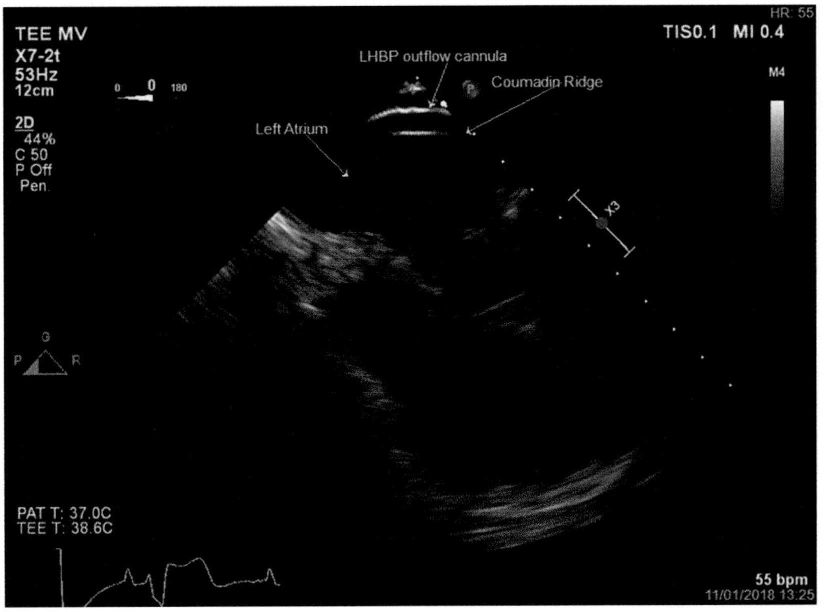

Fig. 14.3 Transesophageal echocardiography. Off-axis view of the outflow cannula joining the left atrium by the inferior left pulmonary vein

associated with a low risk of bleeding due to a mild heparinization [73]. Briefly, the basic circuit for LHBP is composed by an inflow cannula, a centrifugal pump, and an outflow cannula. In the left heart bypass (LHBP), the inflow cannula is placed in the pulmonary vein or left atrial appendage (Fig. 14.3), while the outflow cannula is positioned in the distal aorta or the femoral artery [74]. During the surgical anastomosis of the visceral vessels, perfusion of the abdominal organs is usually guaranteed by a selective catheterization of individual arteries [75, 76]. A flow of 200–300 mL/min of normothermic oxygenated blood for each catheter maintains a visceral perfusion pressure around 70 mmHg. The kidneys are perfused by cold crystalloids or cold Custodiol. Several studies have reported that a cold Ringer lactate solution is superior to normothermic oxygenated blood in terms of prevention of renal dysfunction during selective renal artery perfusion and supraceliac aortic cross-clamp [77–79]. Moreover, Tshomba et al. observed that in patients undergoing TAAA open repair, a selective renal perfusion with histidine-tryptophan-ketoglutarate solution (Custodiol; Dr. Franz-Kohler Chemie GmbH, Bensheim, Germany) significantly decreases the incidence of postoperative renal failure when compared with cold Ringer lactate [80].

There is no agreement on which is an adequate distal perfusion pressure when the LHBP is used. Some authors, for instance, suggest that a flow as high as 40 mL/kg/min is adequate to guarantee an optimal distal perfusion. On the contrary, others report that a flow ranging between 1.5 and 3 L/min with a mean femoral artery pressure of 70 mmHg can be considered sufficient for organ perfusion [81]. As practical rule, during aortic cross-clamping, a distal aortic pressure above 70 mmHg and a proximal perfusion pressure above 90 mmHg can be considered optimal for organ and spinal cord perfusion. Further indices of optimal organs perfusion are renal output above 1 mL/kg/h without diuretics and no lactate production [61].

14.7 Strategy to Prevent Postoperative Organ Dysfunction in Visceral Ischemia

Although the distal perfusion technique mitigates the effects of visceral ischemia, postoperative complications due to organ hypoperfusion remain relatively high [1–4]. Several strategies have shown to be effective in mitigating organ ischemia following aortic clamp.

14.7.1 Renal Protection

Postoperative acute kidney injury (AKI) after vascular surgery is a major cause of morbidity and mortality [33, 82]. The etiology of renal failure in the setting of vascular surgery is multifactorial [83]. Ischemic injury (clamp time), nephrotoxic agents (antibiotics, anesthetic agent, contrast media, diuretics, myoglobin), and pre-existing renal failure are major factors related to the development of acute renal failure after aortic surgery [31, 34, 83–85]. In light of this, the avoidance of nephrotoxic insult, prevention of renal hypoperfusion by adequate cardiac output, and MAP have recently been reported as the only measures effective in decreasing the incidence of AKI [86–88]. On the contrary, the use of drugs such as dopamine and fenoldopam is not able to prevent perioperative renal dysfunction [89–91]. Since methylprednisolone, at a dosage of 30 mg/kg, may be a scavenger of free radicals with immunomodulatory proprieties, some authors have postulated that its administration may prevent renal ischemia/reperfusion injury [92–95]. Unfortunately, the results are elusive [96]. Even mannitol (0.5 g/kg), which theoretically has a favorable profile in terms of renal failure prevention due to the induction of osmotic diuresis, the prevention of tubular obstruction, the decrease of epithelial and endothelial cell swelling, the action of free radical scavenger, and the stimulation of the synthesis of intrarenal prostaglandin with a renal vasodilation effect, has shown to be ineffective in preventing AKI [86, 97]. Moreover side effects such as volume depletion and an increased medullary consumption of O_2 are very well known and may have a detrimental impact on renal function [98].

14.7.2 Spinal Cord Protection

Paraplegia caused by ischemic spinal cord injury is a devastating potential complication of aortic surgery [1, 99, 100]. Patients with SCI have poorer long-term survival compared to those who do not [1]. The position of aortic cross-clamping may affect the spinal cord perfusion, with the highest risk during extent II repair (7–10%) and the lowest risk in extent IV (1%) [1, 54, 55]. During surgery, the maintenance of a spinal cord perfusion pressure (SCPP) above 80 mmHG may prevent the development of paraplegia [101, 102]. Notably, the SCPP is the difference between the MAP and the cerebrospinal fluid (CSF) pressure. Interestingly, CSF pressure is influenced by the central venous pressure (CVP). After surgical occlusion of the spinal arteries, the perfusion of the spinal cord depends on the collateral network fed by hypogastric arteries, internal thoracic arteries, and branches from the subclavian arteries. The SCPP is a balance between the driving pressure affected by MAP, cardiac output, and blood volume and outflow pressure which depends on CSF and venous pressure. An increased CVP is associated with higher pressure in the extensive vertebral venous and impairment of spinal cord outflow. For the reasons mentioned above, the use of LHB, inotropes, and vasopressor, acting on the MAP and CVP, prevents paraplegia. The use of CSF drainage has been shown to decrease the risk of paraplegia reducing the CSFP [103]. In a large randomized controlled clinical trial the CSF drainage strategy in patients undergoing TAAA open surgery has shown an 80% decrease of postoperative paraplegia rate [104]. Recently Tshomba et al. observed that the use of the LiquoGuard automated device (Möller Medical GmbH, Fulda, Germany) during TAAA open repair is safe and effective in maintaining the desired CSF pressure values with a significant reduction in complication rates when compared with a standard catheter connected to a dripping chamber [105].

Somatosensory-evoked potentials are used to monitor the integrity of the posterior (sensory) spinal cord, and motor-evoked potentials (MEPs) are used to monitor dysfunction of the anterior (motor) spinal cord, detecting the spinal cord ischemia during the surgery [106–108]. Hypothermia has protective effects on the spinal cord and central nervous system by reducing both metabolic rate and oxygen requirement [109, 110].

14.7.3 Heart

Aortic surgery is a deeming procedure for the heart due to aortic clamp and large volume shift. Since the driving pressure for organs and apparatus depends on the native cardiac performance, it is crucial to optimize preload, afterload, and contractility. In light of this, TEE is an invaluable tool allowing for quick diagnosis and guiding the use of inotropes/vasopressors [111, 112]. Markers of right ventricle dysfunction are CVP over 12 mmHg, tricuspid annular plane systolic excursion below 16 mm, tissue Doppler index below 10 cm/s, right mid-cavity diameter above 42 mm, and longitudinal diameter longer than 9.2 mm (Figs. 14.4–14.6). With pressure or volume overload, the septum becomes flat and the LV assumes a D shape at the end of the systole or diastole, respectively (Videos 14.1 and 14.2). The RV is particularly sensitive to the increase of the pulmonary vascular resistance secondary to hypercapnia, hypoxia, acidosis, protamine and blood transfusion, and reduction of the pulmonary vascular bed, commonly observed during single-lung ventilation. Therefore, the first-line treatment of the right ventricular dysfunction is gas exchange optimization with high FiO2, moderate hyperventilation, and alkalization (pH > 7.40). Central venous pressure above 15 mmHg affecting SCPP should be treated with aggressive diuretic therapy. For moderate RV dysfunction, dobutamine is the drug of choice, while epinephrine is indicated in the event of poor RV contractility with hypotension associated (or not) to left ventricular failure. When RV failure coexists with low systemic vascular resistance, norepinephrine is effective in maintaining coronary perfusion pressure.

Markers of left ventricle dysfunction are wedge pressure above 15 mmHg, ejection fraction below 50%, and left ventricular outflow tract velocity time integral below 20 cm/s with good RV function. In transgastric midpapillary short-axis view, the TEE allow to identify whether the hypotension depends on low preload (papillary kissing) or poor contractility (increase end-diastolic diameter) (Videos 14.3 and 14.4). Poor contractility is managed with epinephrine or dobutamine. Mean arterial pressure is a critical factor, and it is not unusual to observe a significantly altered ST segment and regional wall motion abnormalities with low MAP that become almost normal with adequate systemic perfusion pressure. When the increased afterload is associated with a systolic ventricular dysfunction, "inodilators" are suggested,

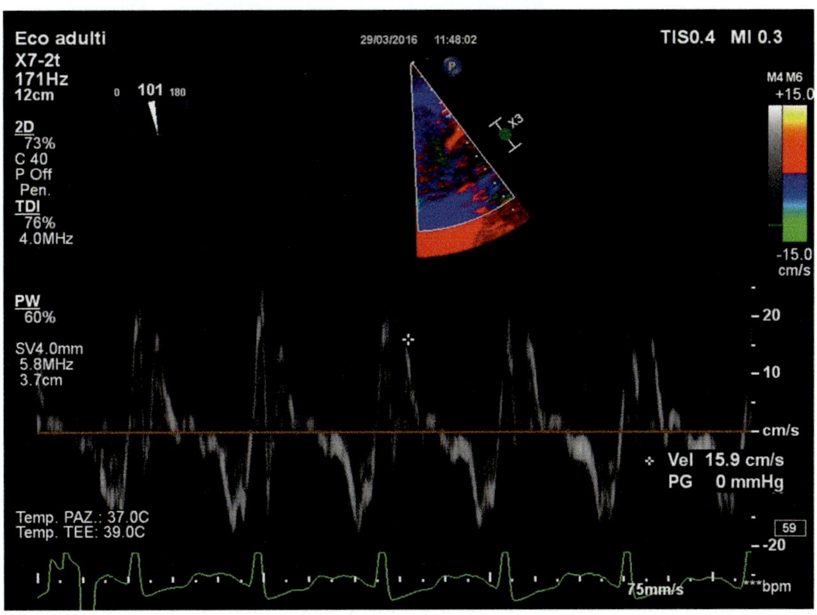

Fig. 14.4 Tissue Doppler index of the right ventricle. A value above 10 cm/s is normal under general anesthesia

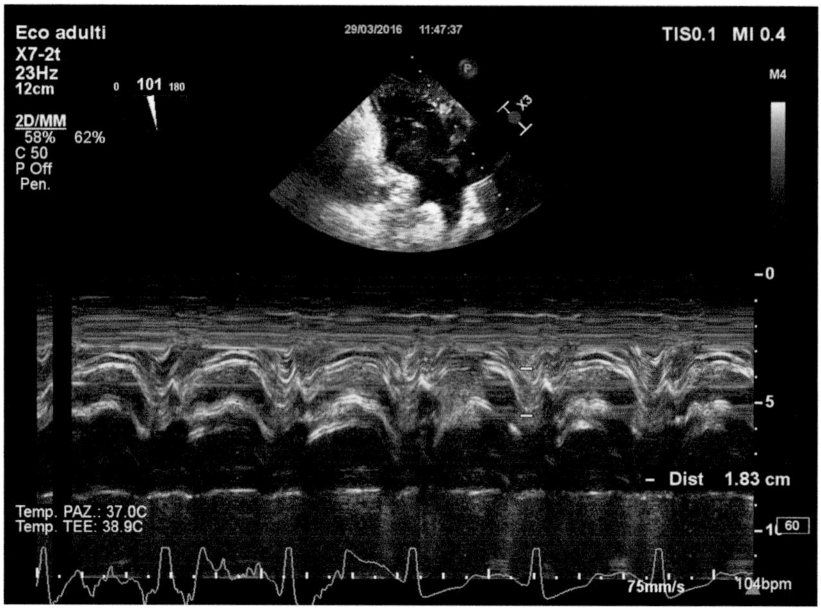

Fig. 14.5 Tricuspid annular plane systolic excursion. A value above 16 mm is normal under general anesthesia

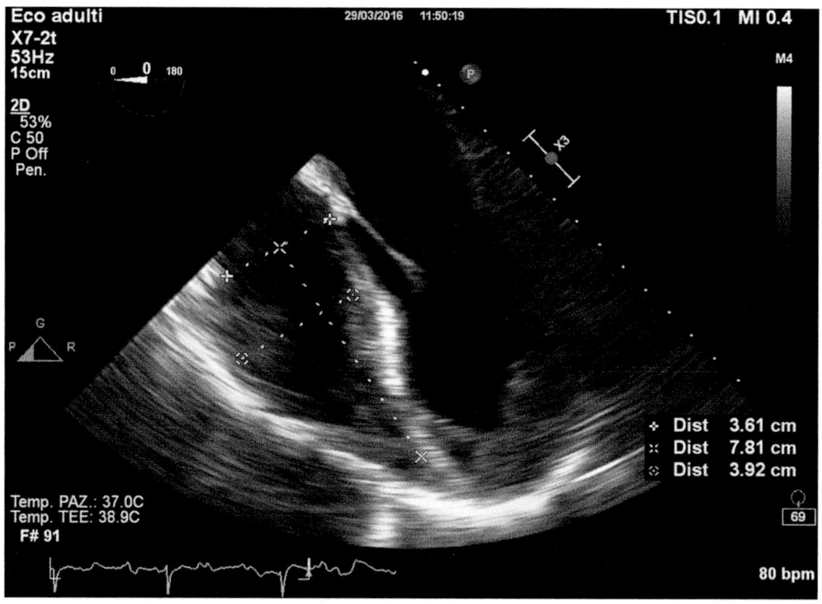

Fig. 14.6 Transesophageal echocardiography. In the midesophageal four-chamber view, the diameters of the right ventricle are best assessed

while with an almost normal systolic contraction brief, acting vasodilator drugs (nitroglycerine) are recommended. As proximal aortic hypotension compromises the perfusion to collateral-dependent tissue beds distal to the aortic clamp, the use of short-term drugs are recommended. Short-acting beta-blockers are preferred agents when a hypertensive episode is associated with tachycardia.

14.7.4 Abdominal Viscera

Surgical occlusion by aortic clamp of the celiac axis and superior and inferior mesenteric leads to hypoxia of the abdominal viscera. The clamping time plays a pivotal role in the development of visceral ischemia, and the adoption of the selective perfusions of the visceral arteries with warm blood mitigates this phenomenon [78]. Even a transitory period of bowel ischemia, affecting the mucosal integrity, promotes the translocation of intestinal bacteria into the circulation promoting systemic infection and sepsis.

With the aortic clamp release, the washout of both the endotoxins produced by intestinal bacteria and the cardio-depressant metabolites from the ischemic area contributes to the systemic vasodilation and hemodynamic instability observed after visceral reperfusion [16]. Therefore, acid-base alterations occurring throughout the surgery should be promptly treated even by the administration of sodium bicarbonate.

In addition, visceral ischemia may be associated with systemic coagulopathy due to increased intestinal permeability, bacterial translocation, hepatic ischemia, and primary fibrinolysis. Therefore, the use of antifibrinolytic such as tranexamic acid or aminocaproic acid is strongly suggested [18].

14.7.5 Lungs

Postoperative pulmonary complications are common after aortic surgery [1, 3]. In addition to surgical trauma, diaphragm incision, and need of the one-lung ventilation (OLA), lung manipulation, blood transfusion, and fluid overload are very well-recognized risk factors. Furthermore, preoperative risk factors, such as COPD and history of smoking, significantly increase the chance of postoperative lung dysfunction. With this in mind, the adoption of a “protective ventilation” with low tidal volume, higher levels of positive end-expiratory pressure, and low plateau pressure is able to decrease the occurrence of acute lung injury [113]. However during the OLV, the priority is to guarantee oxygen saturation above 90%. A drop in oxygen saturation may lead to a significant decrease in the delivery oxygen with relative tissue hypoxia. A parsimoniously administration of blood products contributes to decreasing the risk of transfusion-related acute lung injury and transfusion-related immune modulation. To avoid large-volume transfusion, a ROTEM-guided protocol may be useful. Further studies are needed to confirm this data.

14.8 Conclusion

Visceral ischemia during supraceliac aortic cross-clamp is a multifactorial complex syndrome associated with an increased risk of developing severe postoperative organ dysfunction, requiring therefore an extensive and detailed anesthesiological and surgical workup. Often, visceral ischemia is devious, and only a prompt treatment may avoid severe postoperative complications. For all these reasons, adequate preoperative assessment and risk stratification, a skillful anesthetic technique, a meticulous intraoperative monitoring, and an appropriate postoperative course are all necessary measures to guarantee an uneventful procedure and avoid potentially fatal complications.

References

1. Coselli JS, LeMaire SA, Preventza O, de la Cruz KI, Cooley DA, Price MD, Stolz AP, Green SY, Arredondo CN, Rosengart TK. Outcomes of 3309 thoracoabdominal aortic aneurysm repairs. J Thorac Cardiovasc Surg. 2016;151(5):1323–37.
2. Crawford ES. Thoraco-abdominal and abdominal aortic aneurysms involving renal, superior mesenteric, celiac arteries. Ann Surg. 1974;179:763–72.
3. Deery S, Lancaster R, Baril D, Indes J, Bertges D, Conrad M, Cambria R, Patel V. Contemporary outcomes of open complex abdominal aortic aneurysm repair. J Vasc Surg. 2016;63(5): 1195–200.
4. Katseni K, Chalkias A, Kotsis T, Dafnios N, Arapoglou V, Kaparos G, Logothetis E, Iacovidou N, Karvouni E, Katsenis K. The effect of perioperative ischemia and reperfusion on multiorgan dysfunction following abdominal aortic aneurysm repair. Biomed Res Int. 2015;2015:598980.
5. Welborn MB, Oldenburg HS, Hess PJ, Huber TS, Martin TD, Rauwerda JA, Wesdorp RI, Espat NJ, Copeland EM 3rd, Moldawer LL, Seeger JM. The relationship between visceral ischemia, proinflammatory cytokines, and organ injury in patients undergoing thoracoabdominal aortic aneurysm repair. Crit Care Med. 2000;28(9):3191–7.
6. Eide TO, Aasland J, Romundstad P, Stenseth R, Saether OD, Aadahl P, Myhre HO. Changes in hemodynamics and acid-base balance during cross-clamping of the descending thoracic aorta: a study in patients operated on for thoracic and thoracoabdominal aortic aneurysm. Eur Surg Res. 2005;37(6):330–4.

7. Norwood MGA, Bown MJ, Sayers RD. Ischaemia/reperfusion injury and regional inflammatory responses in abdominal aortic aneurysm repair. Eur J Vasc Endovasc Surg. 2004;28(3):234–45.
8. Lindsay TF, Luo XP, Lehotay DC, et al. Ruptured abdominal aortic aneurysm, a 'two-hit' ischemia/reperfusion injury: evidence from an analysis of oxidative products. J Vasc Surg. 1999;30(2):219–28.
9. Carden DL, Granger DN. Pathophysiology of ischaemia–reperfusion injury. J Pathol. 2000;190:255–66.
10. Aivatidi C, Vourliotakis G, Georgopoulos S, Sigala F, Bastounis E, Papalambros E. Oxidative stress during abdominal aortic aneurysm repair—biomarkers and antioxidant's protective effect: a review. Eur Rev Med Pharmacol Sci. 2011;15(3):245–52.
11. Barry MC, Kelly C, Burke P, Sheehan S, Redmond HP, Bouchier-Hayes D. Immunological and physiological responses to aortic surgery: effect of reperfusion on neutrophil and monocyte activation and pulmonary function. Br J Surg. 1997;84(4):513–9.
12. Galle C, De Maertelaer V, Motte S, et al. Early inflammatory response after elective abdominal aortic aneurysm repair: a comparison between endovascular procedure and conventional surgery. J Vasc Surg. 2000;32(2):234–46.
13. Thompson MM, Nasim A, Sayers RD, Thompson J, Smith G, Lunec J, Bell PR. Oxygen free radical and cytokine generation during endovascular and conventional aneurysm repair. Eur J Vasc Endovasc Surg. 1996;12(1):70–5.
14. Lefer AM, Lefer DJ. The role of nitric oxide and cell adhesion molecules on the microcirculation in ischaemia-reperfusion. Cardiovasc Res. 1996;32(4):743–51.
15. Kubes P, McCafferty DM. Nitric oxide and intestinal inflammation. Am J Med. 2000;109(2):150–8.
16. Suzuki Y, Deitch EA, Mishima S, Lu Q, Xu DZ. Inducible nitric oxide synthase gene knockout mice have increased resistance to gut injury and bacterial translocation after an intestinal ischemia-reperfusion injury. Crit Care Med. 2000;28:3692–6.
17. Ziegenfuß T, Wanner GA, Grass C, et al. Mixed agonistic-antagonistic cytokine response in whole blood from patients undergoing abdominal aortic aneurysm repair. Intensive Care Med. 1999;25(3):279–87.
18. Holzheimer RG, Gross J, Schein M. Pro- and anti-inflammatory cytokine-response in abdominal aortic aneurysm repair: a clinical model of ischemia-reperfusion. Shock. 1999;11(5):305–10.
19. Heller T, Hennecke M, Baumann U, et al. Selection of a C5a receptor antagonist from phage libraries attenuating the inflammatory response in immune complex disease and ischemia/reperfusion injury. J Immunol. 1999;163(2):985–94.
20. Kimura T, Andoh A, Fujiyama Y, Saotome T, Bamba T. A blockade of complement activation prevents rapid intestinal ischaemia-reperfusion injury by modulating mucosal mast cell degranulation in rats. Clin Exp Immunol. 1998;111(3):484–90.
21. Wada K, Montalto MC, Stahl GL. Inhibition of complement C5 reduces local and remote organ injury after intestinal ischemia/reperfusion in the rat. Gastroenterology. 2001;120(1):126–33.
22. Bown MJ, Nicholson ML, Bell PRF, Sayers RD. Cytokines and inflammatory pathways in the pathogenesis of multiple organ failure following abdominal aortic aneurysm repair. Eur J Vasc Endovasc Surg. 2001;22(6):485–95.
23. Maziak DE, et al. The impact of multiple organ dysfunction on mortality following ruptured abdominal aortic aneurysm repair. Ann Vasc Surg. 1998;12(2):93–100.
24. Mallick IH, Yang W, Winslet MC, Seifalian AM. Ischemia-reperfusion injury of the intestine and protective strategies against injury. Dig Dis Sci. 2004;49(9):1359–77.
25. Molmenti EP, Ziambaras T, Perlmutter DH. Evidence for an acute phase response in human intestinal epithelial cells. J Biol Chem. 1993;268(19):14116–24.
26. Soong CV, Blair PH, Halliday MI, McCaigue MD, Campbell GR, Hood JM, Rowlands BJ, Barros D'Sa AA. Endotoxaemia, the generation of the cytokines and their relationship to intramucosal acidosis of the sigmoid colon in elective abdominal aortic aneurysm repair. Eur J Vasc Surg. 1993;7(5):534–9.
27. Black SA, Brooks MJ, Naidoo MN, Wolfe JHN. Assessing the impact of renal impairment on outcome after arterial intervention: a prospective review of 1559 patients. Eur J Vasc Endovasc Surg. 2007;32:300–4.
28. Wahlberg E, Dimuzio PJ, Stoney RJ. Aortic clamping during elective operations for infrarenal disease: the influence of clamping time on renal function. J Vasc Surg. 2002;36:13–8.
29. Kudo FA, Nishibe T, Miyazaki K, et al. Postoperative renal function after elective abdominal aortic aneurysm repair requiring suprarenal aortic cross-clamping. Surg Today. 2004;34:1010–3.
30. Powell RJ, Roddy SP, Meier GH, et al. Effect of renal insufficiency on outcome following infrarenal aortic surgery. Am J Surg. 1997;174:126–30.
31. Dariane C, Coscas R, Boulitrop C, Javerliat I, Vilaine E, Goeau-Brissonniere O, et al. Acute kidney injury after open repair of intact abdominal aortic aneurysms. Ann Vasc Surg. 2017;39:294–300.
32. Drews JD, Patel HJ, Williams DM, Dasika NL, Deeb GM. The impact of acute renal failure on early and late outcomes after thoracic aortic endovascular repair. Ann Thorac Surg. 2014;97(6):2027–33.
33. Jalalzadeh H, Indrakusuma R, Vogt L, van Beek SC, Vahl AC, Wisselink W, et al. Long-term survival after acute kidney injury following ruptured abdominal aortic aneurysm repair. J Vasc Surg. 2017;66(6):1712–8.
34. Kopolovic I, Simmonds K, Duggan S, Ewanchuk M, Stollery DE, Bagshaw SM, et al. Risk factors

and outcomes associated with acute kidney injury following ruptured abdominal aortic aneurysm. BMC Nephrol. 2013;14(1):99.
35. Safi HJ, Harlin SA, Miller CC, et al. Predictive factors for acute renal failure in thoracic and thoracoabdominal aortic aneurysm surgery. J Vasc Surg. 1996;24:338–44.
36. Breckwoldt WL, Mackey WC, Belkin M, O'Donnell TF Jr. The effect of suprarenal cross-clamping on abdominal aortic aneurysm repair. Arch Surg. 1992;127(5):520–4.
37. Chong T, Nguyen L, Owens CD, Conte MS, Belkin M. Suprarenal aortic cross-clamp position: a reappraisal of its effects on outcomes for open abdominal aortic aneurysm repair. J Vasc Surg. 2009;49:873–80.
38. Giulini SM, Bonardelli S, Portolani N, Giovanetti M, Galvani G, Maffeis R, Coniglio A, Tiberio GA, Nodari F, De Lucia M, Lussardi L, Regina P, Scolari F, Tomasoni GSM. Suprarenal aortic cross-clamping in elective abdominal aortic aneurysm surgery. Eur J Vasc Endovasc Surg. 2000;20:286–9.
39. Rothenbach P, Turnage RH, Iglesias J, Riva A, Bartula L, Myers SI. Downstream effects of splanchnic ischemia-reperfusion injury on renal function and eicosanoid release. J Appl Physiol. 1997;82:530–6.
40. Myers SI, Wang L, Liu F, Bartula LL. Suprarenal aortic clamping and reperfusion decreases medullary and cortical blood flow by decreased endogenous renal nitric oxide and PGE2 synthesis. J Vasc Surg. 2005;42(3):524–31.
41. Laufer J, Oren R, Farzam N, Goldberg I, Passwell J. Differential cytokine regulation of complement proteins in human glomerular epithelial cells. Nephron. 1997;76(3):276–83.
42. Schouten O, Sillesen H, Poldermans D. New guidelines from the European society of cardiology for perioperative cardiac care: a summary of implications for elective vascular surgery patients. Eur J Vasc Endovasc Surg. 2010;39:1–4.
43. Abraham N, Lemech L, Sandroussi C, et al. A prospective study of subclinical myocardial damage in endovascular versus open repair of infrarenal abdominal aortic aneurysms. J Vasc Surg. 2005;41:377–80.
44. Kelly RA, Smith TW. Cytokines and cardiac contractile function. Circulation. 1997;95:778–81.
45. Garcia-Dorado D, Oliveras J. Myocardial oedema: a preventable cause of reperfusion injury? Cardiovasc Res. 1993;27:1555–63.
46. Park JL, Lucchesi BR. Mechanisms of myocardial reperfusion injury. Ann Thorac Surg. 1999;68(5):1905–12.
47. Böttiger BW, Motsch J, Böhrer H, Böker T, Aulmann M, Nawroth PP, Martin E. Activation of blood coagulation after cardiac arrest is not balanced adequately by activation of endogenous fibrinolysis. Circulation. 1995;92:2572–8.
48. Paterson IS, Smith FC, Tsang GM, Hamer JD, Shearman CP. Reperfusion plasma contains a neutrophil activator. Ann Vasc Surg. 1993;7(1):68–75.
49. Koyama S, Sato E, Nomura H, Kubo K, Miura M, Yamashita T, Nagai S, Izumi T. Bradykinin stimulates type II alveolar cells to release neutrophil and monocyte chemotactic activity and inflammatory cytokines. Am J Pathol. 1998;153(6):1885–93.
50. Grommes J, Soehnlein O. Contribution of neutrophils to acute lung injury. Mol Med. 2011;17(3–4):293–307.
51. Fanelli V, Vlachou A, Ghannadian S, Simonetti U, Slutsky AS, Zhang H. Acute respiratory distress syndrome: new definition, current and future therapeutic options. J Thorac Dis. 2013;5(3):326–34.
52. Panthee N, Ono M. Spinal cord injury following thoracic and thoracoabdominal aortic repairs. Asian Cardiovasc Thorac Ann. 2015;23(2):235–46.
53. David Rosenthal MD, et al. Spinal cord ischemia after abdominal aortic operation: is it preventable? J Vasc Surg. 1999;30(3):391–7.
54. Etz DC, Luehr M, Aspern KV, et al. Spinal cord ischemia in open and endovascular thoracoabdominal aortic aneurysm repair: new concepts. J Cardiovasc Surg. 2014;55(2 Suppl 1):159–68.
55. Melissano G, Bertoglio L, Rinaldi E, Leopardi M, Chiesa R. An anatomical review of spinal cord blood supply. J Cardiovasc Surg. 2015;56:699–706.
56. Melissano G, Bertoglio L, Mascia D, Rinaldi E, Del Carro U, Nardelli P, Chiesa R. Spinal cord ischemia is multifactorial: what is the best protocol? J Cardiovasc Surg. 2016;57(2):191–201.
57. Yu Q, Huang J, Hu J, Zhu H. Advance in spinal cord ischemia reperfusion injury: blood-spinal cord barrier and remote ischemic preconditioning. Life Sci. 2016;154:34–8.
58. Zammert M, Gelman S. The pathophysiology of aortic cross-clamping. Best Pract Res Clin Anaesthesiol. 2016;30(3):257–69.
59. Gelman S. The pathophysiology of aortic cross-clamping and unclamping. Anesthesiology. 1995;82(4):1026–60.
60. Cuzick LM, Lopez AR, Cooper JR Jr. Pathophysiology of aortic cross-clamping. In: Chiesa R, Melissano G, Zangrillo A, Coselli JS, editors. Thoraco-abdominal aorta: surgical and anesthetic management. Milan: Springer; 2011. p. 65–72.
61. O'Connor CJ, Rothenberg DM. Anesthetic considerations for descending thoracic aortic surgery: part II. J Cardiothorac Vasc Anesth. 1995;9:734–47.
62. Subramaniam K, Caldwell JC. Anesthesia for descending aortic surgery. In: Subramaniam K, Park K, Subramaniam B, editors. Anesthesia and perioperative care for aortic surgery. New York, NY: Springer; 2011.
63. El-Sabrout RA, Reul GJ. Suprarenal or supraceliac aortic clamping during repair of infrarenal abdominal aortic aneurysms. Tex Heart Inst J. 2001;28(4):254–64.
64. Cingolani HE, Pérez NG, Cingolani OH, Ennis IL. The Anrep effect: 100 years later. Am J Physiol Heart Circ Physiol. 2013;304(2):H175–82.

65. Nichols CG, Hanck DA, Jewell BR. The Anrep effect: an intrinsic myocardial mechanism. Can J Physiol Pharmacol. 1988;66(7):924–9.
66. Kahn RA, Stone ME, Moskowitz DM. Anesthetic consideration for descending thoracic aortic aneurysm repair. Semin Cardiothorac Vasc Anesth. 2007;11(3):205–23.
67. Puchakayala MR, Lau WC. Descending thoracic aortic aneurysms. Contin Educ Anaesth Crit Care Pain. 2006;6(2):54–9.
68. Cullen DJ, Eger EI. Cardiovascular effects of carbon dioxide in man. Anesthesiology. 1974;41(4):345–8.
69. McLellan SA, Walsh TS. Oxygen delivery and haemoglobin. Contin Educ Anaesth Crit Care Pain. 2004;4(4):123–6.
70. Di Luozzo G. Visceral and spinal cord protection during thoracoabdominal aortic aneurysm repair: clinical and laboratory update. J Thorac Cardiovasc Surg. 2013;145(3 Suppl):S135–8.
71. Coselli JS, Lemaire SA. Descending and thoracoabdominal aortic aneurysms. In: Cohn LH, editor. Cardiac surgery in the adult., 3rd edn. New York: McGraw-Hill Medical; 2008. p. 1277–98.
72. Crawford ES, Walker HS 3rd. Graft replacement of aneurysm in descending thoracic aorta: results without bypass or shunting. Surgery. 1981;89:73–85.
73. Coselli JS. The use of left heart in the repair of thoracoabdominal aortic aneurysms: current techniques and results. Semin Thorac Cardiovasc Surg. 2003;15:326–32.
74. Hessel EA. Circuitry and cannulation techniques. In: Gravlee GP, Davis RD, Stammers RD, et al., editors. Cardiopulmonary. 3rd ed. Philadelphia: Lippincott Williams & Wilkins; 2008. p. 63–144.
75. Aftab M, Coselli JS. Reprint of: renal and visceral protection in thoracoabdominal aortic surgery. J Thorac Cardiovasc Surg. 2015;149(2 Suppl):S130–3.
76. Aftab M, Coselli JS. Renal and visceral protection in thoracoabdominal aortic surgery. J Thorac Cardiovasc Surg. 2014;148(6):2963–6.
77. Jacobs MJ, Eijsman L. Reduced renal failure following thoracoabdominal aortic aneurysm repair by selective perfusion. Eur J CardiothoracSurg. 1998;14:201–5.
78. Kuniyoshi Y, Koja K, Miyagi K, et al. Selective visceral perfusion during thoracoabdominal aortic aneurysm repair. Ann Thorac Cardiovasc Surg. 2004;10:367–72.
79. Lemaire SA. Randomized comparison of cold blood and cold crystalloid renal perfusion for renal protection during thoracoabdominal aortic aneurysm repair. J Vasc Surg. 2009;49:11–9.
80. Tshomba Y, Kahlberg A, Melissano G, Coppi G, Marone E, Ferrari D, Lembo R, Chiesa R. Comparison of renal perfusion solutions during thoracoabdominal aortic aneurysm repair. J Vasc Surg. 2014;59(3):623–33.
81. De Luca M, De Simone F. Left heart bypass. In: Chiesa R, Melissano G, Zangrillo A, editors. Thoraco-abdominal aorta. Milano: Springer; 2011.
82. Grams ME, Sang Y, Coresh J, Ballew S, Matsushita K, Molnar MZ, et al. Acute kidney injury after major surgery: a retrospective analysis of veterans health administration data. Am J Kidney Dis. 2016;67(6):872–80.
83. Roh GU, Lee JW, Nam SB, Lee J, Choi JR, Shim YH. Incidence and risk factors of acute kidney injury after thoracic aortic surgery for acute dissection. Ann Thorac Surg. 2012;94(3):766–71.
84. Marrocco-Trischitta MM, Melissano G, Kahlberg A, Vezzoli G, Calori G, Chiesa R. The impact of aortic clamping site on glomerular filtration rate after juxtarenal aneurysm repair. Ann Vasc Surg. 2009;23(6):770–7.
85. Wong GT, Lee EY, Irwin MG. Contrast induced nephropathy in vascular surgery. Br J Anaesth. 2016;117 Suppl 2:ii63–73.
86. Kellum JA, Lameire N, KDIGO AKI Guideline Work Group. Diagnosis, evaluation, and management of acute kidney injury: a KDIGO summary (part 1). Crit Care. 2013;17(1):204.
87. Sasabuchi Y, Kimura N, Shiotsuka J, Komuro T, Mouri H, Ohnuma T, et al. Long-term survival in patients with acute kidney injury after acute type a aortic dissection repair. Ann Thorac Surg. 2016;102(6):2003–9.
88. Landoni G, Bove T, Székely A, Comis M, Rodseth RN, Pasero D, et al. Reducing mortality in acute kidney injury patients: systematic review and international web-based survey. J Cardiothorac Vasc Anesth. 2013;27(6):1384–98.
89. Joannidis M, Druml W, Forni LG, Groeneveld ABJ, Honore PM, Hoste E, Ostermann M, Oudemans-van Straaten HM, Schetz M. Prevention of acute kidney injury and protection of renal function in the intensive care unit: update 2017: expert opinion of the working group on prevention, AKI section, European society of intensive care medicine. Intensive Care Med. 2017;43(6):730–49.
90. Bove T, Zangrillo A, Guarracino F, Alvaro G, Persi B, Maglioni E, Galdieri N, Comis M, Caramelli F, Pasero DC, Pala G, Renzini M, Conte M, Paternoster G, Martinez B, Pinelli F, Frontini M, Zucchetti MC, Pappalardo F, Amantea B, Camata A, Pisano A, Verdecchia C, Dal Checco E, Cariello C, Faita L, Baldassarri R, Scandroglio AM, Saleh O, Lembo R, Calabrò MG, Bellomo R, Landoni G. Effect of fenoldopam on use of renal replacement therapy among patients with acute kidney injury after cardiac surgery: a randomized clinical trial. JAMA. 2014;312(21):2244–53.
91. Zangrillo A, Biondi-Zoccai GG, Frati E, Covello RD, Cabrini L, Guarracino F, Ruggeri L, Bove T, Bignami E, Landoni G. Fenoldopam and acute renal failure in cardiac surgery: a meta-analysis of randomized placebo-controlled trials. J Cardiothorac Vasc Anesth. 2012;26(3):407–13.
92. Jongkind V, Yeung KK, Akkersdijk GJM, et al. Juxtarenal aortic aneurysm repair. J Vasc Surg. 2010;52(3):760–7.

93. Chiesa R, Marone EM, Brioschi C, et al. Open repair of pararenal aortic aneurysms: operative management, early results, and risk factor analysis. Ann Vasc Surg. 2006;20(6):739–46.
94. Sasaki T, Ohsawa S, Ogawa M, et al. Postoperative renal function after an abdominal aortic aneurysm repair requiring a suprarenal aortic cross-clamp. Surg Today. 2000;30(1):33–6.
95. Allen BT, Anderson CB, Rubin BG, et al. Preservation of renal function in juxtarenal and suprarenal abdominal aortic aneurysm repair. J Vasc Surg. 1993;17(5):948–59.
96. Girbes AR. Prevention of acute renal failure: role of vaso-active drugs, mannitol and diuretics. Int J Artif Organs. 2004;27(12):1049–53.
97. Yallop KG, Sheppard SV, Smith DC. The effect of mannitol on renal function following cardio-pulmonary bypass in patients with normal pre-operative creatinine. Anaesthesia. 2008;63:576–82.
98. Solomon R, Werner C, Mann D, et al. Effects of saline, mannitol, and furosemide to prevent acute decreases in renal function induced by radiocontrast agents. N Engl J Med. 1994;331:1416–20.
99. Coselli JS, LeMaire SA, Miller CC III, et al. Mortality and paraplegia after thoracoabdominal aortic aneurysm repair: a risk factor analysis. Ann Thorac Surg. 2000;69:409–14.
100. Acher C, Wynn M. Paraplegia after thoracoabdominal aortic surgery: not just assisted circulation, hypothermic arrest, clamp and sew, or TEVAR. Ann Cardiothorac Surg. 2012;1(3):365–72.
101. McGarvey ML, Mullen MT, Woo EY, et al. The treatment of spinal cord ischemia following thoracic endovascular aortic repair. Neurocrit Care. 2007;6:35–9.
102. Cheung AT, Weiss SJ, McGarvey ML, et al. Interventions for reversing delayed-onset postoperative paraplegia after thoracic aortic reconstruction. Ann Thorac Surg. 2002;74(2):413–9.
103. Erbel R, Aboyans V, Boileau C, et al. 2014 ESC guidelines on the diagnosis and treatment of aortic diseases. Eur Heart J. 2014;35:2873–926.
104. Coselli JS, LeMaire SA, Köksoy C, Schmittling ZC, Curling PE. Cerebrospinal fluid drainage reduces paraplegia after thoracoabdominal aortic aneurysm repair: results of a randomized clinical trial. J Vasc Surg. 2002;35:631–9.
105. Tshomba Y, Leopardi M, Mascia D, Kahlberg A, Carozzo A, Magrin S, Melissano G, Chiesa R. Automated pressure-controlled cerebrospinal fluid drainage during open thoracoabdominal aortic aneurysm repair. J Vasc Surg. 2017;66(1):37–44.
106. Liu LY, Callahan B, Peterss S, Dumfarth J, Tranquilli M, Ziganshin BA, Elefteriades JA. Neuromonitoring using motor and somatosensory evoked potentials in aortic surgery. J Card Surg. 2016;31(6):383–9.
107. Keeling B, Chen EP. Reaching the full potential of MEP monitoring during surgery of the thoracoabdominal aorta. J Thorac Cardiovasc Surg. 2016;151(2):518–9.
108. Estrera AL, Sheinbaum R, Miller CC 3rd, Harrison R, Safi HJ. Neuromonitor-guided repair of thoracoabdominal aortic aneurysms. J Thorac Cardiovasc Surg. 2010;140(6 Suppl):S131–5.
109. Martirosyan NL, Patel AA, Carotenuto A, Kalani MY, Bohl MA, Preul MC, Theodore N. The role of therapeutic hypothermia in the management of acute spinal cord injury. Clin Neurol Neurosurg. 2017;154:79–88.
110. Kang J, Albadawi H, Casey PJ, Abbruzzese TA, Patel VI, Yoo HJ, Cambria RP, Watkins MT. The effects of systemic hypothermia on a murine model of thoracic aortic ischemia reperfusion. J Vasc Surg. 2010;52(2):435–43.
111. Fayad A, Shillcutt SK. Perioperative transesophageal echocardiography for non-cardiac surgery. Can J Anaesth. 2018;65(4):381–98.
112. Kristensen SD, Knuuti J, Saraste A, Anker S, Bøtker HE, De Hert S, Ford I, Gonzalez Juanatey JR, Gorenek B, Heyndrickx GR, Hoeft A, Huber K, Iung B, Kjeldsen KP, Longrois D, Luescher TF, Pierard L, Pocock S, Price S, Roffi M, Sirnes PA, Uva MS, Voudris V, Funck-Brentano C, Authors/Task Force Members. 2014 ESC/ESA guidelines on non-cardiac surgery: cardiovascular assessment and management: the joint task force on non-cardiac surgery: cardiovascular assessment and management of the European Society of Cardiology (ESC) and the European Society of Anaesthesiology (ESA). Eur J Anaesthesiol. 2014;31(10):517–73.
113. Şentürk M, Slinger P, Cohen E. Intraoperative mechanical ventilation strategies for one-lung ventilation. Best Pract Res Clin Anaesthesiol. 2015;29(3):357–69.

Tissue Ischemia During Aortic Repair: The Point of View of the Perfusionist

15

De Simone Francesco, Tshiombo Gianbattista, and Colombo Elisa

15.1 Introduction

Thoracoabdominal aortic surgery involves the cross-clamping of the descending thoracic aorta, which causes an abrupt reduction of the blood supply to both viscera and lower limbs. The reduction of blood flow induces the decrease of oxygen and substrates, which are essential for the Krebs cycle and the "respiratory chain." It also lowers the clearance of cellular catabolites, increases the probability of bleeding disorders, and prompts the release of inflammation mediators and free radicals [1–4].

The sudden exclusion of an extensive vascular district generates an immediate and significant increase of heart afterload and blood pressure. Furthermore, it is also associated with an increase in the cerebrospinal fluid (CSF) pressure [1–3, 5–7], which may determine a significant change in the perfusion pressure of the spinal cord (estimated as the gradient between blood pressure and CSF pressure) eventually leading to the collapse of its feeding vessels.

D. S. Francesco (✉)
Department of Extracorporeal Circulation, IRCCS San Raffaele Scientific Institute, Milan, Italy
e-mail: desimone.francesco@hsr.it

T. Gianbattista
Fondazione Cariplo, Milan, Italy

C. Elisa
Vascular Surgery Unit, IRCCS San Raffaele Scientific Institute, Milan, Italy

© Springer Nature Switzerland AG 2019
Y. Tshomba et al. (eds.), *Visceral Vessels and Aortic Repair*, https://doi.org/10.1007/978-3-319-94761-7_15

In the past, strategies such as expeditious surgery [8] or passive shunts [9] have been advocated to prevent these damages, however in more recent times, distal perfusion [7] has emerged as the method of choice.

In consideration of the foregoing, the teamwork of surgeons, anesthesiologists, perfusionists, nursing and allied healthcare professionals must be emphasized.

The aims of using distal perfusion during thoracic aortic cross-clamping are:

- Support of heart function, especially if already compromised [1, 2, 10–12]
- Reduction of end organ ischemia
- Control of proximal hypertension

15.2 Different Methods for Distal Perfusion

15.2.1 Partial and Total Cardiopulmonary Bypass (Fig. 15.1a, b)

During thoracoabdominal aortic surgery, distal perfusion may be obtained either by partial cardiopulmonary bypass (CPB) (Fig. 15.1a, b) [13] or left heart bypass (LHB) (Fig. 15.1c, d). The circuit for CPB consists of a venous cannula placed in a femoral vein or in the right atrium, a pump, an oxygenator, and an arterial cannula positioned in the

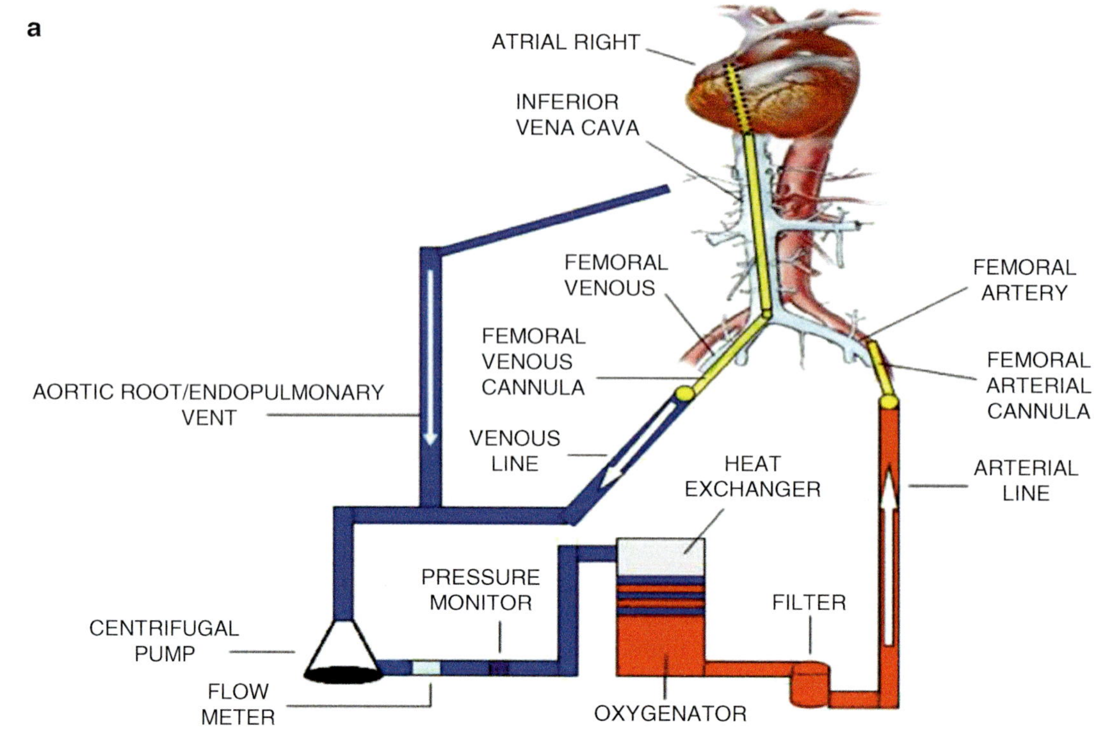

-The circuit for CPBP consists of a venous cannula placed in right atrium through the femoral vein, a pump, an oxygenator, and an arterial cannula positioned in femoral artery or in the distal aorta; a heat exchanger is also usually part of the CPBP circuit.-

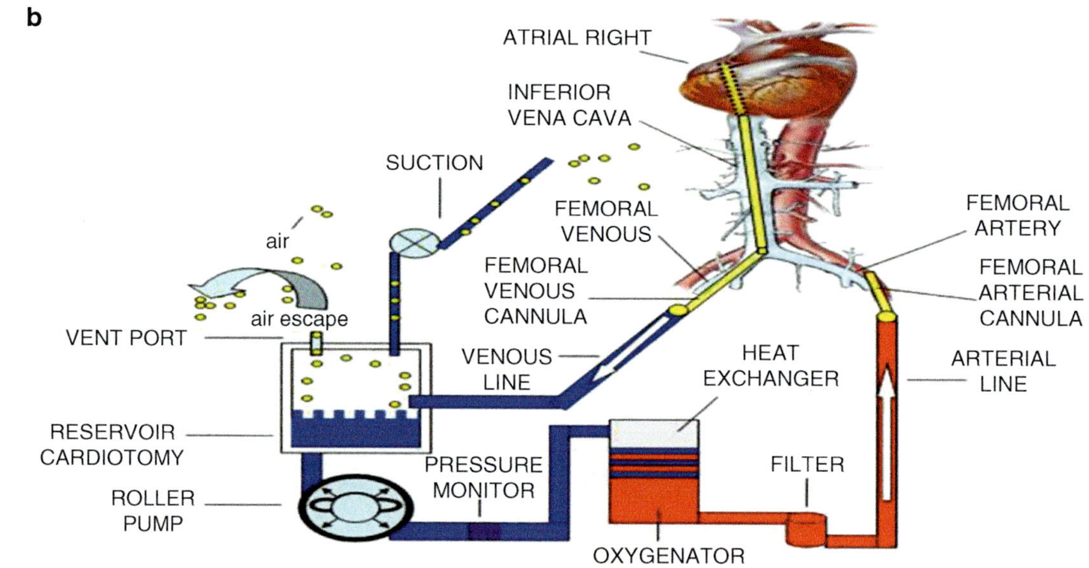

- A circuit for extracorporeal circulation is defined as "closed" when does not involve a contact between air and blood, and "open" when an air/blood interface is present.-

- "Open" systems, include a reservoir for venous blood and blood aspirated from the operative field.-

Fig. 15.1 (**a**) CPBP closed circuit. (**b**) CPBP open circuit. (**c**) Left bypass (LBP). (**d**) Left heart bypass (LHBP)

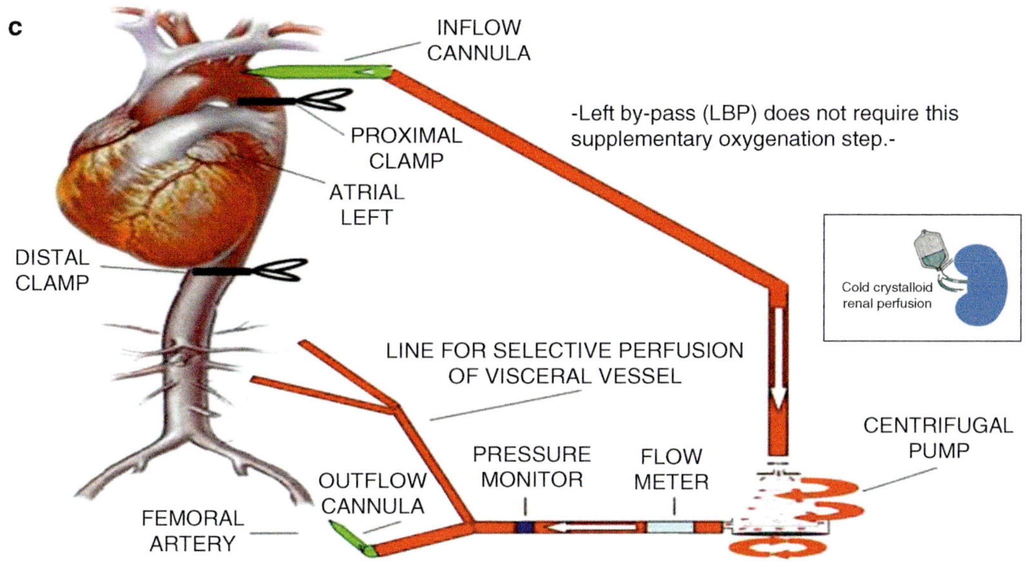

-When a LBP is used, the circuit is composed by an inflow cannula placed in the thoracic aorta proximal to the clamp, a pump, and an outflow cannula placed in the distal aorta or in the femoral artery.-

-A line for selective perfusion of visceral vessels needs to be positioned along outflow line.-

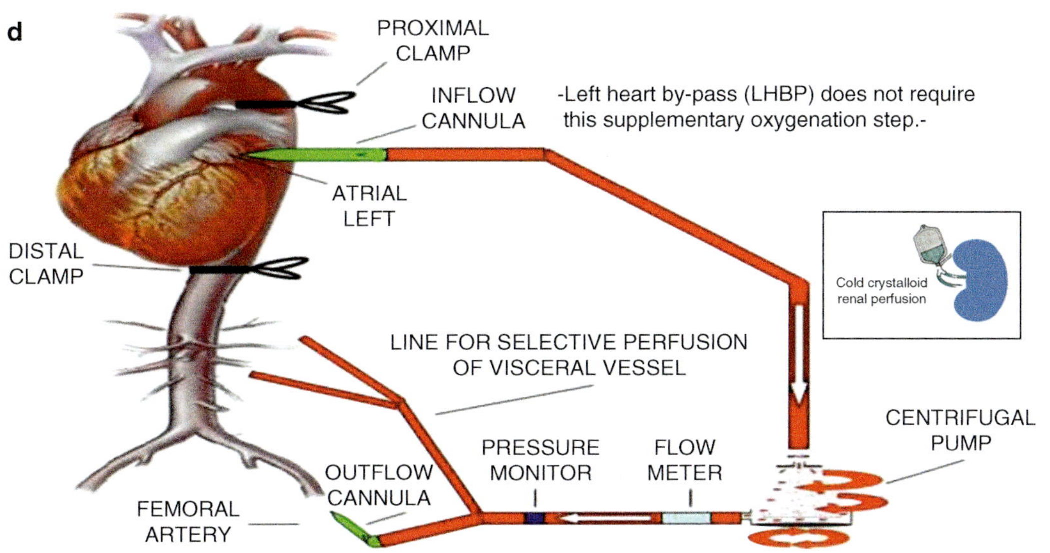

-When a LHBP is used, the circuit is composed by an inflow cannula placed in the pulmonary vein or left atrial appendage, a pump, and an outflow cannula placed in the distal aorta or in the femoral artery.-

-A line for selective perfusion of visceral vessels needs to be positioned along outflow line.-

Fig. 15.1 (continued)

femoral artery or in the distal aorta [13]; usually, a heat exchanger is also part of the CPB circuit. When an LHB is used, the circuit is composed by an inflow cannula placed in the pulmonary vein or left atrial appendage (left heart bypass) (Fig. 15.1d), or in the thoracic aorta proximal to the clamp (left bypass) (Fig. 15.1c), a pump, and an outflow cannula placed in the distal aorta or in the femoral artery [7, 14]. The common goal of both systems is to ensure cardiac support and distal perfusion.

There are several differences between the two methods, each one having advantages and drawbacks (Table 15.1). The mechanism of partial CPB (Fig. 15.1a, b) works by taking a portion of blood from the venous district that is re-infused in the arterial compartment, bypassing the pulmonary circulation. This is why the blood needs to pass through an oxygenator; CPB requires full heparinization. Left bypasses do not require the oxygenation step and a lesser grade heparinization [7, 14].

A significant limitation of both systems is that they do not provide adequate perfusion in the upper body district in case of sudden and severe cardiac dysfunction. This occurs because the outflow cannula is positioned distally to the distal clamp [15]. Partial CPB, however (Fig. 15.1a, b), is more versatile than LHB (Fig. 15.1c, d) and in case of need, it can be converted into a total CPB by adding a second outflow branch with a cannula placed proximally to the aortic clamp.

Total CPB (an open system) (Fig. 15.1b) also offers the possibility to induce (profuse) hypothermia and perform a circulatory arrest. For more extensive operations, hypothermic circulatory arrest can be performed on full cardiopulmonary bypass by reducing the body temperature down to 16 °C to 18 °C. This procedure protects the distal organs during ischemia, even though it is complicated by coagulopathy and the increased complexity of hypothermic cardiac arrest [16].

Total CPB with an interval of hypothermic circulatory arrest is widely used for surgeries on the ascending aorta and aortic arch, but less commonly exploited for operations on the thoracoabdominal aorta. Nevertheless, in these settings it offers several advantages since it requires only minimal dissection of the periaortic tissues, eliminates the need for proximal and sequential aortic clamping, and provides easy access to the distal aortic arch. It also offers a bloodless and quiet surgical field when the circulation is arrested and allows the recollection into the perfusion circuit of all blood lost [17].

Table 15.1 Comparison between different extracorporeal circulation techniques

Method	Pros	Cons
LHB-CPB	• Cardiac support • Proximal arterial pressure control • Distal perfusion	• Heparinization needed • Coagulation cascade • Inflammatory response
LHB	• Low heparin doses	• Cannot replace heart function in case of failure • Hemotransfusion mandatory in case of massive bleeding
CPB closed circuit	• Low heparin doses • If needed it can be switched into a total CPB by adding a second outflow cannula proximally to the aortic clamp	• Oxygenator needed • More expensive • High heparin doses • Need of vasoactive drugs • Hemotransfusion mandatory in case of massive bleeding
CPB open circuit	• No blood loss • Less need of crystalloids supplementation • Less need of plasma and platelets infusion • Better management of VF or congestive heart failure • May be used to induce DHCA	• High heparin doses • More expensive • Need of venous reservoir and aspirators • More difficult hemostasis after protamine administration

Systemic heparinization is a fundamental factor, especially upon extensive surgical accesses or in emergency cases [18, 19]. The need for heparinization is not particularly influenced by the circuit type used (CPB or LBP) (Fig. 15.1a–d), but rather by the use of a "closed" (Fig. 15.1b) [13, 18–20] or "open" circuit. A closed extracorporeal circulation system does not involve a contact between air and blood, whereas it is defined "open" when an air/blood interface is present. Provided that a sufficiently high flow is maintained in order to prevent platelet aggregation in the circuit, a "closed" system requires only a mild anticoagulation [13] (less than 100 u/kg) [1, 2, 20]. "Open" systems require total systemic anticoagulation, with the goal of maintaining the ACT >480 s, because they include a reservoir for venous blood and blood aspirated from the operative field implying contact between air and blood.

15.2.2 Left Bypass and Left Heart Bypass (Fig. 15.1c, d)

In our institution, the preferred method of circulatory assistance during thoracoabdominal aortic surgery is LBP (Fig. 15.1c, d). CPB (Fig. 15.1b), on the other hand, is used in selected cases (for instance, when the surgeon is not sure about the safety of proximal cross-clamping and circulatory arrest may be needed to perform an open proximal anastomosis).

In an LHB or LPB (Fig. 15.1c, d) setup, the heart perfuses everything proximal to the proximal aortic clamp (head and upper limbs). The patient must have both an adequate cardiac function to tolerate the clamping of the descending aorta and the consequent swings in the afterload, as well as good lung function to tolerate single-lung ventilation during a thoracotomy. Generally, the pump used for LBP (Fig. 15.1c, d) is centrifugal [16]: it consists of a bell in which a number of coaxial cones or fins are housed. The bell rests on a rotational magnet, which confers blood velocity with its fast rotary motion. The forced vortex principle ($f = m \times a$) applies to very high fluid velocity: a central area with negative pressure (inflow zone) and a peripheral area with positive pressure (outflow zone) are generated within the bell. The kinetic energy produced by the pump and passed on the blood can overcome the resistance found throughout the circuit. The pump flow is directly proportional to the velocity, and inversely proportional to the resistance. A flowmeter is required because the outflow of the pump changes with the afterload at constant speed of the magnet.

As opposed to roller pumps (positive displacement pumps), centrifugal pumps cannot develop pressures that could be dangerous by breaking the circuit or damaging the vessels. Air embolism is a fairly rare complication, because the lack of mass prevents acceleration.

The main advantage is that this simple circuit can tolerate a lower activated clotting time (ACT) and in some cases no heparin at all [2]. Once LHB or LPB (Fig. 15.1c, d) is established the patient's temperature can be lowered to 32–33 °C. This is because mild hypothermia decreases the risk of hypothermia-induced ventricular fibrillation. Arterial pressure is monitored proximal to the aortic clamp through a radial arterial line and distal to the clamp through a femoral arterial line [2].

Nevertheless, there are major disadvantages. One is the lack of reservoir, which, in the eventuality of massive blood loss does not allow the supply of blood directly to the patient, as it might be in a full CPB (Fig. 15.1b) setup. Then, it is not feasible to conversion to complete CPB (Fig. 15.1b) if the heart fibrillates or in case oxygenation on single-lung ventilation becomes problematic.

15.2.3 Distal Perfusion

The criteria for optimal distal perfusion during aortic cross-clamping are still debated. Some authors propose flows greater than 40 mL/kg/min [21], or flows ranging from 1.5 to 3 L/min [22–25] with a mean femoral artery pressure of 70 mmHg [1, 2, 13, 21–24]. Others advise the use of motor evoked potentials meps.

Diuresis is a practical means for the evaluation of perfusion [26], although the non-pulsatile flow from the pump, the preoperative renal impairment, and hypo-perfusion may play a role in the etiology of anuria [27].

Other criteria for regulation of the pump depend on the area to perfuse (i.e., one or both lower limbs, kidneys, splanchnic vessels, etc.), on the relationship between the pressures developed by the heart (radial pressure), those developed by the pump (femoral pressure) and ventricular volumes monitored through trans-esophageal echocardiographic (tee) examination [1, 2, 10, 12]. As far as distal perfusion is concerned, information on both pressure and flow is available, however concerning the proximal district, only blood pressure can be monitored, thus providing incomplete information on the real perfusion of organs such as the heart and the brain. Furthermore, due to a plethora of variables such as of the position of the patient on the surgical table, the pressure of the retractors and single-lung mechanical ventilation, the interpretation of parameters such as difficult and the importance of tee monitoring during aortic cross-clamping may not be overemphasized, especially in cardiopathic patients [1, 2, 10, 12].

15.2.4 Components

The basic circuit for LBP (Fig. 15.1c) or LHB (Fig. 15.1d) includes an inflow cannula, a pump, and an outflow cannula. A heat exchanger may be included to allow a better management of the patient's temperature by actively cooling organs. Consequently, it reduces the organs' metabolic rate [2, 21, 28] before clamping and re-warming. However, hypothermia does not come without risks, which include cardiac arrhythmias [15] and coagulopathy [26, 27].

In our clinical practice, the heat exchanger is not used, since the patient passively cools down to approximately 34 °C before cross-clamping and LBP (Fig. 15.1c) or LHB (Fig. 15.1d) is discontinued at the time of clamp removal. Afterwards, re-warming is facilitated by warm infusions and a heat-exchange mattress placed beneath the patient.

In the LBP (Fig. 15.1c) or LHB (Fig. 15.1d) circuit, an accessory pathway may be positioned on the inflow line, to allow recirculation of fluids during the priming. In this way, any air bubbles accidentally aspirated in the circuit are eliminated and rapid re-infusion is facilitated. The blood aspirated from the operative field must pass through a cell-saver system and may then be re-infused through the accessory line mentioned above. The immediate restoration of blood volume is fundamental to maintaining stable hemodynamics.

Furthermore, adequate tissue perfusion is based on oxygen availability. Therefore, the preservation of all parameters that guarantee good oxygen supply to tissues, namely a good arterial oxygen saturation and a good level of hemoglobin, is fundamental. This is particularly true in situations where blood flow may not be optimal. The immediate re-infusion of autologous blood collected in the cell-saver also reduces the need of homologous transfusions, which may carry the risk of pulmonary damage [29] and others.

During the surgical anastomosis of the visceral vessels, abdominal organ perfusion may be continued by selective catheterization of the individual arteries. The line for selective perfusion of visceral vessels is to be positioned along the outflow one. Double lumen occlusion/perfusion 9-french catheters are used to cannulate the individual vessels [21, 25, 30, 31]. Flows of 200–300 mL/min for each catheter [32] maintain a visceral perfusion pressure of about 70 mmHg [21, 31] (Fig. 15.1c, d).

Recent studies [33] have shown that perfusion of the renal arteries with cold crystalloid solutions is equally effective to protect the kidneys. In our practice, Custodiol® solution at 4 °C is used for renal perfusion, while the celiac and superior mesenteric arteries are perfused with warm blood from the pump (Fig. 15.1c, d).

15.2.5 Priming of the Circuit

The solutions used for priming vary according to the protocols employed in different centers. Generally, the priming of the circuit is done with 400 mL of crystalloid or colloid solutions, but in special cases (i.e., patients with anemia, or dialysis, etc.), the patient's autologous blood can be exploited. Technically, after the connection of the circuit with the inflow cannula and before the connection to the outflow cannula, it is possible to replace the priming with blood drawn from inflow cannula. When blood has substituted to the crystalloid solution in the circuit, the connection with the inflow cannula is completed. This maneuver induces some degree of hypovolemia that may result in a short period hemodynamic instability, which

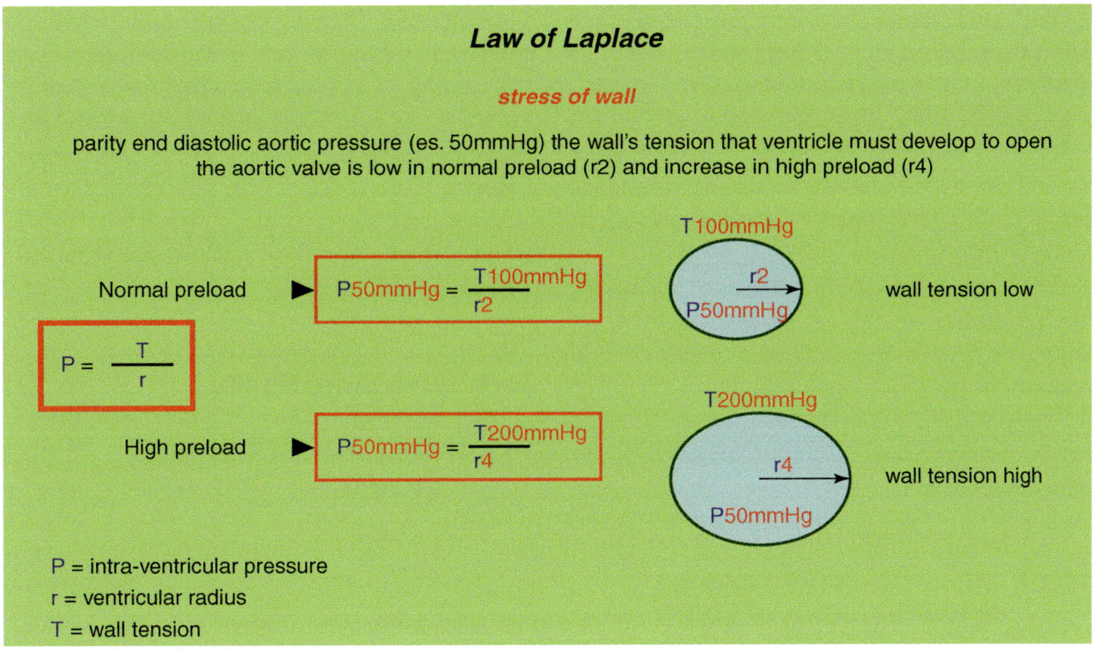

Fig. 15.2 The left ventricular afterload is determined also by the dimension of ventricle in the initial phase of iso-volumetric contraction

can be controlled pharmacologically or with the administration of homologous blood.

15.2.6 Proximal Cannulation/Cardiac Support

During the beginning of isovolumetric contraction, the afterload is influenced by the systemic resistance, related to aortic pressure, and by the preload, determined by ventricular end-diastolic volume. At the aortic cross-clamping, LBP (Fig. 15.1c) or LHB (Fig. 15.1d) supports heart function by reducing cardiac work. The inflow cannula can be positioned in the left atrium (LHB) (Fig. 15.1d) or in the thoracic aorta proximal to the clamp (LBP) (Fig. 15.1c).

15.2.7 Inflow Cannula Positioned in the Left Atrium (LHB) (Fig. 15.1d)

The left ventricular afterload is determined by the dimension of ventricle in the initial phase of isovolumetric contraction; (Laplace $t = p\ r$) in other words the wall tension (t) that the heart will need to develop to increase intra-ventricular pressure will be proportional to preload stand for the left ventricular radius (r). (Fig. 15.2)

Aortic cross-clamping excludes much of systemic circulation, thus the direct effect is an increase of ventricular radius (r) and the wall's tension that ventricle must develop to open the aortic valve (at the same end-diastolic aortic pressure) will be greater.

After aortic clamping, if the inflow cannula is positioned in the left atrium (left heart bypass) (Fig. 15.1d) drainage is made possible, the ventricular radius does not increase and the wall tension that the ventricle must develop to open the aortic valve will not be as high. Therefore, this placement benefits the heart by reducing the left ventricular volume (LVEDP) and oxygen consumption during isovolumetric contraction, by improving coronary perfusion and reducing pulmonary congestion. When the pulmonary stasis is reduced, both gas exchange and right ventricular function are also improved [1, 2, 6, 7, 34].

With atrial cannulation, care must be taken to avoid the aspiration of air from the outside, that would result in systemic embolism. From a surgical point of view, the cannulation of the left atrium may be obtained from either the left atrial appendage or the pulmonary vein. In our clinical practice, the left superior pulmonary vein is favored (Fig. 15.1d).

The surgeon has to be precise in positioning the left atrium cannula. A misplacement of the latter may result in the injection into the circuit of partially oxygenated blood coming in part from the nonventilated lung. This may be masked by a correct blood oxygen saturation measured in the upper body district.

15.2.8 Inflow Cannula Positioned in the Thoracic Aorta (LBP) (Fig. 15.1c)

The positioning of the inflow cannula in the thoracic aorta proximally to the clamp allows a smaller increase in afterload and peripheral resistance (SVR) induced by aortic cross-clamping, the consequence is a reduction of work for the left ventricle during isovolumetric contraction, in fact the ventricle does not need to increase the intracavitary pressure (*p*) because the resistance against which it must work to open the aortic valve is not as high. Being the wall's tension (*t*) directly proportional to the intra-ventricular pressure that the ventricle must develop, when the ventricular wall's tension is moderate the ventricular pressure will be moderate too, as a consequence the myocardial oxygen consumption (MvO2) will be reduced [2].

This cannulation placement is particularly useful for patients with aortic or mitral insufficiency, because the afterload reduction determines the decrease of trans-valvular regurgitation.

15.2.9 Distal Cannulation

LBP (Fig. 15.1c) or LHB (Fig. 15.1d) requires relatively low flows, thus it allows the use of small diameter cannulas (i.e., 14-16-18 fr.). This represents an advantage especially when the inflow cannula is placed in the femoral artery. The cannula is secured with a purse-string suture and the artery is not occluded allowing distal perfusion of the ipsilateral limb. If the aortic cross-clamping time is prolonged, this strategy avoids ischemia/reperfusion damage, which may also be associated with metabolic acidosis and renal failure [35, 36] (Fig. 15.3).

15.3 Biocompatibility

15.3.1 Activation of Biological Circuits (Fig. 15.4)

Blood has a very complex structure, consisting mainly of corpuscles (erythrocytes, leukocytes, and platelets) and plasma proteins. During bypass, blood is circulated via mechanical pump and homeostasis is impaired; intravascular pressures fluctuate outside normal ranges, fluid shifts occur with the extracellular compartment, and capillary permeability increases.

Direct injury to blood elements is produced by contact with synthetic (non-endothelial) surfaces, shear stress, turbulence, cavitation, and osmotic forces. Surface electrical charges are important in the repulsion or attraction of blood elements. The presence or absence of specific chemical groups, the surface tension, wettability of the polymer, and the presence of fillers and plasticizer are all relevant as well. Moreover, the activation of mediators triggers a series of reactions that involve the coagulation cascade, fibrinolysis, the k system, complement, and cytokines. When blood comes into contact with the synthetic materials of the various components of the extracorporeal circulation circuit, plasma proteins (albumin, gamma globulins, fibrinogen) immediately adsorb onto the circuit. This mechanism is determined by the material surface properties, being the plastic hydrophobic and with a high interfacial energy. The protein that initially adheres to the circuit walls is fibrinogen, which causes the adhesion of platelets mediated by the exposure of its hydrophobic residues that interact with the platelets GPIIb and GPIIIa receptors. Slow blood flow

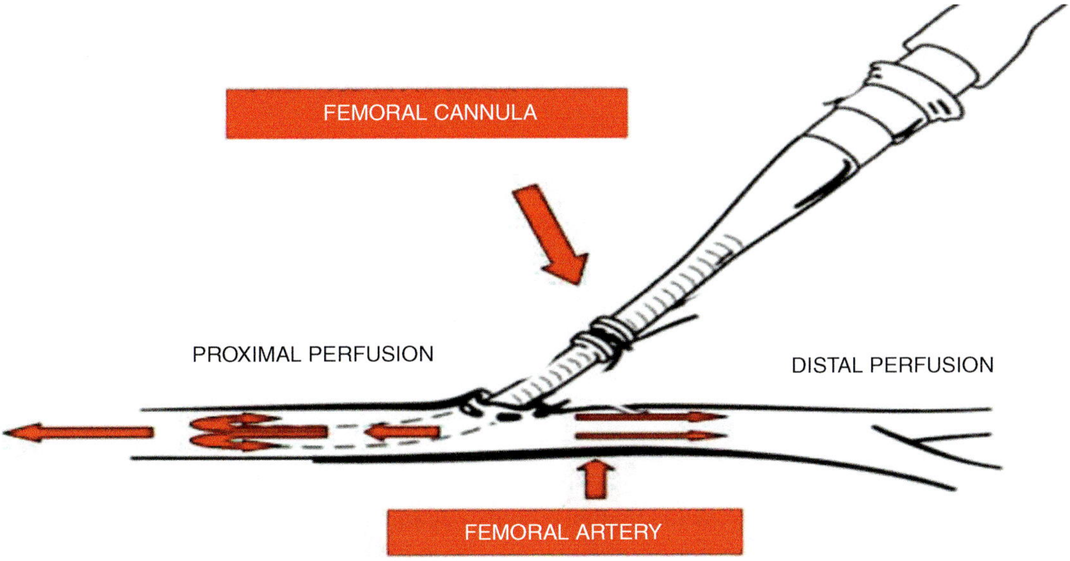

Fig. 15.3 The cannula is secured with a purse-string suture and the artery is not occluded allowing distal perfusion of the ipsilateral limb

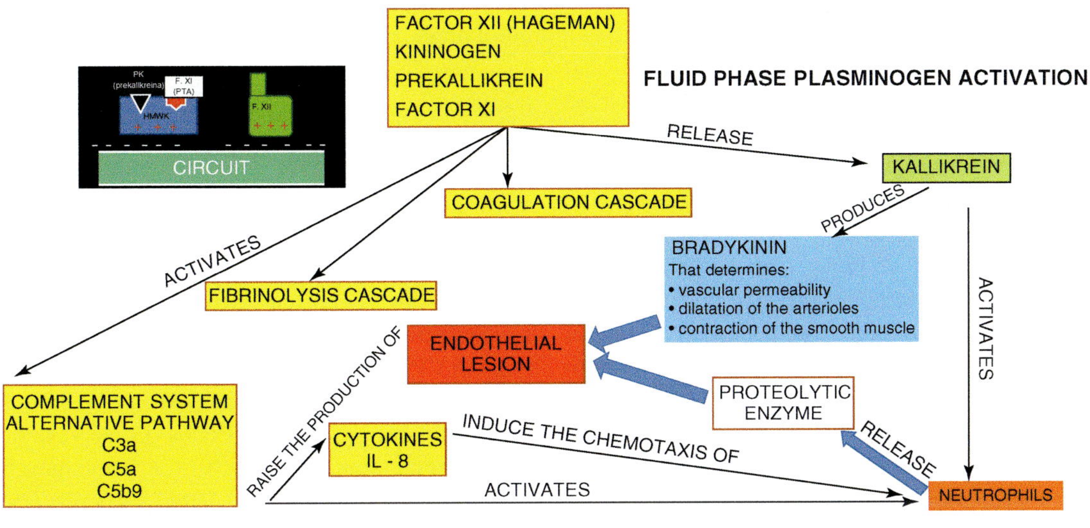

Fig. 15.4 Effects on blood and plasma components baited by extracorporeal bypass

may significantly increase the binding between platelets and foreign materials, this may happen, for instance, in the oxygenator meshes, through heat exchangers and in the filters present along the circuit, especially under hypothermic conditions. Adhesion, aggregation, and subsequent activation of platelets cause the release of granules and potent chemical inflammation mediators (β-thromboglobulin, platelet factor 4 [PF4], etc.), which are an important determinants of postoperative coagulopathy.

By means of the intrinsic and extrinsic coagulation systems, extracorporeal circulation activates factor X, which in turn triggers the common coagulation pathway that leads to clot formation. To avoid clotting, which may be fatal, heparin must be administered. In fact, by binding to antithrombin III, heparin accelerates its function through the inhibition of coagulation factors such as factor X and thrombin. Due to the contact of blood with the non-endothelial surfaces, immediately after starting extracorporeal circulation, the Hageman factor (factor XII) is activated. This factor acts on both the coagulation cascade, and fibrinolysis, the plasmin can further activate prekallikrein, the complement system and again the Hageman factor (Fig. 15.4).

The cascade of kallikrein determines the production of bradykinin, as well as the activation of other mediators, such as the Hageman XII factor or plasminogen [37]. Other factors that were previously underestimated, namely hemodilution, blood contact with air, complex heparin-protamine, etc., may contribute to the activation of the blood components [38].

15.3.2 Metabolic Acid–Base Balance

Metabolic acidosis is associated with CPB, and the management of this complication must be aggressive. However, its pathogenesis is poorly understood because the traditional methods of examining acid–base changes (i.e., Anion Gap Analysis) are lacking in this setting. The effect of the composition of pump priming solution on serum lactate concentration has been studied, and it has been demonstrated that the use of a solution with no lactate significantly limits the increase in serum concentrations of this chemical in the postoperative period.

Metabolic acidosis also tends to develop during CPB, even when apparently adequate flow rates are used [39]. This is probably related to the uneven distribution of flow during CPB, with the consequent development of hypoperfused areas that release lactic acid. Usually, the resultant metabolic acidosis is not severe, and the concentration of lactic acid rarely exceeds 5 mmol/L [3].

Anesthesiologists' expertise is fundamental to face the following responses to cardiopulmonary bypasses techniques: whole-body (nonspecific: neutrophil activation, platelet response) complement activation inflammatory response to use of a pump-oxygenator, humoral response (kallikrein-bradykinin activation, fibrinolytic cascade, coagulation cascade, arachidonic acid cascade, cytokines), cellular response, metabolic response.

15.3.3 Distribution of Blood Flow

15.3.3.1 Brain

During euthermic and moderately hypothermic CPB in adults and elderly patients, cerebral blood flow is not importantly influenced by variations of mean arterial blood pressure [21, 22]. This is similar to what happens to normal awake adult humans, in whom cerebral blood flow does not vary significantly with variations of about 60–150 mmHg in mean arterial blood pressure.

Cerebral blood flow during CPB is affected by arterial carbon dioxide pressure ($PaCO2$). Hypercarbia increases cerebral blood flow and hypocarbia decreases it [23–25]. Usually, when mean blood pressure is lower than 40 mmHg for more than a few minutes during re-warming, anesthesiologists should elevate arterial blood pressure.

Blood flow to the skin is severely reduced during non-pulsatile CPB. The off-pump cardiac surgery patients had less severe, but statistically significant, microcirculatory alterations immediately postoperatively. These alterations improved slightly but persisted after 24 h. Thus, microvascular perfusion presented similar alterations in CPB and off-pump patients 6–24 h after admission to the intensive care unit.

Veins constrict during CPB by an increase in venous tone that may persist for some hours afterward. The mechanism of this vasoconstriction has not been determined with certainty, even if high levels of circulating catecholamines probably play an important role.

15.3.3.2 Kidney

Ischemia stops blood supply to the glomerulus and post glomerular vessels, if it persists more than 10 min acute tubular necrosis, which is the most frequent form of acute renal failure (70%), may result.

Postoperative dialysis-dependent renal failure is associated with a 50–60% mortality risk; thus, the preservation of renal function and the avoidance of dialysis reduce mortality risk and improve long-term survival [30, 40].

From the cellular point of view, the whole tubule can undergo necrosis with the terminal portions of the proximal tubule and the ascending branch of the Henle loop, that are seats of important metabolic processes, having a higher tendency. The cells of these districts receive nourishment from peritubular capillaries. A reduction in perfusion, therefore a drop in the oxygen supply to these cells, leads to the loss of cytoskeletal polymerization with consequent loss of the brush-border and cell polarity. The result is a dislocation of the Na^+/K^+ pump with loss of the resorption capacity of the tubular solutes.

The brush-like orifice disappears, the cell-cell connections are no longer stable, and the cell falls into the tubular lumen, where cellular debris adheres to a protein substance produced by the tubule (Tamm-Horsfall glycoprotein). The outcomes are cylinders occluding the lumen and preventing the passage of urine from the occluded tubule.

The open spaces on the lateral-lateral slope favor the back diffusion of solutes and luminal water (pre-urine) towards the peritubular circulation, where they are reabsorbed and recirculated. The reflux of urinary material in the interstitial space causes acute inflammation with edema.

Perfusion at higher pressures with moderate or deep hypothermia (hypothermic arrest or cold renal perfusion decreasing renal temperature to <20 °C during occlusion) appears to provide effective renal protection, with dialysis rates of 3% or less in most reports whether cold blood or crystalloid is used [31–34] (Fig. 15.1c, d).

15.3.3.3 Viscera

The physiology of splanchnic circulation is complex and not fully understood. Different intrinsic (metabolic and myogenic) and extrinsic (neural and humoral) systems regulating the intestinal blood flow interact with each other. Self-regulation of blood flow pressure, reactive hyperemia, and hypoxic vasodilation are considered intrinsic control mechanisms and are responsible for instantaneous changes in blood flow in the splanchnic district. According to the metabolic theory, the distribution of oxygen has a greater influence than blood flow on variations in the splanchnic circulation. Therefore, an imbalance between oxygen supply and tissue demand will result in a greater concentration of local metabolites such as hydrogen, potassium, carbon dioxide, and adenosine, which will cause vasodilatation and hyperemia. In accordance with the myogenic theory, the voltage receptors of the arterioles regulate the vessel resistance in relation to the transmural pressure. The extrinsic neural factors of regulation of the splanchnic circulation include the α-adrenergic vasoconstrictive fibers, their activation results in vasoconstriction of the small vessels and a reduction of the mesenteric blood flow.

After 35–40 minutes of complete normothermic exclusion from the circulation, liver function is restored without consequences [35]. The time lapse increases to 60 minutes in the case of mild hypothermia (20–22 °C), after which liver function resumes without structural or functional abnormalities [36].

Intestinal hypothermia experimentally induced in rats by maintaining temperature tissue between 15 and 20 °C has been shown to protect intestinal mucosa from damage associated with mesenteric ischemia. Although the mechanism remains not entirely known, protection is likely to be guaranteed by multiple factors: reduced consumption of oxygen and ATP, reduced formation of ROS, and reduced activation of the Nf-kb. [41].

15.3.3.4 Spinal Cord

Hypothermia provides important protection of the spinal cord during ischemic intervals produced by aortic clamping. In a clinical study of hypothermic CPB and circulatory arrest (mean interval of arrest, 38 min; range, 8–62 min) among the 109 survivors with thoracoabdominal aortic disease, early paraplegia occurred in 1 of 36 with Crawford extent I, 0 of 42 with extent II, and 2 of 31 with extent III disease [42].

During surgeries on the descending thoracic and thoracoabdominal aorta on 161 patients, the prevalence of paraplegia or paresis from spinal cord ischemia remained constant and less than 3.5% for ischemic (but hypothermic) intervals of up to 138 min [39].

15.3.4 Biocompatibility of Materials

Modern extracorporeal circulation circuits have an internal biopolymers coating (usually made of heparin or phosphorylcholine) [20, 42]. The coatings mimic the endothelial lining and so reduced the requirement for anticoagulation and decrease the inflammatory response. Nevertheless, the inner surfaces of these circuits are far from complete biocompatibility and do not perfectly replicate the endothelium that is capable of preventing blood elements adhesion clot formation.

As soon as plasma proteins come in contact with the surface, they are adsorbed on to heparinized blood onto all non-endothelial cell surfaces to form a monolayer of bound proteins. For a specific protein, the amount adsorbed depends on its plasma concentration and the intrinsic activity of the artificial surface. The physical and chemical compositions of the polymer determine the proteins, not necessary the most abundant ones, which will likely adhere to that surface. Being every extracorporeal circuit made of a variety of different biomaterials, chemical, physical, and morphological properties of each polymer surface must be considered for the assessment of the adsorbed proteins, which compete for space on the biomaterial surface, are tightly packed, irreversibly bound, and immobile.

Fibrinogen is one of the main proteins adsorbed by most artificial surfaces (it adheres more selectively to hydrophobic rather than hydrophilic materials).

The surfaces constantly change their protein layer as blood flows. Moreover, as proteins adhere to the surface, they can undergo specific conformational changes and expose amino-acid receptor groups recognized by determined blood cells or plasma proteins such as factor XII, complement protein (C3a–C5a etc.), or platelets. Uncontrolled conformational changes of adsorbed protein vary among different biomaterial surfaces and change the reactivity of the adsorbed protein with cells and blood components. In contrast, endothelial cells selectively bind specific proteins using specialized receptors in response to cellular signals that regulate anticoagulants and pro-coagulants mediators. Different biomaterials vary in thrombogenicity, but all eventually simulate clot formation.

15.4 Conclusions

The precise isolation of the individual contributors to better results observed in thoracoabdominal aortic surgery in recent times [41] is not possible. The explanation is multifactorial. In fact, not only the nature of the disease and the characteristics of the operation challenge the integrity and the function of all organs systems, but also many factors contribute to the success or failure of the procedure. Overall, the improvement is likely to be related to the synergism of many small variations in the use of surgical and anesthetic techniques and technological novelties.

According to our experience, it is relevant to underline the substantial contribution of better materials and a more rational use of the existing extracorporeal circulation systems among the many technological improvements that have taken place.

References

1. Kahn RA, Stone ME. Anesthetic consideration for descending thoracic aortic aneurysm repair. Semin Cardiothorac Vasc Anesth. 2007;11(3):205–23.
2. Hessel EA. Techniques for descending thoracic aorta surgery. Semin Cardiothorac Vasc Anesth. 2001;5:293–320.
3. Schepens M, Dossche K. Introduction of adjuncts and their influence on changing results in 402 consecutive thoracoabdominal aortic aneurysm repairs. Eur J Cardiothorac Surg. 2004;25(5):701–7.
4. Pantin EJ, Cheung AT. Thoracic aortic disease. In: Kaplan JA, Reich DL, Lake CL, et al., editors. Kaplan's cardiac anesthesia. 5th ed. Philadelphia: Saunders Elsevier; 2006. p. 723–64.
5. Coselli JS, Lemaire SA. Descending and thoracoabdominal aortic aneurysms. In: Cohn LH, editor. Cardiac surgery in the adult. 3rd ed. New York: McGraw-Hill Medical; 2008. p. 1277–98.
6. Coselli JS. The use of left heart in the repair of thoracoabdominal aortic aneurysms: current techniques and results. Semin Thorac Cardiovasc Surg. 2003;15(4):326–32.
7. Crawford ES, Walker HS. Graft replacement of aneurysm in descending thoracic aorta: results without bypass or shunting. Surgery. 1981;89(1):73–85.
8. Murray GF, Young WG Jr. Thoracic aneurysmectomy utilizing direct left ventriculofemoral shunt (TDMAC–heparin) bypass. Ann Thorac Surg. 1976;21(1):26–9.
9. Fayad A, Sawchuk C. Transesophageal echocardiography in the management of left atrio-femoral during

thoracoabdominal aortic aneurysm repair: a case report. Can J Anaesth. 2002;49(10):1081–3.

10. Suzuki S, Davis CA. Cardiac function predicts mortality following thoracoabdominal and descending thoracic aortic aneurysm repair. Eur. J Cardiothorac Surg. 2003;24(1):119–24.
11. Fayad A, Yang H. Acute diastolic dysfunction in thoracoabdominal aortic aneurysm surgery. Can J Anaesth. 2006;53(2):168–73.
12. Palombo D, Valenti D. Early experience with the minimal extracorporeal circulation system (MECC) during thoracoabdominal aortic aneurysm repair. Eur J Vasc Endovasc Surg. 2004;27(3):324–6.
13. Moore EE, Burch JM. Repair of the torn descending thoracic aorta using the centrifugal pump for partial left heart. Ann Surg. 2004;240(1):38–43.
14. Edwards JT, Brown DM. A versatile extracorporeal circuit for use during repair of descending and thoracoabdominal aortic aneurysms in high-risk patients with cardiac and/or pulmonary dysfunction: a novel approach to a significant perfusion management dilemma. J Extra Corpor Technol. 2004;36(3):245–9.
15. Ziganshin B, Elefteriades JA. Deep hypothermic circulatory arrest. Ann Cardiothorac Surg. 2013;2(3):303–15.
16. Kouchoukos NT. TAAA repair using hypothermic cardiopulmonary bypass and circulatory arrest. Ann Cardiothorac Surg. 2012;1(3):409–11.
17. Leach WR, Sundt TM. Oxygenator support for partial left-heart. Ann Thorac Surg. 2001;72(5):1770–1.
18. Downing SW, Cardarelli MG. Heparinless partial cardiopulmonary for the repair of aortic trauma. J Thorac Cardiovasc Surg. 2000;120(6):1104–9.
19. Tagarakis GI, Tsilimingas NB. Heparin-coated extracorporeal circulation systems in heart surgery. Recent Pat Cardiovasc Drug Discov. 2009;4(3):177–9.
20. Paparella D, Yau TM. Cardiopulmonary induced inflammation: pathophysiology and treatment. An update. Eur J Cardiothorac Surg. 2002;21(2):232–44.
21. Greeley WJ, Ungerleider RM, Kern FH, Brusino FG, Smith LR, Reves JG. Effects of cardiopulmonary bypass on cerebral blood flow in neonates, infants, and children. Circulation. 1989;80:I209.
22. Govier AV, Reves JG, McKay RD, Karp RB, Zorn GL, Morawetz RB, et al. Factors and their influence on regional cerebral blood flow during nonpulsatile cardiopulmonary bypass. Ann Thorac Surg. 1984;38:592.
23. Murkin JM, Farrar JK, Tweed WA, McKenzie KN, Cuirauden G. Cerebral autoregulation and flow/metabolic coupling during cardiopulmonary bypass: the influence of PaCO2. Anesth Analg. 1987;66:825.
24. Prough DS, Stump DA, Roy RC, Gravlee GP, Williams T, Mills SA, et al. Response of cerebral blood flow to changes in carbon dioxide tension during hypothermic cardiopulmonary bypass. Anesthesiology. 1986;64:576.
25. Ataka K, Okada M. Clinical study of optimal flow for temporary with centrifugal pump in surgical treatment of aneurysm of the descending thoracic aorta. Nippon Kyobu Geka Gakkai Zasshi. 1994;42(6):879–85.
26. Szwerc MF, Benckart DH. Recent clinical experience with left heart using a centrifugal pump for repair of traumatic aortic transection. Ann Surg. 1999;230(4):484–90.
27. Cimen B, et al. Pulmonary function tests, aerobic capacity, respiratory muscle strength and endurance of patients with rheumatoid arthritis. Clin Rheumatol. 2001;20:168–73.
28. Jacobs MJ, Mommertz G. Surgical repair of thoracoabdominal aortic aneurysms. J Cardiovasc Surg. 2007;48(1):49–58.
29. Cimen OB, et al. Pulmonary function tests, respiratory muscle strength, and endurance of patients with osteoporosis. South Med J. 2003;96:423–6.
30. Jacobs MJ, et al. Prevention of renal failure in patients undergoing thoracoabdominal aortic aneurysm repair. J Vasc Surg. 2004;40:1067–73. discussion 1073.
31. Kouchoukos NT, et al. Hypothermic bypass and circulatory arrest for operations on the descending thoracic and thoracoabdominal aorta. Ann Thorac Surg. 1995;60:67–76. discussion 76–77.
32. Fehrenbacher JW, et al. Optimal end-organ protection for thoracic and thoracoabdominal aortic aneurysm repair using deep hypothermic circulatory arrest. Ann Thorac Surg. 2007;83:1041–6.
33. Koksoy C, et al. Renal perfusion during thoracoabdominal aortic operations: cold crystalloid is superior to normothermic blood. Ann Thorac Surg. 2002;73:730–8.
34. Huguet C, Nordlinger B, Bloch P, Conard J. Tolerance of the human liver to prolonged normothermic ischemia. Arch Surg. 1978;113:1448.
35. Rittenhouse EA, Mohri H, Reichenbach DD, Merendino KA. Morphological alterations in vital organs after prolonged cardiac arrest at low body temperature. Ann Thorac Surg. 1972;13:564.
36. Hassoun HT, Kozar RA, Kone BC, Safi HJ, Moore FA. Intraischemic hypothermia differentially modulates oxidative stress proteins during mesenteric ischemia/reperfusion. Surgery. 2002;132:369–76.
37. Swaminathan M, Phillips-Bute BG. The association of lowest hematocrit during cardiopulmonary bypass with acute renal injury after coronary artery bypass surgery. Ann Thorac Surg. 2003;76(3):784–91.
38. De Somer F, Van Belleghem Y. Phosphorylcoline coating offers natural platelet preservation during cardiopulmonary bypass. Perfusion. 2002;17(1):39–44.
39. Harris EA, Seelye ER, Barratt-Boyes BG. Respiratory and metabolic acid-base changes during cardiopulmonary bypass in man. Br Anesth. 1970;42:912.
40. Hanssen SJ, Derikx JP. Visceral injury and systemic inflammation in patients undergoing extracorporeal circulation during aortic surgery. Ann Surg. 2008;248(1):117–25.
41. Kouchoukos NT, Masetti P, Rokkas CK, Murphy SF, Blackstone EH. Safety and efficacy of hypothermic ardiopulmonary bypass and circulatory arrest for operations on the descending thoracic and thoracoabdominal aorta. Ann Thorac Surg. 2001;72:699.
42. Brusino FG, Reves JG, Smith LR, Prough DS, Stump DA, McIntyre RW. The effect of age on cerebral blood flow during hypothermic cardiopulmonary bypass. J Thorac Cardiovasc Surg. 1989;97:541.

Perioperative Renal Pharmacological Protection During Cardiovascular Surgery

16

Alessandro Belletti, Margherita Licheri, and Tiziana Bove

16.1 Introduction

Acute kidney injury (AKI), previously known also as acute renal failure, is a syndrome characterized by a rapid decline in kidney function (within hours to days) [1], with associated alterations in metabolic, electrolyte, and fluid homeostasis. It has been estimated that more than 20% of hospitalized patients develop AKI [2–4], and AKI is associated with increased short- and long-term morbidity and mortality, including an increased risk of developing chronic kidney disease (CKD) [5, 6].

Accordingly, AKI is now considered a major health problem worldwide [7, 8], which acquires particular importance considering that several cases of hospital-acquired AKI are iatrogenic [9].

Unfortunately, cardiovascular surgery is considered a major risk factor for AKI development [3, 10, 11]. In this chapter, we will review current definition, epidemiology and available pharmacological strategies to prevent and treat AKI in aortic surgery.

A. Belletti
Department of Anesthesia and Intensive Care, IRCCS San Raffaele Scientific Institute, Milan, Italy

M. Licheri
Department of Medical Sciences and Public Health "M. Aresu", University of Cagliari, Cagliari, Italy

T. Bove (✉)
Department of Medicine, University of Udine, Udine, Italy
e-mail: tiziana.bove@uniud.it

16.2 Acute Kidney Injury: Definition and Epidemiology

Until the last decade, the definition of AKI was highly variable across different studies, yielding to a large heterogeneity in reported incidences and associated outcomes as well as lack of comparative data. In 2004, an international consensus conference developed a standard definition and staging system for AKI based on serum creatinine and urine output, called RIFLE (risk, injury, failure, loss, end-stage kidney disease) classification (Table 16.1) [12]. Later, RIFLE criteria were modified into the AKIN (Acute Kidney Injury Network) criteria [13], to account for the increase in mortality observed for even small increase in serum creatinine [14] (Table 16.1). Finally, RIFLE and AKIN criteria were merged in a single definition proposed by the 2012 Kidney Disease: Improving Global Outcome (KDIGO) clinical practice guidelines on AKI [10–15] (Table 16.1). A standard definition for AKI after endovascular aneurysm repair (EVAR), the Aneurysm Renal Injury Score (ARISe), has also been recently developed [16] (Table 16.2).

Incidence of AKI in aortic surgery is highly variable, depending on surgical technique (open versus endovascular), site (ascending aorta/aortic

© Springer Nature Switzerland AG 2019
Y. Tshomba et al. (eds.), *Visceral Vessels and Aortic Repair*,
https://doi.org/10.1007/978-3-319-94761-7_16

Table 16.1 Diagnostic criteria for acute kidney injury according to RIFLE, AKIN, and KDIGO criteria

RIFLE			AKIN			KDIGO		
	Classification			Classification			Classification	
Stage	*Serum creatinine/GFR*	*Urine output*	Stage	*Serum creatinine/GFR*	*Urine output*	Stage	*Serum creatinine/GFR*	*Urine output*
R	Increased SCr ≥1.5 times the baseline value *or* GFR decrease >25% from baseline value	<0.5 mL/kg/h for at least 6 h	1	Increased SCr ≥1.5–1.9 times the baseline value *or* increase ≥0.3 mg/dL (26.5 μmol/L)	< 0.5 mL/kg/h for at least 6 h	1	Increased SCr ≥1.5–1.9 times the baseline value within 7 days *or* increase ≥0.3 mg/dL (26.5 μmol/L) within 48 h	<0.5 mL/kg/h for at least 6 h
I	Increased SCr ≥2 times the baseline value *or* GFR decrease >50% from baseline value	<0.5 mL/kg/h for at least 12 h	2	Increased SCr ≥2 times the baseline value	<0.5 mL/kg/h for at least 12 h	2	Increased SCr ≥2 times the baseline value	<0.5 mL/kg/h for at least 12 h
F	Increased SCr ≥3 times the baseline value *or* GFR decrease >75% from baseline value *or* SCr ≥ 4 mg/dL (350 μmol/L) in the setting of acute rise ≥ 0.5 mg/dL (44 μmol/L)	<0.3 mL/kg/h for at least 24 h *or* anuria for 12 h	3	Increased SCr ≥3 times the baseline value *or* SCr ≥4 mg/dL (350 μmol/L) in the setting of acute rise ≥0.5 mg/dL (44 μmol/L) *or* need for RRT	<0.3 mL/kg/h for at least 24 h *or* anuria for 12 h	3	Increased SCr ≥3 times the baseline value OR SCr ≥4 mg/dL (350 μmol/L) *or* need for RRT OR in patients <18 years a decrease in GFR to <35 mL/min/1.73 m^2	<0.3 mL/kg/h for at least 24 h *or* anuria for 12 h
L	Need for RRT for >4 weeks	N/A		N/A	N/A		N/A	N/A
E	Need for dialysis for >3 months	N/A		N/A	N/A		N/A	N/A

AKIN Acute Kidney Injury Network, *GFR* glomerular filtration rate, *KDIGO* kidney disease: improving global outcome, *RIFLE* risk, injury, failure, loss, end-stage kidney disease, *RRT* renal replacement therapy, *SCr* serum creatinine

Adapted from Bellomo et al. [12], Mehta et al. [13], and Kellum et al. [10]

Table 16.2 Diagnostic criteria for acute kidney injury according to ARISe criteria

Stage	Classification Creatinine/GFR	Urine output
1	Increased SCr >0.3 mg/dL (26.5 μmol/L) or <50% of baseline within 48 h	<0.5 mL/kg/h for >6 h
2	50% to 99% rise in SCr from the preoperative value within 7 days	
3	>100% rise in serum creatinine from the preoperative value within 7 days	
4	Need for RRT	
5	Permanent RRT	

RRT renal replacement therapy
Adapted from Twine et al. [16]

arch, descending thoracic aorta, suprarenal and infrarenal abdominal aorta), and urgency of the procedure (elective versus urgent). Procedures involved requiring suprarenal aortic cross-clamp and renal ischemia clearly carry the highest risk.

In the largest case series on open thoracoabdominal aortic aneurysm (TAAA) repair, Coselli et al. described outcome of 3309 patients. Of these, 12.3% had acute renal dysfunction (defined as doubling of serum creatinine or need for RRT—roughly corresponding to KDIGO AKI stage ≥2) and 7.6% required postoperative renal replacement therapy (RRT), with 5.6% still requiring dialysis at hospital discharge or at time of in-hospital death [17]. Tshomba et al. performed a propensity-matched study on 84 open TAAA patients, reporting a 42.9% incidence of stage 1 AKI (according to AKIN criteria), with 4.7% patients requiring RRT and no patients requiring dialysis at discharge [18]. In their case series of 455 patients undergoing open TAAA repair, Wynn et al. reported a 17% incidence of RIFLE-R AKI and a 2.7% incidence of AKI requiring renal replacement therapy (RRT). Permanent dialysis was required in three (0.66%) cases [19]. Considering surgery for acute aortic dissection, the incidence of AKI may be more than 50% [20–22], with need for RRT in more than 10% of patients [20, 21]. Dariane and colleagues recently performed a systematic review of AKI incidence in open repair of intact abdominal aortic aneurysm (AAA) [23], including only studies using modern standardized criteria for AKI definition (RIFLE, AKIN, KDIGO, or ARISe). In cases of suprarenal aortic cross-clamp, incidence of AKI may be up to 36.8% and need for RRT up to 3.8%. For infrarenal clamping, incidence of AKI was reported in about 25% of cases, with 0.3% of patients requiring RRT. In patients undergoing surgery for ruptured AAA (rAAA), AKI incidence rises up to 75% of patients [24–26].

Patients undergoing endovascular aortic procedures are also at high risk for postoperative AKI. In thoracic endovascular aortic repair (TEVAR), modern case series using RIFLE criteria to define AKI reported incidences of 14–22%, with RRT required in 0.6–7% of patients [27–29]. A similar incidence was found in TEVAR for type B aortic dissection [30] Incidence of RIFLE-, AKIN-, KDIGO- or ARISe-defined AKI after EVAR is similar, with a 5–19% reported incidence, with most of studies reporting a 0% rate of dialysis [31].

16.3 Identification of Patients at Risk

Risk stratification for postoperative AKI is of utmost importance in order to tailor perioperative management according to patient risk. Risk factors for AKI can be related to patients' baseline comorbidities [10, 32]. Importantly, duration of renal ischemia is a key determinant of postoperative AKI in abdominal aortic procedures.

To aid clinicians in stratifying risk objectively, risk scores for postoperative AKI have been developed [33–40]. Importantly, most of these risk scores have been developed to predict need for RRT after cardiac surgery, while specific scores for vascular surgery are currently lacking [41]. Among the different scores, a recent systematic review identified the Cleveland Clinic Score by Thakar et al. (Table 16.3) to have the

Table 16.3 Cleveland clinic score for acute kidney injury requiring dialysis after cardiac surgery

Risk factor	Score	
Female sex	1	
Congestive heart failure	1	
LVEF <35%	1	
Preoperative need for IABP	2	
COPD	1	
Insulin-dependent diabetes	1	
Previous cardiac surgery	1	
Emergency surgery	2	
Valve surgery only	1	
CABG + valve surgery	2	
Other cardiac surgery	2	
Preoperative SCr 1.2–2.1 mg/dL	2	
Preoperative SCr >2.1 mg/dL	5	
Risk categories	Total score	RRT incidence (%)
1	0–2	0.4
2	3–5	1.8
3	6–8	9.5
4	9–13[a]	21.3

CABG coronary artery bypass graft, *COPD* chronic obstructive pulmonary disease, *IABP* intra-aortic balloon pump, *LVEF* left ventricular ejection fraction, *RRT* renal replacement therapy

Adapted from Thakar et al. [33]

[a]No patient had a score greater than 13 in the original dataset

highest predictive value [42]. Whether this score can also be applied to patients undergoing aortic vascular surgery remains to be determined.

16.3.1 Contrast-Induced Acute Kidney Injury

Administration of intravenous contrast media is common during vascular surgical procedures. It is almost always required during endovascular procedures and is sometimes also used following open surgery to confirm vessel patency (e.g., in the oliguric patient following procedures on renal arteries). As contrast media administration is one of the most common causes of iatrogenic AKI, prevention of CI-AKI remains a key issue in renal protection. Therefore, preoperative risk stratification of patients should also consider the risk of CI-AKI.

Unfortunately, up to now, most studies investigating incidence and risk factors for CI-AKI focus on percutaneous coronary interventions [43]. This setting is clearly different from vascular surgery, as patients undergoing vascular surgery may have a greater number of concomitant kidney insults, such as renal ischemia related to aortic or renal arteries cross-clamp, severe blood loss, and hemodynamic instability. The risk of contrast-induced acute kidney injury (CI-AKI) is considered to become clinically important when the baseline serum creatinine concentration is ≥1.3 mg/dL in men and ≥1.0 mg/dL in women, equivalent to an estimated glomerular filtration rate (eGFR) <60 mL/min [44]. As a general rule, patients may be simply stratified in low, intermediate, and high risk depending on GFR and clinical history [45]. Patients with no history of diabetes, heart failure, or monoclonal gammopathy and eGFR >60 mL/min/1.73 m^2 should be considered at low risk. Patients with eGFR 30–60 mL/min/1.73 m^2 or eGFR 45–60 mL/min/1.73 m^2 together with heart failure or diabetes carry an intermediate risk. Finally, patients with monoclonal gammopathy and eGFR ≤30 mL/min/1.73 m^2 regardless of comorbidities and patients with eGFR ≤45 mL/min/1.73 m^2 together with diabetes or heart failure are all considered at high risk [41].

Mehran et al., after analyzing 8357 patients undergoing percutaneous coronary intervention (PCI), proposed a clinical risk score allowing for immediate identification of the variables accounted for before the procedure and appropriate (and timely) risk allocation. It is based on eight readily available variables: (1) patient-related characteristics (age >75 years, diabetes mellitus, chronic congestive heart failure, or admission with acute pulmonary edema, hypotension, anemia, and chronic kidney disease) and (2) procedure-related characteristics (i.e., the use of elective IABP or increasing volumes of contrast media). Patients scoring positive for at least three risk factors will have a 26% probability

Table 16.4 Clinical risk score for contrast-induced acute kidney injury

Risk factor	Score		
Hypotension (SBP <80 mmHg for at least 1 h requiring inotropic support or IABP in the 24 h before procedure)	5		
IABP use	5		
Congestive heart failure (NYHA class III/IV or history of pulmonary edema)	5		
Age >75 years	4		
Anemia (Hct <39% for men and 36% for women)	3		
Diabetes mellitus	3		
Contrast volume	1/100 mL		
Serum creatinine *or* GFR (use only one parameter)			
• Serum creatinine >1.5 mg/dL *OR*	4		
• GFR			
– 40–60 mL/min/1.73 m^2	2		
– 20–39 mL/min/1.73 m^2	4		
– <20 mL/min/1.73 m^2	6		
Risk categories	Total score	AKI incidence (%)	RRT incidence (%)
Low	≤5	7.5	0.04
Moderate	6–10	14	0.12
High	11–15	26.1	1.09
Very high	≥16	57.3	12.6

AKI acute kidney injury, *GFR* glomerular filtration rate, *Hct* hematocrit, *IABP* intra-aortic balloon pump, *NYHA* New York Heart Association, *RRT* renal replacement therapy
Adapted from Mehran et al. [46]

of developing CI-AKI and a 1% probability of needing dialysis following PCI [46] (Table 16.4).

16.4 Preventive Strategies

Considering the high-risk and prognostic impact of perioperative AKI in cardiovascular surgery, the development of strategies aimed at preventing AKI in this setting has always been a major topic in research. Although a large number of studies investigating several strategies have been conducted, only few demonstrated a clear positive effect, while most led to neutral or controversial results [15, 32, 41, 47, 48]. As outlined by recent guidelines, the most important preventive measures are the maintenance of adequate renal perfusion and avoidance of nephrotoxic drugs [15, 32, 47]. Importantly, a recent expert opinion paper from the European Society of Intensive Care Medicine was able to formulate strong recommendations with high level of evidence only *against* some interventions and none in favor [47].

16.4.1 Primum Non Nocere: Avoiding Nephrotoxins

Unfortunately, AKI is considered to be iatrogenic in several cases [41]. Several drugs can contribute to AKI development, including renin-angiotensin-aldosterone system (RAAS) blockers, nonsteroidal anti-inflammatory drugs (NSAIDs), aminoglycosides, amphotericin B, and contrast media [49]. Some categories of patients have a particularly increased risk of drug-induced AKI, such as older, volume-depleted patients or hemodynamically unstable patients [49]. The first step of AKI prevention is therefore to avoid drugs which can induce or exacerbate AKI as much as possible.

Several patients undergoing cardiovascular surgery are treated with RAAS, and optimal management of these agents in the perioperative period remains controversial. Current guidelines recommend to discontinue angiotensin-converting enzyme inhibitors (ACE-Is) and angiotensin receptors blockers (ARBs) before cardiac surgery, albeit with a low level of evidence [50]. In patients with difficult-to-control hypertension, switching long-acting to short-acting ACE-Is/ARBs should be considered.

Similarly, it is reasonable to avoid NSAIDs in the perioperative period in high-risk patients, using alternative drugs such as opioids or paracetamol (acetaminophen) to treat pain [50, 51].

It is intuitive that antimicrobial agents alternative to aminoglycosides and amphotericin B should be used when feasible [15]. When this is not possible, international guidelines recommend to administer a single daily dose of aminoglycosides rather than multiple-dose daily treatment and to monitor drug levels to avoid excessive dosing [15]. If amphotericin B is deemed necessary, lipid formulation should be used rather than conventional formulation [15].

Finally, it should be remembered that CI-AKI is among the most common causes of iatrogenic AKI. Accordingly, benefits and risk of contrast media administration should be adequately weighted before planning a diagnostic or therapeutic procedure requiring intravenous contrast media administration, especially in high-risk patients (e.g., patients with a Mehran score greater than 16). If a diagnostic procedure requiring IV contrast media is deemed necessary, it might be reasonable to delay subsequent elective high-risk surgery or other procedures requiring contrast media (Table 16.5) for a few days, especially if concomitant nephrotoxic agents are being used. However, some recent studies suggested that the risk of CI-AKI may actually be overestimated [52]. Accordingly, while it is reasonable to search for alternative diagnostic tools or delay procedures in elective cases, urgent and life-saving procedures should not be deferred or denied only because of CI-AKI risk.

Table 16.5 Suggested strategy for contrast-induced acute kidney injury prevention

	Low risk	Intermediate risk	High risk
Stratification	eGFR >60 mL/min/1.73 m^2 and no monoclonal gammopathy	– eGFR 30–60 mL/min/1.73 m^2 and no heart failure – eGFR 45–60 mL/min/1.73 m^2 and diabetes or heart failure	– eGFR <30 mL/min/1.73 m^2 and no heart failure – eGFR <45 mL/min/1.73 m^2 and diabetes or heart failure – Monoclonal gammopathy
Volume expansion	Liberal fluid intake – 1 L over 12 h before contrast administration and 1 L over 12 h after contrast administration	Oral volume expansion schedule – 1 g NaCl + 150 mL of H_2O every hour from 2 h before until 6 h after contrast administration	IV volume expansion schedule with one of these regimens – 1 L NaCl 0.9% over 12 h before and after contrast administration – 1 L glucose 5% + 150 mmol/L bicarbonate 8.4%, 3 mL/kg/h over 1 h before and 1 mL/kg/h during 6 h after contrast administration
General management	– Avoid repetitive contrast administration (<7 days after previous contrast administration) – Reschedule if possible in case of recent (i.e., within 72 h) use of nonsteroidal anti-inflammatory drugs	– Avoid repetitive contrast administration (<7 days after previous contrast administration) – Reschedule if possible in case of recent (i.e., within 72 h) use of nonsteroidal anti-inflammatory drugs	– Avoid repetitive contrast administration (<7 days after previous contrast administration) – Reschedule if possible in case of recent (i.e., within 72 h) use of nonsteroidal anti-inflammatory drugs – Stop metformin 48 h before the procedure and restart 72 h after the procedure

eGFR estimated glomerular filtration rate
Adapted from Vanmassenhove et al. [41]

16.4.2 General Hemodynamic Management: MAP and Fluids

Maintenance of an adequate level of mean arterial pressure (MAP) is a mainstay of AKI prevention. However, the optimal target MAP remains to be determined, particularly for chronically hypertensive patients (who consists a large proportion of patients undergoing vascular surgery). In an observational trial including 33,330 noncardiac surgical procedures, Walsh et al. identified 55 mmHg as a threshold below which patients were at increased risk for both renal and myocardial injury. Importantly, even brief periods (1–5 min) below 55 mmHg MAP were associated with an increased risk [53]. In a recent observational study, Salmasi et al. identified a threshold of 65 mmHg or 20% decrease for 10–15 min from baseline, below which there is an increased risk of AKI and myocardial injury. Not surprisingly, the risk increased with lower thresholds and longer duration of hypotension [54]. The authors, however, found that association based on absolute thresholds was comparable to that based on relative thresholds, and no interaction with preoperative pressure was found. Hence, the authors concluded that anesthetic management should target an absolute MAP value greater than 65 mmHg [54] regardless of baseline pressure. A recent multicenter randomized controlled trial (RCT) in septic shock patients compared two MAP levels (65–70 mmHg and 80–85 mmHg). In the overall population, no differences in mortality or renal outcomes were observed, with a higher incidence of atrial fibrillation in the highest target MAP group [55]. However, the authors found a lower incidence of AKI and need for RRT in chronically hypertensive patients when a MAP of 80–85 mmHg was targeted [55]. As these results are derived from a subgroup analysis in a different clinical setting, generalization to vascular surgery patients remains to be determined. Furthermore, higher MAP levels may be associated with increased bleeding risk and disruption of vascular anastomosis. Hence, the optimal MAP target should be evaluated on a case-by-case basis together with the surgeon and may vary within the same surgical procedure.

Hypovolemia (both relative and absolute) is a well-known risk factor for AKI, and hypovolemic patients should receive adequate volume replacement. Unfortunately, volume overload has been associated to increased risk of AKI development too [56, 57]. A major issue remains therefore to accurately determine patient volume status. It is now well recognized that the absolute value of static parameters such as central venous pressure (CVP) and pulmonary capillary wedge pressure (PCWP) does not reliably predict fluid responsiveness [58], although CVP remains a good marker of preload and a key determinant of pressure gradient for organ perfusion (MAP-CVP) [59]. Dynamic indices of fluid responsiveness have shown better performance in predicting fluid responsiveness, but all have drawbacks which may limit their use in cardiovascular surgery (e.g., the need for absence of arrhythmias, high tidal volumes and lung compliance, closed chest, and continuous cardiac output monitoring) [59].

The choice of fluid to administer is also a critical issue. Fluids can be divided in crystalloids, artificial colloids, and natural colloids [60]. Until recently, it was believed that colloids, compared with crystalloids, had a better volume-expanding capacity (1 L colloid equivalent to 3 L crystalloids), which should theoretically translate in a more sustained hemodynamic effect with a reduced extravascular edema. However, recent trials demonstrated that actual colloid/crystalloid volume expansion ratio is probably less than 1:1.5 [60]. In addition, artificial colloids have been associated to several side effects, including allergic reactions, coagulation impairment, and, above all, nephrotoxicity [47, 61–63]. The largest multicenter RCT (mRCT) performed so far investigated the effect of hydroxyethyl starch (HES) in critically ill patients and showed increased mortality and AKI in HES-treated patients, as compared with crystalloids [64, 65]. Accordingly, use of HES is currently contraindicated by international guidelines, while use of other artificial colloids is discouraged [47]. Some authors, nevertheless, suggest that the use of colloids (including HES) is safe in selected patients and following strict dosing and monitoring protocol [66]. Human albumin is the only colloid that has not been associated with increased risk of AKI, and safety in adults has been assessed in several mRCTs [67, 68], although an increased mortality associated with both 5% human albumin and 0.9% saline fluid bolus in children with sepsis was found [69]. In summary, human albumin remains the most attractive colloid when hypooncotic hypovolemia is suspected, although the high costs may limit its use.

Among crystalloids, it has been suggested that large infusion of 0.9% saline may increase AKI risk due to the high chloride levels and subsequent acid-base and electrolyte equilibrium alterations. Although a clear effect has not been demonstrated in large mRCTs [70], it seems prudent and physiologically more rational to use balanced crystalloid solutions instead of 0.9% saline when large-volume resuscitation is required [32, 47].

16.4.3 Specific Drugs

16.4.3.1 Dopamine

Dopamine is an endogenous catecholamine with different effects on adrenergic receptors depending on dose. At doses ≤3 μg/kg/min, dopamine is considered to stimulate dopaminergic receptors only; between 4 and 10 μg/kg/min, it stimulates β-adrenergic receptors, increasing ino- and chronotropism, and in doses >10 μg/kg/min, it has also α-receptor-mediated vasoconstrictor effect. Low-dose dopamine (≤3 μg/kg/min) has been advocated in the past to preserve renal blood flow through a selective afferent arteriolar vasodilation mediated by dopaminergic receptors [71]. Although low-dose dopamine may actually increase renal plasma flow, GFR, and sodium excretion, this effect seems to be attributable to increase in cardiac output, rather than specific effects on renal hemodynamics [71]. Some authors have even found that low-dose dopamine may actually worsen renal perfusion [72]. Finally both high-quality mRCTs and meta-analyses failed to demonstrate any effect of low-dose dopamine on incidence or clinical course of AKI or mortality [73, 74].

The use of dopamine as a vasopressor in shock has been investigated in a large mRCT comparing dopamine and norepinephrine [75]. Although no difference in mortality was observed between the two groups, dopamine use was associated with an increased risk of arrhythmias and a trend toward increased renal support-free days in the norepinephrine group. Furthermore, a subgroup analysis suggested a survival benefit in patients with cardiogenic shock receiving norepinephrine [75].

Therefore, there is no rationale to support use of low-dose dopamine to prevent or treat AKI, and current evidence also discourages the use of dopamine as first-line inotropic/vasopressor agent [47, 76, 77].

16.4.3.2 Fenoldopam

Fenoldopam is a selective D_1 dopamine receptor agonist which acts as a systemic and renal vasodilator. It has been shown to promote diuresis and natriuresis and to increase renal blood flow. Several meta-analyses of RCTs on fenoldopam use in cardiovascular and major surgery suggested a possible beneficial effect of fenoldopam on AKI development, but not on need for RRT or mortality [78–80]. Notably, most trials included in meta-analyses were small and considered at high risk of bias.

The largest mRCT performed on fenoldopam use so far randomized 667 post-cardiac surgery patients with RIFLE-R AKI to fenoldopam or placebo and found no difference in need for RRT or mortality [81]. Furthermore, fenoldopam use was associated with a higher incidence of hypotension.

Although there still may be room for future investigation on preventive use of fenoldopam (i.e., in high-risk patients before AKI development), current evidence does not support fenoldopam use in patients with or at risk for AKI [47]. This recommendation is further supported by the hypotensive effect of fenoldopam in light of the key role of MAP in kidney protection.

16.4.3.3 Levosimendan

Levosimendan is a calcium sensitizer with positive inotropic, vasodilatory, and cardioprotective effects [82, 83]. It has been suggested that levosimendan may enhance kidney protection through systemic and renal hemodynamics effects, as well as direct anti-ischemic, anti-inflammatory, and anti-apoptotic effects [84]. Promising results were indeed shown in meta-analyses of RCTs in patients with or at risk for AKI receiving levosimendan [85, 86]. However, three recent mRCTs in cardiac surgery setting failed to demonstrate an improvement in renal outcome associated with levosimendan use, either as "prophylactic" measure in high-risk patients [87, 88] or as "therapeutic" measure in patients with established postoperative cardiovascular dysfunction [89].

Accordingly, use of levosimendan to treat or prevent AKI in cardiovascular surgery is currently not supported by randomized evidence. Nevertheless, levosimendan might still have a role in the preoperative optimization of patients with moderate-to-severe myocardial dysfunction. In this case, however, the optimal use would probably be to start levosimendan at least 6 h before surgery and ideally 24 h before.

16.4.3.4 Vasopressin

Vasopressin and its analogue terlipressin are potent non-catecholaminergic vasoconstrictors which improve systemic hemodynamics in catecholamine-resistant vasodilatory shock [90] and may improve GFR through post-glomerular vasoconstriction [91]. A large mRCT in septic patients did not show a beneficial effect on mortality or renal outcome of low-dose vasopressin in septic shock patients, as compared with norepinephrine [92]. However, a post hoc analysis of the same trial suggested that vasopressin could prevent AKI progression in patients with stage 1 AKI at baseline [93]. A subsequent 2 × 2 mRCT on vasopressin and steroids use in early septic shock, however, did not demonstrate a reduction in incidence or progression to stage 3 AKI in vasopressin-treated patients [94]. Need for RRT was reduced but only in non-survivors. Another recent single-center RCT in post-cardiac surgery patients with vasodilatory shock compared vasopressin and norepinephrine as first-line vasopressor agent. Incidence of AKI and need for RRT was reduced in patients receiving vasopressin [95]; however, these findings require confirmation in high-quality mRCTs [47].

In summary, current evidence suggest that early use of vasopressin should be considered in patients requiring high-dose norepinephrine to maintain MAP.

16.4.3.5 Diuretics

Diuretics have been a mainstay of AKI treatment for years [96]. The hypothesized direct beneficial effects of diuretics (loop diuretics in particular) include the prevention of tubular obstruction, increase in renal blood flow, and reduction in oxygen consumption in the renal medulla. In addition, they might have an indirect beneficial effect by reducing volume overload and venous congestion.

Up to now, no perioperative RCT showed a convincing reduction in incidence, severity, or clinical course of AKI with diuretics administration [15, 47, 97–99].

Nevertheless, diuretics could still have a fundamental role in controlling fluid overload, which is associated with venous congestion and increased CVP, conditions that worsen renal perfusion and contribute to renal damage development.

Furthermore, a standardized furosemide stress test to predict AKI severity was recently developed and validated. Urinary output lower than 200 mL/2 h after a 1–1.5 mg/kg furosemide bolus in oliguric patients was found to be associated to AKI progression to more severe stages [100]. Furosemide stress test in the setting of perioperative cardiovascular surgery remains to be validated. However, it is particularly attractive in this setting, especially during procedures involving renal arteries. In an oliguric patient who underwent a procedure on renal arteries, absence of an adequate diuretic response following the test should trigger further diagnostic work-up, such as ultrasound or angiographic assessment of renal vascular bed.

16.4.3.6 Steroids

Steroids are frequently administered in patients at risk for AKI with the aim of reducing inflammatory and ischemia-reperfusion injury. However, recent large mRCTs failed to demonstrate a protective effect of both methylprednisolone and dexamethasone on renal failure following cardiac surgery [101, 102]. Nevertheless, a post hoc analysis of one of the trials showed a reduction in need for RRT in patients receiving 1 mg/kg dexamethasone intraoperatively, particularly when eGFR was lower than 15 mL/min/1.73 m^2 [103]. In addition, subgroup analyses of these trials suggested that steroids may have an age-dependent effect, being beneficial in patients aged <65 years and possibly harmful in patients aged >80 years [104]. However, these preliminary findings need to be confirmed and require further investigation.

16.4.3.7 Statins

Similarly to steroids, statins have anti-inflammatory, antioxidant, and antithrombotic effects (so-called pleiotropic effects) which may have a role in preventing perioperative kidney damage [105, 106]. Accordingly, perioperative administration of statins to improve cardiovascular and renal outcome has been investigated in large number of RCTs, especially in cardiovascular surgery setting. Unfortunately, contrary to expectation, recent trials in cardiac surgery found that perioperative statin administration was associated with an increased risk of AKI, particularly in statin-naïve patients [107–109]. A recent meta-analysis including these recent RCTs found a trend toward increase in mortality in patients receiving statins [110]. In vascular surgery, a recent meta-analysis highlighted lack of definitive evidence of beneficial effects of perioperative statin administration [111], as did a recent mRCT in noncardiac surgery [112]. According to results of these trials, statins should not be administered perioperatively in statin-naïve patients, while the management of statins in patients already receiving chronic therapy remains controversial, especially considering the possible detrimental effect of statin withdrawal due to rebound effect [113, 114]. In the absence of trials addressing this issue, it seems prudent to continue statins perioperatively in patients already receiving a chronic statin therapy.

16.4.3.8 Natriuretic Peptides

Natriuretic peptides include atrial natriuretic peptide (ANP) and b-type natriuretic peptide (BNP), both released by cardiac myocytes in response to acute increase in stretch or pressure [115–117]. Both natriuretic peptides induce dilation of afferent and constriction of efferent arterioles, promotes an increase in glomerular filtration rate and sodium excretion, and has a dose-dependent hypotensive effect.

Several RCTs and meta-analyses of RCTs on perioperative administration of natriuretic peptides to prevent kidney damage have been published [118–122]. These studies found that administration of low-dose ANP might reduce incidence of AKI and RRT in cardiovascular surgery (at expense of a higher incidence of hypotension and arrhythmias), while high-dose ANP and BNP have no effect or may even be detrimental. However, a panel of expert from the European Society of Intensive Care Medicine also highlighted that published trials are of overall small sample size and low quality, and therefore routine perioperative administration of ANP cannot currently be recommended [47]

16.4.3.9 *N*-Acetylcysteine

N-Acetylcysteine (NAC) is a glutathione precursor with antioxidant and free radical-scavenging properties. These properties have been suggested to have a kidney-protective effect from ischemia-reperfusion injury and inflammatory damage. Accordingly NAC has been studied in a large number of RCTs performed in the setting of contrast-induced AKI and cardiac surgery patients [47]. As for many other interventions, RCT on perioperative NAC use in cardiac and vascular surgery showed controversial effects, with some trials reporting some beneficial effects [123, 124] and other a neutral effect [125–128]. If a benefit exists, it is probably limited to patients with a creatinine clearance <60 mL/min [123, 124]. However, quality of evidence is considered low [47]. In addition, NAC is not devoid of side effects, such as anaphylactic and anaphylactoid reactions [129, 130].

16.4.3.10 Future Directions

Due to negative or controversial results of almost all interventions investigated so far, research on pharmacological strategies to treat or prevent AKI is still ongoing. Several agents have been suggested to be of potential benefit in patients with or at risk for AKI, including alkaline phosphatase, endothelin-A receptor antagonist, prostaglandins, and antioxidant vitamins such as vitamins C and E [6, 51]. Some promising results have been suggested in preclinical, observational, or phase II trials, and further trails are likely to be completed in the next years. Alkaline phosphatase at the most advanced stage of clinical investigation is being currently investigated in a phase II mRCT in septic patient (NCT02182440).

16.4.4 Prevention of Contrast-Induced Acute Kidney Injury

A major limitation of current evidence concerning CI-AKI prevention is that most of available trials were performed in the setting of coronary angiography, peripheral angiography, or diagnostic CT scan, which may be slightly different from major endovascular procedures (e.g., branched-fenestrated EVAR). Nevertheless, general recommendations should also apply to vascular surgery patients.

16.4.4.1 Contrast Volume and Type

There is a correlation between the risk of CI-AKI and the volume of iodinated contrast media administered [131]. It has been found that a ratio <1 between grams of iodine (g-I) and eGFR is safe in a patient without multiple risk factors; the risk of CI-AKI in this setting is 3%, while it increase to 25% at a g-I/eGFR ratio ≥1 [132].

Osmolarity of contrast media is also considered to have a role in CI-AKI development. In patients with normal renal function, low- and high-osmolar contrast media are considered to carry the same CI-AKI risk [133]. On the contrary, low-osmolar contrast media are considered less nephrotoxic than high-osmolar contrast in patients with pre-existing kidney function impairment, and in these patients, the use of iso- or low-osmolar contrast media is recommended [15, 43].

16.4.4.2 Volume Expansion

To date, volume expansion remains the only widely recognized strategy to prevent CI-AKI [15, 32, 41, 43]. A common protocol for elective procedures may be administration of 1 mL/kg/h of 0.9% normal saline for 12 h before and 12 h after scheduled contrast administration. Other authors suggest administering 1 L over 12 h independently from patient weight [41]. For urgent procedures, a possible alternative might be 3 mL/kg/h for 1 h before contrast administration and 1 mL/kg/h for 6 h after [134]. Others suggest using a 1 L glucose 5% + 150 mmol/L sodium bicarbonate 8.4% instead of 0.9% normal saline for urgent procedures, with an infusion rate of 3 mL/kg/h (maximal rate 300 mL/h; reduce rate by half in heart failure patients) over 1 h before and 1 mL/kg/h (maximal rate 100 mL/h; reduce rate by half in heart failure patients) for 6 h after contrast administration [41]. Infusion rate should be reduced, and careful monitoring is recommended for patients who may not tolerate excessive volume expansion (e.g., advanced heart failure). Low- and intermediate-risk patients may receive oral fluid administration only [41], although evidence is controversial. On the contrary, high-risk patients should receive intravenous volume expansion [41]. While suggested by some authors, the effectiveness of sodium bicarbonate on CI-AKI in high-risk patients remains uncertain. Accordingly, guidelines from different societies provided different recommendations regarding sodium bicarbonate use as volume expansion [32, 134]. However, two recent mRCT challenged this view, showing no difference in CI-AKI incidence between patients with GRF <60 mL/min receiving intravenous 0.9% normal saline (1 mL/kg/h for 12 h before and after contrast exposure) and patients receiving no hydration [135] and no difference in CI-AKI incidence between patients receiving sodium bicarbonate versus 0.9% normal saline and N-acetylcysteine versus placebo [136].

Recently, some randomized trials have shown some beneficial effect of forced diuresis with furosemide administration and matched hydration using an automated fluid delivery system [137]. In a meta-analysis of RCTs, incidence of CI-AKI and post-procedural need for RRT were reduced when contrast media was administered after a diuresis of 300 mL/h using was achieved [137]. However, all trials included in this meta-analysis were considered at high risk of bias, and further investigation on automated fluid delivery devices is required. Of note, there is agreement that urgent or emergent diagnostic or therapeutic interventions should not be delayed solely to perform volume expansion for CI-AKI prevention.

16.4.4.3 Pharmacological Intervention

A wide number of pharmacological interventions to prevent CI-AKI have been investigated, with only few of them showing high-quality evidence of benefit [41, 43, 47, 138]. The two strategies which showed the most convincing effect are *N*-acetylcysteine (NAC) and statin administration.

A lot of study demonstrated renoprotective effects of NAC prophylaxis once AKI is administered before the onset of renal insult due to the antioxidant properties [139]. In a recent meta-analysis, NAC plus saline showed superior effect as compared with normal saline in patients receiving low-osmolar contrast media [138]. Considering the possible side effects of intravenous NAC, KDIGO guidelines suggest using oral NAC together with saline in patients at high risk for CI-AKI with a very low level of evidence [134], while other authors do not recommend such strategy [32, 41].

We described earlier the possible kidney-protective effects of statins due to their pleiotropic effects. Current evidence from RCTs performed in the setting of coronary angiography suggests that short-term use of atorvastatin or rosuvastatin may reduce incidence of CI-AKI [47]. These findings were confirmed in a meta-analysis of RCT showing beneficial effect in CI-AKI prevention of a regimen of statins plus NAC plus saline over NAC plus saline alone [138]. Accordingly, periprocedural statin administration may be considered in high-risk patients undergoing contrast media administration. However, to further complicate the clinical picture, perioperative statin administration showed detrimental effect in patients undergoing cardiac surgery [137]. Statin administration in statin-naïve patients should be therefore carefully considered in patients undergoing major cardiovascular surgery, even if contrast media administration is planned. On the contrary, patients undergoing diagnostic or therapeutic endovascular procedures may benefit from statins, although these will require further investigation. Notably, most patients scheduled for vascular surgery are likely to already receive statins as part of their chronic medical therapy.

References

1. Bellomo R, Kellum JA, Ronco C. Acute kidney injury. Lancet. 2012;380(9843):756–66. https://doi.org/10.1016/S0140-6736(11)61454-2.
2. Chertow GM, Burdick E, Honour M, Bonventre JV, Bates DW. Acute kidney injury, mortality, length of stay, and costs in hospitalized patients. J Am Soc Nephrol. 2005;16(11):3365–70.
3. Zeng X, McMahon GM, Brunelli SM, Bates DW, Waikar SS. Incidence, outcomes, and comparisons across definitions of AKI in hospitalized individuals. Clin J Am Soc Nephrol. 2014;9(1):12–20. https://doi.org/10.2215/CJN.02730313.
4. Wang HE, Muntner P, Chertow GM, Warnock DG. Acute kidney injury and mortality in hospitalized patients. Am J Nephrol. 2012;35(4):349–55. https://doi.org/10.1159/000337487.
5. Doyle J, Forni L. Acute kidney injury: short-term and long-term effects. Crit Care. 2016;20:188.
6. Bellomo R, Ronco C, Mehta RL, Asfar P, Boisramé-Helms J, Darmon M, et al. Acute kidney injury in the ICU: from injury to recovery: reports from the 5th Paris International Conference. Ann Intensive Care. 2017;7(1):49. https://doi.org/10.1186/s13613-017-0260-y.
7. Lewington AJ, Cerdá J, Mehta RL. Raising awareness of acute kidney injury: a global perspective of a silent killer. Kidney Int. 2013;84(3):457–67. https://doi.org/10.1038/ki.2013.153.
8. Mehta RL, Cerdá J, Burdmann EA, Tonelli M, García-García G, Jha V, et al. International Society of Nephrology's 0by25 initiative for acute kidney injury (zero preventable deaths by 2025): a human rights case for nephrology. Lancet. 2015;385(9987):2616–43. https://doi.org/10.1016/S0140-6736(15)60126-X.
9. Wonnacott A, Meran S, Amphlett B, Talabani B, Phillips A. Epidemiology and outcomes in community-acquired versus hospital-acquired AKI. Clin J Am Soc Nephrol. 2014;9(6):1007–14. https://doi.org/10.2215/CJN.07920713.
10. Kellum JA, Lameire N, KDIGO AKI Guideline Work Group. Diagnosis, evaluation, and management of acute kidney injury: a KDIGO summary (part 1). Crit Care. 2013;17(1):204. https://doi.org/10.1186/cc11454.

11. Grams ME, Sang Y, Coresh J, Ballew S, Matsushita K, Molnar MZ, et al. Acute kidney injury after major surgery: a retrospective analysis of veterans health administration data. Am J Kidney Dis. 2016;67(6):872–80. https://doi.org/10.1053/j.ajkd.2015.07.022.
12. Bellomo R, Ronco C, Kellum JA, Mehta RL, Palevsky P, Acute Dialysis Quality Initiative Work Group. Acute renal failure - definition, outcome measures, animal models, fluid therapy and information technology needs: the second international consensus conference of the acute dialysis quality initiative (ADQI) group. Crit Care. 2004;8(4):R204–12.
13. Mehta RL, Kellum JA, Shah SV, Molitoris BA, Ronco C, Warnock DG, et al. Acute kidney injury network: report of an initiative to improve outcomes in acute kidney injury. Crit Care. 2007;11(2):R31. https://doi.org/10.1186/cc5713.
14. Lassnigg A, Schmidlin D, Mouhieddine M, Bachmann LM, Druml W, Bauer P, et al. Minimal changes of serum creatinine predict prognosis in patients after cardiothoracic surgery: a prospective cohort study. J Am Soc Nephrol. 2004;15(6):1597–605.
15. Kidney Disease: Improving Global Outcomes (KDIGO) Acute Kidney Injury Work Group. KDIGO clinical practice guideline for acute kidney injury. Kidney Int Suppl. 2012;2:1–138.
16. Twine CP, Boyle JR. Renal dysfunction after EVAR: time for a standard definition. J Endovasc Ther. 2013;20(3):331–3. https://doi.org/10.1583/12-4104C.1.
17. Coselli JS, LeMaire SA, Preventza O, de la Cruz KI, Cooley DA, Price MD, et al. Outcomes of 3309 thoracoabdominal aortic aneurysm repairs. J Thorac Cardiovasc Surg. 2016;151(5):1323–37. https://doi.org/10.1016/j.jtcvs.2015.12.050.
18. Tshomba Y, Kahlberg A, Melissano G, Coppi G, Marone E, Ferrari D, et al. Comparison of renal perfusion solutions during thoracoabdominal aortic aneurysm repair. J Vasc Surg. 2014;59(3):623–33. https://doi.org/10.1016/j.jvs.2013.09.055.
19. Wynn MM, Acher C, Marks E, Engelbert T, Acher CW. Postoperative renal failure in thoracoabdominal aortic aneurysm repair with simple cross-clamp technique and 4°C renal perfusion. J Vasc Surg. 2015;61(3):611–22. https://doi.org/10.1016/j.jvs.2014.10.040.
20. Roh GU, Lee JW, Nam SB, Lee J, Choi JR, Shim YH. Incidence and risk factors of acute kidney injury after thoracic aortic surgery for acute dissection. Ann Thorac Surg. 2012;94(3):766–71. https://doi.org/10.1016/j.athoracsur.2012.04.057.
21. Tsai HS, Tsai FH, Chen YC, Wu ML, Chen SW, Chu JJ, et al. Impact of acute kidney injury on one-year survival after surgery for aortic dissection. Ann Thorac Surg. 2012;94:1407–12.
22. Sasabuchi Y, Kimura N, Shiotsuka J, Komuro T, Mouri H, Ohnuma T, et al. Long-term survival in patients with acute kidney injury after acute type a aortic dissection repair. Ann Thorac Surg. 2016;102(6):2003–9. https://doi.org/10.1016/j.athoracsur.2016.05.006.
23. Dariane C, Coscas R, Boulitrop C, Javerliat I, Vilaine E, Goeau-Brissonniere O, et al. Acute kidney injury after open repair of intact abdominal aortic aneurysms. Ann Vasc Surg. 2017;39:294–300. https://doi.org/10.1016/j.avsg.2016.09.010.
24. Kopolovic I, Simmonds K, Duggan S, Ewanchuk M, Stollery DE, Bagshaw SM, et al. Risk factors and outcomes associated with acute kidney injury following ruptured abdominal aortic aneurysm. BMC Nephrol. 2013;14:99. https://doi.org/10.1186/1471-2369-14-99.
25. van Beek SC, Legemate DA, Vahl A, Wisselink W, Barnes M, Fitridge RA, et al. External validation of the Endovascular aneurysm repair Risk Assessment model in predicting survival, reinterventions, and endoleaks after endovascular aneurysm repair. J Vasc Surg. 2014;59(6):1555–1561.e1. https://doi.org/10.1016/j.jvs.2013.12.043.
26. Jalalzadeh H, Indrakusuma R, Vogt L, van Beek SC, Vahl AC, Wisselink W, et al. Long-term survival after acute kidney injury following ruptured abdominal aortic aneurysm repair. J Vasc Surg. 2017;66(6):1712.e2–8.e2. https://doi.org/10.1016/j.jvs.2017.04.049.
27. Piffaretti G, Benedetto F, Menegolo M, Antonello M, Tarallo A, Grego F. Outcomes of endovascular repair for blunt thoracic aortic injury. J Vasc Surg. 2013;6:1483–9. https://doi.org/10.1016/j.jvs.2013.05.096.
28. Drews JD, Patel HJ, Williams DM, Dasika NL, Deeb GM. The impact of acute renal failure on early and late outcomes after thoracic aortic endovascular repair. Ann Thorac Surg. 2014;97(6):2027–33. https://doi.org/10.1016/j.athoracsur.2014.02.045.
29. Jeon YH, Bae CH. The risk factors and outcomes of acute kidney injury after thoracic endovascular aortic repair. Korean J Thorac Cardiovasc Surg. 2016;49(1):15–21. https://doi.org/10.5090/kjtcs.2016.49.1.15.
30. Luo S, Ding H, Luo J, Li W, Ning B, Liu Y, et al. Risk factors and early outcomes of acute renal injury after thoracic aortic endograft repair for type B aortic dissection. Ther Clin Risk Manag. 2017;13:1023–9. https://doi.org/10.2147/TCRM.S131456.
31. Jhaveri KD, Saratzis AN, Wanchoo R, Sarafidis PA. Endovascular aneurysm repair (EVAR)- and transcatheter aortic valve replacement (TAVR)-associated acute kidney injury. Kidney Int. 2017;91(6):1312–23. https://doi.org/10.1016/j.kint.2016.11.030.
32. Ichai C, Vinsonneau C, Souweine B, Armando F, Canet E, Clec'h C, et al. Acute kidney injury in the perioperative period and in intensive care units (excluding renal replacement therapies). Ann Intensive Care. 2016;6(1):48. https://doi.org/10.1186/s13613-016-0145-5.
33. Thakar CV, Arrigain S, Worley S, Yared JP, Paganini EP. A clinical score to predict acute renal failure after cardiac surgery. J Am Soc Nephrol. 2005;16(1):162–8.
34. Mehta RH, Grab JD, O'Brien SM, Bridges CR, Gammie JS, Haan CK, Society of Thoracic Surgeons National Cardiac Surgery Database Investigators,

et al. Bedside tool for predicting the risk of postoperative dialysis in patients undergoing cardiac surgery. Circulation. 2006;114(21):2208–16.. quiz 2208.
35. Chertow GM, Lazarus JM, Christiansen CL, Cook EF, Hammermeister KE, Grover F, et al. Preoperative renal risk stratification. Circulation. 1997;95(4):878–84.
36. Wijeysundera DN, Karkouti K, Dupuis JY, Rao V, Chan CT, Granton JT, et al. Derivation and validation of a simplified predictive index for renal replacement therapy after cardiac surgery. JAMA. 2007;297(16):1801–9.
37. Brown JR, Cochran RP, Leavitt BJ, Dacey LJ, Ross CS, MacKenzie TA, et al. Multivariable prediction of renal insufficiency developing after cardiac surgery. Circulation. 2007;116(11 Suppl):I139–43. https://doi.org/10.1161/CIRCULATIONAHA.106.677070.
38. Pannu N, Graham M, Klarenbach S, Meyer S, Kieser T, Hemmelgarn B, et al. A new model to predict acute kidney injury requiring renal replacement therapy after cardiac surgery. CMAJ. 2016;188(15):1076–83.
39. Palomba H, de Castro I, Neto AL, Lage S, Yu L. Acute kidney injury prediction following elective cardiac surgery: AKICS score. Kidney Int. 2007;72(5):624–31.
40. Jorge-Monjas P, Bustamante-Munguira J, Lorenzo M, Heredia-Rodríguez M, Fierro I, Gómez-Sánchez E, et al. Predicting cardiac surgery-associated acute kidney injury: the CRATE score. J Crit Care. 2016;31(1):130–8. https://doi.org/10.1016/j.jcrc.2015.11.004.
41. Vanmassenhove J, Kielstein J, Jörres A, Biesen WV. Management of patients at risk of acute kidney injury. Lancet. 2017;389(10084):2139–51. https://doi.org/10.1016/S0140-6736(17)31329-6.
42. Kristovic D, Horvatic I, Husedzinovic I, Sutlic Z, Rudez I, Baric D, et al. Cardiac surgery-associated acute kidney injury: risk factors analysis and comparison of prediction models. Interact Cardiovasc Thorac Surg. 2015;21(3):366–73. https://doi.org/10.1093/icvts/ivv162.
43. Wong GT, Lee EY, Irwin MG. Contrast induced nephropathy in vascular surgery. Br J Anaesth. 2016;117(Suppl 2):ii63–73. https://doi.org/10.1093/bja/aew213.
44. Lameire N, Adam A, Becker CR, Davidson C, McCullough PA, Stacul F, et al. Baseline renal function screening. Am J Cardiol. 2006;98(6A):21K–6K. https://doi.org/10.1016/j.amjcard.2006.01.021.
45. Brown JR, McCullough PA, Splaine ME, Davies L, Ross CS, Dauerman HL, et al. How do centres begin the process to prevent contrast-induced acute kidney injury: a report from a new regional collaborative. BMJ Qual Saf. 2012;21(1):54–62. https://doi.org/10.1136/bmjqs-2011-000041.
46. Mehran R, Aymong ED, Nikolsky E, Lasic Z, Iakovou I, Fahy M, et al. A simple risk score for prediction of contrast-induced nephropathy after percutaneous coronary intervention: development and initial validation. J Am Coll Cardiol. 2004;44(7):1393–9.
47. Joannidis M, Druml W, Forni LG, Groeneveld ABJ, Honore PM, Hoste E, et al. Prevention of acute kidney injury and protection of renal function in the intensive care unit: update 2017: expert opinion of the Working Group on Prevention, AKI section, European Society of Intensive Care Medicine. Intensive Care Med. 2017;43(6):730–49. https://doi.org/10.1007/s00134-017-4832-y.
48. Landoni G, Bove T, Székely A, Comis M, Rodseth RN, Pasero D, et al. Reducing mortality in acute kidney injury patients: systematic review and international web-based survey. J Cardiothorac Vasc Anesth. 2013;27(6):1384–98. https://doi.org/10.1053/j.jvca.2013.06.028.
49. Kane-Gill SL, Goldstein SL. Drug-induced acute kidney injury: a focus on risk assessment for prevention. Crit Care Clin. 2015;31(4):675–84. https://doi.org/10.1016/j.ccc.2015.06.005.
50. Sousa-Uva M, Head SJ, Milojevic M, Collet JP, Landoni G, Castella M, et al. 2017 EACTS Guidelines on perioperative medication in adult cardiac surgery. Eur J Cardiothorac Surg. 2018;53:5–33. https://doi.org/10.1093/ejcts/ezx314.
51. Di Tomasso N, Monaco F, Landoni G. Renal protection in cardiovascular surgery. F1000Research. 2016;5:331. https://doi.org/10.12688/f1000research.7348.1.
52. Wilhelm-Leen E, Montez-Rath ME, Chertow G. Estimating the risk of radiocontrast-associated nephropathy. J Am Soc Nephrol. 2017;28(2):653–9. https://doi.org/10.1681/ASN.2016010021.
53. Walsh M, Devereaux PJ, Garg AX, Kurz A, Turan A, Rodseth RN, et al. Relationship between intraoperative mean arterial pressure and clinical outcomes after noncardiac surgery: toward an empirical definition of hypotension. Anesthesiology. 2013;119(3):507–15. https://doi.org/10.1097/ALN.0b013e3182a10e26.
54. Salmasi V, Maheshwari K, Yang D, Mascha EJ, Singh A, Sessler DI, et al. Relationship between intraoperative hypotension, defined by either reduction from baseline or absolute thresholds, and acute kidney and myocardial injury after noncardiac surgery: a retrospective cohort analysis. Anesthesiology. 2017;126(1):47–65.
55. Asfar P, Meziani F, Hamel JF, Grelon F, Megarbane B, Anguel N, et al. High versus low blood-pressure target in patients with septic shock. N Engl J Med. 2014;370(17):1583–93. https://doi.org/10.1056/NEJMoa1312173.
56. Bouchard J, Soroko SB, Chertow GM, Himmelfarb J, Ikizler TA, Paganini EP, et al. Fluid accumulation, survival and recovery of kidney function in critically ill patients with acute kidney injury. Kidney Int. 2009;76(4):422–7. https://doi.org/10.1038/ki.2009.159.
57. Payen D, de Pont AC, Sakr Y, Spies C, Reinhart K, Vincent JL, et al. A positive fluid balance is associated with a worse outcome in patients with acute renal failure. Crit Care. 2008;12(3):R74. https://doi.org/10.1186/cc6916.

58. Marik PE, Cavallazzi R. Does the central venous pressure predict fluid responsiveness? An updated meta-analysis and a plea for some common sense. Crit Care Med. 2013;41(7):1774–81. https://doi.org/10.1097/CCM.0b013e31828a25fd.
59. Monnet X, Cipriani F, Camous L, Sentenac P, Dres M, Krastinova E, et al. The passive leg raising test to guide fluid removal in critically ill patients. Ann Intensive Care. 2016;6(1):46. https://doi.org/10.1186/s13613-016-0149-1.
60. Myburgh JA, Mythen MG. Resuscitation fluids. N Engl J Med. 2013;369(13):1243–51. https://doi.org/10.1056/NEJMra1208627.
61. Pisano A, Landoni G, Bellomo R. The risk of infusing gelatin? Die-hard misconceptions and forgotten (or ignored) truths. Minerva Anestesiol. 2016;82(10):1107–14.
62. Mailloux L, Swartz CD, Capizzi R, Kim KE, Onesti G, Ramirez O, et al. Acute renal failure after administration of low-molecular weight dextran. N Engl J Med. 1967;277(21):1113–8.
63. Laxenaire MC, Charpentier C, Feldman L. Anaphylactoid reactions to colloid plasma substitutes: incidence, risk factors, mechanisms. A French multicenter prospective study. Ann Fr Anesth Reanim. 1994;13(3):301–10.
64. Perner A, Haase N, Guttormsen AB, Tenhunen J, Klemenzson G, Åneman A, et al. Hydroxyethyl starch 130/0.42 versus Ringer's acetate in severe sepsis. N Engl J Med. 2012;367(2):124–34. https://doi.org/10.1056/NEJMoa1204242.
65. Myburgh JA, Finfer S, Bellomo R, Billot L, Cass A, Gattas D, et al. Hydroxyethyl starch or saline for fluid resuscitation in intensive care. N Engl J Med. 2012;367(20):1901–11. https://doi.org/10.1056/NEJMoa1209759.. Erratum. N Engl J Med. 2016;374(13):1298.
66. Meybohm P, Van Aken H, De Gasperi A, De Hert S, Della Rocca G, Girbes AR, et al. Re-evaluating currently available data and suggestions for planning randomised controlled studies regarding the use of hydroxyethyl starch in critically ill patients - a multidisciplinary statement. Crit Care. 2013;17(4):R166. https://doi.org/10.1186/cc12845.
67. Finfer S, Bellomo R, Boyce N, French J, Myburgh J, Norton R. A comparison of albumin and saline for fluid resuscitation in the intensive care unit. N Engl J Med. 2004;350(22):2247–56.
68. Caironi P, Tognoni G, Masson S, Fumagalli R, Pesenti A, Romero M, et al. Albumin replacement in patients with severe sepsis or septic shock. N Engl J Med. 2014;370(15):1412–21. https://doi.org/10.1056/NEJMoa1305727.
69. Maitland K, Kiguli S, Opoka RO, Engoru C, Olupot-Olupot P, Akech SO, et al. Mortality after fluid bolus in African children with severe infection. N Engl J Med. 2011;364(26):2483–95. https://doi.org/10.1056/NEJMoa1101549.
70. Young P, Bailey M, Beasley R, SPLIT Investigators; ANZICS CTG, et al. Effect of a buffered crystalloid solution vs saline on acute kidney injury among patients in the intensive care unit: the SPLIT randomized clinical trial. JAMA. 2015;314(16):1701–10. https://doi.org/10.1001/jama.2015.12334.
71. Jones D, Bellomo R. Renal-dose dopamine: from hypothesis to paradigm to dogma to myth and, finally, superstition? J Intensive Care Med. 2005;20(4):199–211. https://doi.org/10.1177/0885066605276963.
72. Lauschke A, Teichgräber UK, Frei U, Eckardt KU. 'Low-dose' dopamine worsens renal perfusion in patients with acute renal failure. Kidney Int. 2006;69(9):1669–74. https://doi.org/10.1038/sj.ki.5000310.
73. Friedrich JO, Adhikari N, Herridge MS, Beyene J. Meta-analysis: low-dose dopamine increases urine output but does not prevent renal dysfunction or death. Ann Intern Med. 2005;142(7):510–24.
74. Karthik S, Lisbon A. Low-dose dopamine in the intensive care unit. Semin Dial. 2006;19(6):465–71. https://doi.org/10.1111/j.1525-139X.2006.00208.x.
75. De Backer D, Biston P, Devriendt J, Madl C, Chochrad D, Aldecoa C, et al. Comparison of dopamine and norepinephrine in the treatment of shock. N Engl J Med. 2010;362(9):779–89. https://doi.org/10.1056/NEJMoa0907118.
76. Rhodes A, Evans LE, Alhazzani W, Levy MM, Antonelli M, Ferrer R, et al. Surviving sepsis campaign: international guidelines for management of sepsis and septic shock: 2016. Intensive Care Med. 2017;43(3):304–77. https://doi.org/10.1007/s00134-017-4683-6.
77. Møller MH, Claudius C, Junttila E, Haney M, Oscarsson-Tibblin A, Haavind A, et al. Scandinavian SSAI clinical practice guideline on choice of first-line vasopressor for patients with acute circulatory failure. Acta Anaesthesiol Scand. 2016;60(10):1347–66. https://doi.org/10.1111/aas.12780.
78. Landoni G, Biondi-Zoccai G, Marino G, Bove T, Fochi O, Maj G, et al. Fenoldopam reduces the need for renal replacement therapy and in-hospital death in cardiovascular surgery: a meta-analysis. J Cardiothorac Vasc Anesth. 2008;22(1):27–33. https://doi.org/10.1053/j.jvca.2007.07.015.
79. Zangrillo A, Biondi-Zoccai GG, Frati E, Covello RD, Cabrini L, Guarracino F, et al. Fenoldopam and acute renal failure in cardiac surgery: a meta-analysis of randomized placebo-controlled trials. J Cardiothorac Vasc Anesth. 2012;26(3):407–13. https://doi.org/10.1053/j.jvca.2012.01.038.
80. Gillies MA, Kakar V, Parker RJ, Honoré PM, Ostermann M. Fenoldopam to prevent acute kidney injury after major surgery-a systematic review and meta-analysis. Crit Care. 2015;19:449. https://doi.org/10.1186/s13054-015-1166-4.
81. Bove T, Zangrillo A, Guarracino F, Alvaro G, Persi B, Maglioni E, et al. Effect of fenoldopam on use of renal replacement therapy among patients with acute kidney injury after cardiac surgery: a randomized clinical trial. JAMA. 2014;312(21):2244–53. https://doi.org/10.1001/jama.2014.13573.

82. Papp Z, Édes I, Fruhwald S, De Hert SG, Salmenperä M, Leppikangas H, et al. Levosimendan: molecular mechanisms and clinical implications: consensus of experts on the mechanisms of action of levosimendan. Int J Cardiol. 2012;159(2):82–7. https://doi.org/10.1016/j.ijcard.2011.07.022.
83. Farmakis D, Alvarez J, Gal TB, Brito D, Fedele F, Fonseca C, et al. Levosimendan beyond inotropy and acute heart failure: evidence of pleiotropic effects on the heart and other organs: an expert panel position paper. Int J Cardiol. 2016;222:303–12. https://doi.org/10.1016/j.ijcard.2016.07.202.
84. Yilmaz MB, Grossini E, Silva Cardoso JC, Édes I, Fedele F, Pollesello P, et al. Renal effects of levosimendan: a consensus report. Cardiovasc Drugs Ther. 2013;27(6):581–90. https://doi.org/10.1007/s10557-013-6485-6.
85. Bove T, Matteazzi A, Belletti A, Paternoster G, Saleh O, Taddeo D, et al. Beneficial impact of levosimendan in critically ill patients with or at risk for acute renal failure: a meta-analysis of randomized clinical trials. Heart Lung Vessel. 2015;7(1):35–46.
86. Zhou C, Gong J, Chen D, Wang W, Liu M, Liu B. Levosimendan for prevention of acute kidney injury after cardiac surgery: a meta-analysis of randomized controlled trials. Am J Kidney Dis. 2016;67(3):408–16. https://doi.org/10.1053/j.ajkd.2015.09.015.
87. Mehta RH, Leimberger JD, van Diepen S, Meza J, Wang A, Jankowich R, Harrison RW, Hay D, Fremes S, Duncan A, Soltesz EG, Luber J, Park S, Argenziano M, Murphy E, Marcel R, Kalavrouziotis D, Nagpal D, Bozinovski J, Toller W, Heringlake M, Goodman SG, Levy JH, Harrington RA, Anstrom KJ, Alexander JH, LEVO-CTS Investigators. Levosimendan in patients with left ventricular dysfunction undergoing cardiac surgery. N Engl J Med. 2017;376:2032–42. https://doi.org/10.1056/NEJMoa1616218.
88. Cholley B, Caruba T, Grosjean S, Amour J, Ouattara A, Villacorta J, et al. Effect of Levosimendan on low cardiac output syndrome in patients with low ejection fraction undergoing coronary artery bypass grafting with cardiopulmonary bypass: the LICORN randomized clinical trial. JAMA. 2017;318(6):548–56. https://doi.org/10.1001/jama.2017.9973.
89. Landoni G, Lomivorotov VV, Alvaro G, Lobreglio R, Pisano A, Guarracino F, et al. Levosimendan for hemodynamic support after cardiac surgery. N Engl J Med. 2017;376(21):2021–31. https://doi.org/10.1056/NEJMoa1616325.
90. Russell JA. Bench-to-bedside review: Vasopressin in the management of septic shock. Crit Care. 2011;15(4):226. https://doi.org/10.1186/cc8224.
91. Bragadottir G, Redfors B, Nygren A, Sellgren J, Ricksten SE. Low-dose vasopressin increases glomerular filtration rate, but impairs renal oxygenation in post-cardiac surgery patients. Acta Anaesthesiol Scand. 2009;53(8):1052–9. https://doi.org/10.1111/j.1399-6576.2009.02037.x.
92. Russell JA, Walley KR, Singer J, Gordon AC, Hébert PC, Cooper DJ. Vasopressin versus norepinephrine infusion in patients with septic shock. N Engl J Med. 2008;358(9):877–87. https://doi.org/10.1056/NEJMoa067373.
93. Gordon AC, Russell JA, Walley KR, Singer J, Ayers D, Storms MM, et al. The effects of vasopressin on acute kidney injury in septic shock. Intensive Care Med. 2010;36(1):83–91. https://doi.org/10.1007/s00134-009-1687-x.
94. Gordon AC, Mason AJ, Thirunavukkarasu N, Perkins GD, Cecconi M, Cepkova M, et al. Effect of early vasopressin vs norepinephrine on kidney failure in patients with septic shock: the VANISH randomized clinical trial. JAMA. 2016;316(5):509–18. https://doi.org/10.1001/jama.2016.10485.
95. Hajjar LA, Vincent JL, Barbosa Gomes Galas FR, Rhodes A, Landoni G, Osawa EA, et al. Vasopressin versus norepinephrine in patients with vasoplegic shock after cardiac surgery: the VANCS randomized controlled trial. Anesthesiology. 2017;126(1):85–93. https://doi.org/10.1097/ALN.0000000000001434.
96. Bagshaw SM, Delaney A, Jones D, Ronco C, Bellomo R. Diuretics in the management of acute kidney injury: a multinational survey. Contrib Nephrol. 2007;156:236–49. https://doi.org/10.1159/000102089.
97. Ho KM, Power BM. Benefits and risks of furosemide in acute kidney injury. Anaesthesia. 2010;65(3):283–93. https://doi.org/10.1111/j.1365-2044.2009.06228.x.
98. Bagshaw SM, Delaney A, Haase M, Ghali WA, Bellomo R. Loop diuretics in the management of acute renal failure: a systematic review and meta-analysis. Crit Care Resusc. 2007;9(1):60–8.
99. Sampath S, Moran JL, Graham PL, Rockliff S, Bersten AD, Abrams KR. The efficacy of loop diuretics in acute renal failure: assessment using Bayesian evidence synthesis techniques. Crit Care Med. 2007;35(11):2516–24.
100. Koyner JL, Davison DL, Brasha-Mitchell E, Chalikonda DM, Arthur JM, Shaw AD, Tumlin JA, Trevino SA, Bennett MR, Kimmel PL, Seneff MG, Chawla LS. Furosemide stress test and biomarkers for the prediction of AKI severity. J Am Soc Nephrol. 2015;26:2023–31. https://doi.org/10.1681/ASN.2014060535.
101. Dieleman JM, Nierich AP, Rosseel PM, van der Maaten JM, Hofland J, Diephuis JC, et al. Intraoperative high-dose dexamethasone for cardiac surgery: a randomized controlled trial. JAMA. 2012;308(17):1761–7. https://doi.org/10.1001/jama.2012.14144.
102. Whitlock RP, Devereaux PJ, Teoh KH, Lamy A, Vincent J, Pogue J, et al. Methylprednisolone in patients undergoing cardiopulmonary bypass (SIRS): a randomised, double-blind, placebo-controlled trial. Lancet. 2015;386(10000):1243–53. https://doi.org/10.1016/S0140-6736(15)00273-1.

103. Jacob KA, Leaf D, Dieleman J, van Dijk D, Nierich AP, Rosseel PM, et al. Intraoperative high-dose dexamethasone and severe AKI after cardiac surgery. J Am Soc Nephrol. 2015;26(12):2947–51. https://doi.org/10.1681/ASN.2014080840.
104. Dieleman JM, van Dijk D. Corticosteroids for cardiac surgery: a summary of two large randomised trials. Neth J Crit Care. 2016;24:6–10.
105. Kavalipati N, Shah J, Ramakrishan A, Vasnawala H. Pleiotropic effects of statins. Indian J Endocrinol Metab. 2015;19:554–62. https://doi.org/10.4103/2230-8210.163106.
106. Galyfos G, Sianou A, Filis K. Pleiotropic effects of statins in the perioperative setting. Ann Card Anaesth. 2017;20(Supplement):S43–8. https://doi.org/10.4103/0971-9784.197796.
107. Billings FT 4th, Hendricks PA, Schildcrout JS, Shi Y, Petracek MR, Byrne JG, Brown NJ. High-dose perioperative atorvastatin and acute kidney injury following cardiac surgery: a randomized clinical trial. JAMA. 2016;315:877–88. https://doi.org/10.1001/jama.2016.0548.
108. Park JH, Shim JK, Song JW, Soh S, Kwak YL. Effect of atorvastatin on the incidence of acute kidney injury following valvular heart surgery: a randomized, placebo-controlled trial. Intensive Care Med. 2016;42(9):1398–407. https://doi.org/10.1007/s00134-016-4358-8.
109. Zheng Z, Jayaram R, Jiang L, Emberson J, Zhao Y, Li Q, et al. Perioperative rosuvastatin in cardiac surgery. N Engl J Med. 2016;374(18):1744–53. https://doi.org/10.1056/NEJMoa1507750.
110. Putzu A, Capelli B, Belletti A, Cassina T, Ferrari E, Gallo M, et al. Perioperative statin therapy in cardiac surgery: a meta-analysis of randomized controlled trials. Crit Care. 2016;20(1):395. https://doi.org/10.1186/s13054-016-1560-6.
111. Sanders RD, Nicholson A, Lewis SR, Smith AF, Alderson P. Perioperative statin therapy for improving outcomes during and after noncardiac vascular surgery. Cochrane Database Syst Rev. 2013;7:CD009971. https://doi.org/10.1002/14651858.CD009971.pub2.
112. Berwanger O, de Barros E, Silva PG, Barbosa RR, Precoma DB, Figueiredo EL, Hajjar LA, et al. Atorvastatin for high-risk statin-naïve patients undergoing noncardiac surgery: the lowering the risk of operative complications using atorvastatin loading dose (LOAD) randomized trial. Am Heart J. 2017;184:88–96. https://doi.org/10.1016/j.ahj.2016.11.001.
113. Pineda A, Cubeddu LX. Statin rebound or withdrawal syndrome: does it exist? Curr Atheroscler Rep. 2011;13(1):23–30. https://doi.org/10.1007/s11883-010-0148-x.
114. Le Manach Y, Godet G, Coriat P, Martinon C, Bertrand M, Fléron MH, et al. The impact of postoperative discontinuation or continuation of chronic statin therapy on cardiac outcome after major vascular surgery. Anesth Analg. 2007;104(6):1326–33.. table of contents.
115. Swärd K, Valsson F, Sellgren J, Ricksten SE. Differential effects of human atrial natriuretic peptide and furosemide on glomerular filtration rate and renal oxygen consumption in humans. Intensive Care Med. 2005;31(1):79–85.
116. Houben AJ, van der Zander K, de Leeuw PW. Vascular and renal actions of brain natriuretic peptide in man: physiology and pharmacology. Fundam Clin Pharmacol. 2005;19(4):411–9. https://doi.org/10.1111/j.1472-8206.2005.00336.x.
117. Kuhn M. Endothelial actions of atrial and B-type natriuretic peptides. Br J Pharmacol. 2012;166(2):522–31. https://doi.org/10.1111/j.1476-5381.2012.01827.x.
118. Nigwekar SU, Navaneethan SD, Parikh CR, Hix JK. Atrial natriuretic peptide for preventing and treating acute kidney injury. Cochrane Database Syst Rev. 2009;4:CD006028. https://doi.org/10.1002/14651858.
119. Mitaka C, Kudo T, Haraguchi G, Tomita M. Cardiovascular and renal effects of carperitide and nesiritide in cardiovascular surgery patients: a systematic review and meta-analysis. Crit Care. 2011;15(5):R258. https://doi.org/10.1186/cc10519.
120. Xiong B, Wang C, Yao Y, Huang Y, Tan J, Cao Y, et al. The dose-dependent effect of nesiritide on renal function in patients with acute decompensated heart failure: a systematic review and meta-analysis of randomized controlled trials. PLoS One. 2015;10(6):e0131326. https://doi.org/10.1371/journal.pone.0131326.
121. Mori Y, Kamada T, Ochiai R. Reduction in the incidence of acute kidney injury after aortic arch surgery with low-dose atrial natriuretic peptide: a randomised controlled trial. Eur J Anaesthesiol. 2014;31(7):381–7. https://doi.org/10.1097/EJA.0000000000000035.
122. Sezai A, Nakata K, Iida M, Yoshitake I, Wakui S, Hata H, et al. Early results of human atrial natriuretic peptide infusion in non-dialysis patients with chronic kidney disease undergoing isolated coronary artery bypass grafting: the NU-HIT trial for CKD-II. Ann Thorac Cardiovasc Surg. 2014;20(3):217–22.
123. Sisillo E, Ceriani R, Bortone F, Juliano G, Salvi L, Veglia F, et al. N-acetylcysteine for prevention of acute renal failure in patients with chronic renal insufficiency undergoing cardiac surgery: a prospective, randomized, clinical trial. Crit Care Med. 2008;36(1):81–6. https://doi.org/10.1097/01.CCM.0000295305.22281.1D.
124. Wijeysundera DN, Beattie WS, Rao V, Granton JT, Chan CT. N-acetylcysteine for preventing acute kidney injury in cardiac surgery patients with preexisting moderate renal insufficiency. Can J Anaesth. 2007;54(11):872–81. https://doi.org/10.1007/BF03026790.
125. Macedo E, Abdulkader R, Castro I, Sobrinho AC, Yu L, Vieira JM Jr. Lack of protection of N-acetylcysteine (NAC) in acute renal failure related to elective aortic aneurysm repair-a randomized controlled trial. Nephrol Dial Transplant. 2006;21(7):1863–9. https://doi.org/10.1093/ndt/gfl079.

126. Adabag AS, Ishani A, Koneswaran S, Johnson DJ, Kelly RF, Ward HB, et al. Utility of N-acetylcysteine to prevent acute kidney injury after cardiac surgery: a randomized controlled trial. Am Heart J. 2008;155(6):1143–9. https://doi.org/10.1016/j.ahj.2008.01.013.
127. Song JW, Shim JK, Soh S, Jang J, Kwak YL. Double-blinded, randomized controlled trial of N-acetylcysteine for prevention of acute kidney injury in high risk patients undergoing off-pump coronary artery bypass. Nephrology. 2015;20(2):96–102. https://doi.org/10.1111/nep.12361.
128. Fraga CM, Tomasi CD, Damasio DC, Vuolo F, Ritter C, Dal-Pizzol F. N-acetylcysteine plus deferoxamine for patients with prolonged hypotension does not decrease acute kidney injury incidence: a double blind, randomized, placebo-controlled trial. Crit Care. 2016;20(1):331. https://doi.org/10.1186/s13054-016-1504-1.
129. Lynch RM, Robertson R. Anaphylactoid reactions to intravenous N-acetylcysteine: a prospective case controlled study. Accid Emerg Nurs. 2004;12(1):10–5.
130. Sandilands EA, Bateman DN. Adverse reactions associated with acetylcysteine. Clin Toxicol. 2009;47(2):81–8. https://doi.org/10.1080/15563650802665587.
131. Cigarroa RG, Lange RA, Williams RH, Hillis LD. Dosing of contrast material to prevent contrast nephropathy in patients with renal disease. Am J Med. 1989;86(6 Pt 1):649–52.
132. Nyman U, Björk J, Aspelin P, Marenzi G. Contrast medium dose-to-GFR ratio: a measure of systemic exposure to predict contrast-induced nephropathy after percutaneous coronary intervention. Acta Radiol. 2008;49(6):658–67. https://doi.org/10.1080/02841850802050762.
133. Barrett BJ, Carlisle EJ. Metaanalysis of the relative nephrotoxicity of high- and low-osmolality iodinated contrast media. Radiology. 1993;188(1):171–8. https://doi.org/10.1148/radiology.188.1.8511292.
134. Lameire N, Kellum JA, KDIGO AKI Guideline Work Group. Contrast-induced acute kidney injury and renal support for acute kidney injury: a KDIGO summary (part 2). Crit Care. 2013;17(1):205. https://doi.org/10.1186/cc11455.
135. Nijssen EC, Rennenberg RJ, Nelemans PJ, Essers BA, Janssen MM, Vermeeren MA, et al. Prophylactic hydration to protect renal function from intravascular iodinated contrast material in patients at high risk of contrast-induced nephropathy (AMACING): a prospective, randomised, phase 3, controlled, open-label, non-inferiority trial. Lancet. 2017;389(10076):1312–22. https://doi.org/10.1016/S0140-6736(17)30057-0.
136. Weisbord SD, Gallagher M, Jneid H, Garcia S, Cass A, Thwin SS, et al. Outcomes after angiography with sodium bicarbonate and acetylcysteine. N Engl J Med. 2018;378:603–14. https://doi.org/10.1056/NEJMoa1710933.
137. Putzu A, Boscolo Berto M, Belletti A, Pasotti E, Cassina T, Moccetti T, et al. Prevention of contrast-induced acute kidney injury by furosemide with matched hydration in patients undergoing interventional procedures: a systematic review and meta-analysis of randomized trials. JACC Cardiovasc Interv. 2017;10(4):355–63. https://doi.org/10.1016/j.jcin.2016.11.006.
138. Subramaniam RM, Suarez-Cuervo C, Wilson RF, Turban S, Zhang A, Sherrod C, et al. Effectiveness of prevention strategies for contrast-induced nephropathy: a systematic review and meta-analysis. Ann Intern Med. 2016;164(6):406–16. https://doi.org/10.7326/M15-1456.
139. Anderson SM, Park ZH, Patel RV. Intravenous N-acetylcysteine in the prevention of contrast media-induced nephropathy. Ann Pharmacother. 2011;45(1):101–7. https://doi.org/10.1345/aph.1P275.

17 Renal Perfusion During Aortic Surgery: Looking for the Ideal Substrate

Curitiba Trial Investigators

Y. Tshomba, E. Simonini, E. Colombo, V. Ardita, L. Apruzzi, E. Rinaldi, L. Pasin, T. Cambiaghi, B. Catenaccio, R. Castellano, M. Venturini, G. Landoni, P. Nardelli, M. Leopardi, E. Espinar, S. Salvati, R. Lembo, D. Baccellieri, L. Bertoglio, A. Kahlberg, S. Bossi, G. Melissano, and Roberto Chiesa

17.1 Pathogenesis of Ischemic Acute Tubular Necrosis During Aortic Surgery

The kidneys are the body's natural blood filters, eliminating around 1.5 l per day of urine [1–4]. The reabsorption of fluids after filtration in the renal tubule is the crucial process in maintaining body intravascular volume, in adjusting electrolytes and acid-base balance, and in concentrating toxic metabolites in the urine. Fluid reabsorption is mainly driven by Na^+ transport from the tubular lumen into the peritubular capillaries by the Na^+/K^+-ATPase pump in the basolateral membrane

Y. Tshomba (✉)
Unit of Vascular Surgery, Fondazione Policlinico Universitario A. Gemelli IRCCS, Università Cattolica del Sacro Cuore, Rome, Italy

Unit of Vascular Surgery, San Raffaele Scientific Institute, Vita-Salute University, Milan, Italy
e-mail: y.tshomba@hsr.it

A. Kahlberg · G. Melissano
Vascular Surgery Unit, IRCCS San Raffaele Scientific Institute, Milan, Italy

Vita-Salute San Raffaele University of Milan, Milan, Italy

E. Simonini · E. Colombo · V. Ardita · L. Apruzzi
E. Rinaldi · T. Cambiaghi · B. Catenaccio
R. Castellano · M. Leopardi · E. Espinar · S. Salvati
L. Bertoglio · S. Bossi
Vascular Surgery Unit, IRCCS San Raffaele Scientific Institute, Milan, Italy

D. Baccellieri
Unit of Vascular Surgery, San Raffaele Scientific Institute, Milan, Italy

L. Pasin · P. Nardelli · R. Lembo
Department of Anesthesia and Intensive Care, IRCCS San Raffaele Scientific Institute, Milan, Italy

M. Venturini
Department of Radiology, IRCCS San Raffaele Scientific Institute, Milan, Italy

G. Landoni
Vita-Salute San Raffaele University of Milan, Milan, Italy

Department of Anesthesia and Intensive Care, IRCCS San Raffaele Scientific Institute, Milan, Italy

R. Chiesa
Unit of Vascular Surgery, San Raffaele Scientific Institute, Vita-Salute University, Milan, Italy

© Springer Nature Switzerland AG 2019
Y. Tshomba et al. (eds.), *Visceral Vessels and Aortic Repair*,
https://doi.org/10.1007/978-3-319-94761-7_17

of the epithelial cells. This enzyme pumps three sodium ions out of the cell for every two potassium ions taken in. Both ions are moved against their concentration gradients, and since both have equal ionic charges, their movement creates an electrochemical gradient between the cell and its exterior. So this pumping is active and determines the essential energy consumption of the kidney because electrochemical gradient requires continuous energy supply from ATP to be maintained.

When surgical techniques require temporary interruption of renal blood flow, less Na^+ is transported within the tubular space, and Na^+/K^+-ATPase pump activity diminishes with a drop in ATP consumption. This process should lead to a theoretically high ischemic tolerance, but the range of safe ischemic time is largely variable. Laboratory studies indicate that most animals exhibit fatal renal failure for ischemic time longer than 2 h. Rats can survive after a thoracic aortic occlusion of 2 h [5]; dogs also tolerate 2 h of aortic occlusion with only a temporary and slight reduction in renal function [6], while rabbits did not survive with renal failure following 1 h of renal ischemia [7].

The safe duration of renal ischemia in humans is variable, even if, based on a study prospectively analyzing renal artery clamping in patients undergoing partial nephrectomy, human kidneys seem to safely tolerate 30–60 min of clamp ischemia if other nephrologic insults are not present [8]. It is however a common experience during aortic surgery that even suprarenal aortic clamping of less than 30 min is usually associated with some degree of renal damage in most patients. Hence, the crucial question is "why is a tissue with the energy consumption mainly related to Na^+ reabsorption so vulnerable to ischemia when the processes of reabsorption are inactivated?"

To answer this question, we have to keep in mind that, even if open TAAA repair is the most investigated clinical setting of renal ischemia/reperfusion injury, the pathophysiology of postoperative renal dysfunction is complex and still only partially known. Several intraoperative mechanisms typically affect tubular renal cells, among these, hemodynamic instability and anemia related to massive blood loss, embolism, vasospasm, increased myoglobin for lower limbs muscles ischemia, massive overall body fluid shifting, medications given, and hypoxia. Furthermore, many additional intraoperative nephrotoxic insults such as those related to the extracorporeal circulation may be involved, including activation of inflammatory mediators, oxygen free radicals systemic release, red blood cell damage, and activation of the coagulation cascade, fibrinolytic system, and complement chain.

We should also keep in mind that in the kidney, the workload is markedly inhomogeneous and fluid reabsorption occurs for approximately 70% of the total amount in the proximal convolute tubule. Hence, histology and cytological building of such an active tissue is complex with lush brush border carpets in the tubular lumen and lateral cellular processes largely interdigitating each other to expand the membrane surface. The surface of the basal tubular membrane is also amplified by extensive membrane infolding, creating numerous tiny feet. So, there is a non-negligible baseline ATP needed to preserve such an expanded and biologically active tubular epithelial surface, even when reabsorption processes are inactivated.

Additionally, the renal cortex, where proximal convoluted tubules are involved, in a normal condition is the most vascularized tissue of the entire human body in proportion to its weight. It receives far higher blood flow than would be required to nourish it, having 98–99% of the 1200 ml of oxygenated blood that every minute perfuses the kidneys in a subject of 70 kg. So, in the hypervascularized tissue of renal cortex, only oxygen-linked processes such as aerobic glycolysis and fatty acids beta-oxidation are used. But in ischemic tissues, the anaerobic glycolysis is the only cellular process able to produce the ATP providing energy enough for preparing sufficient postischemic function. Therefore, in the proximal tubule cells in case of poor oxygenation, block of cellular respiration, critical intracellular ATP reduction, and increase in lactate are early. At this point, a variety of factors can promote the development of cell injury, including the intracellular accumulation of calcium,

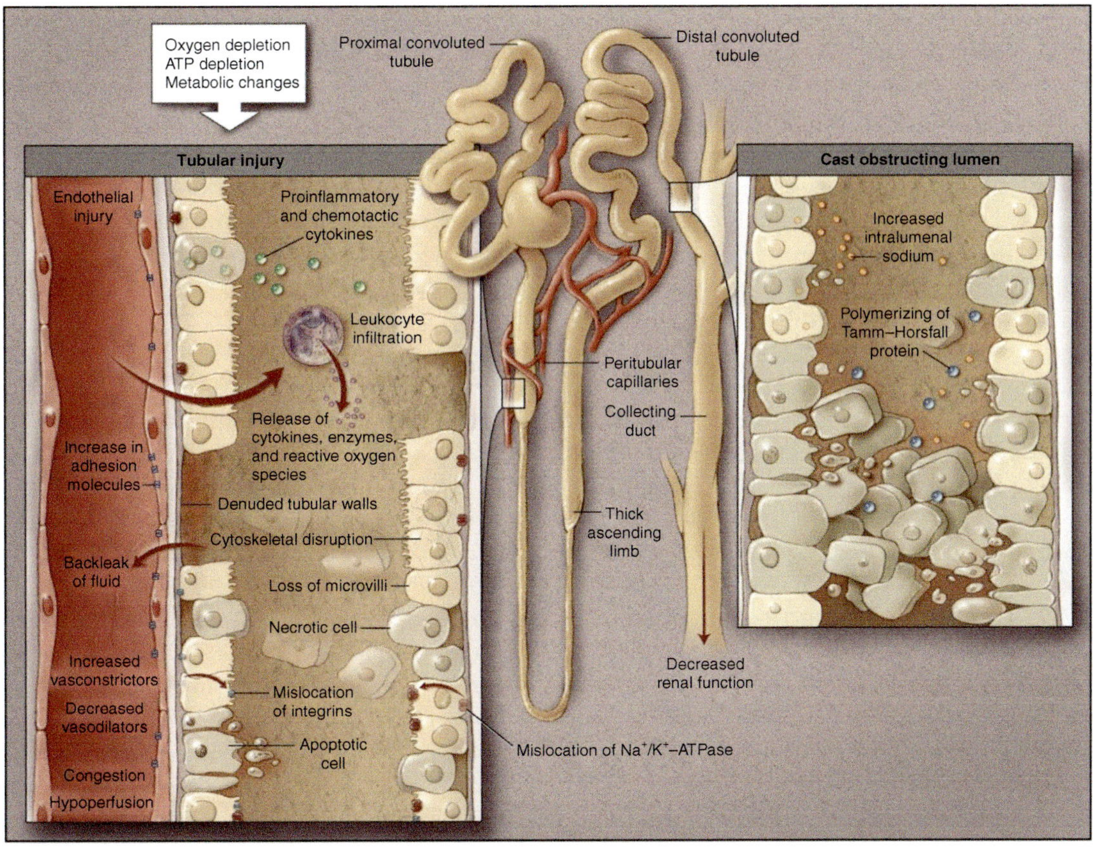

Fig. 17.1 Illustration showing the mechanisms of acute tubular necrosis. The major histologic changes are loss of proximal tubule brush border and patchy loss of proximal tubule cells by impairment of normal cell-to-basement membrane adhesion. This process leads to multiple areas of denudation of the basement membrane. Obstructing distal tubule casts of viable cells might also be observed and focal areas of proximal tubule dilatation appear. Intratubular obstruction by cells and cellular debris is an important component of acute tubular necrosis; the intraluminal casts are composed, in part, of Tamm-Horsfall protein, which is converted to a gel-like polymer in the setting of high local luminal sodium concentrations that is characteristic of acute tubular necrosis. Tubules from multiple nephrons drain into a single collecting tubule; as a result, obstruction in a relatively small number of collecting tubules may lead to failure of filtration in a large number of nephrons. In addition to observable tubule obstruction, complement activation is another early event underlying ischemic injury and influences the recruitment of neutrophils and directly damages the endothelium and surrounding cells. This process leads to back leak of filtered tubular fluid into the vascular space across the damaged tubule epithelium and peritubular capillaries congestion by leukocyte accumulation that impairs local renal blood flow. After revascularization, the combination of continued glomerular filtration and impaired proximal and loop reabsorptive function leads to increased sodium chloride delivery to the macula densa in individual nephrons. This activates the tubuloglomerular feedback mechanism, causing afferent arteriolar constriction, which lowers the GFR in an attempt to reduce tubule flow rate (Abuelo JG. Normotensive ischemic acute renal failure. N Engl J Med. 2007; 357(8):797–805. With permission of Massachusetts Medical Society. All rights reserved)

the generation of reactive oxygen species, and activation of phospholipases and proteases.

In the hypoxic areas, the net effect is the *so-called* acute tubular necrosis with either necrotic or apoptotic processes leading to cell death that is usually restricted to the proximal tubule and thick ascending limb of the loop of Henle.

The acute tubular necrosis is a direct consequence of metabolic pathways activated by ischemia, but it is potentiated by inflammation with a wide variety of pro-inflammatory molecules released in response to ischemic injury. This disorder is initially characterized by a decline in the glomerular filtration rate that is usually more prominent than the severity of the histologic changes (Fig. 17.1).

The urine volume may be reduced, and the early rising of plasma creatinine concentration is usually associated to a characteristic set of laboratory changes including elevation in specific urine and serum biomarkers that are indicative of tubular injury.

Eventually, according to the severity and duration of ischemia, histologic changes might recover with restored areas of cellular regeneration. In particular when preoperative renal function is good and kidneys are not exposed to adjunctive nephrotoxic agents and harmful conditions, renal function might stabilize back to baseline.

17.2 Surgical Strategies for Renal Perfusion

The most encouraging approaches in renal protection are currently based on surgical techniques focused on the reduction of ischemic time, together with renal artery perfusion.

Over the last 50 years, several strategies have been developed for selective renal artery perfusion during the repair of the visceral aorta, including blood perfusion with passive shunts and extracorporeal circulation (Fig. 17.2).

Warm selective blood perfusion of the renal arteries is, in theory, the nearest approach to physiology preventing cell membrane injury and intracellular swelling, thanks to a continuous delivery of oxygen and buffers.

However, the protective effects of local renal cooling against ischemia/reperfusion injury have been established as well for almost six decades [4]. In the randomized trial of Köksoy, acute renal dysfunction in patients who underwent TAAA repair under renal artery selective perfusion with cold crystalloid was 21%, compared to the 63% reported for warm blood [9].

Cold blood, combining the benefits of hypothermia and blood substrates, has also been used in clinical settings. However, in the retrospective study of Hassoun, in which 359 patients underwent open TAAA repair with either warm or cold visceral perfusion, cold blood did not provide any significant advantage in postoperative renal

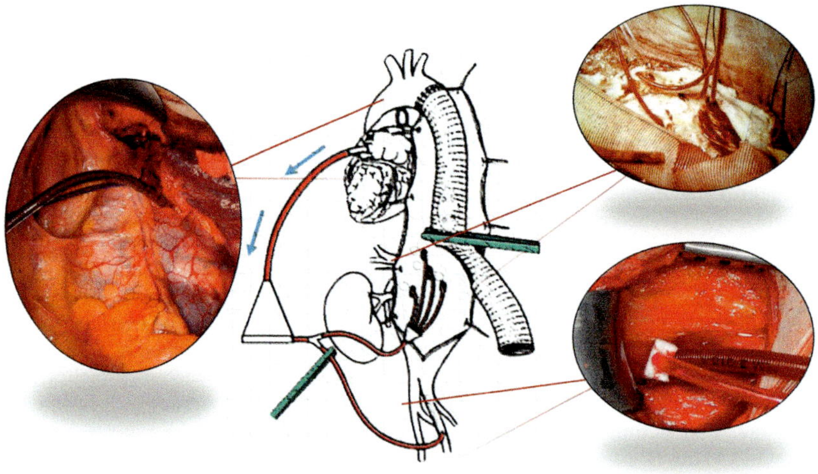

Fig. 17.2 Schematic drawing and surgical pictures showing an open TAAA repair performed with sequential clamping and distal aortic perfusion with a centrifugal pump. The circuit in-flow site is usually the left atrium, and intraoperative picture on the left shows left atrium cannulation through the left superior pulmonary vein. After proximal aortic anastomosis and reattachment of the intercostal arteries, the visceral segment of the aorta is opened, and coeliac trunk, superior mesenteric artery, and renal arteries are cannulated with occlusion-perfusion balloon catheters for selective hematic perfusion. Intraoperative picture in the upper right corner shows hematic visceral artery perfusion during repair of visceral aorta. Intraoperative picture in the lower right corner shows nonocclusive cannulation of the left common femoral artery for distal lower limbs and visceral perfusion during proximal aortic clamping

dysfunction and recovery compared to warm blood [10].

Even compared to cold crystalloid, cold blood failed to provide any significant superiority. In the prospective trial from Lemaire, 155 patients were randomized, receiving intermittent renal perfusion with 4 °C lactated Ringer's solution or 4 °C blood. No significant difference was reported in postoperative renal dysfunction score or in subclinical injury, measured with changes of specific renal biomarkers [11].

Cold blood properties have not been fully studied at 4 °C, and several arguments may justify the reported lack of superiority, including oxyhemoglobin dissociation curve shift to the left that reduces its ability to release oxygen. Cold blood perfusion also requires adjunctive lines and issues in extracorporeal blood circuits. Some authors advocated that the concept of selective blood renal perfusion technique should be questioned because non-pulsatile hypotensive perfusion is not effective [12, 13]. Kalder has recently focused on the effectiveness and safety of selective renal artery blood perfusion in porcine model, thus in animals with similar vascular vessel diameters and hemodynamic parameters compared to humans [13]. In his study, despite an acceptable blood pressure in the target vessels, the selective roller pump failed to supply sufficient perfusion volume to the renal arteries. Elevated NGAL levels were also measured in renovenous blood and in urinary samples together with significantly increased serum free hemoglobin. The study concluded that selective organ perfusion system induces kidney tubule injury and erythrocyte damage [13]. However, these disappointing results with roller pump are in contrast with those reported by Idu, again in a porcine model, with selective renal blood perfusion instituted with a centrifugal pump [14]. In this study, adequate renal perfusion volumes without significant hemolysis and effective renal tissue oxygenation were reported during supraceliac aortic cross-clamping [14].

In the debated area of selective blood perfusion, the concept proposed by Jacobs in the clinical setting is of special interest [15]. The author states that selective renal blood perfusion is an effective measure to protect renal function during open TAAA repair, but only if perfusion is provided with adequate volume and pressure. In a series of 279 consecutive TAAA repairs, selective visceral perfusion was instituted with centrifugal pump and renal volume flow was assessed with ultrasound. Pressure channels were placed in the perfusion catheters, enabling real-time-controlled perfusion of the kidneys. Repeated adjustments of renal artery perfusion pressure were performed as a dynamic process increasing arterial pressure in the renal catheters by diminishing flow and pressure to the femoral or the visceral arteries based on urinary output. The volume flow in the catheters for the renal arteries varied between 80 and 500 ml/min; intrarenal mean arterial pressure is between 60 and 112 mmHg. Uninterrupted urine output during aortic cross-clamping, irrespective of clamp time, and good postoperative renal outcomes were reported. Unfortunately, we are not allowed to consider these results as evidence because the article has been retracted for unresolvable issues in data collection [16].

The dispute regarding the effectiveness of blood perfusion is still unsolved; however, until today, both warm and cold blood have failed to support the hypothesis that blood perfusion is undoubtedly more effective in renal protection than cold crystalloid [9, 11]. Due to debated results and technical troubles and drawbacks issued with blood, current clinical practice has been mainly addressed to crystalloid perfusion, an easier and effective strategy based on an independent roller pump or even a simple dripping chamber (Fig. 17.3).

As far as the substrate is concerned, crystalloid has come to mean lactated Ringer's solution because most of the studies in this area are Ringer's solution-based. Whynn recently reported a retrospective analysis of postoperative renal function in 55 patients treated for TAAA with simple cross-clamp technique and profound renal cooling with crystalloid perfusion [12]. The renal perfusion was done by infusing 300 ml of lactated Ringer's solution at 4 °C containing mannitol 12.5 g and heparin 1000 units/l under moderate pressure into each renal artery. Very low rates of renal complications were reported with acute kidney injury in 7.6% of patients, acute renal failure in 4%, temporary dialysis in 2%, and permanent dialysis in 0.66% .

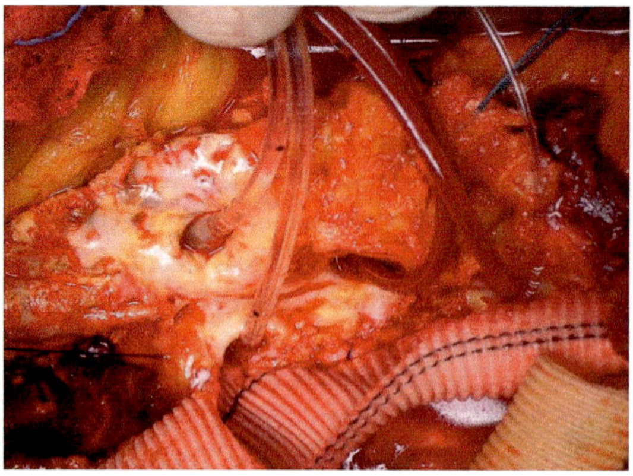

Fig. 17.3 Intraoperative image showing visceral artery reattachment in a visceral patch during an open TAAA repair. Of note, occlusion-perfusion balloon catheters into coeliac trunk, superior mesenteric artery for selective hematic perfusion, and occlusion-perfusion balloon catheters into renal arteries for selective cold crystalloid perfusion

However, we must be aware that renal damage with lactated Ringer's solution is still non-negligible and acute kidney injury may be found in the majority of patients [9, 11, 12].

Alternative crystalloids should be evaluated, and those developed over time for cardioplegia and organ preservation during transplantation are especially appealing in this research area.

17.3 Custodiol Solution: The Rationale, Results, and Future Perspectives

Custodiol or histidine-tryptophan-ketoglutarate (HTK) or Bretschneider's solution is a buffered crystalloid solution produced by Dr. Franz-Kohler Chemie GmbH, Bensheim, Germany. It was originally developed as cardioplegic agent by the German surgical research pioneer Hans Jürgen Bretschneider in 1964, with histidine added in 1975. It was soon registered as drug/medical product in several European countries.

The solution was developed with the aim of protecting the heart through the inactivation of organ function by withdrawal of extracellular sodium and calcium, together with intensive buffering of the extracellular space by means of histidine. Custodiol also contains high concentrations of the amino acids tryptophan and α-ketoglutarate that support membrane integrity and the osmotic agent mannitol. As far as the effectiveness of Custodiol as cardioplegic agent is concerned, the solution has successfully been applied for many years worldwide as a routine method, and it has been shown that even high doses (25 ml/kg) perfused in the heart are safe [17].

Furthermore, Custodiol was found to have the potential to exert its protective effect not only in the heart, but it has also become a standard perfusion/preservation solution of several organs during donor transplantation including the liver, kidney, pancreas, and lungs (Fig. 17.4). This indication has been approved by many countries, with the inclusion of the United States (FDA 510(k) approval).

In ex vivo application during renal transplant surgery, particularly encouraging results have been reported in renal function preservation. The donor kidney perfusion with Custodiol has been shown to maintain organ vitality during cold ischemic times of longer than 20 h, and the reduced rate of delayed graft function even compared to other solutions has been confirmed in meta-analysis, systematic review, and randomized trials [18–20].

This led to the question of whether the working principles of Custodiol can also be applied for direct in vivo perfusion in an organ as different from the heart as the kidney, where the aerobic metabolism and function are distinctly different.

The most used and investigated solution for in vivo direct renal perfusion is lactated Ringer's solution that is considered the benchmark substrate for the comparison of any other and that is totally different in concept and composition compared to Custodiol (Table 17.1).

Off-label in vivo Custodiol perfusion was reported in 1995 in a series of 11 patients undergoing renal tumor resection [21]. Continuous Custodiol perfusion was performed in all patients, the mean cold ischemia time was 62.1 min (range 18–88), and mean perfusion volume was 2875 cm^3. The kidneys resumed excretion within an average of 16.8 min (range 0–60) and no patient required dialysis. Postoperative renal function was unimpaired in all patients without changes in serum electrolyte levels and no disorders of cardiac conduction.

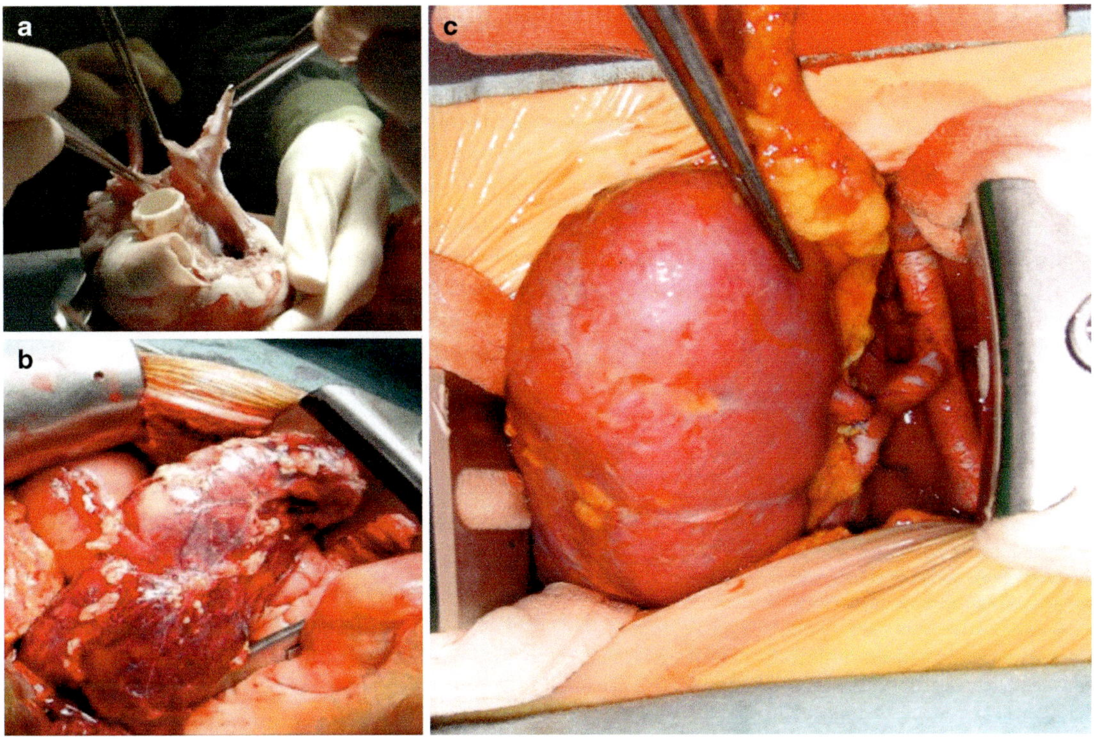

Fig. 17.4 Custodiol solution is a crystalloid solution approved for cardioplegia in open heart surgical procedures (**a**) as well as for the preservation of several organs in non-heart-beating donor transplantation including the pancreas (**b**) and kidney (**c**). During hypothermic storage and transportation to the recipient, the solution is left in the organ vasculature and is not currently indicated for continuous perfusion. The solution is ready to use, and the low potassium content makes preflushing from the organ unnecessary prior to implantation (courtesy of Dr. Carlo Socci)

Furthermore, several series with off-label use of Custodiol with direct renal arteries perfusion during suprarenal aortic clamping were reported, but, until 2014, no comparative studies were performed.

In 2014, Tshomba and Chiesa reported a retrospective comparative study to assess effectiveness in renal protection of Custodiol when compared with lactated Ringer's solution [22].

Study primary endpoints were acute kidney injury (AKI) according to the KDIGO guidelines criteria and postoperative eGFR calculated by using the Chronic Kidney Disease Epidemiology Collaboration (CKD-EPI) formula [23]. Study provided statistical evidence of reduction of AKI incidence of almost 25% in the Custodiol group compared to Ringer, with a reduction of AKI rate in each AKI class, with a halved rate of AKI class II (Fig. 17.5). Furthermore, Custodiol renal perfusion resulted as the only independent intraoperative predictor of freedom from AKI and was associated with a significantly improved perioperative trend of eGFR. Interestingly, these improved renal outcomes were reported despite longer total renal ischemic time and increased transfusion requirements in Custodiol group.

Study findings support the hypothesis that Custodiol perfusion has the potential to be more effective than lactated Ringer's solution in preserving renal function. However, several limitations affect the study, including its retrospective nature and temporal bias related to the different periods in which the patients of the two study groups were treated.

A prospective trial has been designed specifically to resolve these issues. "CUstodiol and Ringer: whaT Is the Best Agent?" (CURITIBA) trial (ClinicalTrials.gov Identifier: NCT02327611) is a monocentric phase IV double-blinded randomized trial with parallel groups

Table 17.1 Different electrolyte concentrations in Custodiol and Ringer's lactated solutions

	Ringer (mmol/l)	Custodiol (mmol/l)
Sodium chloride	130.0	15.0
Potassium chloride	4.0	9.0
Magnesium chloride $6H_2O$	0.0	4.0
Histidine hydrochloride H_2O	0.0	18.0
Potassium hydrogen 2-Ketoglutarate	0.0	1.0
Histidine	0.0	180.0
Tryptophan	0.0	2.0
Mannitol	0.0	30.0
Calcium chloride $2H_2O$	2.7	0.015
Sodium lactate	28.0	0.0

Custodiol is a crystalloid solution with electrolyte concentrations similar to the intracellular environment, containing lower levels of sodium, calcium, potassium, and magnesium compared to a standard isotonic solution used for intravenous systemic infusion, such as Ringer, in which several salts are dissolved

Compared to extracellular solutions, organ perfusion with Custodiol should reduce the cellular swelling, toxicity, and damage caused by the ischemic insults. Custodiol solution also contains a high hydrogen ion buffer level that reduces acidosis associated with ongoing anaerobic metabolism. Custodiol solution is also enriched with three main factors: histidine/histidine hydrochloride (an amino acid buffering agent), tryptophan, and α-ketoglutarate enhancing the buffering and protecting capacity of the solution during the ischemic-induced acidosis

Alpha-ketoglutarate is also a key intermediate in the Krebs cycle, coming after isocitrate and before succinyl CoA and contributing in immediate intracellular ATP production, that is, the ultimate determinant of respiratory pathways, when oxygen is still available after ischemic time

aimed at comparing the effects of selective renal perfusion with Custodiol versus lactated Ringer's solution in patients undergoing open TAAA repair with renal artery crystalloid perfusion. The primary endpoint is the incidence of AKI; secondary endpoints are the eGFR trend during the hospital stays, together with the mortality rate at 30 days from the surgery and at 1 year. Also, serum cystatine C and urinary submarkers of renal injury including albumin (uALB), retinol-binding protein (uRBP), and neutrophil gelatinase-associated lipocalin (uNGAL) will be measured in order to evaluate more precisely filtration failure, protein reabsorption failure, and proximal and distal tubular injury. The trial results are still unpublished but, when available, will contribute to bridging the gap of our current knowledge about the real safety and effectiveness of Custodiol in vivo renal perfusion.

Currently, several new research lines and horizons might be imagined, among these, solutions specifically aimed at protecting hypothermic tissues from reperfusion damage. An interesting mechanism of cell damage after cardiac arrest in heart surgery has been found to be induced by hypothermia leading to cold-induced increase of iron-dependent formation of highly reactive oxygen species [24]. Custodiol-N, is a chloride- and histidine-poor cardioplegic solution based on Custodiol and supplemented by cytoprotective amino acids: LK614 and deferoxamine. LK614 is a lipophilic, membrane-permeable intracellular free iron chelator. Deferoxamine is a well-known extracellular iron chelator. Histidine has proven to be an excellent buffer and has therefore been introduced into Custodiol, but this protective buffer itself can be the origin of cytotoxity, and its concentration is reduced in Custodiol-N [25]. A study comparing the efficacy and safety of Custodiol-N with Custodiol in a model of heterotopic heart transplantation in the rat reported improved myocardial and endothelial function during the critical phase of reperfusion after heart transplantation, and this solution could also be assessed in hypothermic renal protection [26].

In the fascinating research area of organ protection during reperfusion, and especially in the area of renal protection, it has been also shown that several adhesion molecules, such as ICAM-1, may participate in the development of ischemic acute tubular necrosis [27]. The administration of anti-ICAM-1 antibodies preserves renal function and mitigates cell injury in experimental models of acute tubular necrosis, even if given as long as 2 h after the ischemic insult. In addition, mutant mice without ICAM-1 are almost completely protected against ischemic renal injury [28]. However, in human trials, the administration of anti-ICAM-1 monoclonal antibody did not prevent acute tubular necrosis in deceased-donor kidney transplant recipients following ischemia [29].

Several studies have also suggested a role for other adhesion molecules, such as E- and

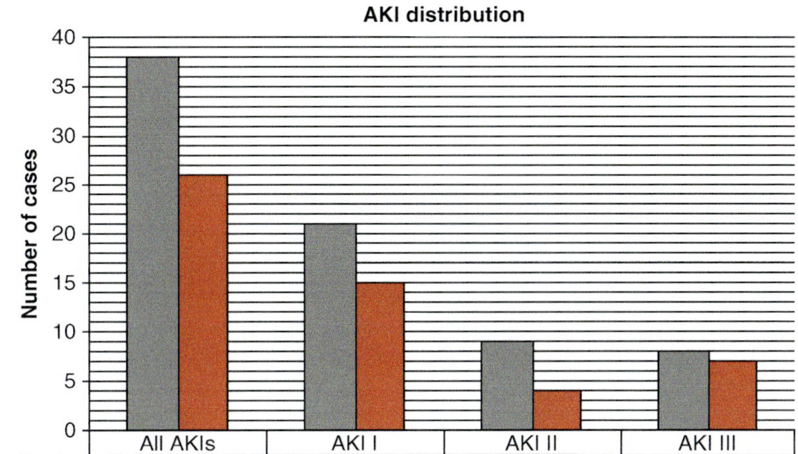

	All AKIs	AKI I	AKI II	AKI III
Ringer	38	21	9	8
Custodiol	26	15	4	7

Fig. 17.5 Acute kidney injury (AKI) distribution in two groups of patients who underwent open TAAA repair with direct renal artery perfusion either with Custodiol or lactated Ringer's solution [22]

P-selectins and integrins, and in an animal model, the use of specific monoclonal antibody reduced ischemia/reperfusion injury [30].

17.4 Conclusions

The prognostic value of reduction of any class of postoperative AKI is priceless because acute kidney injury, even if often temporary and totally reversible, is a strong postoperative determinant of mortality after open TAAA repair. Patients with AKI type I have more than three times the in-hospital mortality rate of patients without AKI. Similarly, patients with AKI type II have close to twice the mortality rate of patients with AKI type I, and patients with AKI type III have 10 times the mortality rate of patients without AKI [31].

Every effort and research focused on full understanding of mechanisms of postoperative AKI and on the development of strategies specifically addressed to reduce both its occurrence and severity should be strongly supported.

Various molecules with the potential to contrast harmful processes of renal ischemia/reperfusion injury may be investigated for a direct in vivo perfusion. Furthermore, the efficacy of different strategies of arterial perfusion together with the effects of different temperatures of perfusion substrates should be carefully evaluated.

In this research area, 4 °C Custodiol renal perfusion, even if currently considered off-label, is simple and provides excellent protection, even in prolonged times of renal ischemia and during complex operations.

Larger comparative series, randomized trials, and the use of new biomarkers able to detect even subclinical renal injury together with continuous evaluation of new substrates are needed for an incessant renal outcomes improvement.

References

1. Tang Y, Chen J, Huang K, Luo D, Liang P, Feng M, Chai W, Fung E, Lan HY, Xu A. The incidence, risk factors and in-hospital mortality of acute kidney injury in patients after abdominal aortic aneurysm repair surgery. BMC Nephrol. 2017;18(1):184.
2. Wong DR, Parenti JL, Green SY, Chowdhary V, Liao JM, Zarda S, et al. Open repair of thoracoabdominal aortic aneurysm in the modern surgical era: contemporary outcomes in 509 patients. J Am Coll Surg. 2011;212(4):569–79.
3. Hiratzka LF, Bakris GL, Beckman JA, Bersin RM, Carr VF, Casey DE Jr, American College of Cardiology Foundation/American Heart Association Task Force on Practice Guidelines; American Association for Thoracic Surgery; American College of Radiology; American Stroke Association; Society of Cardiovascular Anesthesiologists; Society for Cardiovascular Angiography and Interventions; Society of Interventional Radiology; Society of Thoracic Surgeons; Society for Vascular Medicine, et al. 2010 ACCF/AHA/AATS/ACR/ASA/SCA/

SCAI/SIR/STS/SVM guidelines for the diagnosis and management of patients with thoracic aortic disease: a report of the American College of Cardiology Foundation/American Heart Association Task Force on Practice Guidelines, American Association for Thoracic Surgery, American College of Radiology, American Stroke Association, Society of Cardiovascular Anesthesiologists, Society for Cardiovascular Angiography and Interventions, Society of Interventional Radiology, Society of Thoracic Surgeons, and Society for Vascular Medicine. Circulation. 2010;121(13):e266–369.
4. Semb G, Krog J, Johansen K. Renal metabolism and blood flow during local hypothermia, studied by means of renal perfusion in situ. Acta Chir Scand Suppl. 1960;253:196–202.
5. Koletsky S. Effects of temporary interruption of renal circulation in rats. Arch Pathol. 1954;58:592.
6. Hamilton PB, Phillips RA, Hiller A. Duration of renal ischemia required to produce uraemia. Am J Phys. 1949;152:517.
7. Badenoch AW, Darmady EM. Effects of temporary occlusion of the renal artery in rabbits and its relationship to traumatic uraemia. J Pathol Bacteriol. 1947;4:79.
8. Parekh DJ, Weinberg JM, Ercole B, Torkko KC, Hilton W, Bennett M, Devarajan P, Venkatachalam MA. Tolerance of the human kidney to isolated controlled ischemia. J Am Soc Nephrol. 2013;24(3):506–17. https://doi.org/10.1681/ASN.2012080786.
9. Köksoy C, LeMaire SA, Curling PE, Raskin SA, Schmittling ZC, Conklin LD, et al. Renal perfusion during thoracoabdominal aortic operations: cold crystalloid is superior to normothermic blood. Ann Thorac Surg. 2002;73:730–8.
10. Hassoun HT, Miller CC 3rd, Huynh TT, Estrera AL, Smith JJ, Safi HJ. Cold visceral perfusion improves early survival in patients with acute renal failure after thoracoabdominal aortic aneurysm repair. J Vasc Surg. 2004;39(3):506–12.
11. Lemaire SA, Jones MM, Conklin LD, Carter SA, Criddell MD, Wang XL, Raskin SA, Coselli JS. Randomized comparison of cold blood and cold crystalloid renal perfusion for renal protection during thoracoabdominal aortic aneurysm repair. J Vasc Surg. 2009;49(1):11–9.
12. Wynn MM, Acher C, Marks E, Engelbert T, Acher CW. Postoperative renal failure in thoracoabdominal aortic aneurysm repair with simple cross-clamp technique and 4°C renal perfusion. J Vasc Surg. 2015;61(3):611–22. https://doi.org/10.1016/j.jvs.2014.10.040.
13. Kalder J, Kokozidou M, Keschenau P, Tamm M, Greiner A, Koeppel TA, Tolba R, Jacobs MJ. Selective renal blood perfusion induces renal tubules injury in a porcine model. J Vasc Surg. 2016;63(3):778–87.
14. Idu MM, Heintjes RJ, Scholten EW, Balm R, de Mol BA, Legemate DA. Visceral and renal tissue oxygenation during supraceliac aortic crossclamping and left heart bypass with selective organ perfusion. Eur J Vasc Endovasc Surg. 2004;27:138–44.
15. Jacobs MJ, van Eps RG, de Jong DS, Schurink GW, Mochtar B. Prevention of renal failure in patients undergoing thoracoabdominal aortic aneurysm repair. J Vasc Surg. 2004;40(6):1067–73.
16. Jacobs MJ, van Eps RG, de Jong DS, Schurink GW, Mochtar B. Regarding "Prevention of renal failure in patients undergoing thoracoabdominal aortic aneurysm repair". J Vasc Surg. 2006;43(2):428–9.
17. Viana FF, Shi WY, Hayward PA, Larobina ME, Liskaser F, Matalanis G. Custodiol versus blood cardioplegia in complex cardiac operations: an Australian experience. Eur J Cardiothorac Surg. 2013;43(3):526–31.
18. Ounissi M, Cherif M, Abdallah TB, Bacha M, Hedri H, Abderrahim E, et al. Risk factors and consequences of delayed graft function. Saudi J Kidney Dis Transpl. 2013;24(2):243–6.
19. O'Callaghan JM, Knight SR, Morgan RD, Morris PJ. Preservation solutions for static cold storage of kidney allografts: a systematic review and meta-analysis. Am J Transplant. 2012;12:896–906.
20. Klaus F, Castro DB, Bittar CM, Bittar AE, Keitel E, Seelig DC, Goldani JC, Meinne MH, Garcia VD. Kidney transplantation with Belzer or Custodiol solution: a randomized prospective study. Transplant Proc. 2007;39(2):353–4.
21. Gschwend JE, de Petriconi R, Maier S, Kleinschmidt K, Hautmann RE. Continuous in situ cold perfusion with histidine tryptophan ketoglutarate solution in nephron sparing surgery for renal tumors. J Urol. 1995;154(4):1307–11.
22. Tshomba Y, Kahlberg A, Melissano G, Coppi G, Marone E, Ferrari D, Lembo R, Chiesa R. Comparison of renal perfusion solutions during thoracoabdominal aortic aneurysm repair. J Vasc Surg. 2014;59(3):623–33.
23. Stevens LA, Coresh J, Greene T, Levey AS. Assessing kidney function—measured and estimated glomerular filtration rate. N Engl J Med. 2006;354:2473–83.
24. Rauen U, Petrat F, Li T, De Groot H. Hypothermia injury/cold-induced apoptosis—evidence of an increase in chelatable iron causing oxidative injury in spite of low O_2-/H_2O_2 formation. FASEB J. 2000;14(13):1953–64.
25. Rauen U, Klempt S, de Groot H. Histidine-induced injury to cultured liver cells, effects of histidine derivatives and of iron chelators. Cell Mol Life Sci. 2007;64(2):192–205.
26. Loganathan S, Radovits T, Hirschberg K, Korkmaz S, Koch A, Karck M, Szabó G. Effects of Custodiol-N, a novel organ preservation solution, on ischemia/reperfusion injury. J Thorac Cardiovasc Surg. 2010;139(4):1048–56.
27. Molitoris BA, Marrs J. The role of cell adhesion molecules in ischemic acute renal failure. Am J Med. 1999;106(5):583–92.
28. Kelly KJ, Williams WW Jr, Colvin RB, Meehan SM, Springer TA, Gutierrez-Ramos JC, Bonventre

JV. Intercellular adhesion molecule-1-deficient mice are protected against ischemic renal injury. J Clin Invest. 1996;97(4):1056–63.
29. Salmela K, Wramner L, Ekberg H, Hauser I, Bentdal O, Lins LE, Isoniemi H, Bäckman L, Persson N, Neumayer HH, Jørgensen PF, Spieker C, Hendry B, Nicholls A, Kirste G, Hasche G. A randomized multicenter trial of the anti-ICAM-1 monoclonal antibody (enlimomab) for the prevention of acute rejection and delayed onset of graft function in cadaveric renal transplantation: a report of the European Anti-ICAM-1 Renal Transplant Study Group. Transplantation. 1999;67(5):729–36.
30. Dehnadi A, Benedict Cosimi A, Neal Smith R, Li X, Alonso JL, Means TK, Arnaout MA. Prophylactic orthosteric inhibition of leukocyte integrin CD11b/CD18 prevents long-term fibrotic kidney failure in cynomolgus monkeys. Nat Commun. 2017;8:13899.
31. Uchino S, Bellomo R, Goldsmith D, Bates S, Ronco C. An assessment of the RIFLE criteria for acute renal failure in hospitalized patients. Crit Care Med. 2006;34:1913–7.

Thoracoabdominal Aortic Aneurysm Open Repair: Visceral Arteries Reattachment Strategies

18

Luca Bertoglio, Alessandro Grandi, Tommaso Cambiaghi, Cilli Giuseppe, and Apruzzi Luca

18.1 Introduction

One of the crucial steps during thoracoabdominal aortic aneurysm open repair is the management of the visceral and renal vessels. Different techniques are available to obtain the same revascularization, but they vary in a few details and can have different indications and outcomes. Historically, the first proposed was the inclusion technique that consists in direct reimplantation of the origin of the celiac trunk, superior mesenteric artery, and renal arteries onto the graft [1].

However, associated atherosclerotic disease might complicate the reimplantation of the ostia of the visceral arteries. The presence of flow-limiting stenosis, calcifications, or thrombus apposition can increase the risk of reimplanted vessel occlusion and end-organ ischemia. Traditionally, in complex situations, open endarterectomy and graft bypass interposition were employed. Nowadays, different ancillary techniques have been proposed such as direct open stenting, sutureless anastomosis, and multibranched graft reimplantations. The aim of this chapter is to illustrate the different techniques used today.

L. Bertoglio (✉) · A. Grandi · T. Cambiaghi
C. Giuseppe · A. Luca
Division of Vascular Surgery, "Vita – Salute" University, Scientific Institute H. San Raffaele, Milan, Italy
e-mail: bertoglio.luca@hsr.it; alex@eenet.it; cilli.giuseppe@hsr.it; apruzzi.luca@hsr.it

18.2 Inclusion Techniques

The most common revascularization technique employed is the inclusion technique: the anastomosis onto the surgical graft of a button of the aortic wall from which visceral vessels arise. This has the advantage of requiring only one anastomosis compared to single-artery reimplantation, thus reducing the end-organ damage and visceral ischemic time. The aortic patch can include a variable number of visceral vessels ostia so that sovrannumerary renal or splanchnic vessel can be reimplanted all together in case of anomalous vessel origin.

18.2.1 Carrel Patch

The first configuration used was the Carrel patch into which the origins of all the renal and splanchnic vessels are included. The major downside of this revascularization technique is the amount of pathologic aortic wall left that could be prone to further degeneration and subsequent further dilation into what is now referred to as visceral aortic patch (VAP) aneurysm [2]. Eventual management of VAP aneurysms is extremely challenging, with consequent high morbidity and mortality associated with redo open treatment [3, 4].

© Springer Nature Switzerland AG 2019
Y. Tshomba et al. (eds.), *Visceral Vessels and Aortic Repair*,
https://doi.org/10.1007/978-3-319-94761-7_18

18.2.2 Undersized Patch (Three Vessels) and Left Renal Artery Direct Reimplantation: 3+1 Patch

If the four ostia are too far away from each other, and to minimize the amount of aortic wall left in place, three (celiac trunk, superior mesenteric artery, and right renal artery) of the four vessels can be reimplanted with an aortic wall button/island, and the remaining one, usually the left renal artery, can be reattached selectively with different techniques (Fig. 18.1).

18.2.3 Direct Reimplantation

Direct reimplantation of any visceral artery on the surgical graft is a feasible option to reduce the amount of aortic tissue used for the reimplantation (Fig. 18.2); however, it can be technically demanding when the original anatomy is distorted by the aneurysm and the available vessel length does not allow a reimplantation in the desired position.

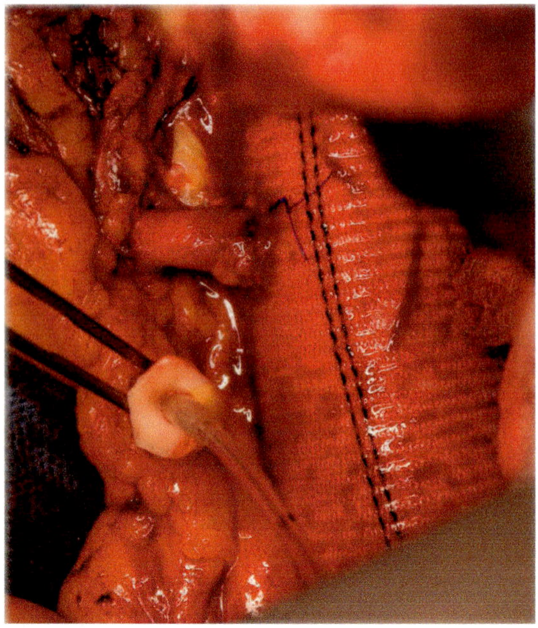

Fig. 18.2 Intraoperative capture of a direct reimplant of the superior mesenteric artery during a thoracoabdominal repair

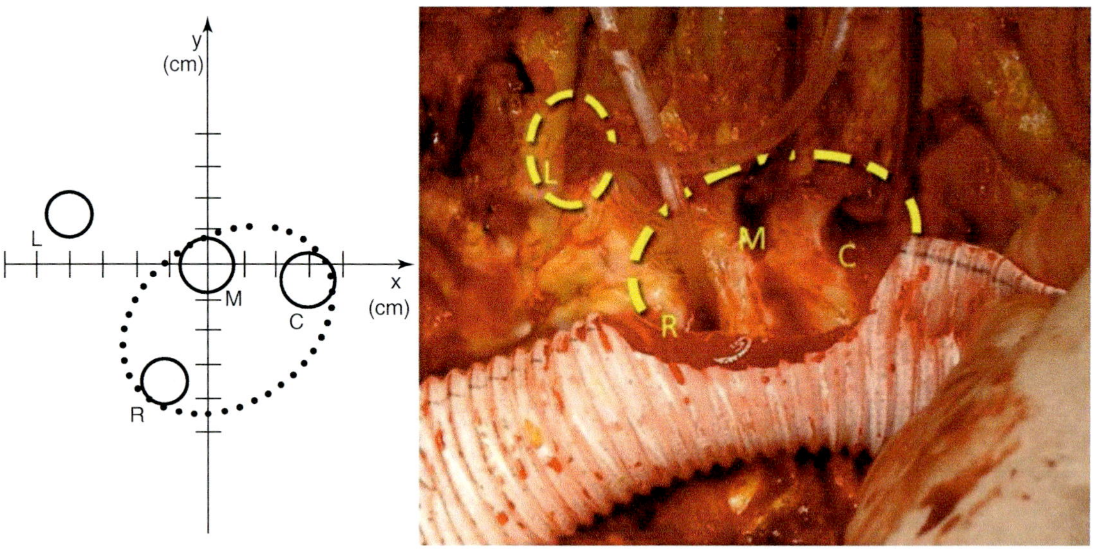

Fig. 18.1 Undersized patch to include three vessels and separately reimplant the left renal artery

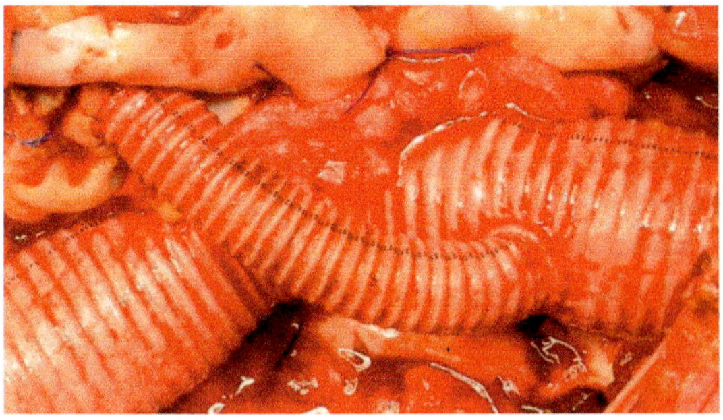

Fig. 18.3 Graft interposition to revascularize the left renal artery

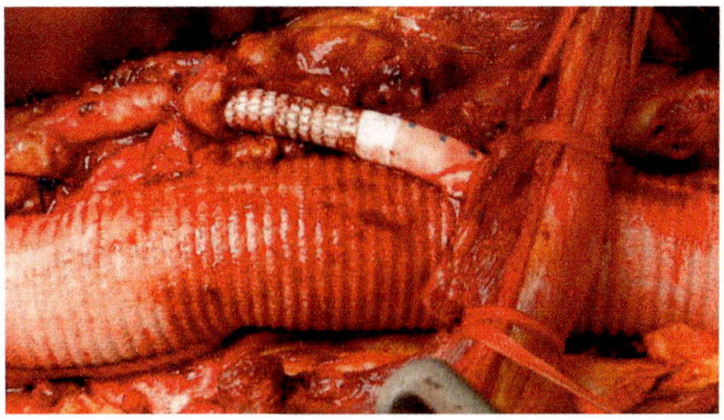

Fig. 18.4 Revascularization of the left renal artery with a sutureless graft

18.2.4 Surgical Graft Interposition

In these cases, or when the origin of the target vessel is pathologic (stenotic, dissected, aneurysmatic), a small-diameter (6–8 mm) prosthetic graft can be used to perform a bypass in between the aortic surgical graft and the visceral vessel (Fig. 18.3). This technique also allows shortening of the vessel, kinking correction, and possible excision of the ostial aortic disease (stenosis or aneurysmatic dilation). The drawback of this technique is the possible kinking and occlusion of the graft and therefore of the vessel.

18.2.5 Gore Hybrid Graft

The Gore Hybrid is an ePTFE vascular graft, constructed with an extremity joint to a self-expandable nitinol-covered stent, which allows the possibility of "sutureless" vascular anastomosis. A recent study by our group [5] described the first application of this graft for revascularization of visceral arteries in open TAAA repair. The advantage of this new graft lies in the requirement of an anastomosis only on the free end of the bypass, while the stented end can be fixed only with a couple of stitches as the stent holds the graft in place. The results show that this technique is feasible even in the most tortuous anatomies and allows a new time-saving strategy of reperfusion of target vessels (Fig. 18.4).

18.2.6 Multibranched Graft

If the ostia of the visceral and renal arteries are too far apart, or no diseased aortic wall is to be spared, single reimplantation of the target vessel can be performed directly on the graft. Youssef et al. reported a better outcome at 5 and 10 years for selective reimplantation compared to patch inclusion with a patency of 100% vs 94.2% and 100% vs 81.3%, respectively [6]. Single-vessel revascularization reduces the amount of aortic tissue left, but it also allows to tailor the intraoperative strategy during the repair.

A four-branch synthetic graft can be used for extensive TAAA aneurysm where the surgeon needs to reattach individually the celiac trunk, the superior mesenteric artery, and the two renal arteries without leaving any aortic wall in place [7]. Single-/multivessel revascularization gives the ability to freely dictate whether or not to firstly revascularize the visceral vessels or perform the distal anastomosis.

Prioritization between visceral vessel revascularization and distal anastomosis can be done by using intraoperative motor and somatosensory evoked potentials to understand how the patient is reacting to the distal reperfusion and the aortic cross-clamping [8].

The use of this type of graft is ideal especially in two situations: when the patient is affected by a genetic collagenopathy such as Marfan, Loeys-Dietz, or Ehlers-Danlos syndromes, in these patients, indeed, any portion of native aortic tissue left in place is a potential site of further dilation, or when the origins of the visceral vessels are so distant that an inclusion technique is contraindicated (Fig. 18.5).

18.3 Ancillary Techniques for Vessel Management

18.3.1 Ostial Endarterectomy

Branch vessel stenosis in TAAA patents is most often related to atherosclerotic occlusive disease but can also be caused by aortic dissection. The visceral artery lesions are frequently proximal extensions of aortic atherosclerosis. In these cases, endarterectomy can be performed to remove the stenosis (Fig. 18.6). It is a feasible and safe technique that can be safely performed without exponentially increasing the operative time and yielding good results. However, it has important limitations, including the risks of vessel thrombosis related to an unsatisfactory endpoint and perforation of the thinned outer, fragile vessel wall [9, 10]. The friable endarterectomized wall also increases the risk of vessel perforation during the insertion of balloon catheters that are commonly used to deliver renal perfusion. Bypasses to the branch vessels—the traditional alternative to endarterectomy—increase the end-organ ischemic times and may be associated with increased morbidity. The success of percutaneous visceral arterial stenting, combined with the associated technological advances, has created an opportunity to apply these techniques during open surgery [11].

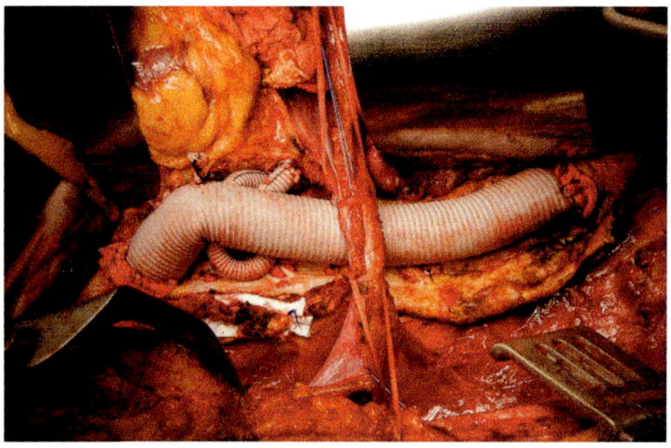

Fig. 18.5 Multibranched reimplantation of all the visceral arteries during a TAAA repair in a Marfan patient

18.3.2 Direct Stenting

Balloon expandable stents can be a useful adjunct for optimizing the visceral reconstruction during open TAAA repair. Direct stenting of ostial stenosis can greatly reduce operative time, and as reported by Coselli et al., patients who underwent visceral stenting had a low incidence of postoperative renal failure despite their high prevalence of preoperative renal insufficiency, renal occlusive disease, acute presentation, advanced age, and other risk factors [10].

Safe deployment requires that the stents are positioned precisely within the proximal portion

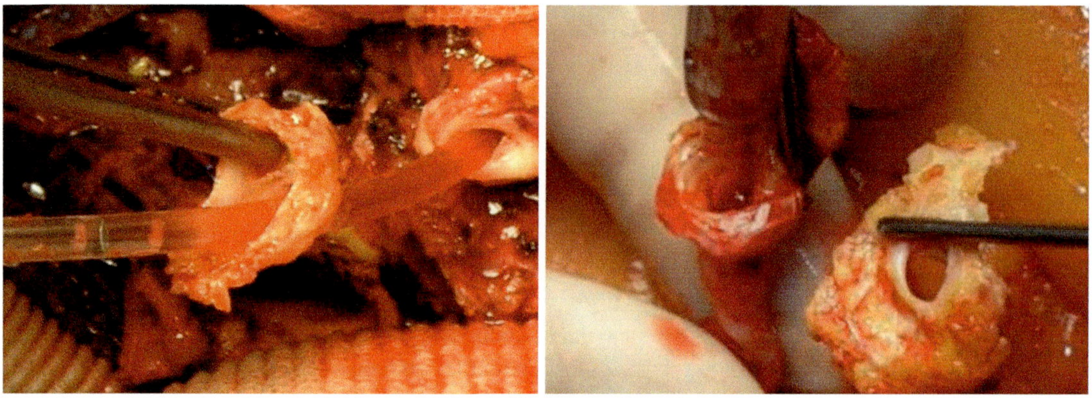

Fig. 18.6 Left renal artery endarterectomy before the reimplant to ease the suture and reimplant

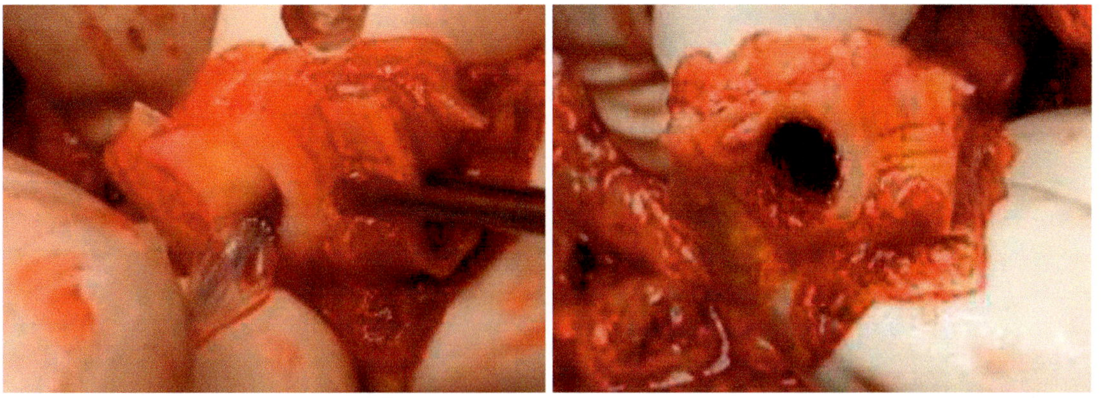

Fig. 18.7 Direct stenting of a stenotic renal artery before reimplant

of the vessel and expanded under direct visualization; insertion into a vessel lumen that is not well visualized should be strictly avoided (Fig. 18.7).

References

1. Coselli JS, LeMaire SA, Preventza O, de la Cruz KI, Cooley DA, Price MD, et al. Outcomes of 3309 thoracoabdominal aortic aneurysm repairs. J Thorac Cardiovasc Surg. 2016;151(5):1323–37. https://doi.org/10.1016/j.jtcvs.2015.12.050.
2. Dardik A, Perler BA, Roseborough GS, Williams GM. Aneurysmal expansion of the visceral patch after thoracoabdominal aortic replacement: an argument for limiting patch size? J Vasc Surg. 2001;34(3):405–9. discussion 410.
3. Bertoglio L, Mascia D, Cambiaghi T, Kahlberg A, Melissano G, Chiesa R. Fenestrated and branched endovascular treatment of recurrent visceral aortic patch aneurysm after open thoracoabdominal repair. J Vasc Interv Radiol. 2018;29(1):72–77.e2. https://doi.org/10.1016/j.jvir.2017.08.012.
4. Bertoglio L, Mascia D, Cambiaghi T, Kahlberg A, Tshomba Y, Gomez JC, Melissano G, Chiesa R. Management of recurrent of visceral aortic patch aneurysms after thoracoabdominal repair: open, hybrid and endovascular approach. J Vasc Surg. 2018;67:41S–3S.
5. Chiesa R, Kahlberg A, Mascia D, Tshomba Y, Civilini E, Melissano G. Use of a novel hybrid vascular graft for sutureless revascularization of the renal arteries during open thoracoabdominal aortic aneurysm repair. J Vasc Surg. 2014;60(3):622–30. https://doi.org/10.1016/j.jvs.2014.03.256.
6. Youssef M, Neufang A, Jungmann F, Vahl CF, Dorweiler B. Patency of renal and visceral vessels after open thoracoabdominal aortic replacement. J Vasc Surg. 2015;62(3):594–9. https://doi.org/10.1016/j.jvs.2015.04.386.
7. de la Cruz K, LeMaire SA, Weldon SA, Coselli JS. Thoracoabdominal aortic aneurysm repair with a branched graft. Ann Cardiothorac Surg. 2012;1(3):381–93. https://doi.org/10.3978/j.issn.2225-319X.2012.08.05.
8. Keyhani K, Miller CC, Estrera AL, Wegryn T, Sheinbaum R, Safi HJ. Analysis of motor and somatosensory evoked potentials during thoracic and thoracoabdominal aortic aneurysm repair. J Vasc Surg. 2009;49(1):36–41. https://doi.org/10.1016/j.jvs.2008.08.005.
9. Stoney RJ, Messina LM, Goldstone J, Reilly LM. Renal endarterectomy through the transected aorta: a new technique for combined aortorenal atherosclerosis—a preliminary report. J Vasc Surg. 1989;9:224–33.
10. Clair DG, Belkin M, Whittemore AD, Mannick JA, Donaldson MC. Safety and efficacy of transaortic renal endarterectomy as an adjunct to aortic surgery. J Vasc Surg. 1995;21:926–34.
11. LeMaire SA, Jamison AL, Carter SA, Wen S, Alankar S, Coselli JS. Deployment of balloon expandable stents during open repair of thoracoabdominal aortic aneurysms: a new strategy for managing renal and mesenteric artery lesions. Eur J Cardiothorac Surg. 2004;26(3):599–607. https://doi.org/10.1016/j.ejcts.2004.04.035.

Renal and Visceral Sutureless Anastomosis During Thoracoabdominal Aortic Repair

19

Andrea Kahlberg, Matteo Bossi, Daniele Mascia, Enrico Rinaldi, Yamume Tshomba, Germano Melissano, and Roberto Chiesa

19.1 Introduction

In spite of multiple technical improvements in the surgical treatment of thoracoabdominal aortic aneurysm (TAAA) that lead to significant morbidity and mortality reduction, visceral and renal ischemic complications are still frequent, even in the most specialized centers [1].

As a matter of fact, perioperative acute kidney dysfunction still complicates up to 70% of these procedures, and the consequences of postoperative renal failure are remarkable. They represent the strongest predictor of early mortality and are associated with permanent long-term chronic kidney disease [2, 3].

Multiple etiopathological factors are supposed to be involved in perioperative visceral and renal dysfunction: the most important, following many authors' opinions, are the time of organ ischemia during artery reattachment and the associated atherosclerotic vessel disease, such as ostial stenosis or dissection. These factors account for a significant increase in technical difficulty, prolonged time of anastomosis, and increased global risk of intraoperative organ injury.

In the past, the first "sutureless anastomoses" performed on visceral aortic branches (including visceral and renal arteries) were performed during debranching procedures, using covered self-expanding stents [4]. The goal was to obviate the need for technically demanding vessel exposure and challenging anastomoses, thus obtaining reduction of flow interruption and simplifying the performance of complex aortic repair.

The Gore Hybrid Vascular Graft (GHVG; WL Gore and Associates, Flagstaff, Ariz) represents the linear evolution of this technique: a novel expanded polytetrafluoroethylene (ePTFE) vascular prosthesis is associated with a nitinol-reinforced covered self-expanding section at one of its extremities that allows to perform "sutureless" endovascular anastomosis at one side and a standard surgical suture on the other side of the prosthesis.

Electronic Supplementary Material The online version of this chapter (doi:10.1007/978-3-319-94761-7_19) contains supplementary material, which is available to authorized users.

A. Kahlberg (✉) · M. Bossi · D. Mascia · E. Rinaldi
G. Melissano
Vascular Surgery, Vita-Salute University
School of Medicine, San Raffaele Scientific Institute, Milan, Italy
e-mail: kahlberg.andrea@hsr.it

Y. Tshomba
Unit of Vascular Surgery, Fondazione Policlinico Universitario A. Gemelli IRCCS, Università Cattolica del Sacro Cuore, Rome, Italy

Unit of Vascular Surgery, San Raffaele Scientific Institute, Vita-Salute University, Milan, Italy

R. Chiesa
Unit of Vascular Surgery, San Raffaele Scientific Institute, Vita-Salute University, Milan, Italy

© Springer Nature Switzerland AG 2019
Y. Tshomba et al. (eds.), *Visceral Vessels and Aortic Repair*,
https://doi.org/10.1007/978-3-319-94761-7_19

In this chapter, we describe this novel device and our experience with this graft for renal and visceral revascularization during TAAA open repair, in order to assess the safety and short-term results of this technique as compared to standard revascularization strategies.

19.2 General Considerations

Open surgical repair for thoracoabdominal aortic disease, such as atherosclerotic aneurysms or dissection, is durable with well-defined and acceptable long-term survival [5]. With open surgical procedures, the widest range of aortic anatomies and diseases can be covered. In spite of specific renal and visceral protection strategies, acute kidney dysfunction still remains one of the most serious complications of TAAA open repair, with around 6–10% of patients requiring postoperative hemodialysis [2, 6]. Considering lesser grades of postoperative kidney injury, an up to 50% elevation in baseline creatinine level may be observed in more than 70% of patients [1] who underwent open surgical repair of TAAA.

In this regard, an important consideration must be undertaken: in a recent study reviewing all the published data of the past decade (2000–2010) for open TAAA surgical repair [7], the rate of postoperative renal complications did not seem to decrease if compared with a similar review published in 1995, regardless of medical and surgical advances [8].

Major causes of intraoperative renal damage include temporary ischemia during aortic cross-clamping and visceral vessels repair, arterial embolism, and stenosis or dissection of the reattached renal vessel [9–11]. These harmful mechanisms are known to develop especially when the quality of the arterial wall is poor, with severe atherothrombotic vessel degeneration, and when the surgical reattachment of the renal artery is demanding because of its anatomical location.

Methods usually employed for renal artery revascularization during TAAA open repair include direct reattachment on the aortic graft using the "Carrel patch technique," described by Crawford et al. (usually together with other visceral vessels or even by direct single-vessel reimplantation) [12], or the use of a single aorto-renal bypass.

The inclusion of many vessels in a visceral aortic patch (VAP) is relatively simple and carries two important advantages: decreasing the global number of anastomoses and, most of all, the duration of organ ischemia. However, a fragile aortic wall (such as in dissected patients or in Marfan's) can cause difficulties with bleeding control, the suture line may become too long in case of considerable distances between the visceral arterial ostia, and the aortic patch tissue may result in subsequent aneurysmal degeneration in time [13]. The latter is considered the main disadvantage of the VAP technique: we previously demonstrated that a large VAP including four visceral vessels is associated with VAP aneurysm formation [13] and that consequent corrective surgery is associated with high morbidity and mortality [14].

To obtain a reduction in VAP size, separate reattachment of distant visceral vessels must be considered, directly or with the interposition of a graft. The vessel is usually indicated for a separated reattachment in the left renal artery. A single aorto-renal/visceral graft interposition allows better bleeding control, may accommodate several anatomies, and presents reduced risk of late aneurysmal degeneration. Its major disadvantage is that two anastomoses are required for each vessel revascularization, often making this option time-consuming and occasionally challenging. Alternatively, the use of presewn aortic branched grafts carries the advantage of reducing the number of total anastomoses to be performed, consequently decreasing operative times [15]. The negative aspect of this graft is that branches are presewn to the aortic graft in a fixed position and may not adapt well to the patient's anatomy leading to subsequent kinking or twisting after viscera derotation.

Finally, customized branched aortic graft may be employed, in which prosthetic ramifications are sewn during the operation prior to aortic cross-clamping, considering the variable anatomy of each single patient [16]. Although this strategy may theoretically represent a valuable alternative in order to reduce the visceral ischemic time (but definitely increasing total operative time), it is quite difficult to predict a priori how the aortic graft will arrange after performing the proximal, distal, and intercostal patch anastomoses.

In relation to atherosclerotic disease, or caused by aortic dissection, patients with TAAAs often present an occlusive disease involving the visceral branches. The presence of calcification and thrombus at the origin of the renal or visceral arteries is associated with a high risk of plaque disruption and dissection during vessel reattachment, leading to visceral malperfusion [17], and still represents a significant predictor of renal or visceral complications after TAAA repair [18]. Despite the fact that artery endarterectomy may be required before revascularization to improve patency rates, it represents a high-risk maneuver with important limitations, including the risk of vessel thrombosis, distal dissection, and vessel perforation due to the friable endarterectomized wall [19].

To overcome these difficulties, several groups started using bare stents during TAAA open repair, positioned and expanded within the artery under direct vision, in order to both treat arterial stenosis or dissection avoiding endarterectomy and also to tack down an unsatisfactory endpoint after visceral endarterectomy [20–22].

The use of covered self-expanding stents for "sutureless anastomoses" in challenging anatomies has been reported by several authors. First among all, Lachat et al. reported the concept of a Viabahn-assisted (WL Gore and Associates, Flagstaff, Ariz) sutureless anastomosis in the so-called "VORTEC" technique. The author proposed this technique for visceral revascularization during debranching procedures in hybrid complex aortic repair [4]. The distal end of the covered stent was inserted over a guidewire into the visceral vessel, and the proximal end was sutured end to side directly with the main graft or was fixed into an interposition branch graft on the main bypass. In 2009, the same group published the results of 58 patients submitted to hybrid repair of TAAA or pararenal aortic aneurysm, using the VORTEC technique to revascularize 98 renal and 15 visceral arteries, reporting an overall primary patency rate of 97% at 22 months [23]. They also applied this technique to debranching procedures of supra-aortic trunks, reporting a midterm 91% patency rate without implantation-related complications [24]. Another setting in which this technique can be employed, as described by several groups, is for femoropopliteal revascularization [25, 26].

The GHVG represents the natural evolution of these procedures with a tubular heparin-bounded ePTFE graft pre-connected to the nitinol stent-reinforced section, guaranteeing in-line flow while avoiding flow turbulence. Excluding the literature regarding hemodialysis access, just three case reports have been published to date reporting the use of this novel graft: Levack et al. reported its use for rapid left common carotid revascularization during aortic arch debranching [27], Nigro et al. used the GHVG to perform a sutureless distal anastomosis during surgery for a high-lying internal carotid artery aneurysm [28], and Bornak et al. reported a modified use for celiac trunk and superior mesenteric artery revascularization during a visceral debranching procedure, with satisfying early patency [29].

In our experience of TAAA open repair with the use of GHVG for remote or hostile vessels, many advantages must be underlined:

1. The ability to perform the aorto-renal bypass in a faster and easier manner, reducing ischemic renal time during cold perfusion
2. Low-risk rate and less time to access to remote ostium locations, typically the right renal artery, avoiding extensive preparation and reducing connected complications
3. Possibility to obtain high conformability of the graft, resulting in less kinking or twisting of the revascularized vessels upon viscera derotation
4. Helpful in cases of stenotic or dissected vessels, avoiding the need for additional surgical (endarterectomy) or endovascular procedures (bare stenting)
5. Great applicability for all the visceral and renal vessels (also for the celiac trunk), as long as they respect minimum requirements in length and diameter
6. Possibility to obtain a customized reconstruction in complex anatomy
7. Direct flow into the vessel, with high reduction in turbulence of the blood flow

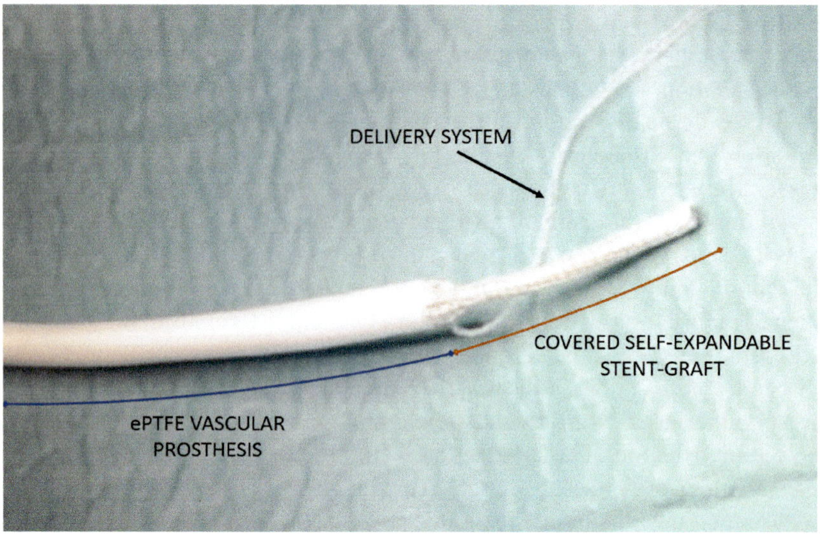

Fig. 19.1 The Gore Hybrid Vascular Graft (GHVG). To notice: the ePTFE standard vascular prosthesis associated with a closed covered self-expandable stent-graft and the linear delivery system

19.3 Device Description

The Gore Hybrid Vascular Graft (GHVG) is an expanded polytetrafluoroethylene (ePTFE) vascular prosthesis that has a distal section reinforced with nitinol. The nitinol-reinforced section is partially constrained to allow for easy insertion and deployment into a vessel. The graft has a continuous lumen bonded with the CARMEDA® BioActive Surface, consisting of a stable covalently bonded reduced molecular weight heparin of porcine origin. An embedded low-permeability film provides a barrier to ultrafiltration.

This graft received the United States (US) Food and Drug Administration (FDA) approval on March 2010 and obtained the CE mark in July 2012. This device is currently commercially available in the USA, Europe, Russia, and few Middle Eastern countries. At the time of writing, this device is approved in the European market for hemodialysis access, lower-limb bypass grafting, aortic arch debranching, and visceral revascularization [30].

The prosthesis is available with the vascular graft section length of 50 cm and a fixed diameter of 6 mm; the nitinol-reinforced section instead presents length of 5 and 10 cm with diameter of 6, 7, 8, and 9 mm.

The delivery system consists of a line that, once pulled, releases the constrained graft. Deployment of the nitinol-reinforced section will occur from the tip of the constraint graft toward the non-nitinol section. Correct deployment of the nitinol-reinforced section does not entail a shortening of the graft. Once deployment has started, repositioning of the nitinol section should not be attempted (Fig. 19.1).

19.4 Indications and Contraindications

In the initial part of our experience, indication for the use of the GHVG was generally limited to renal vessels. Once the real efficacy of these devices had been verified, their use has been expanded to other visceral vessels, both in open and hybrid TAAA surgical reconstructions.

Generally, our indications to the use of the GHVG are:

- Vessels which were not considered suitable for inclusion in an aortic patch, because of their anatomical location or the poor quality of the surrounding aortic wall
- Anatomical location of the artery ostium considered challenging for performing a conventional anastomosis with a standard single bypass
- Severe atherosclerotic disease of the proximal tract of the artery (including the presence of highly calcified or disrupted plaque, critical stenosis, or local dissection)

The choice to use the GHVG was guided by the intention to decrease technical complexity and duration of the distal anastomosis, reduce accidental damage to the arterial wall, concurrently treat stenotic or dissected arteries, and prevent early kinking of bypassed renal vessels during viscera derotation.

Anatomical contraindications for the use of the GHVG do exist: target artery larger than 9 mm or smaller than 5 mm, the presence of anomalous major collaterals of the target artery originating in its proximal tract, and the presence of a severe stenosis of the distal tract of the target artery.

19.5 Operative Technique

With the patient positioned in a right lateral decubitus, thoraco-phreno-laparotomy is performed, and the thoracoabdominal aorta is exposed following our standard surgical technique [20]. After institution of LHBP and with a sequential clamping technique, proximal anastomosis is performed, and then critical intercostal arteries are reattached. The distal clamp is then moved below the renal arteries and the visceral aorta is opened. Using 9 Fr irrigation-occlusion catheters (LeMaitre Vascular) into the celiac trunk and the superior mesenteric artery, visceral normothermic hematic perfusion is then restored by the pump (400 mL/min). Finally, selective perfusion of the renal arteries is performed with cold (4 °C) crystalloid solution enriched with histidine-tryptophan-ketoglutarate (Custodiol) [31]. When a separate reattachment for the visceral arteries is not required, they are usually reimplanted first by means of a Carrel patch. Then, the distal aortic anastomosis is performed, and the aortic clamps are removed.

After identification of the GHVG-target vessel, the perfusion catheter is temporarily removed. A flexible steerable J tip guidewire (usually 0.035″) is inserted into the renal artery, and then the constrained stented segment of the GHVG is gently placed into the artery for 2–3 cm, with respect to the distances measured at preoperative CTA (Fig. 19.2).

Sizing of the nitinol-reinforced section was performed using a 10–20% oversizing compared to the real diameter of the target renal vessel, as measured at preoperative CTA and confirmed by intraoperative finding. The distance between the origin and the bifurcation of the renal artery is always measured at preoperative CTA, in order to avoid unintentional coverage of renal artery branches during GHVG deployment.

The deployment line is maintained facing upward. The stent is released pulling the deployment line parallel to the vascular graft section. Great attention must be taken during these phases to hold the stented portion fixed in the correct position, avoiding to pull it deeply into the artery or retracting the graft leaving an inadequate overlapping with the artery.

Stent post-dilatation is always performed after GHVG distal segment deployment, using a 5 or 6 mm non-compliant balloon advanced on the guidewire through the graft. After ballooning, a

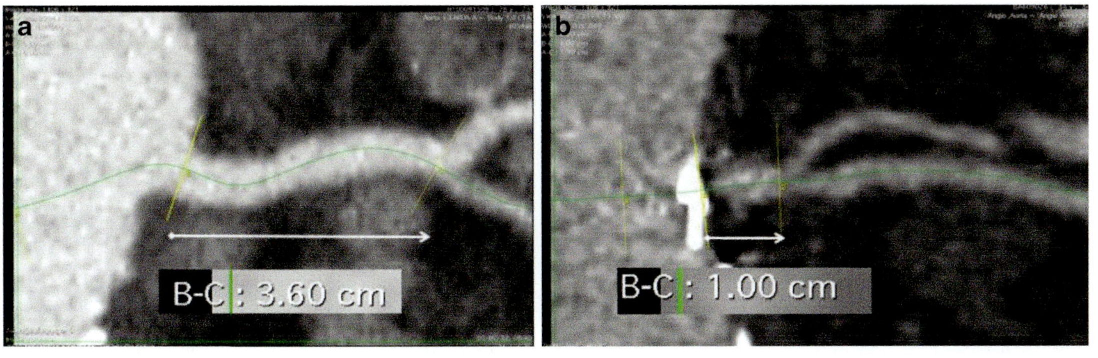

Fig. 19.2 CT scan measurement of the length of the renal artery, before the origin of a main collateral vessel. (**a**) Straight renal artery for 3.6 cm, available for GHVG employment; (**b**) early collateral vessel, arising 1 cm from the ostium, not suitable for GHVG

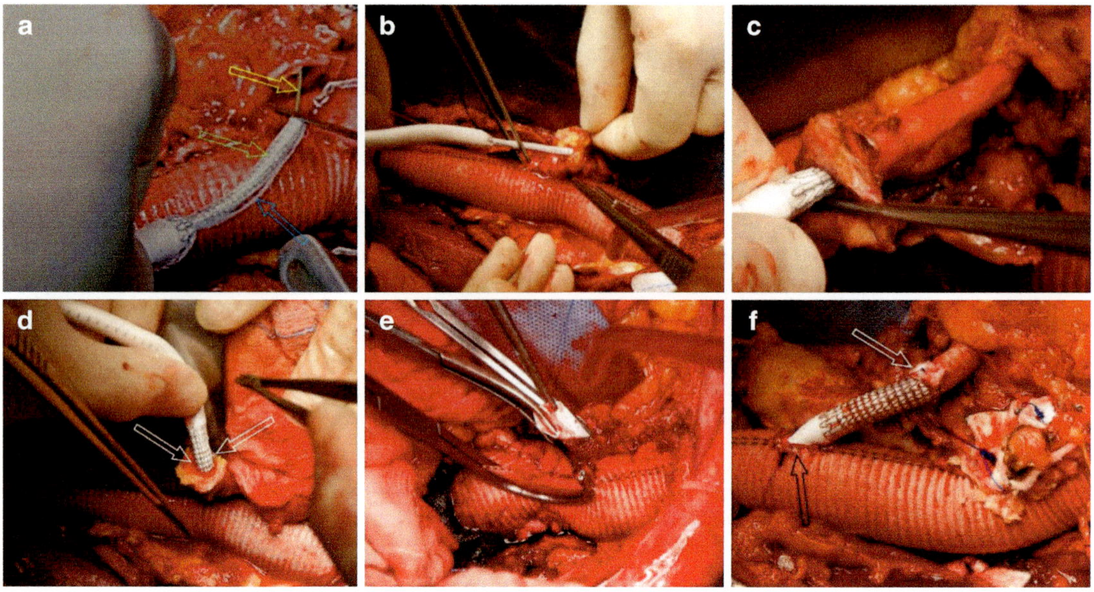

Fig. 19.3 Sequence of GHVG deployment to perform revascularization of a left renal artery. (**a**) Under vision, a 0.035″ flexible steerable J tip guidewire (yellow arrow) facilitates the insertion of the nitinol-reinforced segment of the GHVG (green arrow) into the renal artery; (**b**) the nitinol-reinforced segment is gently placed into the artery for the appropriate length; (**c**) the stent is released pulling the deployment line (blue arrow—(**a**)); (**d**) after the release, the nitinol-reinforced segment is fixed sewing to the artery with two or four circumferential stiches (white arrows); (**e**) after tangential cross-clamp of the main aortic graft, the proximal anastomosis is performed; (**f**) final result of renal revascularization with GHVG: to notice the distal fixing stiches (white arrow) and the proximal anastomosis on the main aortic graft (black arrow)

cold renal perfusion catheter is then immediately reinserted into the graft to reduce renal ischemia. To avoid accidental retraction or dislodgment of the stented portion, the GHVG is then sewn in place with at least four single circumferential monofilament polypropylene stitches. Finally, proximal anastomosis to the main aortic graft is completed in the usual fashion after cutting the proximal unstented section of the graft at the proper length. Particular care must be taken by choosing the length of the graft and the position of the proximal anastomosis to avoid kinking or compression of the unstented segment.

After blood flow restoration, protamine is administered to completely reverse heparin. Red blood cells, platelets, and plasma transfusions are aggressively used to correct severe thrombocytopenia and coagulation derangements. Anastomoses are carefully checked for bleeding and reinforced as needed. Mild initial bleeding from ePTFE needle holes usually resolved spontaneously after few minutes. In case of major suture-hole bleeding, hemostasis is obtained by manual compression with surgical gauze and oxidized cellulose pads (Fig. 19.3).

Antiplatelet therapy (usually aspirin) is routinely initiated by the third postoperative day, if not contraindicated. Double antiplatelet therapy (adding ticlopidine or clopidogrel) is then started by the tenth postoperative day and continued after discharge for at least 1 month.

19.6 San Raffaele Hospital Experience

A series of 146 consecutive patients who underwent elective TAAA open repair, including revascularization with the GHVG of at least 1 of the celiac trunk (CT), the superior mesenteric artery (SMA), and the right renal (RRA) or left renal artery (LRA) between September 2012 and September 2017, was included in this analysis. During this period, 288 other patients were submitted to TAAA open repair using standard renal or visceral revascularization (SRVR) techniques (such as inclusion in the Carrel patch or as a selective revascularization with a Coselli graft or an isolated standard bypass graft), because the GHVG was deemed contraindicated or not necessary by the operating surgeon (Table 19.1).

At preoperative CTA, all GHVG patients had patent CT and SMA, 140 patients had 2 functioning kidneys with both patent renal arteries, while 6 patients had only 1 functioning kidney, for a total of 578 patent visceral vessels in this group. Visceral artery stenosis was defined as a >50% lesion as documented by CTA. Acute renal failure was defined as both a doubling of serum creatinine level and an absolute value greater than 3.0 mg/dL [32] (Fig. 19.4).

Table 19.1 Other main preoperative characteristics of 146 patients submitted to TAAA open repair, including at least one vessel revascularization with the GHVG

Variables	Patients *N* (%)
Total	146
Gender (male)	105 (72%)
Age, y, mean ± SD	66.7 ± 8.2
Etiology	
Atherosclerotic/degenerative	95 (65%)
Chronic type B dissection	45 (31%)
Para-anastomotic pseudoaneurysm	6 (4%)
Connective tissue disorder	0 (0%)
Classification of aneurysms[a]	
TAAA extent I	10 (7%)
TAAA extent II	61 (42%)
TAAA extent III	32 (22%)
TAAA extent IV	40 (27%)
TAAA extent V	3 (2%)
Aneurysm maximum diameter, mm, mean ± SD	65 ± 21
Pararenal aortic diameter, mm, mean ± SD	58 ± 18
CKD stages	
Stage I	45 (31%)
Stage II	63 (43%)
Stage III	29 (20%)
Stage IV	9 (6%)
Stage V	0 (0%)
ASA score ± SD	3.5 ± 0.5

[a]According to the Crawford-Safi revised TAAA extent classification

TAAA thoracoabdominal aortic aneurysm, *GHVG* Gore Hybrid Vascular Graft, *SD* standard deviation, *CKD* chronic kidney disease, *ASA* American Society of Anesthesiologists

All CTAs performed after the operation were carefully reviewed in order to ascertain patency of the visceral vessels and of the implanted grafts and identify graft migration, stenosis, kinking or twisting, stent fractures, and instances of bleeding or renal/bowel infarctions.

In the analyzed period, at least one GHVG was used for revascularization in 33.6% of patients submitted to TAAA open repair. In this group of patients, among the 286 patent renal arteries, 134 were revascularized with the GHVG (96 left and 38 right), and 152 using standard surgical techniques (110 by means of Carrel patch reimplantation and 42 by means of conventional aorto-renal bypass, including Coselli graft technique). Among 140 patent CTs and 140 patent SMAs, 9 CTs and 11 SMAs were revascularized with the GHVG, respectively; the others were all

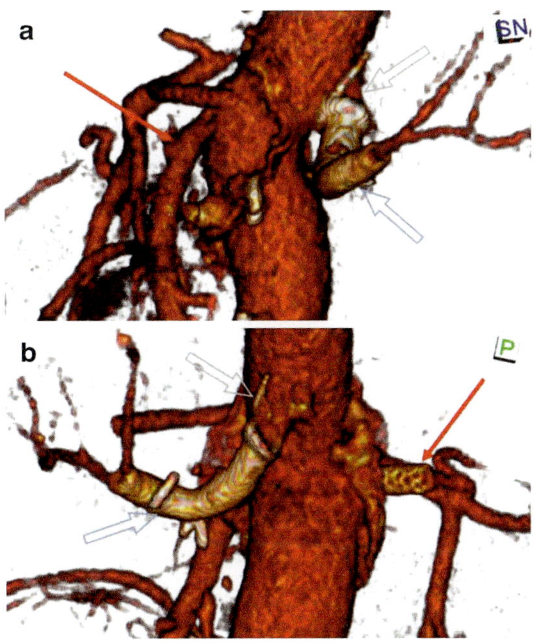

Fig. 19.4 Three-dimensional reconstruction of follow-up CT scan following TAAA open repair associated with aorto-left renal artery bypass using the GHVG. In this left view (**a**) and posterior view (**b**) of a 3D reconstruction, we should notice the ePTFE segment (gray arrow) of the GHVG, anastomosed to the main aortic graft, and the nitinol-reinforced segment (blue arrow) into the left renal artery. The small red arrow shows a bare metal stent into the right renal artery, included in Carrel patch

included in a Carrel patch or revascularized with a Coselli graft (68% and 32%, respectively).

Indications to the use of the GHVG included intraoperative detection of a remote location of the ostium of the visceral artery (76% of cases); poor-quality vessel walls, such as severe atherosclerotic degeneration or dissection (52% of cases); and visceral artery stenosis (20% of cases).

All intended target vessels were treated without technical concerns with the GHVG. No significant bleeding from ePTFE needle holes or from the graft anastomoses was observed. Total surgical and total renal ischemic times were 250 ± 79 min and 49 ± 23 min, respectively. Cold renal perfusional time resulted 27 ± 11 min. No additional unplanned endovascular or surgical procedures were required on the GHVG-treated vessels. Prior to revascularization, a balloon-expandable stent was directly implanted at the ostium of 26 visceral arteries (6.3% of non-GHVG revascularized visceral arteries).

In the GHVG group, 30-day mortality was 5.4% (eight patients), including one patient who died on postoperative day 6 due to myocardial infarction, two patients who died due to coagulopathy and bleeding, and five other patients who suffered from multi-organ failure. Perioperative peak decrease of the eGFR was significantly lower in the GHVG group (26 ± 18 mL/min/1.73 m^2 vs 37 ± 22 mL/min/1.73 m^2, $P = 0.034$).

Perioperative complications included acute renal failure, occurring in 13 patients (8%) and requiring dialysis in 5 (temporary dialysis in 4 cases and permanent dialysis in 1). Occlusion of the GHVG at subsequent CTA was found to be the main causative factor of renal failure in four of these patients. In one case, early thrombosis of a right renal GHVG was found on postoperative day 8 and then successfully treated by means of urgent endovascular recanalization with stenting PTA of the distal endpoint. No cases of GHVG-related bowel ischemia were observed in our series (Table 19.2).

Follow-up was performed with CTA scan and clinical investigation. Patency rate at mean 22 months was 92% (141 grafts) for the aorto-renal grafts performed with the GHVG, 91% for the contralateral renal arteries revascularized with standard techniques in the same group, and 92% for revascularized renal vessels in the SRR group. The observed 13 occluded GHVGs were most of all left aorto-renal bypass grafts (12 graft for LRA and 1 for RRA). A kinking/twisting of the non-stented segment was observed in eight cases, and a compressed/narrowed lumen of the stented segment was observed in five cases. No areas of renal infarction were observed in patients with patent aorto-renal grafts.

No other GHVG-related complications, re-intervention, or cases of new-onset renal failure requiring dialysis were reported at follow-up in available patients.

Table 19.2 Short-term outcomes of GHVG patients

Variables	Patients *N* (%)
Total	146
Perioperative peak decrease of eGFR, mL/min/1.73 m^2, mean ± SD	26 ± 18
Acute renal failure	13 (8%)
Temporary hemodialysis	4 (3%)
Dialysis at discharge	1 (1%)
Respiratory insufficiency	69 (47%)
Paraplegia/paraparesis	13 (8%)
Cardiac complication	13 (8%)
Bleeding requiring re-intervention	3 (2%)
Operative mortality	0 (0%)
In-hospital mortality	7 (5%)
30-day mortality	7 (5%)

GHVG Gore Hybrid Vascular Graft, *SD* standard deviation, *eGFR* estimated glomerular filtration rate

19.7 Gore Hybrid Vascular Graft in Hybrid Treatment

For TAAA treatment, in addition to the standard open surgical approach and the most innovative total endovascular solution, a third option may exist: the hybrid intervention merges open surgery with endovascular options.

This procedure consists of the creation of the distal neck to allow the delivery of a thoracic endoprosthesis with the rerouting of the visceral and renal vessels through multiple selective bypasses; after an abdominal access, selective and retrograde bypasses for each abdominal vessel are created, starting from the iliac vessels or from the distal part of the abdominal aorta.

The main advantage of this intervention is to avoid thoracotomy with a consequent reduction of respiratory complications and heart overload due to proximal aortic cross-clamping.

As written above, Lachat describes firstly his experience with VORTEC technique in the hybrid treatment of TAAAs. The natural evolution of this procedure is the use of the hybrid graft, in order to reduce the invasiveness of the procedure.

Placement of the GHVG may occur in all of the visceral and renal vessels, provided that the dimensional criteria are respected and the GHVG placement did not undergo occlusion of the early origin collateral vessels. Most of all, the renal artery and superior mesenteric artery are involved in this aspect: intentional coverage of a collateral renal artery that arises close to the aortic renal ostium may cause variable loss of renal functional parenchyma; furthermore, the middle colic artery and inferior pancreaticoduodenal artery arising in the first 2 cm of SMA still represent a contraindication to the use of the GHVG in order to avoid bowel hypoperfusion.

Usefulness of GHVG is represented by:

- Lack of need for extensive vessel exposure
- Faster anastomosis, even in uncomfortable anatomic situations
- Reduction of complications connected to the extensive vessel exposure (such as pancreatitis, venous or biliary tract lesions)
- Reduction of cross-clamping time and, accordingly, reduction of ischemic time

The course of GHVG into the abdomen is variable, in order to avoid kinking or compression of the graft upon viscera derotation.

Proximal anastomosis on the aortoiliac segment may be obtained with single and selective graft suture to the in-flow segment or through the creation of bifurcated/trifurcated graft with a common origin.

19.8 Conclusions

The specific indications to the use of GHVG included the "most feared" situations of the renal and splanchnic arteries (remote access to the ostium, poor quality of the vessel wall, ostial stenosis, or dissection), leading to the use of this device in about one third of TAAA-operated patients.

A well-known problem with ePTFE grafts, the potential prolonged needle-hole bleeding from the anastomosis, may be exacerbated by heparin, hypothermia, thrombocytopenia, and coagulopathy in TAAA open repair. Suture-line bleeding has been reported to potentially increase operative time, overall blood loss, and risk of infective complications and may require the use of a variety of topical hemostatic agents or sealants [33]. In our experience, mild initial bleeding from ePTFE needle holes resolved spontaneously after few minutes in most cases. In cases of major bleeding, we rapidly obtained hemostasis by manual compression with surgical gauze and oxidized cellulose pads. At the same time, complete reversal of heparin and aggressive transfusions are required to correct thrombocytopenia and coagulation derangements.

Our currently updated experience confirmed that technical feasibility and short-term patency rate of the GHVG for renal and visceral revascularization during TAAA open repair were satisfactory, and we hope that this novel graft will represent an additional step forward in the fight against kidney perioperative injury. Our initial results indicate that this technique is feasible also in challenging anatomies, with several potential technical advantages. Short-term clinical and radiological outcomes were satisfactory. Larger series and longer follow-up are needed to confirm the safety and durability of the proposed technique.

References

1. Lemaire SA, Jones MM, Conklin LD, Carter SA, Criddell MD, Wang XL, et al. Randomized comparison of cold blood and cold crystalloid renal perfusion for renal protection during thoracoabdominal aortic aneurysm repair. J Vasc Surg. 2009;49(1):11–9.
2. Bensley RP, Curran T, Hurks R, Lo RC, Wyers MC, Hamdan AD, et al. Open repair of intact thoracoabdominal aortic aneurysms in the American College of Surgeons National Surgical Quality Improvement Program. J Vasc Surg. 2013;58:894. https://doi.org/10.1016/j.jvs.2013.03.037.

3. van Kuijk JP, Flu WJ, Chonchol M, Hoeks SE, Winkel TA, Verhagen HJ, et al. Temporary perioperative decline of renal function is an independent predictor for chronic kidney disease. Clin J Am Soc Nephrol. 2010;5(7):1198–204.
4. Lachat M, Mayer D, Criado FJ, Pfammatter T, Rancic Z, Genoni M, et al. New technique to facilitate renal revascularization with use of telescoping self-expanding stent grafts: VORTEC. Vascular. 2008;16(2):69–72.
5. Fehrenbacher JW, Corvera JS. Best surgical option for thoracoabdominal aneurysm repair - the open approach. Ann Cardiothorac Surg. 2012;1(3):334–8.
6. Schepens MA, Heijmen RH, Ranschaert W, Sonker U, Morshuis WJ. Thoracoabdominal aortic aneurysm repair: results of conventional open surgery. Eur J Vasc Endovasc Surg. 2009;37(6):640–5.
7. Piazza M, Ricotta JJ 2nd. Open surgical repair of thoracoabdominal aortic aneurysms. Ann Vasc Surg. 2012;26(4):600–5.
8. Panneton JM, Hollier LH. Nondissecting thoracoabdominal aortic aneurysms: part I. Ann Vasc Surg. 1995;9(5):503–14.
9. Svensson LG, Crawford ES, Hess KR, Coselli JS, Safi HJ. Experience with 1509 patients undergoing thoracoabdominal aortic operations. J Vasc Surg. 1993;17(2):357–68; discussion 368–70.
10. Back MR, Bandyk M, Bradner M, Cuthbertson D, Johnson BL, Shames ML, et al. Critical analysis of outcome determinants affecting repair of intact aneurysms involving the visceral aorta. Ann Vasc Surg. 2005;19(5):648–56.
11. Dubois L, Durant C, Harrington DM, Forbes TL, Derose G, Harris JR. Technical factors are strongest predictors of postoperative renal dysfunction after open transperitoneal juxtarenal abdominal aortic aneurysm repair. J Vasc Surg. 2013;57(3):648–54.
12. Crawford ES, Snyder DM, Cho GC, Roehm JO Jr. Progress in treatment of thoracoabdominal and abdominal aortic aneurysms involving celiac, superior mesenteric, and renal arteries. Ann Surg. 1978;188(3):404–22.
13. Tshomba Y, Melissano G, Civilini E, Setacci F, Chiesa R. Fate of the visceral aortic patch after thoracoabdominal aortic repair. Eur J Vasc Endovasc Surg. 2005;29(4):383–9.
14. Tshomba Y, Bertoglio L, Marone EM, Melissano G, Chiesa R. Visceral aortic patch aneurysm after thoracoabdominal aortic repair: conventional vs hybrid treatment. J Vasc Surg. 2008;48(5):1083–91.
15. Kulik A, Castner CF, Kouchoukos NT. Patency and durability of presewn multiple branched graft for thoracoabdominal aortic aneurysm repair. J Vasc Surg. 2010;51(6):1367–72.
16. Black JH 3rd. Technique for repair of suprarenal and thoracoabdominal aortic aneurysms. J Vasc Surg. 2009;50(4):936–41.
17. Clouse WD, Marone LK, Davison JK, Dorer DJ, Brewster DC, LaMuraglia GM, et al. Late aortic and graft-related events after thoracoabdominal aneurysm repair. J Vasc Surg. 2003;37(2):254–61.
18. Svensson LG, Crawford ES, Hess KR, Coselli JS, Safi HJ. Thoracoabdominal aortic aneurysms associated with celiac, superior mesenteric, and renal artery occlusive disease: methods and analysis of results in 271 patients. J Vasc Surg. 1992;16:378–90.
19. Clair DG, Belkin M, Whittemore AD, Mannick JA, Donaldson MC. Safety and efficacy of transaortic renal endarterectomy as an adjunct to aortic surgery. J Vasc Surg. 1995;21:926–34.
20. Chiesa R, Melissano G, Civilini E, Bertoglio L, Rinaldi E, Marone EM, et al. Video-atlas of open thoracoabdominal aortic aneurysm repair. Ann Cardiothorac Surg. 2012;1(3):398–403.
21. LeMaire SA, Jamison AL, Carter SA, Wen S, Alankar S, Coselli JS. Deployment of balloon expandable stents during open repair of thoracoabdominal aortic aneurysms: a new strategy for managing renal and mesenteric artery lesions. Eur J Cardiothorac Surg. 2004;26(3):599–607.
22. Patel R, Conrad MF, Paruchuri V, Kwolek CJ, Cambria RP. Balloon expandable stents facilitate right renal artery reconstruction during complex open aortic aneurysm repair. J Vasc Surg. 2010;51(2):310–5.
23. Donas KP, Lachat M, Rancic Z, Oberkofler C, Pfammatter T, Guber I, et al. Early and midterm outcome of a novel technique to simplify the hybrid procedures in the treatment of thoracoabdominal and pararenal aortic aneurysms. J Vasc Surg. 2009;50(6):1280–4.
24. Donas KP, Rancic Z, Lachat M, Pfammatter T, Frauenfelder T, Veith FJ, et al. Novel sutureless telescoping anastomosis revascularization technique of supra-aortic vessels to simplify combined open endovascular procedures in the treatment of aortic arch pathologies. J Vasc Surg. 2010;51(4):836–41.
25. Bonvini S, Ricotta JJ, Piazza M, Ferretto L, Grego F. ViPS technique as a novel concept for a sutureless vascular anastomosis. J Vasc Surg. 2011;54(3):889–92.
26. Greenberg G, Szendro G, Mayzler O, Ginzburg V, Leytzin A. Use of ViaBahn open revascularisation technique for above-knee femoro-popliteal anastomosis: a technical note. Eur J Vasc Endovasc Surg. 2011;42(2):202–5.
27. Levack MM, Bavaria JE, Gorman RC, Gorman JH 3rd, Ryan LP. Rapid aortic arch debranching using the Gore hybrid vascular graft. Ann Thorac Surg. 2013;95(6):e163–5.
28. Nigro G, Gatta E, Pagliariccio G, Grilli C, Carbonari L. Use of the Gore Hybrid Vascular Graft in a challenging high-lying extracranial carotid artery aneurysm. J Vasc Surg. 2014. https://doi.org/10.1016/j.jvs.2013.04.044.
29. Bornak A, Goldstein LJ, Rey J, Medina A, Yang JK, Velazquez OC, et al. Aortic aneurysmal repair with surtureless visceral revascularization using novel

hybrid vascular graft and a gradual funneling technique. Vasc Endovasc Surg. 2012;46(3):258–61.
30. W. L. Gores & Associates. Instructions for use for Gore Hybrid Vascular Graft. http://www.goremedical.com/resources/dam/assets/AP3350ML3.HYVG.US_IFU.pdf.
31. Tshomba Y, Kahlberg A, Melissano G, Coppi G, Marone E, Ferrari D, et al. Comparison of renal perfusion solutions during thoracoabdominal aortic aneurysm repair. J Vasc Surg. 2014;59:623–33.
32. Kashyap VS, Cambria RP, Davison JK, L'Italien GJ. Renal failure after thoracoabdominal aortic surgery. J Vasc Surg. 1997;26(6):949–55; discussion 955–7.
33. Saha SP, Muluk S, Schenk W 3rd, Dennis JW, Ploder B, Grigorian A, Presch I, Goppelt A. A prospective randomized study comparing fibrin sealant to manual compression for the treatment of anastomotic suture-hole bleeding in expanded polytetrafluoroethylene grafts. J Vasc Surg. 2012;56(1):134–41.

Long-Term Patency of Visceral Vessels After Thoracoabdominal Aortic Repair

20

Andrea Kahlberg, Vincenzo Ardita, Angela M. R. Ferrante, Luca Bertoglio, Daniele Mascia, Domenico Baccellieri, Germano Melissano, and Roberto Chiesa

20.1 Introduction

Open repair of thoracoabdominal aortic aneurysms (TAAAs) is an extraordinary challenge for both vascular surgeons and patients. Consistent outcome data have been reported by high-volume centers with 30-day mortality rates lower than 10% and improved long-term survivals [1]. The development of devices and techniques have allowed total endovascular treatment of TAAA with fenestrated (FEVAR) or branched (BEVAR) endografts [2–6]. Early results are encouraging; a recent meta-analysis has reported a 30-day mortality rate of 8.6%, spinal cord ischemia in 17.3% of cases with permanent consequences in 4.9%, and renal failure in 25.4%. However, anatomic feasibility of BEVAR/FEVAR is still limited, manufacturing times for custom devices are lengthy, and open repair remains the only viable strategy in a number of specific conditions, such as emergency cases, infections, and patients affected by connective tissue disorders.

Recent publications on FEVAR/BEVAR series have highlighted the fate of revascularized visceral vessels (VVs), reporting a progressive loss of stented visceral branches [7]. In addition, a comparison of long-term results with those observed in conventional open repair is still unachievable for such recent technology, which is currently performed in few specialized centers on relatively small groups of patients.

Surprisingly, few data have been reported in the recent literature about the late fate of visceral arteries after open repair of TAAAs [8, 9]. In 2010, Kulik et al. [10] reviewed their TAAA repair experience using a presewn aortic branched graft. Between March 2003 and December 2008, 52 patients with Crawford extent II and III TAAAs underwent surgical repair using a presewn aortic branched graft. The patency rate of the branches to the visceral and renal arteries was 100% and 98%, at 1 and 5 years, respectively. Of the 148 graft branches, two became occluded and four developed stenosis (two patients). One patient

A. Kahlberg (✉) · V. Ardita · L. Bertoglio · D. Mascia
G. Melissano
Vascular Surgery, Vita-Salute University School of Medicine, San Raffaele Scientific Institute, Milan, Italy
e-mail: kahlberg.andrea@hsr.it; ardita.vincenzo@hsr.it; bertoglio.luca@hsr.it; mascia.daniele@hsr.it; melissano.germano@hsr.it

A. M. R. Ferrante
Unit of Vascular Surgery, Fondazione Policlinico Universitario A. Gemelli IRCCS, Università Cattolica del Sacro Cuore, Rome, Italy
e-mail: Angela.Ferrante@unicatt.it

D. Baccellieri
Unit of Vascular Surgery, San Raffaele Scientific Institute, Milan, Italy
e-mail: baccellieri.domenico@hsr.it

R. Chiesa
Unit of Vascular Surgery, San Raffaele Scientific Institute, Vita-Salute University, Milan, Italy
e-mail: chiesa.roberto@hsr.it

© Springer Nature Switzerland AG 2019
Y. Tshomba et al. (eds.), *Visceral Vessels and Aortic Repair*,
https://doi.org/10.1007/978-3-319-94761-7_20

required percutaneous stenting of three stenosed branches, and one patient died after acute occlusion of two branches and stenosis of a third. During the follow-up period that extended to 6.3 years, there were ten late deaths. Six patients required reoperation on the aortic graft or contiguous aorta, but no reoperations were required on the visceral abdominal aorta or its branches. The authors concluded that the use of a presewn aortic branched graft is a safe and suitable option for TAAA repair. Another study performed by Shahverdyan et al. [11], in 2013, showed outcomes of long-term bypass graft patency after visceral hybrid repair of thoracoabdominal aortic aneurysms (TAAAs). Between July 2004 and September 2012, 46 patients (67.5 years in median; range 35–88) with TAAAs underwent to the visceral hybrid procedure (164 grafts). The inflow sites of visceral revascularization originated either from the native artery or from aortic prosthetic grafts. The 30-day primary patency of all grafts was 87.9%. The long-term patency remained 87.9 ± 2.7%, 86.1 ± 3.2%, and 86.1 ± 3.2% after 1, 3, and 5 years, respectively. The patency of all hepatic grafts was 100%. The patency of grafts to the superior mesenteric artery was 88.8 ± 4.8% after 1, 3, and 5 years. The patency was 87.2 ± 6%, 87.2 ± 6%, and 87.2 ± 6% for the left renal artery and 76 ± 7%, 69.6 ± 8.8%, and 69.6 ± 8.8% for the right renal artery after 1, 3, and 5 years, respectively. The authors concluded that hybrid repair demonstrates excellent results regarding long-term bypass graft patency of renovisceral arteries except for the right renal artery. In 2015 Youssef et al. [9] showed data of 62 patients (mean age is 66 ± 10 years, 40 men) who had been operated on for TAAA of Crawford types I (8), II (13), III (13), and IV (24) and Safi type V (4). A total of 181 vessels were revascularized by either patch inclusion (n = 147) or selective revascularization (bypass or transposition, n = 34); 48 survived the procedure, resulting in a number of vessels available for follow-up of 154 (patch, 126; selective revascularization, 28). The patency rates for overall, patch, and selective revascularization were 95.2%, 94.2%, and 100% at 5 years and 83.7%, 81.3%, and 100% at 10 years, respectively. The patency rates for the celiac trunk, superior mesenteric artery, and left and right renal artery were 100%, 97.5%, 92.3%, and 90.3% at 5 years. More recently, Kouchoukos et al. [12] showed their experience of 298 branch grafts to the celiac, superior mesenteric, and renal arteries performed in a total of 99 of 130 patients undergoing open thoracoabdominal aortic aneurysm repair. The authors showed a freedom from occlusion of 98%, 97%, and 93%, at 1, 5, and 10 years of follow-up, respectively.

20.2 San Raffaele Hospital Experience

Between January 2009 and July 2015, 382 patients underwent open TAAA repair at our institution. Patients were selected from a prospectively maintained computerized database and retrospectively reviewed. Demographics and perioperative risk factors are reported in Table 20.1.

An adequate preoperative assessment of physiological reserve of cardiac, pulmonary, and renal function was used to evaluate operative risks, to plan the best operative strategy, and to consider additional perioperative organ protection strategies. A coronary computed tomography was performed in selected patients with a history of coronary artery disease from 2009 to 2012 and in all elective patients since 2013. A preoperative study was conducted on all patients by a computed tomography angiography (CTA) scan of the thoracoabdominal aorta.

The anatomical extent of the aneurysm was defined according to the Crawford classification [13]. Chronic obstructive pulmonary disease (COPD) included all patients with a grade ≥2 in the GOLD score system [14]. Patients were stratified by chronic kidney disease (CKD) stages according to the NKF-KDOQI (National Kidney Foundation's Kidney Disease Outcomes Quality Initiative) guidelines [15]. Cerebrovascular disease included all cases with a history of TIA, minor or major stroke, or carotid occlusive disease.

Details of the surgical technique for open repair of TAAAs at our institution have been previously described [12]. The strategy for VV revascularization was customized (Fig. 20.1) according to the following principles: Inclusion in a "beveled" aortic anastomosis or in Carrel patch was favored in

Table 20.1 Demographics and preoperative risk factors of 382 TAAA patients

Variable	Definition	No.	(%)
Age	Years (mean ± SD)	66 ± 10	
Gender	Male	284	(74%)
Coronary artery disease	Yes	76	(20%)
COPD	Yes	134	(35%)
History of smoking	Yes	186	(49%)
Hypertension	Yes	302	(79%)
Diabetes mellitus	Yes	28	(7%)
Dyslipidemia	Yes	96	(25%)
Cerebrovascular disease	Yes	114	(30%)
Renal function	CKD stage 1	207	(54%)
	CKD stage 2	119	(31%)
	CKD stage 3	43	(11%)
	CKD stage 4	10	(3%)
	CKD stage 5	3	(1%)
TAAA extent	Type I	78	(20%)
	Type II	122	(32%)
	Type III	103	(27%)
	Type IV	79	(21%)
TAAA maximum diameter	mm (mean ± SD)	66 ± 13	
Etiology	Atherosclerosis	312	(82%)
	Dissection	46	(12%)
	Connective tissue disorder	24	(6%)
Previous surgery	TAA open	19	(5%)
	TEVAR	33	(9%)
	AAA	64	(17%)
Presentation	Symptomatic	65	(17%)
	Ruptured	12	(3%)

TAAA thoracoabdominal aortic aneurysm, *COPD* chronic obstructive pulmonary disease, *CKD* chronic kidney disease, *TAA* thoracic aortic aneurysm, *TEVAR* thoracic endovascular aortic repair, *AAA* abdominal aortic aneurysm

case of short distance between the VV ostia; when the aneurysm included the visceral aortic segment, no more than three VVs were normally reimplanted together in a single Carrel patch to avoid the risk of late aneurysm recurrence [16]. A VV originating far from the others was usually reconstructed separately by direct reimplantation on the main aortic graft or by individual graft interposition (6-mm heparin-bonded Dacron or ePTFE). Since 2012, the Gore Hybrid Vascular Graft (W.L. Gore and Associates, Flagstaff, AZ) has been selectively used to perform separate revascularization of one or two VVs allowing for distal sutureless anastomosis. The specific operative technique for this device has been previously described in detail [12]. A separate revascularization of all VVs has always been preferred—in most cases accomplished with presewn multibranched grafts (Coselli graft, Vascutek Terumo, Renfrewshire, UK, or Hemashield Platinum TAAA graft, Maquet, Sunderland, UK)—in case of large aneurysms with excessive distance between all VV ostia, in the event of recurrent aneurysmal disease after previous TAAA surgery, or in patients affected by connective tissue disorders.

Intraoperative details included techniques used for VV revascularization and postoperative outcome variables. The follow-up protocol included a physical exam and CTA at 3 and 12 months postoperatively and yearly thereafter. Patients unable to comply with the follow-up protocol were contacted by phone interviews and asked to provide digital supports of their imaging studies when available. Patients not responding to two consecutive attempts of phone interviews were considered lost to follow-up. Restenosis was defined as >50% reduction of the vessel lumen on both arterial and late-phase scans.

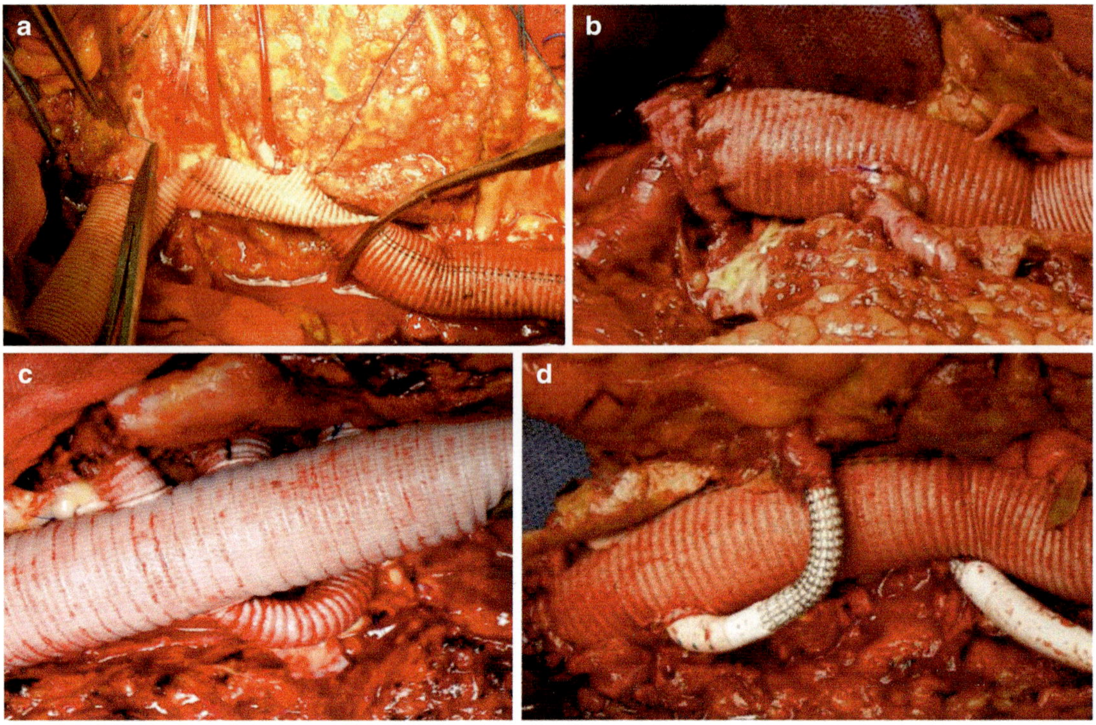

Fig. 20.1 Intraoperative views of different techniques for VV reconstruction: (**a**) Carrel patch including CT (C), SMA (M), and RRA (R). (**b**) Direct reimplantation of the LRA on the main aortic graft. (**c**) Revascularization of all VVs using a presewn multibranched graft. (**d**) Bilateral renal artery revascularization using two Gore Hybrid Vascular Grafts with sutureless distal anastomosis

Table 20.2 Techniques used for reconstruction of visceral vessels in 382 TAAA patients

	CT	SMA	RRA	LRA
Inclusion (Carrel patch/beveled anast.)	321	349	319	175
Direct reimplantation	1	0	0	18
Single bypass (conventional)	5	2	6	67
Single bypass (sutureless)	5	3	21	91
Multibranched graft	26	25	20	22
Associated endarterectomy	3	1	10	30
Associated direct stenting	9	4	19	37

CT celiac trunk, *SMA* superior mesenteric artery, *RRA* right renal artery, *LRA* left renal artery

Cerebrospinal fluid drainage (CSFD) was used in 343 patients, and left heart bypass (LHBP) in 332. Overall, revascularization involved 1476 VVs: 358 celiac trunks (CT), 379 superior mesenteric arteries (SMA), 366 right renal arteries (RRA), and 373 left renal arteries (LRA). Techniques of VV reconstruction and associated procedures—endarterectomy or stenting—are reported in Table 20.2.

Perioperative results are summarized in Table 20.3. The in-hospital mortality was 7.6% (29 patients), including five intraoperative deaths. Complications occurred in 26.8% of patients (n = 102). Among 353 early-surviving patients, 15 were lost to follow-up. The mean length of follow-up was 22 ± 17 months.

General survival was 87% at 1 year, 84% at 2 years, 75% at 3 years, and 65% at 5 years

(Fig. 20.2). No instances of bowel ischemia were recorded during follow-up. Eight patients developed late- onset renal failure requiring dialysis. Estimates for reintervention on VVs were 1.2%, 6.3%, and 17% at 1, 3, and 5 years, respectively (Fig. 20.3). All patients requiring reinterventions on VVs presented with asymptomatic restenosis and were treated by means of percutaneous stenting.

Of 338 patients available at follow-up, 247 had adequate imaging studies for analysis of VV patency. Among these, 952 VVs were analyzed (229 CT, 245 SMA, 238 RRA, and 240 LRA). Overall patency of analyzed VVs was 98% at 1 year, 95% at 3 years, and 94% at 5 years. An analysis of available images provided the following patency rate of individual vessels at 1, 3, and 5 years: 99%, 98%, and 98% for CT; 100%, 100%, and 100% for SMA; 100%, 96%, and 96% for RRA; and 91%, 87%, and 82% for LRA (Fig. 20.4a). Compared with other VVs, the LRA showed a trend of significantly reduced patency in time (log rank [Mantel-Cox] test, $P < 0.0001$). Freedom from restenosis or occlusion at 1, 3, and 5 years was 98%, 94%, and 94% for CT; 100%, 99%, and 99% for SMA; 99%, 93%, and 90% for RRA; and 91%, 82%, and 77% for LRA (log rank [Mantel-Cox] test, $P < 0.0001$, Fig. 20.4b).

The group of 247 patients with available follow-up imaging was divided into three subgroups according to the VV reconstruction technique: patients with all VVs included in Carrel patch or in a "beveled" anastomosis (Group A, 94 patients), patients with 2 or 3 VVs included in Carrel patch and 1 separately reimplanted (Group B, 127 patients), and patients with all VVs reimplanted with separate revascularization (Group C, 26 patients). Freedom from any VV occlusion at 1 and 3 years was 95% and 87% for Group A, 89% and 79% for Group B, and 92% and 92% for Group C ($P = 0.13$, Fig. 20.5).

Table 20.3 Perioperative results in 382 TAAA patients

Variables	No.	(%)
Intraoperative mortality	5	(1.3%)
In-hospital mortality	29	(7.6%)
ICU stay (hours, median, IQR)	23 (18–62)	
LOS (days, mean ± SD)	11 ± 9	
Paraparesis	12	(3.1%)
Paraplegia	19	(5.0%)
Cerebral hemorrhage	5	(1.3%)
Stroke	6	(1.6%)
Bleeding requiring reintervention	9	(2.4%)
Bowel ischemia	6	(1.6%)
Renal failure requiring dialysis	14	(3.7%)
Respiratory failure	57	(15%)
Cardiac complications	18	(4.7%)

ICU intensive care unit, *LOS* length of hospital stay

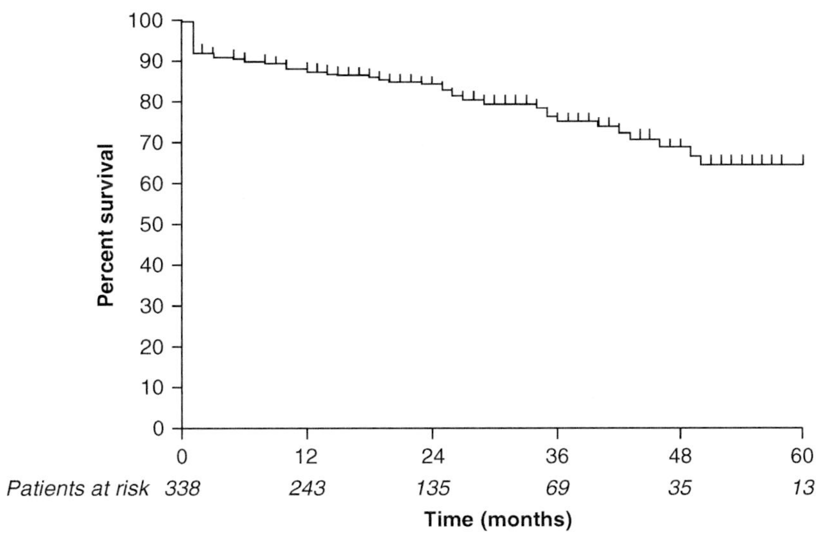

Fig. 20.2 Kaplan-Meier curve of overall survival in 338 patients

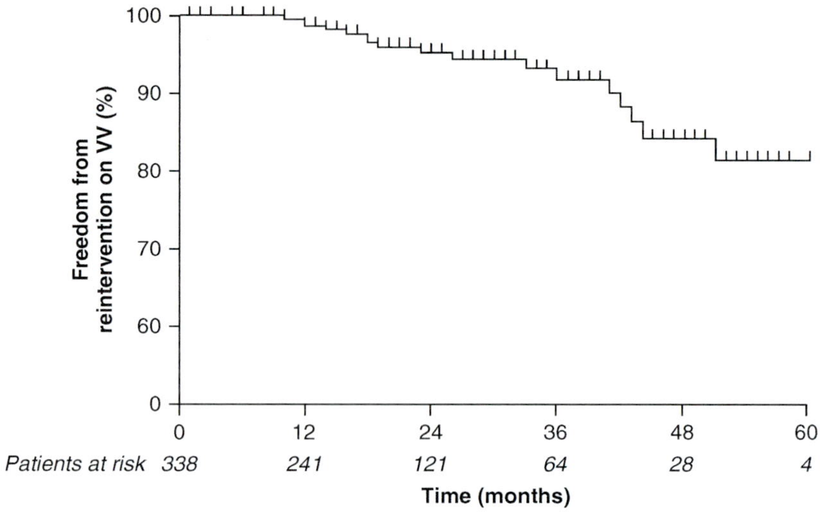

Fig. 20.3 Kaplan-Meier curve of freedom from reinterventions on VVs in 338 patients

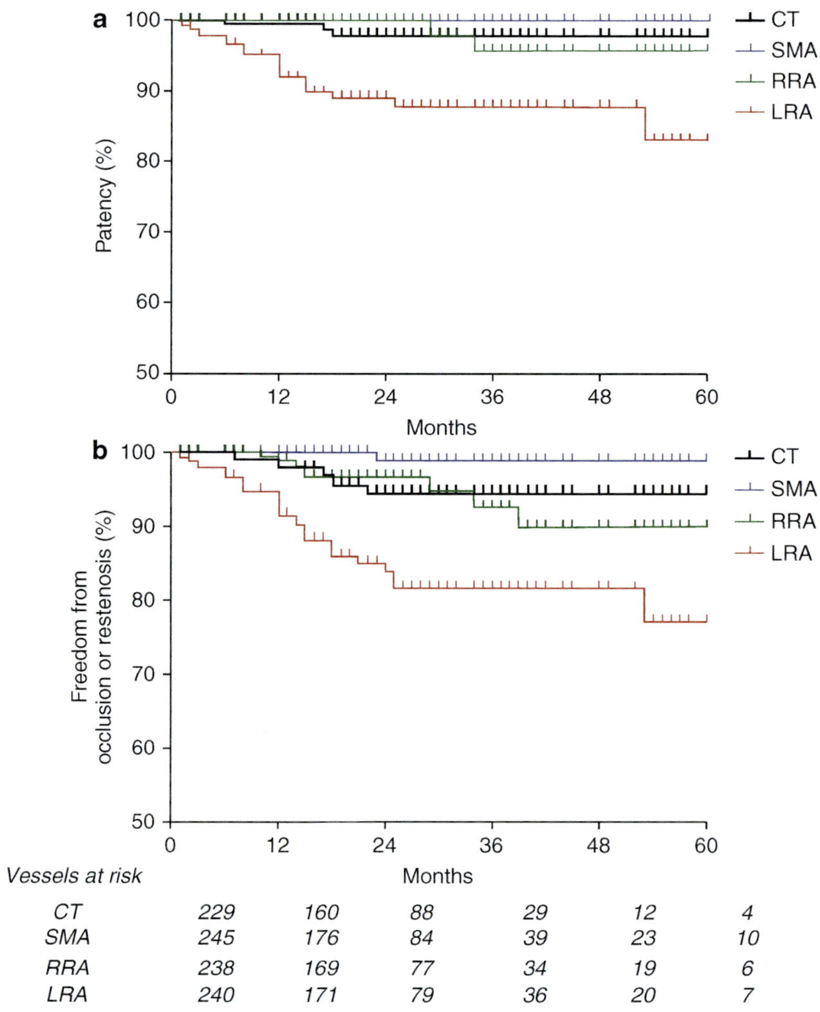

Fig. 20.4 Kaplan-Meier curves of (**a**) VV patency and (**b**) VV freedom from restenosis/occlusion in 247 patients

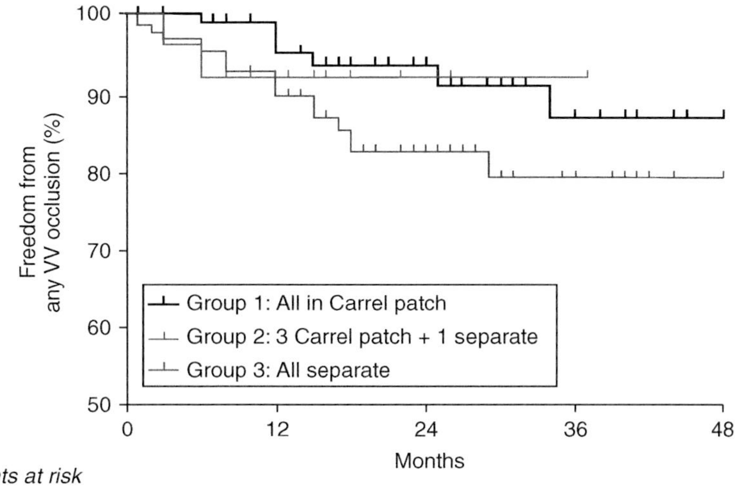

Fig. 20.5 Kaplan-Meier curves of freedom from any VV occlusion based on reconstructive techniques in 247 patients

Patients at risk					
Group 1	*94*	*75*	*43*	*20*	*13*
Group 2	*127*	*91*	*38*	*18*	*10*
Group 3	*26*	*11*	*5*	*3*	*1*

20.3 Discussion

Open repair has historically been considered the gold standard for treatment of TAAAs. Due to severe surgical trauma and early complication rates—even in experienced hands—total endovascular repair and hybrid techniques have been proposed as alternative options in patients considered at unacceptable high risk for conventional surgery.

Hybrid approach (surgical debranching of the abdominal aorta with retrograde bypass and stent grafting) has been proposed as an alternative option to patients who are unfit for surgery [15]. Although such a procedure avoids thoracolaparotomy, single-lung ventilation, aortic cross-clamping, and extracorporeal perfusion, early results of several series reported mortality rates ranging between 2.3% and 24% [13, 14] with significant morbidity (spinal cord ischemia up 8.4% and renal failure requiring dialysis up to 26.2%) [13]. Moreover, the obstruction of visceral bypass is a relevant event in the midterm, affecting almost one third of cases with heavy clinical consequences, namely, emergency reintervention for bowel ischemia or permanent dialysis [13].

In recent years, the development of devices and techniques have allowed total endovascular treatment of TAAA with fenestrated (FEVAR) or branched (BEVAR) endografts [17, 18]. Early results are encouraging; a recent meta-analysis has reported a 30-day mortality rate of 8.6%, spinal cord ischemia in 17.3% of cases with permanent consequences in 4.9%, and renal failure in 25.4% [18].

However, anatomic feasibility of BEVAR/FEVAR is still limited, manufacturing times for custom devices are lengthy, and open repair remains the only viable strategy in a number of specific conditions, such as emergency cases, infections, and patients affected by connective tissue disorders. Moreover, conventional surgery has yielded durable results, and a reliable comparison with long-term results of such recent endovascular techniques is still unachievable [19–22].

Moreover, although total endovascular repair has been performed since 2005 and there are centers with vast experience, long-term data about target vessel patency are still lacking. With a composite end point of branch instability (occlusion, migration, need for secondary intervention), results from the Cleveland Clinic have shown a rate of 70% at 5 years after fenestrated and branched endovascular repair of TAAA [23]. For hybrid TAAA repair, patency rates reported are in the range of 97% at 1 year [15] and 96%

at 3 years [24]. Bianchini Massoni et al. performed a multicenter study providing patency data extending up to 4 years, and there, a patency of 79% was noted [19].

Our findings confirm that, in high-volume centers, perioperative mortality and morbidity rates are acceptable, and open surgery results are durable with high survival rates also at midterm follow-up.

The reconstruction strategy of VV represents a critical point in TAAA surgical repair, often requiring complex technical skills. Early failure of reconstructed branches may result in catastrophic outcomes. A number of techniques for VV reconstruction were described in the past by several authors. Inclusion in a visceral aortic patch (VAP) is the most commonly used strategy to obtain simultaneous revascularizations of multiple VVs, decreasing the global number of anastomoses. Separate reattachment is frequently required when VV ostia are distant, and this particularly applies to the LRA. Separate reattachment of VVs may be performed by direct reimplantation on the main aortic graft or by graft interposition. Recently, we have reported the use of "hybrid" grafts allowing to perform distal sutureless anastomosis as a useful tool for VV revascularization during TAAA open repair [25]. Alternatively, the use of presewn aortic branched grafts allows to separately revascularize each VV, and, for this reason, it is considered the preferred choice in most young patients affected by connective tissue disorders [10]. There are very few data available from the literature about the fate of reconstructed VV and the possible effects of the surgical technique used. Our overall late patency results (94% at 5 years) favorably compare with other series reporting a total patency of the reimplanted vessels of 95.4% and 97% at 5 years [8, 9].

In our experience, late patency rates were not apparently biased by the technique adopted. Interestingly, our study showed that the LRA has a significantly lower patency at all time points as compared to the other VVs. The cause of this finding is not clear, but it can be hypothesized that the intraoperative visceral rotation and subsequent repositioning may play a crucial role leading to kinking or angulation of the revascularized artery. Moreover, the LRA was most often involved by adjunctive procedures, such as endarterectomy or direct stenting.

Late patency of visceral branches following total endovascular TAAA repair (FEVAR and/or BEVAR) is an open issue. Different groups reported excellent early patency rates, followed in the midterm by a slow but progressive loss of visceral branches [1, 26, 27]. Late occlusion involves VVs at different rates, with a significant prevalence of renal arteries compared to other vessels. Renal branch occlusion has been observed in 8–9.6% of cases at midterm follow-up [7, 28]. Along with the high individual anatomic variability of the renal artery angle compared with other VVs, additional factors—e.g., respiratory motion and small vessel size—could have an adjunctive stress effect on stents.

The possible role of different devices employed in VV endovascular reconstruction has not been confirmed in a multicentric series [7], while the mean artery length and anatomic location were considered more likely associated with a poor branch outcome, and this finding could be a touchpoint with possible mechanical factors influencing observed late fate of LRA after open repair—particularly when presewn grafts are used [28].

Further studies are required to evaluate long-term survival and patency rates of visceral branches after total endovascular TAAA repair. Our series of 382 consecutive patients treated with open surgical repair provided early results in line with other high-volume centers and remarkable late patency rates for VV reconstruction. Based on a group of 247 patients and 952 VV available for imaging study, this is, to the best of our knowledge, the largest series of surgical TAAA patients with long-term imaging evaluation of VV. This could be a useful benchmark for comparisons with future endovascular results.

References

1. Hu Z, Li Y, Peng R, Liu J, Jia X, Liu X, et al. Multibranched stent-grafts for the treatment of thoracoabdominal aortic aneurysms: a systematic review and meta-analysis. J Endovasc Ther. 2016;23:626–33.

2. Coselli JS, LeMaire SA, Preventza O, de la Cruz KI, Cooley DA, Price MD, et al. Outcomes of 3309 thoracoabdominal aortic aneurysm repairs. J Thorac Cardiovasc Surg. 2016;151:1323–38.
3. Amiot S, Haulon S, Becquemin JP, Magnan PE, Lermusiaux P, Goueffic Y, et al. Fenestrated endovascular grafting: the French multicentre experience. Eur J Vasc Endovasc Surg. 2010;39:537–4.
4. Mastracci TM, Eagleton MJ, Kuramochi Y, Bathurst S, Wolski K. Twelve-year results of fenestrated endografts for juxtarenal and group IV thoracoabdominal aneurysm. J Vasc Surg. 2015;61:355–64.
5. Dias NV, Sonesson B, Kristmundsson T, Holm H, Resch T. Short-term outcome of spinal cord ischemia after endovascular repair of thoracoabdominal aortic aneurysms. Eur J Vasc Endovasc Surg. 2015;49:403–9.
6. Verhoeven ELG, Katsargyris A, Bekkema F, Oikonomou K, Zeebregts CJ, Ritter W, et al. Editor's choice – ten-year experience with endovascular repair of thoracoabdominal aortic aneurysms: results from 166 consecutive patients. Eur J Vasc Endovasc Surg. 2015;49:524–31.
7. Verzini F, Loschi D, De Rango P, Ferrer C, Simonte G, Coscarella C, et al. Current results of total endovascular repair of thoracoabdominal aortic aneurysms. J Cardiovasc Surg. 2014;55:9–19.
8. Mastracci TM, Carrell T, Constantinou J, Dias N, Martin-Gonzales T, Katsargyris A, et al. Editor's choice – effect of branch stent choice on branch-related outcomes in complex aortic repair. Eur J Vasc Endovasc Surg. 2016;51:536–42.
9. Youssef M, Neufang A, Jungmann F, Vahl C-F, Doweiler B. Patency of renal and visceral vessels after open thoracoabdominal aortic replacement. J Vasc Surg. 2015;62:594–9.
10. Kulik A, Kastner CF, Kouchoukos NT. Patency and durability of presewn multiple branched graft for thoracoabdominal aortic aneurysm repair. J Vasc Surg. 2010;51:1367–72.
11. Shahverdyan R, Gawenda M, Brunkwall J. Five year patency rates of renal and visceral bypasses after abdominal debranching for thoraco-abdominal aortic aneurysms. Eur J Vasc Endovasc Surg. 2013;45(6):648–56.
12. Kouchoukos NT, Kulik A, Castner C. Branch graft patency after open repair of thoracoabdominal aortic aneurysms. J Thorac Cardiovasc Surg. 2017;153:S14.
13. Chiesa R, Kahlberg A, Mascia D, Tshomba Y, Civilini E, Melissano G. Use of a novel hybrid vascular graft for sutureless revascularization of the renal arteries during open thoracoabdominal aortic aneurysm repair. J Vasc Surg. 2014;60:622–30.
14. Crawford ES, Crawford JL, Safi HJ, Coselli JS, Hess KK, Brooks B, et al. Thoracoabdominal aortic aneurysms: preoperative and intraoperative factors determining immediate and long-term results of operations in 605 patients. J Vasc Surg. 1986;3:389–404.
15. National Kidney Foundation. K/DOQI clinical practice guidelines for chronic kidney disease: evaluation, classification, and stratification. Am J Kidney Dis. 2002;39(suppl.1):S1–266.
16. Chiesa R, Melissano G, Civilini E, Bertoglio L, Rinaldi E, Marone EM, et al. Video-atlas of open thoracoabdominal aortic aneurysm repair. Ann Cardiothorac Surg. 2012;1:398–403.
17. Quinones-Baldrich WJ, Panetta TF, Vescera CL, Kashyap VS. Repair of type IV thoracoabdominal aneurysm with combined endovascular and surgical approach. J Vasc Surg. 1999;30:555–60.
18. Lin PH, Kougias P, Bechara CF, Wakley SM, Bakaeen FG, Lemaire SA, et al. Clinical outcome of staged versus combined treatment approach of hybrid repair of thoracoabdominal aortic aneurysm with visceral vessel debranching and aortic endograft exclusion. Perspect Vasc Surg Endovasc Ther. 2012;24:5–13.
19. Bianchini Massoni C, Geisbüsch P, Gallitto E, Hakimi M, Gargiulo M, Böckler D. Follow-up outcomes of hybrid procedures for thoracoabdominal aortic pathologies with special focus on graft patency and late mortality. J Vasc Surg. 2014;59:1265–73.
20. Verhoeven EL, Tielliu IF, Bos WT, Zeebregts CJ. Present and future of branched stent grafts in thoracoabdominal aortic aneurysm repair: a single-centre experience. Eur J Vasc Endovasc Surg. 2009;38:155–61.
21. Guillou M, Bianchini A, Sobocinski J, Maurel B, D'Elia P, Tyrrell M, et al. Endovascular treatment of thoracoabdominal aortic aneurysms. J Vasc Surg. 2012;56:65–73.
22. Lachat M, Veith FJ, Pfammatter T, Glenck M, Bettex D, Mayer D, et al. Chimney and periscope grafts observed over 2 years after their use to revascularize 169 renovisceral branches in 77 patients with complex aortic aneurysms. J Endovasc Ther. 2013;20:597.
23. Mastracci TM, Greenberg RK, Eagleton MJ, Hernandez AV. Dura-bility of branches in branched and fenestrated endografts. J Vasc Surg. 2013;57:926–33.
24. Moulakakis KG, Mylonas SN, Avgerinos ED, Kakisis JD, Brunkwall J, Liapis CD. Hybrid open endovascular technique for aortic thoracoabdominal pathologies. Circulation. 2011;124:2670–80.
25. Tshomba Y, Melissano G, Civilini E, Setacci F, Chiesa R. Fate of the visceral aortic patch after thoracoabdominal aortic repair. Eur J Vasc Endovasc Surg. 2005;29:383–9.
26. Perrin D, Demanget N, Badel P, Avril S, Orgéas L, Geindreau C, et al. Deployment of stent grafts in curved aneurysmal arteries: toward a predictive numerical tool. Int J Numer Method Biomed Eng. 2015;31:e02698.
27. Premprabha D, Sobel J, Pua C, Chong K, Reilly LM, Chuter TAM, et al. Visceral branch occlusion following aneurysmal repair using multibranched thoracoabdominal stent-grafts. J Endovasc Ther. 2014;21:783–90.
28. Kamohara K, Furukawa K, Itoh M, Morokuma H, Tanaka H, Hayashi N, et al. Evaluation of the optimal visceral branch configuration in open thoracoabdominal aortic repair by computed tomography. Ann Thorac Cardiovasc Surg. 2015;21:59–65.

Hybrid Repair of Thoracoabdominal Aortic Aneurysm with Rerouting of Visceral Arteries

21

Luca Apruzzi, Vincenzo Ardita, Andrea Melloni, Yamume Tshomba, and Roberto Chiesa

21.1 Introduction

The treatment of thoracoabdominal aortic aneurysms (TAAA) is currently the most challenging operation for vascular and cardiovascular surgeons. In most cases, conventional open repair of TAAA represents the best treatment for patients deemed fit for surgery.

In the last few decades, technical advances in surgery, anesthesiology, and intensive care have improved clinical outcomes of TAAA open repair with 30-day mortality of less than 10% in selected series [1]. In larger series of patients, these results are not duplicated with overall mortality from 20 to 25%, even higher in subgroups of older patients [2]. Apart from mortality, neurological complications, in particular represented by spinal cord ischemia, remain the critical issue for the outcome of patient treated with open repair. Thus, in order to treat that proportion of patients with severe comorbidities or with prior aortic surgery, a less-invasive approach is needed. Hybrid TAAA treatment consists of the debranching of aortic collaterals and the exclusion of aortic aneurysms with a straight aortic endograft.

21.2 Surgical Procedure

Hybrid TAAA repair consists in a two-staged procedure: the first is the open visceral and renal debranching and the second is the aortic endografting.

The first stage is usually achieved through midline laparotomy; in fact, in the absence of prior abdominal surgery or laparotomy, this approach allows a contemporary exposure of the proximal segment of visceral and renal arteries as well as the iliac arteries.

Celiac trunk (CT) isolation can be achieved in the omental bursa above the pancreas (Fig. 21.1).

CT revascularization can be accomplished via an end-to-side bypass to the common hepatic artery. By revascularizing the hepatic artery but ligating the celiac trunk, the left gastric and splenic arteries can continue to be perfused by retrograde flow from the proximal hepatic artery. In the case

L. Apruzzi (✉) · V. Ardita · A. Melloni
Scientific Institute H. San Raffaele, Vita-Salute University School of Medicine, Milan, Italy
e-mail: apruzzi.luca@hsr.it; ardita.vincenzo@hsr.it; melloni.andrea@hsr.it

Y. Tshomba
Unit of Vascular Surgery, Fondazione Policlinico Universitario A. Gemelli IRCCS, Università Cattolica del Sacro Cuore, Rome, Italy

Unit of Vascular Surgery, San Raffaele Scientific Institute, Vita-Salute University, Milan, Italy
e-mail: yamume.tshomba@unicatt.it

R. Chiesa
Unit of Vascular Surgery, San Raffaele Scientific Institute, Vita-Salute University, Milan, Italy
e-mail: chiesa.roberto@hsr.it

© Springer Nature Switzerland AG 2019
Y. Tshomba et al. (eds.), *Visceral Vessels and Aortic Repair*,
https://doi.org/10.1007/978-3-319-94761-7_21

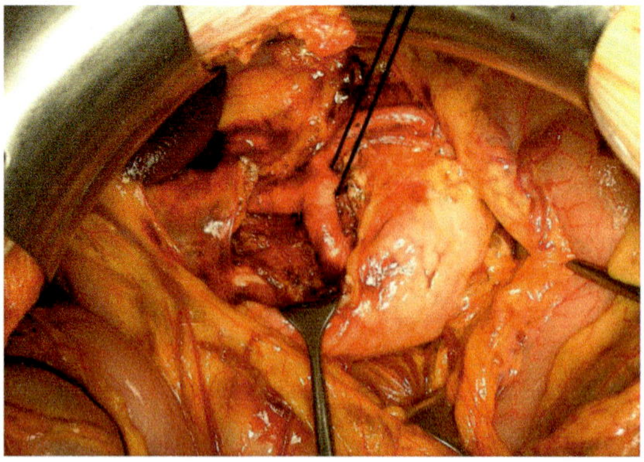

Fig. 21.1 Intraoperative image showing celiac trunk exposure. The greater omentum is divided and the stomach moved down and to the left side, exposing the pancreas. The origin of celiac trunk (under a vessel loop) is just behind the pancreas which can be carefully moved down to gain enough space for the anastomosis

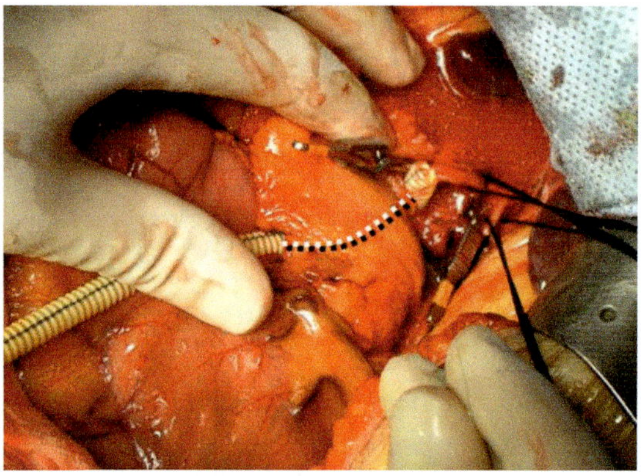

Fig. 21.2 The prosthetic branch to celiac trunk can be routed behind the pancreas as shown by the dashed line

of anastomosis directly to the celiac trunk, an end-to-end anastomosis is usually preferred in a position which allows the vessel to be ligated after completion of the bypass. The bypass can be routed in retropancreatic position, but antepancreatic routing especially in cases of anastomosis on the common hepatic artery can avoid the risk of pancreatic damages due to tunneling (Fig. 21.2).

An end-to-end anastomosis is usually preferred for the superior mesenteric artery (SMA) in the omental bursa behind the pancreas. The SMA can be easily identified at the base of the transverse mesocolon and vascularized by an end-to-side anastomosis with a ligation just proximally to the graft (Figs. 21.3 and 21.4).

Both renal arteries can be easily isolated proximally as they branch from the abdominal aorta, and also in this case, an end-to-end bypass is preferred.

In cases in which a distal isolation of the right renal artery is needed, it can be achieved with Kocher's maneuver consisting in medial mobilization of the duodenum (Fig. 21.5).

During visceral reconstruction, organ ischemia can be managed using Pruitt-Inahara catheters positioned in vessels' ostia in order to permit contemporary clamping and perfusion (Fig. 21.6).

The visceral arteries can be perfused with cold perfusion (Ringer's solution 4 °C); in cases requiring a longer renal clamping, a renal perfusion with a bolus of 4 °C 300 mL of lactated Ringer's solution supplemented with mannitol 18% (70 mL) and 6-methylprednisolone (500 mg) or Custodiol® solution can be used.

In all reconstruction the grafted vessels are dissected over adequate distances to allow for secure management and ligation. Prosthetic bypass grafts are used for revascularization. Commercially available grafts designed for abdominal debranching can be used, but in addition, different custom-made configurations for visceral bypasses can be obtained with a variety of straight or bifurcated Dacron or e-PTFE prostheses.

In most cases, bypasses are constructed in a retrograde fashion. The choice of inflow site is based on the TAAA extension, the presence of prior aortoiliac surgery, and the quality of the walls of native vessels. In fact, the proximal anastomosis is usually placed on the common iliac arteries, but the infrarenal aorta, in the absence of aneurysms, can be used as inflow site. In cases of infrarenal and iliac aneurysms, it is possible to replace infrarenal aorta with a tube or bifurcated prosthesis and then use the graft as the inflow site for visceral bypasses (Fig. 21.7).

In these cases, attention must be taken to leave enough native aorta or graft to ensure a good distal landing zone to place the planned endograft. Rarely, in selected cases, the thoracic aorta can be used as inflow site for visceral debranching constructing the bypasses in anterograde fashion (Fig. 21.8).

Target vessels can be revascularized individually or in a series with jump grafts. Finally, in the majority of cases, the proximal stump of the target arteries was ligated to avoid retrograde perfusion of the aneurysm.

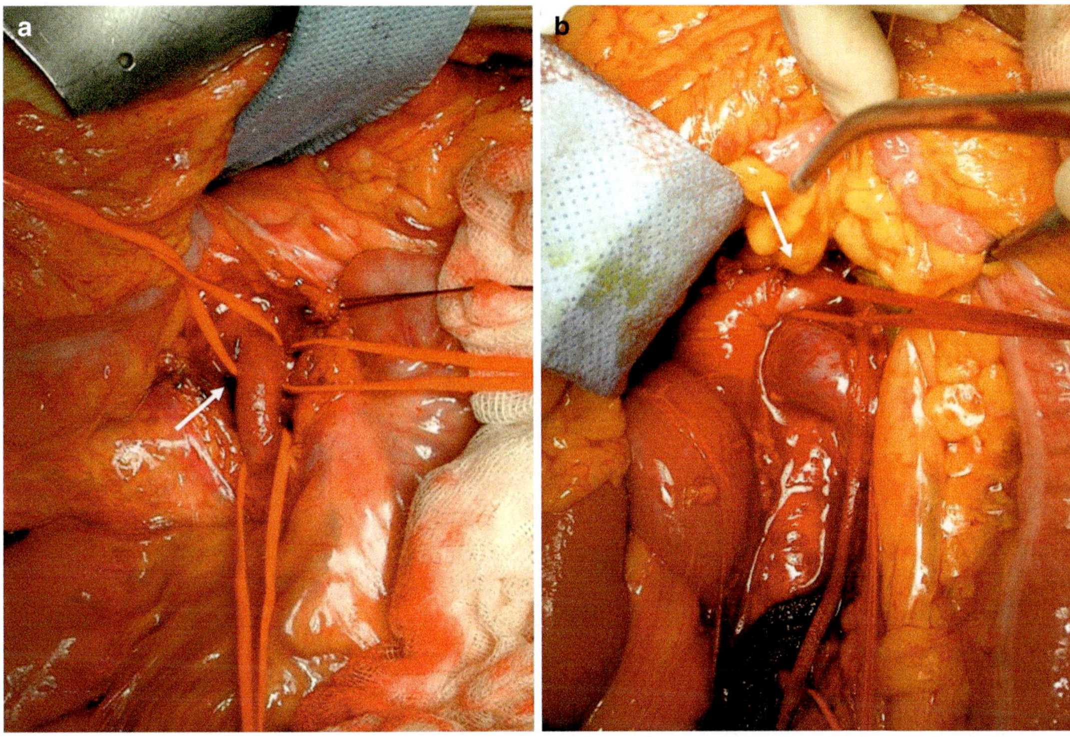

Fig. 21.3 Vascular access for the superior mesenteric artery (white arrow) can be achieved via the omental bursa at its origin from the aorta (A) or at the base of the mesocolon just cranially to the left renal vein

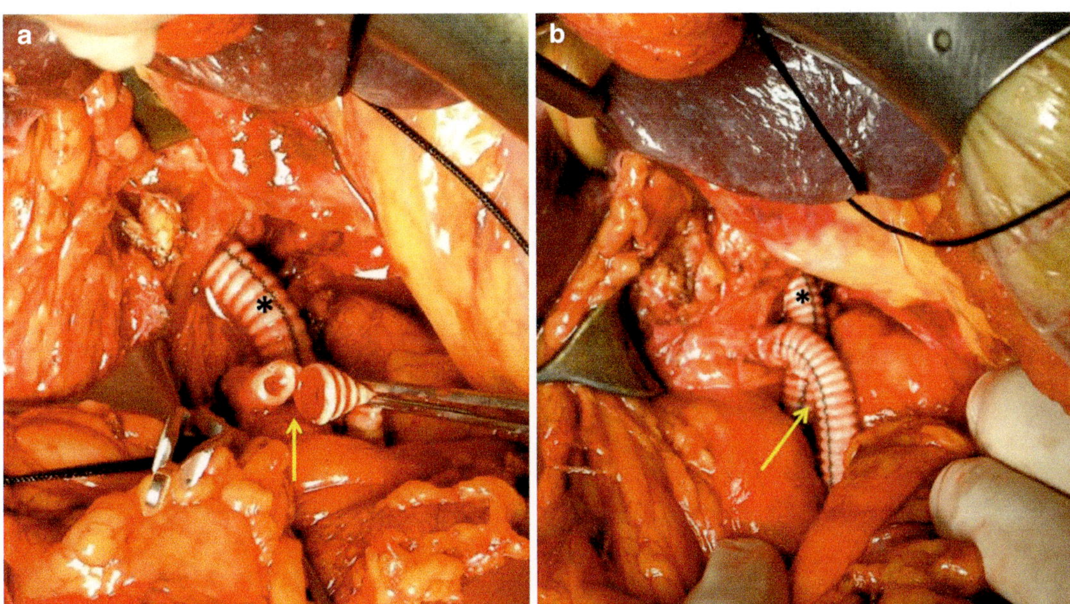

Fig. 21.4 Intraoperative image showing distal SMA separated from its origin and is exposed nearby the graft (yellow arrow) to perform the distal end-to-end anastomosis. After the completion of the suture, the graft to the SMA is positioned in the omental bursa nearby the graft to the celiac trunk (asterisk)

Recently, the use of sutureless anastomosis techniques has been proposed for the reconstruction of visceral vessels (Chap. 22). The VORTEC (Viabahn Open Revascularization TEChnique) [3] is a less-invasive prosthetic graft anastomotic technique that uses self-expanding stent grafts (W.L. Gore & Associates, Inc., Flagstaff, AZ, USA) that are "telescoped" into aortic vessels, and the end of the stent graft outside of the target artery is sutured end to side directly with the inflow vessel. The main morphological indications to perform the VORTEC are diameter of the renal or superior mesenteric artery >4 mm, distal landing zone of >1 cm, and absence of relevant branches of the artery in the landing zone.

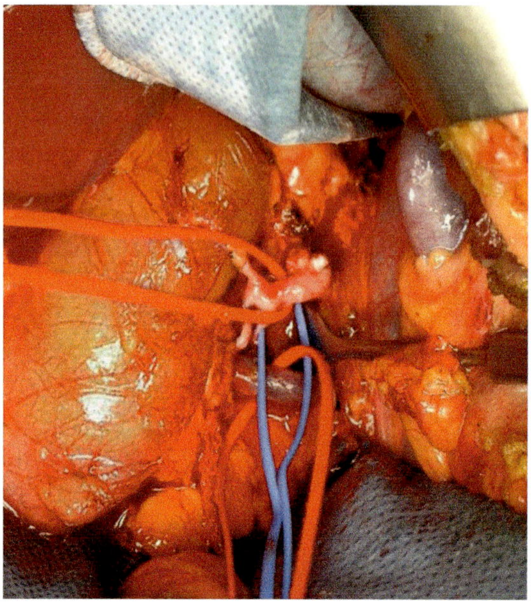

Fig. 21.5 Intraoperative image showing complete skeletonization of the renal hilum with renal vessels suspended by red vessel loops. By a surgical dissection of the duodenum, it can be reflected to the left (Kocher's maneuver) giving access to distal right renal artery

The use of Gore Hybrid Vascular Graft (W.L. Gore & Associates, Inc., Flagstaff, AZ, USA) may represent a significant advantage in reducing vessel dissection and organ ischemia during revascularization [4]. As described for the VORTEC, the use of this graft in most cases is limited to renal arteries (Fig. 21.9) which usually have enough space for the deployment of the covered stent before the origin of its first side branches.

After the completion of renovisceral bypasses, when possible, they should be covered with retroperitoneum or omental flaps to avoid direct contact with the bowel.

The second stage of the hybrid repair consists of aortic endografting to exclude the aneurysm. It can be performed concomitantly or in a staged fashion. A staged approach allows the patient to recover from the surgical stress of laparotomy and from visceral and renal debranching, but on the other hand, the waiting for a subsequent aortic endograft leaves the patient at risk of interval rupture [5].

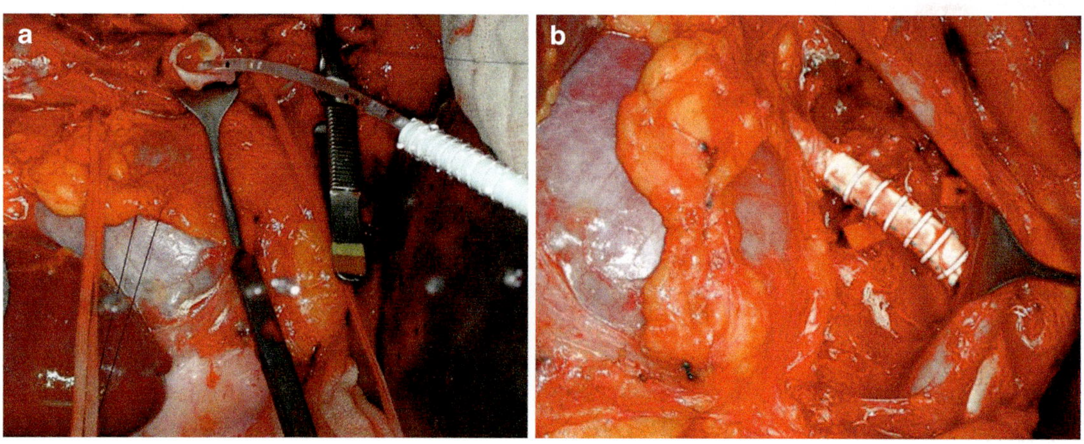

Fig. 21.6 Intraoperative images of a right renal artery reconstruction. A Pruitt-Inahara catheter is positioned into the artery to achieve endo-clamping and contemporary perfusion with cold solution (**a**). In this case the ringed e-PTFE graft is routed behind the inferior cava vein (**b**) which in the image is moved left under the retractor

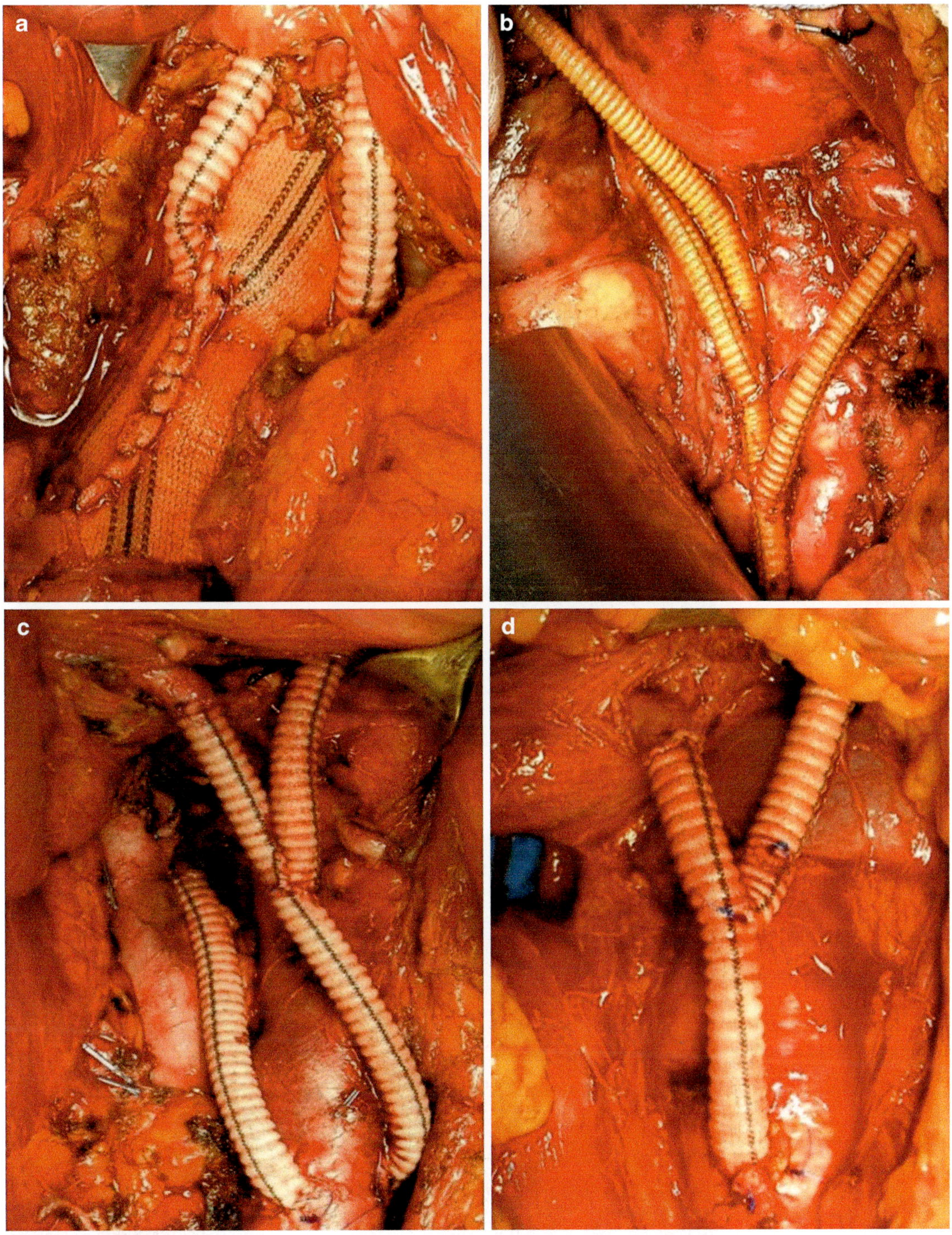

Fig. 21.7 Intraoperative images of different graft configurations for visceral and renal revascularization. (**a**) After infrarenal aortic replacement, aortic graft is used as inflow site for visceral bypasses. In absence of aneurysms, the common iliac artery (**b**) or infrarenal aorta (**c**, **d**) could be an option to seat the proximal anastomosis of bypasses. Visceral and renal vessels can be vascularized individually (**a**) or in series with bifurcated grafts (**b**–**d**)

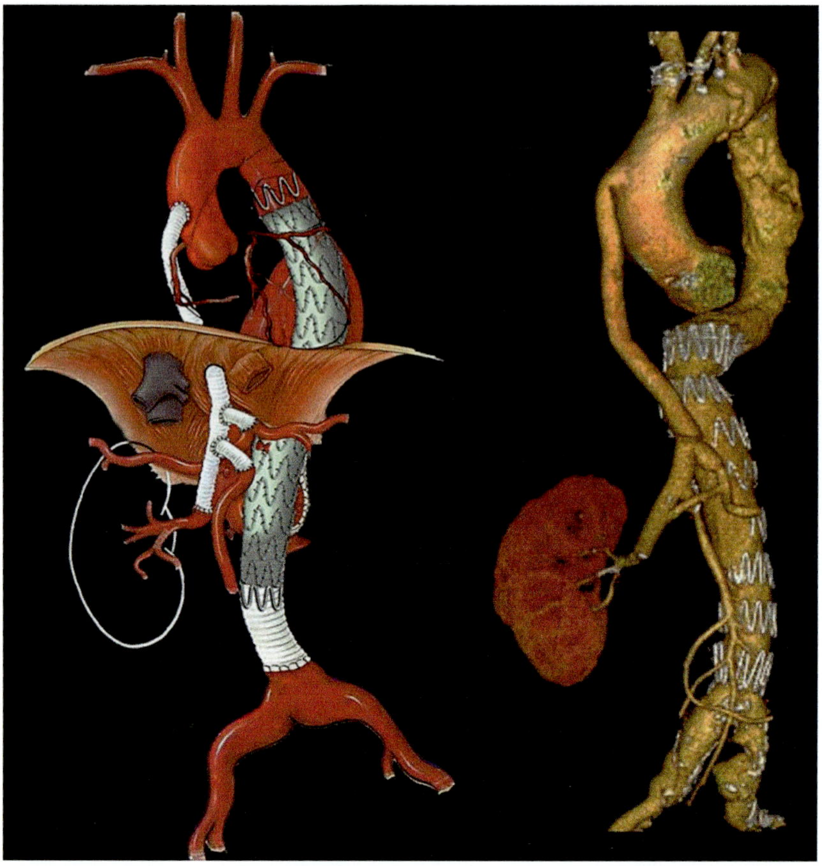

Fig. 21.8 An anatomical drawing and a CT scan 3D reconstruction of an atypical debranching for visceral and renal arteries. In this case, the inflow site used for bypasses is the ascending aorta with the prosthesis routed through the diaphragm

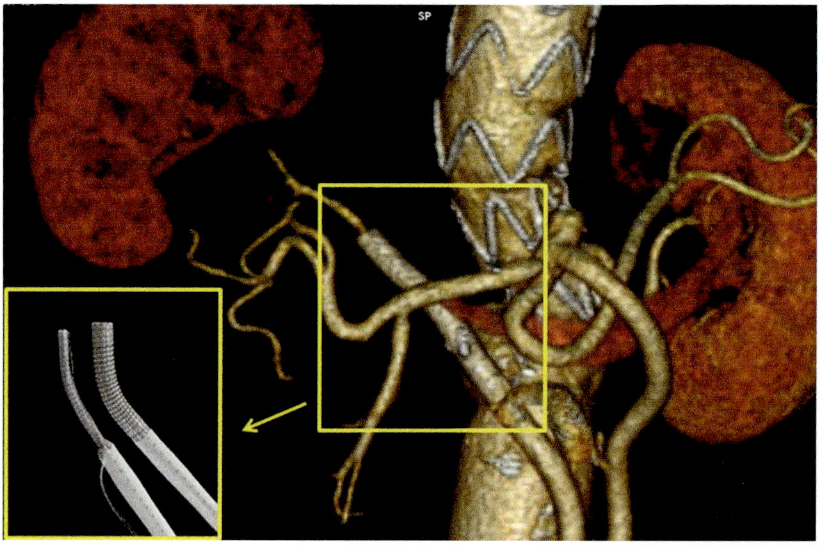

Fig. 21.9 A postoperative CT angiography showing reconstruction of the right renal artery with Gore Hybrid Vascular Graft. In the right yellow box, the reconstructed renal artery is marked, compared with the left yellow box which shows a sample of a Gore Hybrid Vascular Graft

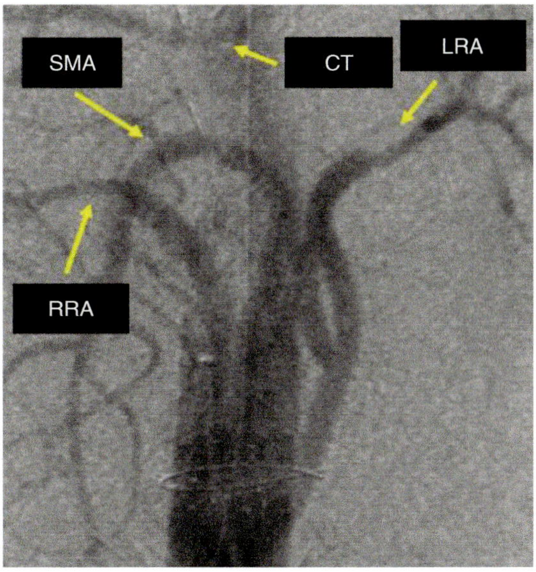

Fig. 21.10 An intraoperative angiography after deployment of the endograft showing the patency of visceral graft to the celiac trunk (CT), superior mesenteric artery (SMA), and left and right renal artery (LRA, RRA)

Different combinations of thoracic endografts can be used to achieve TAAA exclusion. A femoral approach, percutaneous or with a surgical exposure of the artery, is usually preferred. In selected cases, iliac artery or a prosthetic conduit attached or pre-sewn to aortic vascular graft can be used as an access site for the endograft. The choice of endovascular device should be based on surgeon experience and preference and patient anatomy. Completion angiography must always be performed after deploying the graft to ensure the effective aneurysm exclusion and to check the patency of visceral bypasses (Fig. 21.10). Due to the extension of aortic coverage, especially for Crawford's type I to III TAAA, spinal drain and somatosensory evoked potential (SSEP) monitoring might be used for spinal cord protection.

21.3 Clinical Outcome

The hybrid approach to TAAA should have the theoretic advantage to reduce major complications. The possibility to treat a complex aortic pathology with a standard median laparotomy and endovascular repair remains appealing. In scientific literature, many studies have been published reporting ambiguous results with a big heterogeneity in terms of mortality and morbidities (Table 21.1).

In 2012 a meta-analysis published by Moulakakis et al. [27] confirmed such controversial outcomes. The authors analyzed 14 studies with a total of 528 patients and mean follow-up time of 34.2 months. The 30-day mortality rate was 14.3%; the symptomatic spinal cord ischemia, irreversible paraplegia, permanent renal failure, and mesenteric ischemia were 7%, 4.4%, 7%, and 4.5%, respectively. Pooled estimates for primary technical success and visceral graft patency were 95.4% and 96.5%, respectively. Furthermore, the authors reported that better results with lower complication rates are achieved in high-volume aortic centers.

21.4 Discussion

There are currently three options for the treatment of TAAA. Open surgical TAAA repair (Chap. 19) is demonstrated to represent a durable option [28, 29], but in older patients with significant comorbidities, it may not be tolerated for the exposure of two cavities, left heart bypass and aortic cross-clamping. The search for less stressful procedures has been proposed to treat high-risk populations who are not deemed fit for open surgery. Total endovascular approaches with branched or fenestrated endografts (Chap. 24) have been described as very promising options [30] but are not widely available and require a degree of endovascular skills that not all centers possess. Furthermore, in some cases, the waiting time for the production of custom-made devices may expose patients to the risk of aneurysm rupture.

The hybrid TAAA repair, first described by Quinones-Baldrich in 1999 [31], is associated to less surgical stress with a technique that can even be applied in patients with several limitations. By avoiding thoracotomy, hybrid repair may be considered in patients with previous thoracic surgery. In fact, a redo left-side thoracotomy in a "frozen chest" could be technically complicated, and

Table 21.1 Published studies reporting TAAA experience with at least more than five patients (ND, not described or not reported)

Author	*n*	30-day mortality (%)	Paraplegia (%)	Graft patency rate (%)	Endoleaks (%)	Mean follow-up (months)
Fulton et al. [6]	10	0	0	100	10	8.7
Resch et al. [7]	13	23	15	ND	ND	ND
Zhou et al. [8]	31	3.2	0	98	6	16
Gawenda et al. [9]	6	0	0	94.7	0	ND
Lee et al. [10]	17	24	0	96	12	8
Van de Mortel et al. [11]	16	31	0	95	13	13
Böckler et al. [12]	28	14.3	4	86	17.8	22
Quinones-Baldrich et al. [13]	20	0	6.6	100	30	17
Donas et al. [14]	58	8.6	3.4	97	17	22
Biasi et al. [15]	18	16.7	5.6	98.1	38.9	23
Drinkwater et al. [16]	107	15	8.4	87	33	ND
Patel et al. [17]	23	17	4	90	23	6
Kabbani et al. [18]	36	8.3	0	93	39	6
Muehling et al. [19]	16	31.2	6.2	ND	37.5	12
Kuratani et al. [20]	86	2.3	0	99	17	88
Wolf and Eckstein [21]	20	10	10	ND	30	6
Smith et al. [22]	24	12.5	8.3	99	12	12
Hughes et al. [23]	58	9	4	95	ND	26
Tshomba et al. [24]	52	14	1.9	93	7.7	24
Rossett et al. [25]	76	34	11	99	3	30
Massoni et al. [26]	45	24	13	79	ND	26

aortic exposure in a scarred operatory field can increase both intraoperative complications such as bleeding and organ injuries and postoperative complications like respiratory failure [32, 33].

The choice of simultaneous or staged procedure is a debated issue. The one-stage strategy has the advantage to eliminate the risk of interoperative rupture [16] and in cases of inadequate femoral arteries can be an advantage to prompt availability of aortic or iliac access for the endograft deployment. In cases of staged procedure and unavailability of femoral access, a prosthetic conduit implanted on the abdominal aorta may be a solution. The staged approach offers the advantage of shortening the overall procedural time, thus reducing organ ischemic time and the risk of renal injury [4].

Postoperative renal failure remains a major complication after TAAA repair [5]. The hybrid approach does not eliminate the risk of renal injury that remains higher than 60%, especially in patients treated with a single-staged intervention [34]. In fact, the combination of renal ischemia during debranching and the administration of contrast right after renal revascularization can significantly increase the risk of renal failure, especially in patients with preexisting lower renal function. The use of sutureless techniques or new graft configuration [3, 4] for the revascularization of renal arteries showed a reduction of renal injury after renal revascularization due to the shortening of surgical and ischemia time. Tshomba et al. [35] recently proposed the use of Custodiol® solution for renal artery perfusion during open TAAA repair, demonstrating a reduction of acute kidney injury and improving perioperative renal function compared with cool lactated Ringer's solution.

The problem of spinal cord ischemia (SCI) has not been eliminated by hybrid TAAA repair, due to the requirement of extensive coverage of thoracoabdominal aorta [36]. In fact, Gravereaux et al. [37] demonstrated a significant association between a longer stent graft length and the incidence of neurological symptoms. Of course, the avoidance of aortic cross-clamping could lead to a major intraoperative and postoperative hemodynamic stability with reduction of risk of SCI [38]. The use of simultaneous adjuncts such as PESS

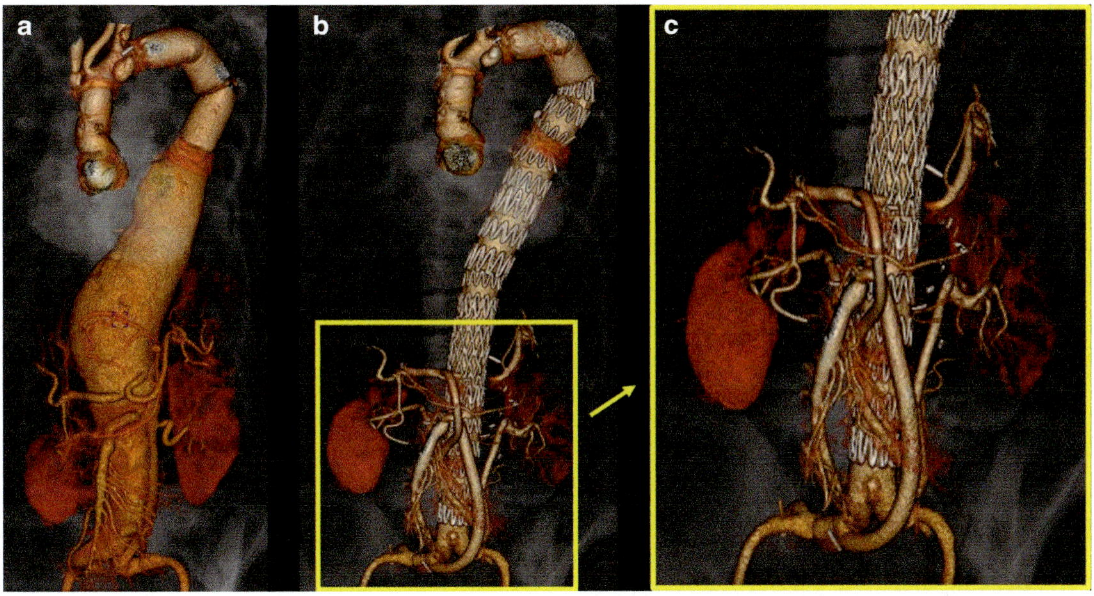

Fig. 21.11 Preoperative (**a**) and 1-year CT angiography (**b**) after a Crawford's type II TAAA hybrid repair. Note in the zoomed image (**c**) the aneurysm exclusion and patency of visceral and renal arteries after repair

and MES monitoring and cerebrospinal fluid drainage can reduce the incidence of SCI especially for Crawford's type II TAAA or in case of prior aortic repairs [39].

The patency and related complications of visceral bypasses are another matter of concern. Visceral graft occlusion may be the cause of devastating complications, such as pancreatitis and bowel ischemia. A safe routing of visceral graft must always be performed, as mentioned above, an antepancreatic routing of celiac trunk graft should be preferred in order to reduce pancreatic injuries. Therefore the risk of enteric erosion or fistulization must be monitored in the follow-up. A postoperative angiogram both in not-staged and in staged procedures can show technical defects of the anastomosis or visceral vessel dissection that can be promptly corrected. In particular for the SMA, vessel angulation can be a risk factor for a graft occlusion evidenced after bowel repositioning, kinked anastomosis, or twisted grafts can be corrected with a self-expandable stent.

A limitation of hybrid TAAA repair involves endoleaks probably secondary to aortic remodeling over time and long-segment endografts implanted for aneurysm exclusion [40]. In scientific literature, the incidence of endoleaks is variable in different series (Table 21.1) but is a matter of concern because it may expose patients to future reintervention and may leave them at risk of aneurysm rupture. Especially in cases of type Ia endoleak, the treatment may be challenging in cases of inadequate proximal landing zone nearby supra-aortic vessels.

A postoperative surveillance of patients, in particular for Crawford's type II TAAA, should be maintained with contrast CT scans at scheduled follow-up intervals of 1, 6, and 12 months and yearly thereafter, given to their risk for endoleak and for visceral graft occlusion (Fig. 21.11).

21.5 Conclusion

Open conventional repair represents the gold standard for the treatment of TAAA for patients considered fit for surgery. Hybrid repair for TAAA remains an appealing technique, but many issues about this approach remain unsolved such as the outcome of visceral bypasses, long-term durability of the endograft materials, and the fate of excluded aneurysm in terms of endoleaks.

Complete abdominal aortic debranching and endovascular aneurysm exclusion remains a good option for selected elderly, high-risk patients in high-volume centers with expertise in management of visceral revascularization. Nowadays, fenestrated and branched endografts are developing as a less-invasive alternative for treating complex aortic aneurysms with good results.

The question of whether hybrid repair leads to improve outcomes compared to open or total endovascular repair still remains controversial, and larger study cohorts with longer follow-up are needed.

References

1. LeMaire SA, Price MD, Green SY, et al. Results of open thoracoabdominal aortic aneurysm repair. Ann Cardiothorac Surg. 2012;1(3):286–92. https://doi.org/10.3978/j.issn.2225-319X.2012.08.16.
2. Cowan JA Jr, Dimick JB, Henke PK, et al. Surgical treatment of intact thoracoabdominal aortic aneurysms in the United States: hospital and surgeon volume-related outcomes. J Vasc Surg. 2003;37:1169–74.
3. Lachat M, Mayer D, Criado FJ, et al. New technique to facilitate renal revascularization with use of telescoping self-expanding stent grafts: VORTEC. Vascular. 2008;16:69–72.
4. Chiesa R, Kahlberg A, Mascia D, et al. Use of a novel hybrid vascular graft for sutureless revascularization of the renal arteries during open thoracoabdominal aortic aneurysm repair. J Vasc Surg. 2014;23(14):670–3.
5. Canaud L, Karthikesalingam A, Jackson D, et al. Clinical outcomes of single versus staged hybrid repair for thoracoabdominal aortic aneurysm. J Vasc Surg. 2013 Nov;58(5):1192–200.
6. Fulton JJ, Farber MA, Marston WA, et al. Endovascular stent-graft repair of pararenal and type IV thoracoabdominal aortic aneurysms with adjunctive visceral reconstruction. J Vasc Surg. 2005;41(2):191–8.
7. Resch TA, Greenberg RK, Lyden SP, et al. Combined staged procedures for the treatment of thoracoabdominal aneurysms. J Endovasc Ther. 2006;13:481–9.
8. Zhou W, Reardon M, Peden EK, et al. Hybrid approach to complex thoracic aortic aneurysms in high-risk patients: surgical challengers and clinical outcome. J Vasc Surg. 2006;44:688–93.
9. Gawenda M, Aleksic M, Heckenkamp J, et al. Hybrid-procedures for the treatment of thoracoabdominal aortic aneurysms and dissections. Eur J Vasc Endovasc Surg. 2007;33:71–7.
10. Lee WA, Brown MP, Martin TD, et al. Early results after staged hybrid repair of thoracoabdominal aortic aeurysms. J Am Coll Surg. 2007;205:420–31.
11. Van de Mortel RHW, Vahl AC, Balm R, et al. Collective experience with hybrid procedures for suprarenal and thoracoabdominal aneurysms. Vascular. 2008;16:140–6.
12. Böckler D, Kotelis D, Geisbusch P, et al. Hybrid procedures for thoracoabdominal aortic aneurysms and chronic aortic dissections – a single center experience in 28 patients. J Vasc Surg. 2008;47:724–32.
13. Quinones-Baldrich W, Jimenez JC, DeRubertis B, et al. Combined endovascular and surgical approach (CESA) to thoracoabdominal aortic pathology: a 10-year experience. J Vasc Surg. 2009;49:1125–34.
14. Donas KP, Lachat M, Rancic Z, et al. Early and mid-term outcome of a novel technique to simplify the hybrid procedures in the treatment of thoracoabdominal and pararenal aortic aneurysms. J Vasc Surg. 2009;50:1280–4.
15. Biasi L, Ali T, Loosemore T, et al. Hybrid repair of complex thoracoabdominal aortic aneurysms using applied endovascular strategies combined with visceral and renal revascularization. J Thorac Cardiovasc Surg. 2009;138:1331–8.
16. Drinkwather SL, Böckler D, Eckstein H, et al. The visceral hybrid repair of thoraco-abdominal aortic aneurysms - a collaborative approach. Eur J Vasc Endovasc Surg. 2009;38:578–85.
17. Patel R, Conrad MF, Paruchuri V, et al. Thoracoabdominal aneurysm repair: hybrid versus open repair. J Vasc Surg. 2009;50:15–22.
18. Kabbani LS, Criado E, Upchurch JR, et al. Hybrid repair of aortic aneurysms involving the visceral and renal vessels. Ann Vasc Surg. 2010;24:219–24.
19. Muehling BM, Bischoff G, Schelzig H, et al. Hybrid procedures for complex thoracoabdominal aortic aneurysms: early results and secondary interventions. Vasc Endovasc Surg. 2010;44:110–5.
20. Kuratani T, Kato M, Shirakawa Y, et al. Long-term results of hybrid endovascular repair for thoracoabdominal aortic aneurysms. Eur J Cardiotorac Surg. 2010;38:299–304.
21. Wolf O, Eckstein HH. Combined open and endovascular treatment of thoracoabdominal aneurysms and secondary expanding aortic dissections: early and mid-term results from a single center series. Ann Vasc Surg. 2010;24:167–77.
22. Smith TA, Gatens S, Andres M, et al. Hybrid repair of thoracoabdominal aortic aneurysms involving the visceral vessels: comparative analysis between number of vessels reconstructed, conduit, and gender. Ann Vasc Surg. 2011;25:64–70.
23. Hughes GC, Andersen ND, Hanna JM, et al. Thoracoabdominal aortic aneurysm: hybrid repair outcomes. Ann Cartiothorac Surg. 2012;1:311–9.
24. Tshomba Y, Melissano G, Logaldo D, et al. Clinical outcomes of hybrid repair for thoracoabdominal aortic aneurysms. Ann Cardiotorac Surg. 2012;1: 293–303.
25. Rosset E, Ben Ahmed S, Galvaing G, et al. Editor's choice – Hybrid treatment of thoracic, thoracoabdominal, and abdominal aortic aneurysms: a multi-

center retrospective study. Eur J Vasc Endovasc Surg. 2014;47:470–8.
26. Massoni CB, Geisbsoch P, Gallitto E, et al. Follow-up outcomes of hybrid procedures for thoracoabdominal aortic pathologies with special focus on graft patency and late mortality. J Vasc Surg. 2014;59:1265–73.
27. Moulakakis KG, Mylonas SN, Antonopoulos CN, et al. Combined open and endovascular treatment of thoracoabdominal aortic pathologies: a systematic review and meta-analysis. Ann Cardiothorac Surg. 2012;1(3):267–76.
28. Wong DR, Parenti JL, Green SY, et al. Open repair of thoracoabdominal aortic aneurysm in the modern surgical era: contemporary outcomes in 509 patients. J Am Coll Surg. 2011;212:569–79. discussion: 579–81.
29. Coselli JB, LeMaire SA. Open surgical repair of 2286 thoracoabdominal aortic aneurysms. Ann Thorac Surg. 2007;83:S862–4. discussion: S890–2.
30. Clough RE, Modarai B, Bell RE, et al. Total endovascular repair of thoracoabdominal aortic aneurysms. Eur J Vasc Endovasc Surg. 2012;43:262–7.
31. Quiñones-Baldrich WJ, Panetta TF, Vescera CL, et al. Repair of type IV thoracoabdominal aneurysm with a combined endovascular and surgical approach. J Vasc Surg. 1999;30(3):555–60.
32. Kawaharada N, Morishita K, Fukada J, et al. Thoracoabdominal aortic aneurysm repair through redo left-sided thoracotomy. Ann Thorac Surg. 2004;77:1304–8.
33. Menard MT, Nguyen LL, Chan RK, et al. Thoracovisceral segment aneurysm repair after previous infrarenal abdominal aortic aneurysm surgery. J Vasc Surg. 2004;39:1163–70.
34. Lin PH, Kougias P, Bechara CF, et al. Clinical outcome of staged versus combined treatment approach of hybrid repair of thoracoabdominal aortic aneurysm with visceral vessel debranching and aortic endograft exclusion. Perspect Vasc Surg Endovasc Ther. 2012;24(1):5–13.
35. Tshomba Y, Kahlberg A, Melissano G, et al. Comparison of renal perfusion solutions during thoracoabdominal aortic aneurysm repair. J Vasc Surg. 2016;59:623–33.
36. Dias NV, Sonesson B, Kristmundsson T, et al. Short-term outcome of spinal cord ischemia after endovascular repair of thoracoabdominal aortic aneurysms. Eur J Vasc Endovasc Surg. 2015;49:403–9.
37. Gravereaux EC, Faries PL, Burks JA, et al. Risk of spinal cord ischemia after endograft repair of thoracic aortic aneurysms. J Vasc Surg. 2001;34:997–1003.
38. Chiesa R, Melissano G, Marrocco-Trischitta MM, et al. Spinal cord ischemia after elective stent-graft repair of the thoracic aorta. J Vasc Surg. 2005;42(1):11–7.
39. Chiesa R, Tshomba Y, Melissano G, et al. Hybrid approach to thoracoabdominal aortic aneurysms in patients with prior aortic surgery. J Vasc Surg. 2007;45:1128–35.
40. Benrashid E, Wang H, Andersen ND, et al. Complementary roles of open and hybrid approaches to thoracoabdominal aortic aneurysm repair. J Vasc Surg. 2016;64:1228–38.

Toward an Entirely Endovascular World for Thoracoabdominal Aortic Disease: Myth or Reality?

22

Piergiorgio Cao and Ciro Ferrer

22.1 Introduction

Endovascular repair (ER) is currently the first-line treatment for the overwhelming majority of aortic disease, and its applicability is expanding to the whole aorta in light of evolving technologies. Whereas with the introduction of new devices developed to overcome common anatomical limitations, techniques of infrarenal (EVAR) and descending thoracic endovascular aneurysm repair (TEVAR) have reached a plateau; the debate is still open on thoracoabdominal aortic aneurysm (TAAA).

Despite continuous intra- and postoperative improvements, open repair (OR) of TAAA is still associated with significant mortality and morbidity, mainly due to the invasiveness of the surgical access and the hemodynamic instability, following proximal aortic clamping and massive blood loss. As the population ages and diagnostic capabilities improve, elderly patients with multiple comorbidities and limited physiological reserve are increasingly referred for treatment of TAAAs. The need to further reduce morbidity and mortality associated with open surgery has made the endovascular approach particularly attractive.

P. Cao (✉)
Mater Dei Hospital, Rome, Italy

C. Ferrer
Department of Surgery "Pietro Valdoni", Sapienza University of Rome, Rome, Italy

Fenestrated stent grafts were originally developed to extend the area suitable for proximal sealing in short-neck abdominal aortic aneurysms (AAAs). Once it was established that the presence of fenestrations did not jeopardize the integrity of the proximal sealing zone or incorporated arteries, clinicians began to extend repairs to more complex aneurysms using covered stents to bridge fenestrations to target vessels.

However, it soon became evident that a fenestrated solution was not adequate to cope with extensive TAAA in which the luminal diameter within the visceral segment of the aorta was much larger than the aortic stent graft. Thus, the concept of a side-arm branched graft, in which a fabric cuff is attached to the main body, was developed, leaving the fenestrated solutions to cases where the aortic internal lumen does not leave enough room for branched stent graft. Considerable progress has been made over the last few years to refine this technique. The introduction of off-the-shelf devices, which sufficiently met anatomical variability, has partially solved the problem of long manufacturing time of custom-made stent grafts. Parallel grafts, as well, play a complementary role in emergency situations where custom-made devices are not available. Staging of extensive repairs is widely adopted to prevent symptoms of spinal cord ischemia (SCI), as well as the full relining of bridged target vessels with bare-metal stents, in order to increase branch stability. Finally, preloaded systems allow for wider anatomic eligibility for complex aortic repair.

© Springer Nature Switzerland AG 2019
Y. Tshomba et al. (eds.), *Visceral Vessels and Aortic Repair*,
https://doi.org/10.1007/978-3-319-94761-7_22

In this scenario, endovascular repair for thoracoabdominal aortic disease with fenestrated (FEVAR) and branched (BEVAR) stent grafts plays a leading role with excellent short-term results and promising long-term durability.

This chapter focuses on clinical and technical aspects involved in the decision-making for the management of TAAA, endovascular anatomical feasibility, and outcome evaluation and tries to determine whether the concept of an entirely endovascular world for thoracoabdominal aortic disease is conceivable.

22.2 Endovascular Feasibility

Total endovascular repair of thoracoabdominal aortic disease depends on the assessment of specific morphological criteria, including landing zones, aortic internal lumen diameter, aortic tortuosity, visceral vessel orientation, and quality of access vessels. Computed tomographic angiography (CTA) of the aorta and branch vessels and three-dimensional reconstruction and post-processing image manipulation software are essential tools when advanced endovascular techniques are being utilized [1]. Multiplanar reconstructions according to the center lumen line are essential for accurate evaluation and planning, including the assessment of proximal and distal landing zones, the relationship of the aneurysm to the aortic arch and supra-aortic vessels, the degree of aortic tortuosity, and the size and quality of the access vessels (Fig. 22.1).

22.2.1 Proximal Landing Zone

The identification of a suitable proximal landing zone is one of the first factors to take in account to determine whether the endovascular technique is applicable. The proximal landing zone must be accurately measured. It is generally recommended to have at least 2 cm of proximal sealing to prevent distal migration. The tendency of the stent graft to follow the greater curvature and the natural tortuosity of the aorta often leads to an underestimation of the coverage length. For this reason, in cases of severe angulation, calcification, or thrombus, it may be necessary to extend the seal zone length. In approximately 20% of cases, the proximal sealing zone can only be achieved by extending across the left subclavian artery (LSA) ostium [2]. Current Society for Vascular Surgery guidelines recommend preoperative LSA revascularization in elective cases and watchful waiting in acute settings, though this remains an area of debate [3]. The presence of a left dominant vertebral artery or a left internal mammary coronary artery bypass graft is a strong indication to consider preemptive LSA revascularization. It should also be noted that the LSA can be an important input to the collateral network feeding the anterior spinal artery, and as such, if other inputs are diseased or excluded, direct revascularization should be strongly considered.

The proximity of the aneurysm to supra-aortic vessels implies to cope with arch TEVAR and the potential neurologic complications related to.

Approaches to complex TAAA with aortic arch involvement, regardless of the technique, cannot be achieved without risk. Treatment options range from open arch repair with elephant trunk or frozen elephant trunk, hybrid repair with total or partial debranching procedures, or total endovascular repair with fenestrated, branched, and scalloped devices, or parallel stent grafts (Fig. 22.2). For open aortic arch replacement, an operative mortality ranging from 0.9 to 9.3% has been reported in single series from high-volume centers [4–6].

However, according to data from the National Inpatient Sample database [7, 8] and the Medicare Provider Analysis and Review [9, 10], reflecting the real-world experience, operative mortality as high as 15% to 20% has been shown.

A variety of debranching procedures could be applied in patients with TAAA and arch involvement. In our published experience on 104 patients who underwent debranching and TEVAR for thoracic aortic disease extended to the arch, mortality was 5.8%, and stroke and SCI rates were 3.8% and 2.9%, respectively. Nevertheless, proximal extent of arch disease is a major determinant of outcome. Total arch debranching was confirmed in our study as an important independent predictor of 30-day mortality [11].

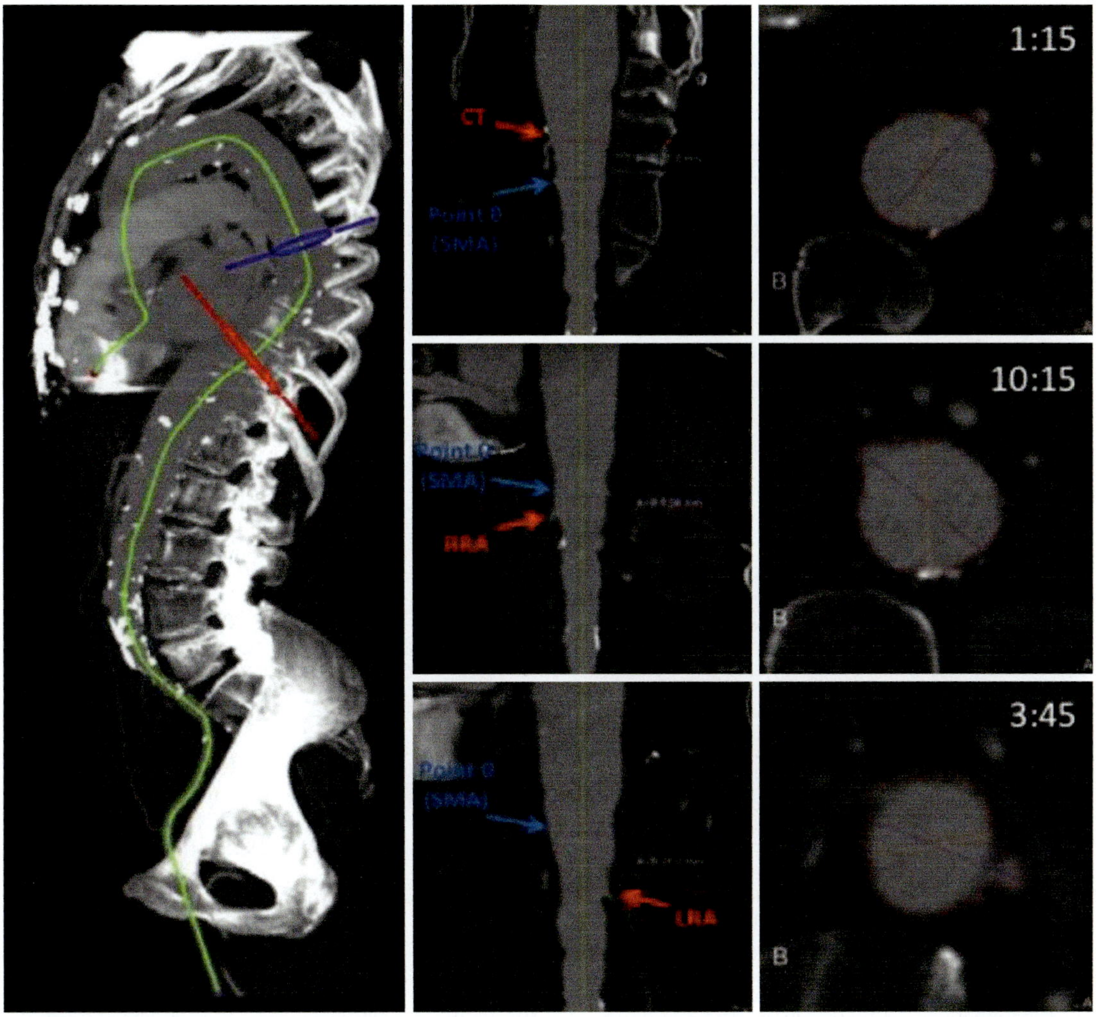

Fig. 22.1 Multiplanar reconstruction according to center lumen line for preoperative evaluation of FEVAR/BEVAR applicability (*CT* celiac trunk, *SMA* superior mesenteric artery, *RRA* right renal artery, *LRA* left renal artery)

The recent availability of new endovascular solutions to avoid these hybrid adjuncts, limiting the invasiveness of the surgical access, may be a valid alternative to decrease intraoperative mortality.

Total endovascular therapeutic options to extend proximal landing zones in extensive TAAA range from off-the-shelf branched solutions equipped with a single branch for LSA revascularization to custom-made devices equipped with up to three fenestrations or inner branches for extension of disease to the ascending aorta (Fig. 22.3) [12, 13].

Spear and co-authors recently reported three cases of post-dissection aortic arch aneurysm treated by totally endovascular means, using a three-inner branched custom-made stent graft. The two proximal branches were antegrade for innominate and the left common carotid artery revascularization, while the third was retrograde and preloaded for LSA perfusion. Technical success was achieved in each case of this small series, and after 6 months, no patient died and no target vessel lost its patency [14].

Chimney and snorkel techniques may be applied in selected cases [15]. Such alternative procedures provide supra-aortic trunks perfusion by parallel fashion, actually representing a valid option mostly in emergent cases

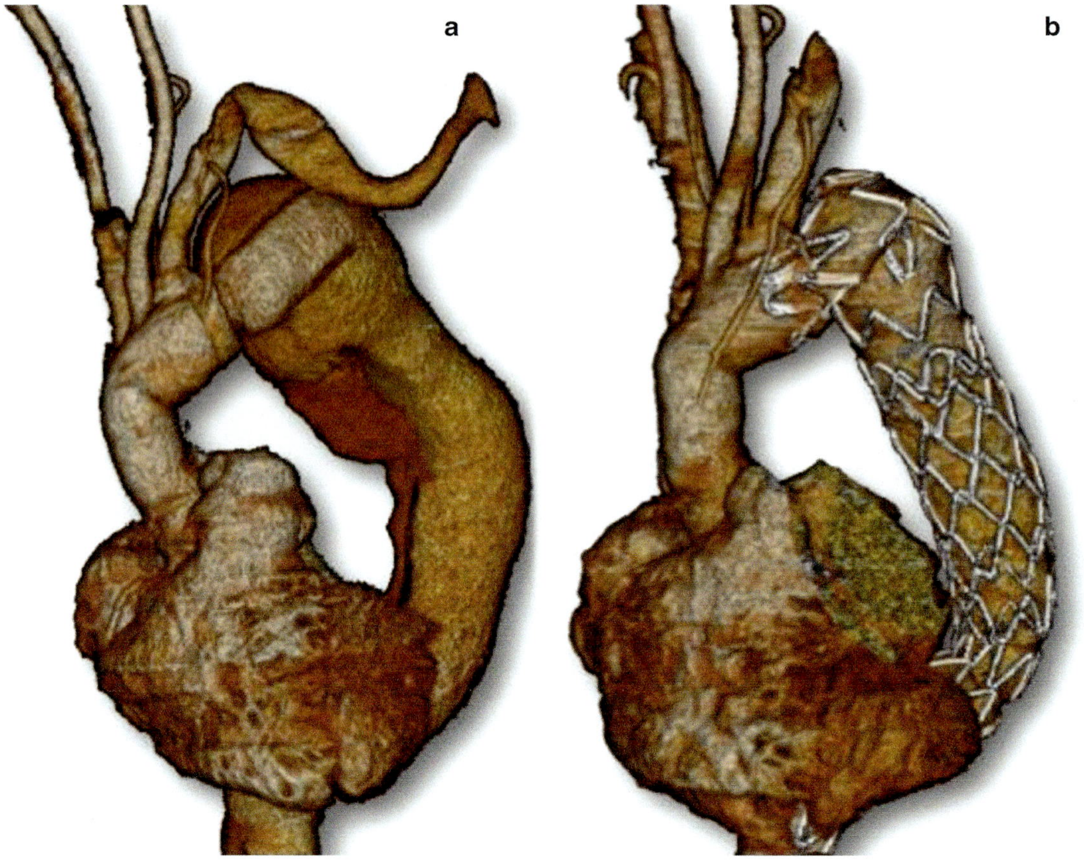

Fig. 22.2 TEVAR completion (**b**) after open arch repair with elephant trunk technique (**a**) for post-dissection TAAA with aortic arch involvement

(Fig. 22.4). Scalloped stent grafts represent another strategy in overcoming the problem of short proximal landing zone. These custom-made stent grafts are equipped with a proximal scallop designed to accommodate the origin of a supra-aortic vessel. In most cases, the proximal scallop is intended for LSA preservation only, although it can be useful in particular cases where left vertebral artery arises directly from the aortic arch.

Nevertheless, the high cost and considerable time delay associated with custom-made devices have paved the way for the development of more versatile on-site modifications of stent grafts. Recently, some reports evaluated the efficacy and safety of needle, laser, or radiofrequency punctures of the aortic stent graft to create retrograde in situ fenestration for LSA or other supra-aortic trunk reperfusion [16–18]. Kasprzak et al. reported the outcome of a patient with aortic arch aneurysm treated by TEVAR and in situ fenestration for the innominate and the left common carotid artery, with in situ stented vessels still patent without any endoleak after 5 years [19].

22.2.2 FEVAR/BEVAR Applicability

Evaluation of anatomical applicability for endovascular TAAA repair obviously goes through the assessment of specific morphological criteria strictly related to thoracoabdominal portion of the aorta, such as aortic angulation, internal lumen diameter, visceral vessel orientation, and

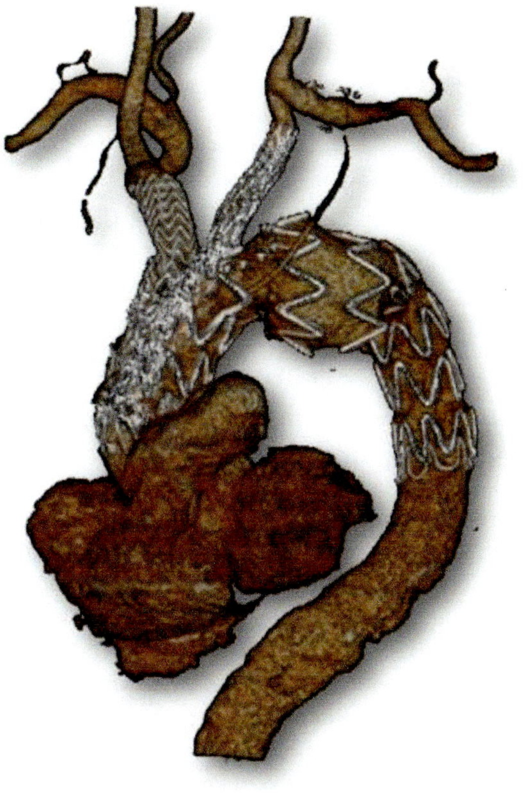

Fig. 22.3 Double inner branch device for the treatment of aortic arch aneurysm

their possible early bifurcation. These features are needed to determine absolute endovascular feasibility and, in particular, whether a solution with fenestrations, branches, or a combination of the two is the most appropriate to fit the patient's anatomy.

Two companies currently provide thoracoabdominal branched stent grafts with tailored design: Cook (Cook Medical, Brisbane, Queensland, Australia) and JOTEC (JOTEC GmbH, Hechingen, Germany). A branched stent graft with custom features, in terms of length and proximal size, aims to reduce the aortic coverage as much as possible, with important advantages in terms of SCI. By designing the side branches close to the ostium of target vessels, the length of bridging stents is significantly reduced with benefits in terms of vessel patency. However, the custom-made design has a considerable limitation due to the relatively long manufacturing time.

This excludes cases where waiting time is not allowed as in very large, symptomatic, or ruptured TAAAs, which have to be repaired through conventional surgery or other off-the-shelf techniques, such as chimney or sandwich [20].

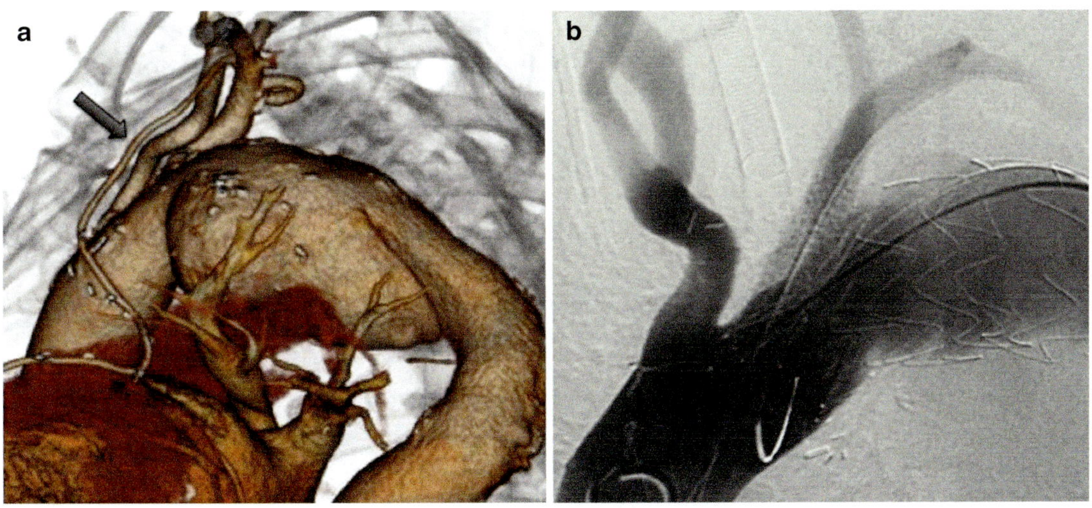

Fig. 22.4 Symptomatic distal arch aneurysm (**a**) in a patient with a previous coronary artery bypass graft from left internal mammary artery (arrow), treated in emergency with TEVAR and double chimney (left common carotid artery and left subclavian artery) technique (**b**)

To overcome these limitations, an off-the-shelf multibranched device (t-Branch; Cook Medical, Bloomington, Ind, USA) has been designed. The main characteristic is the fixed position of the branches, suitable for at least 50% of TAAAs treated with a custom-made device [21]. The device consists of a proximal branched component, a distal bifurcated component, and iliac limb extensions. For extensive aortic disease, proximal thoracic aortic segments may be needed. The branches are oriented downward allowing catheterization only from axillary or brachial artery.

t-Branch use is considered feasible under the following conditions: (1) aortic diameter is >25 mm at the region of the branches, (2) there are no more than four target vessels, (3) the celiac artery (CA) and superior mesenteric artery (SMA) are 6–10 mm in diameter, (4) the renal arteries are 4–8 mm in diameter, (5) all target vessels are accessible from above, (6) the distance between each branch and the corresponding arterial ostium is no longer than 50 mm, and (7) the line between the branch and the ostium deviates by no more than 45° from the main axis of the aorta.

Unused branches could be closed using an occluder plug, expanding the applicability of off-the-shelf branched devices also in cases with less than four visceral arteries.

A recently published paper on the comparison between custom-made and off-the-shelf multibranched stent grafts showed excellent technical success rates for both devices [22]. The t-Branch is theoretically applicable in >50% of patients with TAAAs, and this suggests that not only symptomatic or urgent cases can be treated immediately, but also elective cases are not compelled to wait for the manufacturing of the custom-made stent graft or bear the risk of aneurysm rupture during waiting. The comparable efficacy, however, does not automatically mean that the off-the-shelf stent graft should replace the custom-made device. There are some morphological features that, despite the suitability of the t-Branch, require the performance of adjuvant procedures as additional proximal thoracic endografting or use of longer bridging stents than in custom-made device, which may lead to additional morbidity [22].

These challenges can be successfully solved by means of a custom-made device. The branches in the custom-made stent grafts are usually placed at the most optimal position above the target vessels, facilitating their catheterization. Besides, in TAAAs with a proximal landing zone >32 mm in diameter, the custom-made device can be manufactured with a proximal diameter of 38 mm or larger. In contrast, the t-Branch device, with its fixed diameter of 34 mm, should require a proximal extension with an additional thoracic stent graft.

Another additional disadvantage of the t-Branch is the fixed distal diameter of 18 mm making the bifurcated stent graft almost always necessary.

In other words, the use of custom-made devices leads to less coverage of the aorta, facilitates the catheterization of the target vessels, and often requires fewer implanted materials.

Specific contraindications for the current models of branched devices, such as internal aortic lumen <25 mm, as often happens in post-dissection TAAA, and a lack of brachial or axillary access for branch catheterization, may require the use of a custom-made fenestrated stent graft, although the use of reverse cranially oriented branches, possibly customizable with inner design, may represent a valid option. These reverse branches may be useful also in cases of target vessels with severe upward orientation (Fig. 22.5).

The Gore TAMBE off-the-shelf branched endograft (W.L. Gore & Associates, Flagstaff, Az, USA) features four inner branches, two antegrade and two retrograde. This characteristic leaves more room between the stent graft and the ostia of target vessels, possibly making catheterization maneuvers easier and expanding the applicability of branched stent grafts for TAAA with small internal lumen. The staged deployment of this new design branched stent graft, consisting first in the opening of the proximal and distal endpoints and then of the visceral docking area, may allow a full catheterization of the four target vessels before the complete expansion of the branched stent graft. The four inner branches,

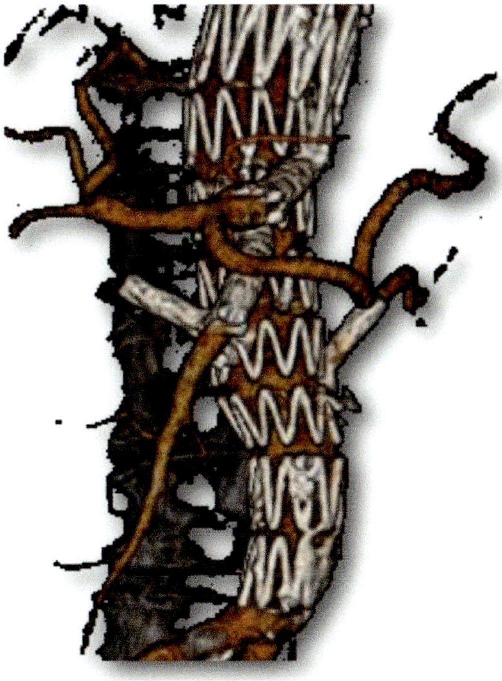

Fig. 22.5 Custom-made stent graft for type III TAAA with two branches for celiac artery and superior mesenteric artery and two fenestrations for cranially oriented renal arteries

two antegrade for CA and SMA and two retrograde for renal arteries, are pre-cannulated with two through-and-through catheters, allowing the catheterization of the four target vessels (CA and SMA from above and renals from below) with the branched stent graft still partially constricted.

The graft has only been used in very few cases, and all these features need to be tested in a reasonable number of patients.

A fenestrated stent graft is custom-made to fit patient anatomy in terms of length, number, and position of fenestrations. In cases of extensive aortic disease, proximal tubular components may be needed. There are two types of fenestrations that can be manufactured in the fenestrated component, including small and large fenestrations. Small fenestrations have dimensions of 6 × 6 mm or 6 × 8 mm. Large fenestrations measure 8–12 mm in diameter. A nitinol ring reinforces all fenestrations.

Contraindications to the use of fenestrated devices often relate to the angulation of visceral aorta and the possible severe internal lumen narrowing, as sometimes happens at renal artery removal. The choice of a fenestrated stent graft in these conditions may result in a twisting during the deployment with unpredictable misalignment of the fenestrations and dramatic consequences on target vessel reperfusion. The presence of a previous surgical infrarenal graft may limit the ability to adjust the stent graft position during and after the deployment. For this reason, single or double diameter-reducing ties are usually placed along the posterior aspect of fenestrated stent grafts in order to limit the initial expansion of the graft after sheath withdrawal, thereby reducing the device profile and increasing longitudinal and axial maneuverability.

22.2.3 Access Vessels

In the planning path of TAAA endovascular repair, once the proximal landing zone has been identified and branched/fenestrated feasibility established, ascertaining suitable access vessels is the final hurdle for endovascular applicability. Whereas hydrophilic sheaths have reduced trauma to iliofemoral axes, the inadequate size of the access vessels, especially in women or calcified and tortuous arteries, may represent a contraindication for TAAA endovascular treatment. The passage of large-caliber devices precludes safe transfemoral TEVAR in up to 30% of patients [23]. In some cases, an iliac or aortic conduit may be needed, increasing the risk of hemorrhage and hemodynamic instability and possibly leading to increased mortality and morbidity, including SCI. Published series of TEVAR report a 9–22% incidence of access vessel complications, contributing to perioperative morbidity in patients who are often elderly and fragile [24–26].

Arnaoutakis et al. reported the outcomes of TEVAR procedures from the American College of Surgeons National Surgical Quality Improvement Program database. A total of 649 patients were evaluated in this report. The 279 women who were included were more likely to require iliac artery access when compared with men (18% vs

7%; $P < 0.001$), and this alternative approach was identified as an independent predictor of 30-day mortality (relative risk, 4.42; 95% confidence interval, 2.07–9.44; $P < 0.001$) [27]. In a series of 164 patients, as reported by Lee et al., an iliac conduit resulted in a 2.6-fold increase in blood loss, 82% longer procedure time, 1.5 additional hospitalization days, and a 1.8-fold higher rate of perioperative complications [28]. Current limitations in TEVAR have recently been addressed with new design, low-profile thoracic stent grafts. Melissano and co-authors reported their initial experience with the Cook Alpha low-profile thoracic stent graft (Cook Medical, Bloomington, Ind, USA) in 42 patients with descending thoracic aortic disease. In this series, including 11 patients with concomitant aortoiliac occlusive disease (TransAtlantic Inter-Society Consensus type B and C), technical success in terms of safe and effective deployment of the thoracic stent graft was 100%, and no access-related complications were recorded. Furthermore, in patients with associated aortoiliac disease, no adjunctive procedures for device insertion, except for predilation with balloon angioplasty in two cases, were required [29].

Although the graft material alterations employed to achieve lower profile could theoretically lead to limited durability, mid-term results seem to be promising. In a series of 70 consecutive patients treated with the Zenith Alpha stent graft published by Torsello and co-workers, just three cases of type Ia endoleak (4.3%), two cases of type Ib endoleak (2.9%), and one case of aneurysm sac enlargement (1.4%) were recorded at a follow-up period of 22.3 ± 15.9 months. Re-intervention was necessary in only one case (1.4%) and no stent fracture was reported in this study group [30].

Low-profile technology was soon applied to multibranched thoracoabdominal devices (Fig. 22.6). Ramanan et al. published a comparative study on 134 pararenal or TAAA treated with standard (97) and low-profile (37) multibranched stent graft. Main outcomes were similar between the two groups. However, a combined outcome of conduit use or access artery injury occurred at a lower rate in the low-profile than in the standard-profile group (16% vs 36%; $P = 0.03$). Furthermore, women experienced significantly higher rates of conduit use and access artery injury than men after repair with standard-profile (64% vs 26%, respectively; $P = 0.001$) but similar rates after repair with low-profile branched stent graft (25% vs 14%, respectively; $P = 0.45$) [31].

The possibility of today applying total endovascular solutions for TAAA with devices loaded onto introducing sheath of 18–20 F in outer diameters makes the percutaneous approach particularly appealing. Although the use of percutaneous technique for TAAA endovascular repair is still debated, this approach is theoretically associated with lower blood loss from the groins, contributing to a more stable hemodynamic status of the patient during the entire procedure. Furthermore, sheath withdrawal from the iliac arteries immediately after deploying the aortic device and before bridging the visceral vessels, with consequent early restoration of blood flow to the pelvis and lower limbs, has proven to be effective in terms of SCI prevention [32].

de Souza et al. reported a 95% of technical success for total percutaneous endovascular aortic repair for thoracic, fenestrated, and branched stent grafts. In this series of 170 femoral arteries approached with ≥20-F-diameter sheaths, access-related complications occurred in 5% of cases within 30 days, and no late access-related events were reported [33].

22.3 Outcome Evaluation

22.3.1 Open Repair

Open repair of TAAAs is still associated with high rates of postoperative mortality and morbidity. Studies on national data report mortality rates as high as 20% after open surgical repair [8, 34], whereas large single-institution reviews report mortality rates as low as 5–8% [35–37]. Although increasing surgical and hospital volume have been associated with improved outcomes after open surgical repair, postoperative complications remain common and include

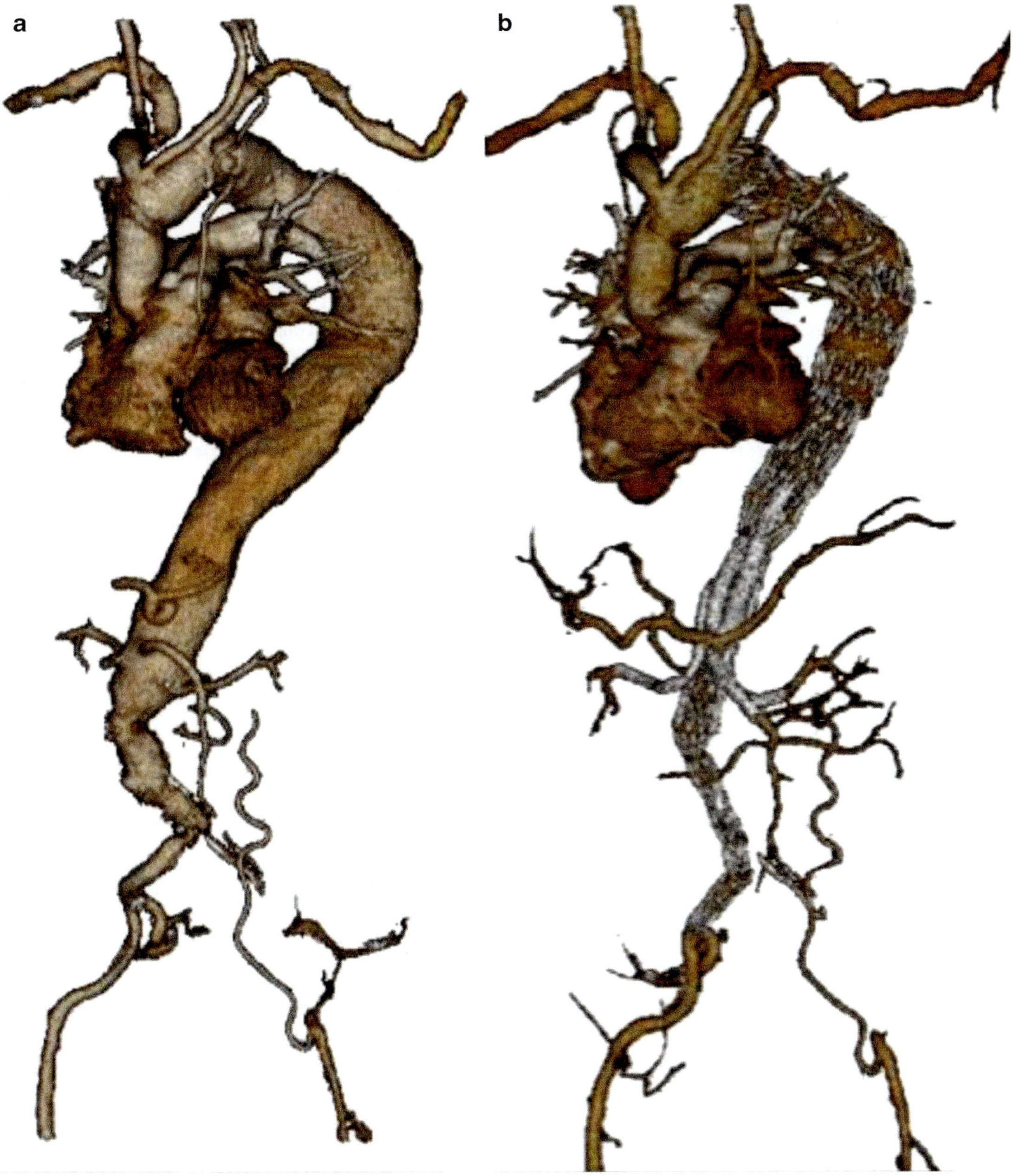

Fig. 22.6 Type II TAAA (**a**) treated with low-profile multibranched stent graft and aorto-uni-iliac distal extension for concomitant left iliac axis chronic occlusion (**b**)

pulmonary, cardiac, and renal complications, as well as spinal cord ischemia (SCI). Perioperative management of patients undergoing TAAA surgery has evolved substantially during the past two decades, resulting in improved early survival and decreased morbidity. The fact that the results are influenced by the caseload was already evident from historical reports like that by Svensson et al. on Houston's experience. In this series of 1509 patients undergoing TAAA open repair from 1960 to 1991, the reported 30-day mortality and SCI rates were 8% and 16%, respectively

[37]. As there is no support from current strategies on organ protection, these values must be considered more than acceptable. Over the last few years, a variety of operative approaches and protective adjuncts have been introduced to minimize organ dysfunction and, in particular, SCI. Conrad et al. reported on 445 consecutive TAAA open repairs with 30-day mortality of 8.2%, with a SCI of any severity of 13.2%, of which 9.5% sustained permanent paraplegia. Predictors of SCI included extent I/II aneurysms, epidural cooling, urgent/emergent operation, intraoperative hypotension, total aortic cross-clamp time, and postoperative pulmonary complications. Late survival rates in this series were 54.4%, 28.7%, and 20.5% at 5, 10, and 15 years, respectively [35]. Coselli et al. in one of the largest published series reported 30-day mortality, SCI, and renal failure requiring hemodialysis of 5%, 3.8%, and 5.6%, respectively. Intraprocedural adjuncts used were segmental arteries reattachment in 61.3% of patients, cerebral spinal fluid drainage in 26.9%, and left heart circulatory support in 39.8% [36].

Data from the National Surgical Quality Improvement Program on 450 patients undergoing TAAA open repair showed a 30-day mortality and morbidity rate of 10% and 51.6%, respectively. Pulmonary complications were the most common, occurring in 45.1% of patients. Cardiac complications were observed in 6.4% of cases. Renal failure requiring hemodialysis occurred in 10.7% of patients, while neurologic complications were more common in emergent than in elective cases (12.5% vs 1.4%; $p = 0.003$) [38]. Many advances have been done also in techniques for renal protection during TAAA open repair. Tshomba et al., in a comparative study on 111 TAAA patients propensity matched according to the type of intraoperative renal perfusion, found that the use of Custodiol provided improved perioperative renal function compared with lactated Ringer's solution [39].

Despite these improvements, the management of patients affected by TAAA remains challenging, and subjects with comorbidities and extensive aneurysms remain at high risk for postoperative complications.

22.3.2 Endovascular Repair

22.3.2.1 FEVAR and BEVAR

Since the first case of branched stent graft for TAAA reported by Chuter et al. in 2001 [40], following the progressive diffusion of this technology worldwide, several case series have been published over the last few years with satisfactory results in terms of short-term mortality and morbidity. The less-invasive nature of the endovascular approach is intended to diminish the magnitude of the repair by limiting groin incisions, avoiding aortic cross-clamping, and minimizing perioperative end-organ ischemia, blood loss, fluid shifts, and injury to the cardiac and respiratory systems. However, there is no evidence of decreased incidence of SCI. Furthermore, late complications, such as endoleaks, stent fractures, or migration, unknown for open repair, can affect the long-term durability of endovascular treatment and should be balanced with the late complications and re-intervention occurring after open repair [35].

One of the largest experiences with endovascular treatment of TAAAs has been provided by the Cleveland Clinic on a series of 406 patients enrolled in a prospective study with 2-year follow-up data. Perioperative mortality was 12.5% for type I, 5.2% for type II or III, and 2.3% for type IV TAAA according to Crawford's classification. Symptoms of SCI were noted in 4.3% of the overall endovascular group (also including 227 AAAs in addition to the 406 TAAAs). Overall survival at 2 years was 70% for type I, 74% for types II and III, and 82% for type IV TAAA [41].

More recently, Eagleton and co-authors published a series of 354 high-risk patients, again from Cleveland Clinic, treated with FEVAR or BEVAR for type II and III TAAA. Thirty-day mortality occurred in 17 patients (4.8%), permanent signs of SCI were observed in 14 patients (4%), and renal failure requiring hemodialysis occurred in 10 (2.8%). Eighty endoleak repairs were performed in 67 patients from this series, including 55 branch-related endoleaks. At 36 months, freedom from aneurysm-related death was 91% (95% CI, 0.88–0.95), and freedom from all-cause mortality was 57% (95% CI,

0.50–0.63). The authors found that extent type II TAAA ($P < 0.01$), age ($P < 0.01$), and chronic obstructive pulmonary disease ($P < 0.05$) negatively affected survival [42].

There is evidence that continuous refinements with the endovascular technique based on accumulated experience have decreased risk of SCI after FEVAR and BEVAR. The French experience of 204 endovascular TAAA repairs using custom-made devices manufactured with branches and fenestrations from 2004 to 2013 reported favorable outcomes after the implementation of an innovative protocol since 2010 that included optimization of the device implantation technique (early restoration of arterial flow to the pelvis and lower limbs, staged approach) and the systematic application of the proactive spinal cord protective protocol. The authors found that the introduction of the new protocol allowed a significant decrease of SCI risk from 14.0% to 1.2% ($p < 0.01$) and a benefit in halving the 30-day mortality from 11.6% to 5.6%, even though it was not statistically relevant ($p = 0.09$). The benefit was particularly evident in reducing the rates of SCI after type I to type III TAAA ER (excluding type IV): 25.0% (6/24 patients) before the protocol and 2.1% (2/95 patients) after the protocol ($p < 0.01$) [32].

Data supporting that endovascular repair of TAAA has today reached a state of maturity with early results at least comparable with open surgery are reported also from Mayo Clinic. Oderich and his group reported a 30-day mortality of 4.3% for a group of 185 patients with TAAA, including mortality of 1.8% for extent IV and 8.2% for extent I to III ($P = 0.03$). The authors underlined that overall mortality decreased in the second half of their clinical experience from 7.5% to 1.2%. SCI occurred in two patients (1.8%) with type IV TAAA and four (3.2%) with extent I-III. At 5 years, primary patency of stented target vessels was 93% [43].

Similar results also came out of high-volume European centers [44].

Verhoeven et al. described the outcomes of 166 patients with TAAA treated with fenestrated or branched devices, reporting a perioperative mortality of 7.8% and SCI of 9% (of which 1.2% leading to permanent paraplegia) and an estimated survival at 1, 2, and 5 years of 83%, 78%, and 66%, respectively [45].

The same group showed one of the largest experiences with the use of fenestrated or branched devices in post-dissection TAAA. Oikonomou and colleagues described the outcome of 31 patients treated with FEVAR or BEVAR for aneurysmal degeneration of chronic dissection. Technical success was 93.5% and 30-day mortality 9.6%. No case of permanent paraplegia was reported, and the seven late deaths recorded in a mean follow-up of 17 months were all unrelated to aneurysms (Fig. 22.7) [46].

Some centers have published information about the durability of complex endovascular repair, especially with regard to re-intervention and branch-related events.

Reilly et al. described their experience with 81 patients who underwent repair with branched stent graft [47]. The overall mortality in this series was 6.2% over a mean follow-up of 21 months. The rate of SCI was 3.7%; however, paraparesis was observed in 20% of cases.

Intraoperative injury of target vessels occurred in 4.6% of branches, the majority of which were treated immediately, with only one requiring occlusion to treat bleeding. Over the course of follow-up, stenosis developed in five patients (renal branches in four and the SMA branch in one). Of the 81 patients, 4 demonstrated aneurysm enlargement. Two of these patients required intervention and extension of the stent graft. An additional ten patients required intervention for persistent endoleaks. Only two endoleaks developed after the 1-month CTA. In total, 32 patients underwent 42 re-interventions over 21 months.

In another publication focusing on the durability of FEVAR and BEVAR, the authors analyzed a cohort of 650 patients undergoing endovascular repair with combined branch and fenestrated devices [48]. The mean follow-up was 3 years (standard deviation = 2.3), and during the 9 years of maximum follow-up, secondary procedures were required for 6% of right renal artery, 5% of left renal artery, 0.6% of CA, and 4% of SMA branches. The need for re-intervention was bimodal but on average appeared at 237 days

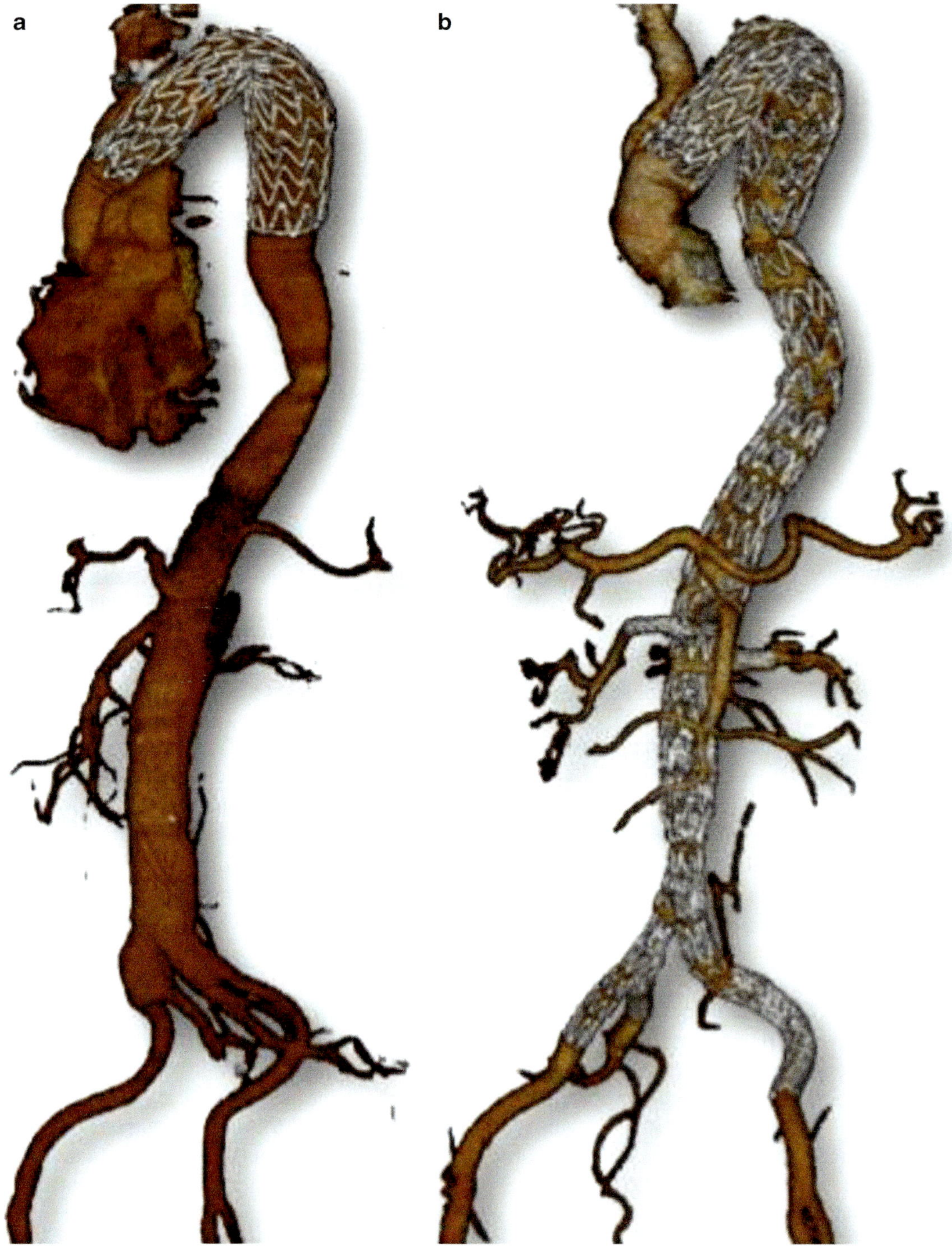

Fig. 22.7 Staged repair with custom-made fenestrated stent graft and iliac branch device (**b**) for post-dissection type II TAAA (**a**)

after index repair. Death from branch stent complications occurred in three patients, all involving the SMA.

The authors recommend that a composite outcome of branch instability, which includes branch occlusion, device migration affecting a branch, branch-related growth, and the need for any secondary intervention in a branch, is to the best metric to assess the durability of repair.

More recently, again from Cleveland Clinic, long-term outcomes of 1091 FEVAR/BEVAR patients were published. Non-risk-adjusted survival at 30 days, 1 year, and 5 years was 96.8%, 85.1%, and 46%, respectively. It is of interest that freedom from aneurysm-related death was 96.8%, 95.2%, and 94.0% at 30 days, 1, and 5 years, respectively. The authors also found that older age, heart failure, chronic obstructive pulmonary disease, renal disease, anemia, and coagulation disorders were risk factors for late mortality [49].

22.3.2.2 Parallel Endografting

Parallel stent grafts, including the chimney, snorkel, and sandwich techniques, are a proposed strategy for increasing the applicability of endovascular repair to aneurysms involving branch vessels. One major disadvantage of this strategy is the imperfect nature of the seal, which is inherent to having multiple side-by-side stent grafts. In fact, the major objection against a chimney-based procedure is the gutter (the channel between the parallel grafts), which can prevent immediate sealing and exclusion of the aneurysm. The sandwich technique was introduced to offer an endovascular off-the-shelf solution to patients with TAAA as an alternative to a custom-made device [50, 51]. Initially described in the treatment of aortoiliac disease, it combines the principles of a chimney graft with aneurysm exclusion by using several aortic stent grafts overlapped [52]. A chimney graft runs parallel to an aortic stent graft into the visceral or renal vessel, and there is a direct contact between the chimney graft and the aortic wall. The limitation in length of the chimney grafts does not permit endovascular exclusion of TAAA. In a sandwich procedure, the parallel stents run into the space created by two aortic stent grafts [53].

The first report about parallel endografting, published by Lobato et al., included patients with complex aortic aneurysm that did not fulfill the requirements for standard endovascular repair. They included patients with aortoiliac, TAAA, and aortic arch disease [50].

Schwierz et al., focusing on patients with TAAA, reported their experience on 104 chimney grafts implanted with sandwich technique in 32 patients with TAAA [54]. Indication for the procedure in 43% was an acute onset of symptoms, including two patients with a rupture and a retroperitoneal hematoma. Two patients died postoperatively because of the operation. Major adverse events were recorded in five patients, including one patient with persistent paraplegia and two with permanent renal failure requiring dialysis. The incidence of chimney graft occlusion was higher in patients with three or four parallel grafts than in those with two chimney grafts only. Patients with chronic dissections had a 12-times higher incidence of chimney graft occlusion than aneurysm patients. Type I or III endoleak was more common in the group with three or four parallel grafts [54]. Sandwich technique requires advanced endovascular techniques and imaging comparable to the deployment of any fenestrated or branched device. The presence and the size of the gutters between the chimney stents and the aortic stent grafts have always been an issue since the first publication of this technique. In a recent report, de Bruin et al. showed experimentally that balloon-expanding stents had larger gutters compared with self-expanding branches [55], and the compression of the main grafts increased with the size of the chimney grafts. Promising results were obtained in an experimental study with endostaples that were used to reduce the size of the gutters [56].

If the sandwich technique requires advanced endovascular techniques and imaging comparable to FEVAR and BEVAR on the one hand, it exposes patients to higher risk of endoleak on the other. For this reason, in our opinion, the use of this technique should not be routine, but reserved to those cases in which fenestrated or branched solutions are not available or definitely not applicable.

22.3.3 Open Versus Endovascular Repair

The decision about which therapy is appropriate for a particular patient is an evolving aspect of care of these complicated patients. Only three industry-sponsored trials comparing surgical and endovascular repair of thoracic aortic aneurysms were published [57–60], and no randomized, controlled prospective trial comparing open and endovascular TAAA repair exists. In addition, comparative studies including only pure TAAA are very few.

The largest series comparing open versus endovascular treatment for TAAA was published by Cleveland's group in 2008 [61]. A total of 372 patients were included in the OR group and 352 in the ER group. Patients treated with ER were on average 8.6 years older (71.3 ± 12 versus 62.7 ± 13 years, $p < 0.001$) than those treated with OR. In this study the 30-day mortality rate was 8.3% in OR and 5.7% in ER patients ($p = 0.2$) and 1-year mortality 15.9% and 15.6%, respectively ($p = 0.9$). SCI was detected in 15 ER patients (4.3%) and 28 OR patients (7.5%; log-rank $p = 0.08$), but at univariable and multivariable analysis, and after propensity score adjustment, the repair technique used was not associated with the presentation of SCI. In contrast, the extent of aneurysm repair was strongly associated with the development of SCI regardless of statistical adjustments. In both these groups, the occurrence of SCI was highest for type II aneurysms, followed by types I, III, and then IV. The severity of the SCI and the potential for recovery did not differ between treatment modalities. In their experience, the authors noted that SCI was more commonly observed immediately after OR (29% versus 13%) and in a delayed presentation (up to 6 days) after ER. A prior distal aortic operation results at the univariable analysis as a risk factor for the development of SCI ($p = 0.004$) in ER patients.

We recently published the results of a comparative analysis of outcome after OR and ER for patients with TAAA referred to three vascular centers from 2007 to 2014 [62]. Patients in the OR group were matched to patients in the ER group on the basis of propensity score. The model included all the baseline characteristics that were reliably measured and were clinically relevant in driving the endovascular or open treatment assignment. The aim of this method was to generate two groups of patients with correction of all differences in baseline characteristics. On the basis of our results, the 65 patients included in the ER and OR groups had similar rates of perioperative mortality (7.7% vs 6.2%) and renal complications (9.2% vs 12.3%). The incidence of SCI was 12.3% in the ER group and 20% in the OR group, a difference that was not statistically significant and disappeared when only rates of permanent paraplegia were considered (9.2% vs 10.8% in ER and OR, respectively). However, OR exposed the patients to a major overall morbidity burden as shown by the two times higher rate of a composite endpoint (including any SCI, renal and respiratory insufficiency) compared with the ER group: 36.9% vs 18.5% after ER and OR, respectively. Furthermore, as expected, the 30-day rate of respiratory insufficiency was significantly lower in ER (0% vs 12.3%; $p = 0.006$) [62]. These findings may help in selecting the open versus endovascular treatment for TAAA tailored to the single patient, specifically with regard to the effect of OR on respiratory function.

In our comparative study, at a median follow-up of 21.6 months, all-cause survival at 24 and 42 months was 82.8% in ER and 84.9% in OR ($p = 0.9$). No aorta-related late deaths occurred after ER, whereas one patient in the OR group died of sepsis secondary to an aortobronchial fistula. Freedom from re-intervention rates was 91.0% in ER vs 89.7% in OR at 24 months and 80.0% in ER vs 79.9% in OR ($p = 0.3$) at 42 months. Our data on re-interventions are partially in disagreement with previous studies showing uncertainty about the durability of ER and reporting a need for re-intervention as high as 26% at a mean follow-up of 2 years after the endovascular procedure for complex aortic disease even though most re-interventions were required for type III endoleak, similar to other reports [63–65]. This divergence may in part be explained by the inclusion, in the previous study, of both juxta-renal and thoracoabdominal aneurysms, causing differences in patient and anatomy selection.

The findings of our study should be interpreted with caution; propensity analysis did not allow a totally balanced comparison as by a randomized trial and resulted in a well-matched but small subset of TAAA patients. This may explain different findings reported by other studies. In a combined French and American institutional experience, the comparison of 147 open and 42 fenestrated repairs for juxta-renal aneurysms with propensity score matching showed unsatisfying results for the endovascular approach. Mortality (9.2% vs 2%; $p = 0.05$) and procedural complications (24% vs 7%; $p < 0.01$) were significantly higher in the endovascular than in the open repairs. Despite the fact that the comparison was focused on patients with juxta-renal aneurysms and TAAAs were excluded, reflecting less challenging diseases to be treated, the endovascular approach was independently associated with fivefold increased 30-day mortality risk (odds ratio, 5.1; 95% CI, 1.1–24; $p = 0.04$). These worse results with fenestrated devices may likely be explained by the older timing of the study ranging from 2001, reflecting the effect of developing training and techniques [66].

To encompass the variability of TAAA patients in the real world, we suggest that open and endovascular repair should not be offered at random, but it is more likely that the choice should be individualized to achieve the best outcomes in different patients. This message may be important also because fenestrated and branched stent grafts, although initially designed to treat only high-risk patients with complex aortic aneurysms, are today increasingly applied in average-risk patients as a less invasive alternative to open repair.

In conclusion, it is reasonable to state that TAAA repair is today performed with respectable results mainly in high-volume centers, regardless of the technique. Even though longer assessment is required to confirm the stability and durability of fenestrated and branched stent grafts, the reduced early morbidity associated with ER may have an impact on decision-making for older and high-risk as well as for young and lower-risk patients.

22.4 Conclusion

The myth of an entirely endovascular world for thoracoabdominal aortic disease should today be considered reality. The unbridled development of FEVAR and BEVAR and the incessant technique refinement, with combination of custom-made and off-the-shelf solutions, made endovascular repair widely applicable, with results at least comparable to a well-defined treatment like open surgery.

However, re-intervention rate after endovascular repair is not negligible. The issue of increased cost (initial cost of the stent grafts, multiple CT scans in follow-up, secondary procedures) will also need to be figured into the equation in considering which therapy is the most appropriate for a particular patient. Furthermore, late survival is poor but is caused mostly by nonaneurysm-related deaths, underlying the short life expectancy of a population of elderly patients with poor preoperative status.

With this in mind, it is today more clear that FEVAR and BEVAR should be further evaluated in low- to average-risk patients who will likely experience better long-term survival.

References

1. Mastracci TM, Greenberg RK. Complex aortic disease: changes in perception, evaluation and management. J Vasc Surg. 2008;48(Suppl 6):17S–23S. discussion 23S.
2. Cheng D, Martin J, Shennib H, et al. Endovascular aortic repair versus open surgical repair for descending thoracic aortic disease a systematic review and meta-analysis of comparative studies. J Am Coll Cardiol. 2010;55(10):986–1001.
3. Matsumura JS, Rizvi AZ, Society for Vascular Surgery. Left subclavian artery revascularization: Society for Vascular Surgery Practice Guidelines. J Vasc Surg. 2010;52(Suppl 4):65S–70S.
4. Patel HJ, Nguyen C, Diener AC, Passow MC, Salata D, Deeb GM. Open arch reconstruction in the endovascular era: analysis of 721 patients over 17 years. J Thorac Cardiovasc Surg. 2011;141:1417–23.
5. Iba Y, Minatoya K, Matsuda H, Sasaki H, Tanaka H, Kobayashi J, et al. Contemporary open aortic arch repair with selective cerebral perfusion in the era of endovascular aortic repair. J Thorac Cardiovasc Surg. 2013;145(3 Suppl):S72–7.

6. Thomas M, Li Z, Cook DJ, Greason KL, Sundt TM. Contemporary results of open aortic arch surgery. J Thorac Cardiovasc Surg. 2012;144:838–44.
7. Sachs T, Pomposelli F, Hagberg R, Hamdan A, Wyers M, Giles K, et al. Open and endovascular repair of type B aortic dissection in the Nationwide Inpatient Sample. J Vasc Surg. 2010;52:860–6.
8. Cowan JA, Dimick JB, Henke PK, Huber TS, Stanley JC, Upchurch GR. Surgical treatment of intact thoracoabdominal aortic aneurysms in the United States: hospital and surgeon volume-related outcomes. J Vasc Surg. 2003;37:1169–74.
9. Patel VI, Mukhopadhyay S, Ergul E, Aranson N, Conrad MF, Lamuraglia GM, et al. Impact of hospital volume and type on outcomes of open and endovascular repair of descending thoracic aneurysms in the United States Medicare population. J Vasc Surg. 2013;58:346–54.
10. Chikwe J, Cavallaro P, Itagaki S, Seigerman M, Diluozzo G, Adams DH. National outcomes in acute aortic dissection: influence of surgeon and institutional volume on operative mortality. Ann Thorac Surg. 2013;95:1563–9.
11. De Rango P, Cao P, Ferrer C, Simonte G, Coscarella C, Cieri E, et al. Aortic arch debranching and thoracic endovascular repair. J Vasc Surg. 2014;59: 107–14.
12. Haulon S, Greenberg RK, Spear R, Eagleton M, Abraham C, Lioupis C, et al. Global experience with an inner branched arch endograft. J Thorac Cardiovasc Surg. 2014;148:1709–16.
13. Spear R, Haulon S, Ohki T, Tsilimparis N, Kanaoka Y, Milne CP, Debus S, Takizawa R, Kölbel T. Subsequent results for arch aneurysm repair with inner branched endografts. Eur J Vasc Endovasc Surg. 2016;51:380–5.
14. Spear R, Clough RE, Fabre D, Roeder B, Hertault A, Martin Gonzalez T, Azzaoui R, Sobocinski J, Haulon S. Total endovascular treatment of aortic arch disease using an arch endograft with 3 inner branches. J Endovasc Ther. 2017;24(4):534–8.
15. Moulakakis KG, Mylonas SN, Dalainas I, Sfyroeras GS, Markatis F, Kotsis T, et al. The chimney-graft technique for preserving supra-aortic branches: a review. Ann Cardiothorac Surg. 2013;2(3):339–46.
16. McWilliams RG, Murphy M, Hartley D, et al. In situ stent graft fenestration to preserve the left subclavian artery. J Endovasc Ther. 2004;11:170–4.
17. Manning BJ, Ivancev K, Harris PL. In situ fenestration in the aortic arch. J Vasc Surg. 2010;52:491–4.
18. Redlinger RE, Ahanchi SS, Panneton JM. In situ laser fenestration during emergent thoracic endovascular aortic repair is an effective method for left subclavian artery revascularization. J Vasc Surg. 2013;58:1171–7.
19. Kasprzak PM, Kobuch R, Schmid C, Kopp R. Long-term durability of aortic arch in situ stent graft fenestration requiring lifelong surveillance. J Vasc Surg. 2017;65(2):538–41.
20. Bisdas T, Donas KP, Bosiers M, Torsello G, Austermann M. One-year follow-up after total endovascular repair of a contained-ruptured thoracoabdominal aortic aneurysm with the sandwich technique. J Vasc Surg. 2013;58:673–8.
21. Bisdas T, Donas KP, Bosiers M, Torsello G, Austermann M. Anatomical suitability of the t-branch stent graft in patients with thoracoabdominal aortic aneurysms treated using custom-made multibranched endografts. J Endovasc Ther. 2013;20:672–7.
22. Bisdas T, Donas KP, Bosiers MJ, Torsello G, Austermann M. Custom-made versus off-the-shelf multibranched endografts for endovascular repair of thoracoabdominal aortic aneurysms. J Vasc Surg. 2014;60:1186–95.
23. Criado FJ, McKendrick C, Criado FR. Technical solutions for common problems in TEVAR: managing access and aortic branches. J Endovasc Ther. 2009;16(suppl 1):I63–79.
24. Rockman C. Reducing complications by better case selection: anatomic considerations. Semin Vasc Surg. 2004;17:298–306.
25. Garcia-Toca M, Eskandari MK. Regulatory TEVAR clinical trials. J Vasc Surg. 2010;52(4 suppl):22S–5S.
26. Fernandez JD, Craig JM, Garrett HE Jr, et al. Endovascular management of iliac rupture during endovascular aneurysm repair. J Vasc Surg. 2009;50:1293–300.
27. Arnaoutakis GJ, Schneider EB, Arnaoutakis DJ, et al. Influence of gender on outcomes after thoracic endovascular aneurysm repair. J Vasc Surg. 2014;59:45–51.
28. Lee WA, Berceli SA, Huber TS, et al. Morbidity with retroperitoneal procedures during endovascular abdominal aortic aneurysm repair. J Vasc Surg. 2003;38:459–63. discussion 464–5.
29. Melissano G, Tshomba Y, Rinaldi E, Chiesa R. Initial clinical experience with a new low-profile thoracic endograft. J Vasc Surg. 2015;62(2):336–42. https://doi.org/10.1016/j.jvs.2015.02.049.
30. Torsello GF, Inchingolo M, Austermann M, Torsello GB, Panuccio G, Bisdas T. Durability of a low-profile stent graft for thoracic endovascular aneurysm repair. J Vasc Surg. 2017;66(6):1638–43.
31. Ramanan B, Fernandez CC, Sobel JD, Gasper WJ, Vartanian SM, Reilly LM, Chuter TA, Hiramoto JS. Low-profile versus standard-profile multibranched thoracoabdominal aortic stent grafts. J Vasc Surg. 2016;64(1):39–45.
32. Maurel B, Delclaux N, Sobocinski J, Hertault A, Martin-Gonzalez T, Moussa M, Spear R, Le Roux M, Azzaoui R, Tyrrell M, Haulon S. The impact of early pelvic and lower limb reperfusion and attentive perioperative management on the incidence of spinal cord ischemia during thoracoabdominal aortic aneurysm endovascular repair. Eur J Vasc Endovasc Surg. 2015;49(3):248–54.
33. de Souza LR, Oderich GS, Banga PV, Hofer JM, Wigham JR, Cha S, Gloviczki P. Outcomes of total percutaneous endovascular aortic repair for thoracic, fenestrated, and branched endografts. J Vasc Surg. 2015;62(6):1442.e3–9.e3.

34. Derrow AE, Seeger JM, Dame DA, Carter RL, Ozaki CK, Flynn TC, Huber TS. The outcome in the United States after thoracoabdominal aortic aneurysm repair, renal artery bypass, and mesenteric revascularization. J Vasc Surg. 2001;34(1):54–61.
35. Conrad MF, Crawford RS, Davison JK, Cambria RP. Thoracoabdominal aneurysm repair: a 20-year perspective. Ann Thorac Surg. 2007;83(2):S856–61. discussion S890–2.
36. Coselli JS, Bozinovski J, LeMaire SA. Open surgical repair of 2286 thoracoabdominal aortic aneurysms. Ann Thorac Surg. 2007;83(2):S862–4. discussion S890–2.
37. Svensson LG, Crawford ES, Hess KR, Coselli JS, Safi HJ. Experience with 1509 patients undergoing thoracoabdominal aortic operations. J Vasc Surg. 1993;17(2):357–68. discussion 368–70.
38. Bensley RP, Curran T, Hurks R, Lo RC, Wyers MC, Hamdan AD, Chaikof EL, Schermerhorn ML. Open repair of intact thoracoabdominal aortic aneurysms in the American College of Surgeons National Surgical Quality Improvement Program. J Vasc Surg. 2013;58(4):894–900.
39. Tshomba Y, Kahlberg A, Melissano G, Coppi G, Marone E, Ferrari D, Lembo R, Chiesa R. Comparison of renal perfusion solutions during thoracoabdominal aortic aneurysm repair. J Vasc Surg. 2014;59(3):623–33.
40. Chuter TA, Gordon RL, Reilly LM, Goodman JD, Messina LM. An endovascular system for thoracoabdominal aortic aneurysm repair. J EndovascTher. 2001;8(1):25–33.
41. Greenberg R, Eagleton M, Mastracci T. Branched endografts for thoracoabdominal aneurysms. J Thorac Cardiovasc Surg. 2010;140(6 Suppl):S171–8.
42. Eagleton MJ, Follansbee M, Wolski K, Mastracci T, Kuramochi Y. Fenestrated and branched endovascular aneurysm repair outcomes for type II and III thoracoabdominal aortic aneurysms. J Vasc Surg. 2016;63(4):930–42.
43. Oderich GS, Ribeiro M, Reis de Souza L, Hofer J, Wigham J, Cha S. Endovascular repair of thoracoabdominal aortic aneurysms using fenestrated and branched endografts. J Thorac Cardiovasc Surg. 2017;153(2):S32.e7–41.e7.
44. Verzini F, Loschi D, De Rango P, Ferrer C, Simonte G, Coscarella C, Pogany G, Cao P. Current results of total endovascular repair of thoracoabdominal aortic aneurysms. J Cardiovasc Surg. 2014;55:9–19.
45. Verhoeven EL, Katsargyris A, Bekkema F, Oikonomou K, Zeebregts CJ, Ritter W, Tielliu IF. Ten-year experience with endovascular repair of thoracoabdominal aortic aneurysms: results from 166 consecutive patients. Eur J Vasc Endovasc Surg. 2015;49(5):524–31.
46. Oikonomou K, Kopp R, Katsargyris A, Pfister K, Verhoeven EL, Kasprzak P. Outcomes of fenestrated/branched endografting in post-dissection thoracoabdominal aortic aneurysms. Eur J Vasc Endovasc Surg. 2014;48(6):641–8.
47. Reilly LM, Rapp JH, Grenon SM, Hiramoto JS, Sobel J, Chuter TA. Efficacy and durability of endovascular thoracoabdominal aortic aneurysm repair using the caudally directed cuff technique. J Vasc Surg. 2012;56(1):53–63. discussion 63–4.
48. Mastracci TM, Greenberg RK, Eagleton MJ, Hernandez AV. Durability of branches in branched and fenestrated endografts. J Vasc Surg. 2013;57(4):926–33. https://doi.org/10.1016/j.jvs.2012.09.071.
49. Beach JM, Rajeswaran J, Parodi FE, Kuramochi Y, Brier C, Blackstone E, Eagleton MJ. Survival affects decision making for fenestrated and branched endovascular aortic repair. J Vasc Surg. 2017;67(3):722.e8–34.e8.
50. Lobato AC, Camacho-Lobato L. Endovascular treatment of complex aortic aneurysms using the sandwich technique. J Endovasc Ther. 2012;19: 691–706.
51. Lobato AC. Sandwich technique for aortoiliac aneurysms extending to the internal iliac artery or isolated common/internal iliac artery aneurysms: a new endovascular approach to preserve pelvic circulation. J Endovasc Ther. 2011;18:106–11.
52. Yoshida R, Yoshida WB, Kolvenbach R, Vieira PR. Modified "stent-graft sandwich" technique for treatment of isolated common iliac artery aneurysm in patient with Marfan syndrome. Ann Vasc Surg. 2012;26:419.
53. Kolvenbach RR, Yoshida R, Pinter L, Zhu Y, Lin F. Urgent endovascular treatment of thoraco-abdominal aneurysms using a sandwich technique and chimney graftsda technical description. Eur J Vasc Endovasc Surg. 2011;41:54–60.
54. Schwierz E, Kolvenbach RR, Yoshida R, Yoshida W. Experience with the sandwich technique in endovascular thoraco- abdominal aortic aneurysm repair. J Vasc Surg. 2014;59:1562e9.
55. de Bruin JL, Yeung KK, Niepoth WW, Lely RJ, Cheung Q, de Vries A, et al. Geometric study of various chimney graft configurations in an in vitro juxtarenal aneurysm model. J Endovasc Ther. 2013;20:184–90.
56. Niepoth WW, de Bruin JL, Yeung KK, Lely RJ, Devrome AN, Wisselink W, et al. A proof-of-concept in vitro study to determine if EndoAnchors can reduce gutter size in chimney graft configurations. J Endovasc Ther. 2013;20:498–505.
57. Makaroun MS, Dillavou ED, Kee ST, Sicard G, Chaikof E, Bavaria J, Williams D, Cambria RP, Mitchell RS. Endovascular treatment of thoracic aortic aneurysms: results of the phase II multicenter trial of the GORE TAG thoracic endoprosthesis. J Vasc Surg. 2005;41(1):1–9.
58. Bavaria JE, Appoo JJ, Makaroun MS, Verter J, Yu ZF, Mitchell RS, Gore TAG Investigators. Endovascular stent grafting versus open surgical repair of descending thoracic aortic aneurysms in low-risk patients: a multicenter comparative trial. J Thorac Cardiovasc Surg. 2007;133(2):369–77.

59. Matsumura JS, Cambria RP, Dake MD, Moore RD, Svensson LG, Snyder S, TX2 Clinical Trial Investigators. International controlled clinical trial of thoracic endovascular aneurysm repair with the Zenith TX2 endovascular graft: 1-year results. J Vasc Surg. 2008;47(2):247–57. discussion 257.
60. Fairman RM, Criado F, Farber M, Kwolek C, Mehta M, White R, Lee A, Tuchek JM, VALOR Investigators. Pivotal results of the medtronic vascular talent thoracic stent graft system: the VALOR trial. J Vasc Surg. 2008;48(3):546–54.
61. Greenberg RK, Lu Q, Roselli EE, Svensson LG, Moon MC, Hernandez AV, Dowdall J, Cury M, Francis C, Pfaff K, Clair DG, Ouriel K, Lytle BW. Contemporary analysis of descending thoracic and thoracoabdominal aneurysm repair: a comparison of endovascular and open techniques. Circulation. 2008;118(8):808–17. https://doi.org/10.1161/CIRCULATIONAHA.108.769695.
62. Ferrer C, Cao P, De Rango P, Tshoma Y, Verzini F, Melissano G, et al. A propensity-matched comparison for endovascular and open repair of thoracoabdominal aortic aneurysms. J Vasc Surg. 2016;63:1201e7.
63. Austermann M, Donas KP, Panuccio G, Troisi N, Torsello G. Pararenal and thoracoabdominal aortic aneurysm repair with fenestrated and branched endografts: lessons learned and future directions. J Endovasc Ther. 2011;18:157–60.
64. Haulon S, Greenberg RK. Part two: treatment of type IV thoracoabdominal aneurysmsd fenestrated stent-graft repair is now the best option. Eur J Vasc Endovasc Surg. 2011;42:4–8.
65. Troisi N, Donas KP, Austermann M, Tessarek J, Umscheid T, Torsello G. Secondary procedures after aortic aneurysm repair with fenestrated and branched endografts. J Endovasc Ther. 2011;18:146–53.
66. Raux M, Patel VI, Cochennec F, Mukhopadhyay S, Desgranges P, Cambria RP, et al. A propensity-matched comparison of outcomes for fenestrated endovascular aneurysm repair and open surgical repair of complex abdominal aortic aneurysms. J Vasc Surg. 2014;60:858–63.

23 Total Endovascular Repair of Thoracoabdominal Aortic Aneurysm: Lessons Learned

D. Loschi, B. Fiorucci, T. Cambiaghi, E. Centonza, and F. Verzini

23.1 The Origins of Total Endovascular Repair of Complex Aortic Aneurysms

Fenestrated endovascular aneurysm repair (fEVAR) has been introduced into the clinical practice to treat patients with abdominal aortic aneurysms (AAAs) with inadequate infrarenal neck, where visceral vessels need to be included in the endovascular reconstruction. The first fenestrated repair has been described by Park in 1996 using a device modification to incorporate an accessory renal artery, in a patient with infrarenal aortic aneurysm [1]. Since these pioneeristic experiences, the technique has dramatically evolved over time. The main body of the endograft was improved after bifurcated endografts for the endovascular treatment of AAAs were proposed in the late 1990s by Stelter and afterward widely adopted. The success of these experiences led to the development of a tubular upper module associated to a separate distal bifurcated component, similar to the contemporary unibody, to treat inadequate aortic necks. Gold radiopaque markers were added to highlight fenestration margins under fluoroscopy and facilitate identification and alignment of the fenestrations with their respective target vessels. The openings in the graft material were reinforced with nitinol rings around the fenestrations to create a more stable and durable connection with the stent. To facilitate endograft alignment, diameter-reducing ties were added to partially constrain the graft following unsheathing, to avoid adhesion of the graft to the aortic wall and allow rotation of the device along the vertical axis and movement to a more proximal/distal level.

Also covered stents available for bridging of visceral arteries have been significantly upgraded to improve stability within fenestrations and avoid endoleaks which could occur between the aortic wall and the fenestrated endograft. Anderson et al. published in 2001 a case series of 13 patients treated by means of fEVAR with implantation of balloon-expandable stents for the superior mesenteric artery (SMA) and renal arteries [2]. Technical success was achieved in all cases and no conversion to open surgery was needed. This permitted to demonstrate the feasibility and safety of a fenestrated endograft design to achieve adequate proximal sealing in case of inadequate neck.

With the increasing expertise and with developments of new technologies, more and

D. Loschi · T. Cambiaghi
Division of Vascular Surgery, IRCCS San Raffaele Scientific Institute, Milan, Italy

B. Fiorucci · E. Centonza
Unit of Vascular and Endovascular Surgery, Hospital S. M. Misericordia, University of Perugia, Perugia, Italy

F. Verzini (✉)
Vascular Surgery Unit, Department of Surgical Sciences, Turin University, A.O.U. Città della Salute e della Scienza, Molinette Hospital, Turin, Italy

© Springer Nature Switzerland AG 2019
Y. Tshomba et al. (eds.), *Visceral Vessels and Aortic Repair*,
https://doi.org/10.1007/978-3-319-94761-7_23

more proximal segments of the aorta have been involved in the reconstruction with management of all visceral vessels in the treatment of thoracoabdominal aneurysms (TAAAs). Nevertheless, TAAAs with a large lumen at the level of visceral arteries would require long bridging stents in fenestrated designs, which could impair stability and long-term patency. For this reason, multibranched devices (branched endovascular repair, bEVAR) have been developed. The first experience with a multibranched endograft has been reported by Chuter in 2001, who implanted in a TAAA an on-table-modified four-vessel-branched endograft [3]. bEVAR designs consist of a tubular endograft with downward-oriented side branches to be extended into visceral vessels with self-expanding stents. The branches need to be accessed from an upper extremity access, either the axillary or the brachial artery.

23.2 Current Endografts

23.2.1 Custom-Made Grafts

Several endograft designs have been proposed by different companies for the management of thoracoabdominal aneurysms. Whenever construction time is not an issue (i.e., elective repairs), most operators rely on custom-made devices (CMDs): just like physician-modified grafts were created to fit patient anatomy, CMDs are designed and built based on aneurysm morphology (aortic neck diameters, lengths, and especially visceral vessel origin and orientation) identified at preoperative CT angiography.

The currently available custom-made endograft is commercialized by Cook (Zenith Fenestrated), Vascutek (Fenestrated Anaconda), and Jotec (E-Xtra Design).

23.2.1.1 Cook Zenith Fenestrated

Intro: The Cook Zenith custom-made fenestrated and branched endografts have been introduced in the European market in 2005 [4]. The whole device consists of a proximal main component with scallops, fenestrations, and/or branches for the visceral vessels, to be completed by a distal bifurcated component (and related iliac limb). The proximal portion of the main component has a bare metal stent for proximal fixation and one or two Z-stents long (27–54 mm) sealing component (Ø 24–36 mm) tapering distally to a diameter of 22 mm to achieve sealing with the 24 mm distal bifurcated component.

Regardless of the branched/fenestrated design, the graft includes gold markers at the proximal edge of the fabric, a check/tick marker (✔) to assess anteroposterior orientation, and three anterior vertical markers which combined to three posterior horizontal markers aid in identifying correct rotation with respect to C-arm position (Fig. 23.1). Each fenestration is identified by four radiopaque markers, at the top, bottom, and both sides of the opening. The branches instead have three markers on the proximal por-

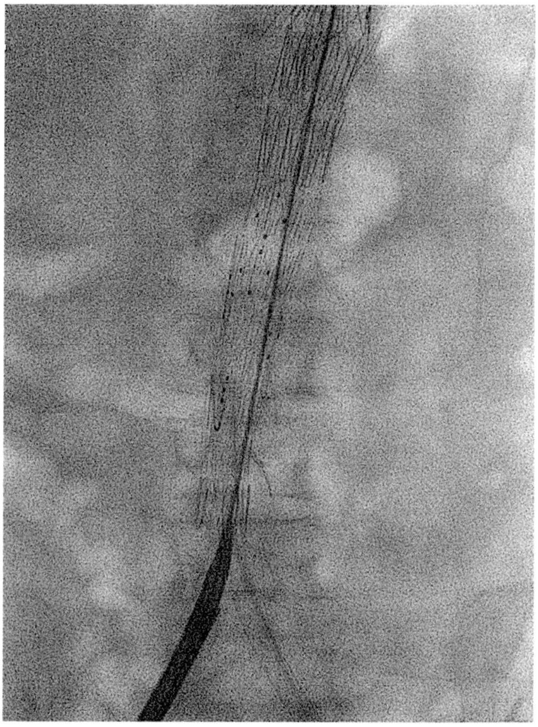

Fig. 23.1 Intraoperative fluoroscopy demonstrating the markers of a fenestrated EVAR. Fenestrations are shown through four small gold markers. Gold markers at the proximal edge of the fabric, a check/tick marker at the distal edge to assess anteroposterior orientation, and three anterior vertical markers combined to three posterior horizontal markers are used to identify correct orientation of the graft

tion, on the inner side (closer to main graft fabric), and two markers at the distal end on the outer side (closer to the aortic wall).

Small fenestrations (6 × 6 mm and 6 × 8 mm), because of constructional constraints, need to be placed at least 15 mm lower than the proximal edge of the fabric, while large fenestrations can be designed >10 mm from the edge. On the European market, all fenestrations are reinforced and without struts crossing the opening (contrary from the US FDA-approved version).

The novel helical branches were proposed to increase mating length with the bridging stents and provide less sharp entry angles into the visceral vessels, while inner branches can be designed to deal with small residual aortic lumen (i.e., dissection or thrombotic wall apposition) when fenestrations are not preferred (Fig. 23.2).

In patients with a renal artery arising too close to the aortic bifurcation (e.g., prior EVAR or aortoiliac graft), a distal bifurcated component with an inverted iliac limb can be requested in order to deploy it lower onto the bifurcation.

Manufacturer: Cook Medical Inc., Bloomington, IN

Platform: Zenith Flex

Stent material: self-expanding stainless steel

Graft material: woven polyester

Available designs: downward/upward branches (Ø 6 mm and 8 mm, 18/21 mm long), fenestrations (Ø 6 × 6 mm, 6 × 8 mm, 8 × 8 mm, 10 × 10 mm, 12 × 12 mm), scallops (10 mm wide, 6–12 deep), helical branches, and inner branches

Application: thoracoabdominal, pararenal, and juxtarenal aneurysms

Available diameters: 24–36 mm

Delivery system diameter: 20 Fr (up to 34 mm Ø) and 22 Fr (36 mm Ø)

Peculiarities: diameter-reducing ties (single, double), preloaded catheters/sheaths, and free-flow

Limitations: construction time 4–6 weeks

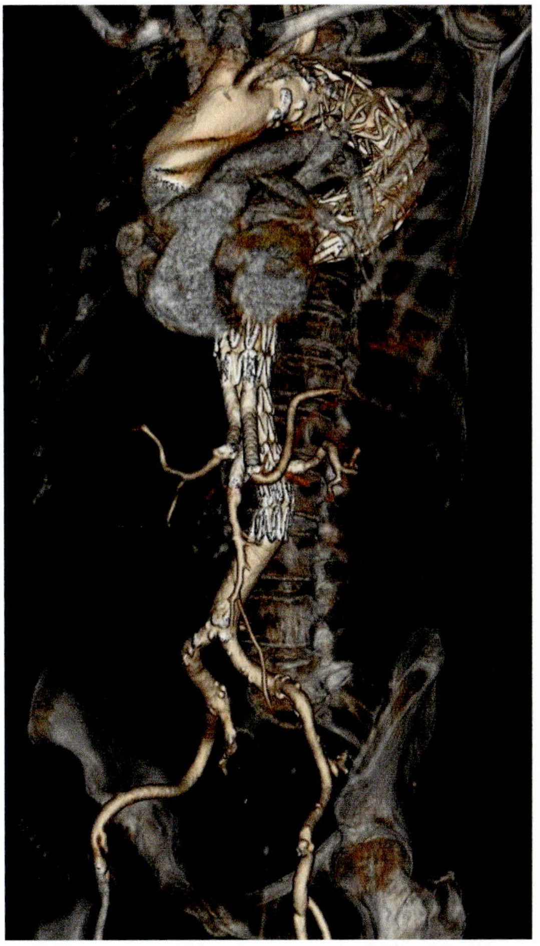

Fig. 23.2 Postoperative computed tomography angiography (CTA) of a patient treated with a combined fenestrated and branched endograft for a thoracoabdominal aneurysm

23.2.1.2 Vascutek Fenestrated Anaconda

Intro: The Fenestrated Anaconda endograft was released on the market in 2011 and is significantly different from other available grafts in many aspects. The bifurcated nature of this graft requires completion only by iliac extensions, but the lack of dedicated proximal thoracic components limits its application in extensive thoracoabdominal aneurysms since its sealing within currently available thoracic endografts has been reported to be suboptimal.

Manufacturer: Vascutek, Renfrewshire, Scotland

Platform: Anaconda AAA

Stent material: nitinol

Graft material: woven polyester

Available designs: fenestrations and augmented valley (comparable to a scallop)

Application: extent IV TAAA and pararenal and juxtarenal aneurysm

Available diameters: up to 34 mm

Delivery system diameter: 20–23 Fr

Peculiarities: repositionable, flexible (no supporting metal stents), no top cap (facilitates access from the upper extremities), magnetic iliac gate cannulation, and case rehearsal with 3D model and prototype

Restrictions: lack of dedicated proximal thoracic component for management of extensive thoracoabdominal aneurysms and construction time 3 weeks

The key characteristic of the graft is the lack of metal stents along the middle portion, where fenestrations are located, which confers extreme flexibility and conformability to tortuous anatomies and, we can assume, would be more forgiving in case of misalignment between fenestration and target ostium.

Proximal sealing is achieved by two circular nitinol rings, which can be collapsed after deployment to allow complete repositioning of the device at any stage before bridging of the visceral vessels.

The "fish-mouth" shape of the proximal component can be exploited to include an additional vessel as its valley can be employed as a scallop (Fig. 23.3).

The Anaconda graft has no top cap (i.e., Cook free-flow), and this can facilitate cannulation from an upper extremity access.

Lastly, the Vascutek Fenestrated Anaconda graft kept the magnetic cannulation tool present in the AAA device, facilitating access to the iliac gate and easing the challenge to access the fenestration from a femoral access which could be presented by the fixed bifurcated design (when compared to other straight tubular grafts).

23.2.1.3 Jotec E-Xtra Design Engineering

Intro: The Jotec E-Xtra Design Engineering graft has a tubular main body with branches/fenestrations placed in the middle portion which is tapered down to a diameter of 16 mm and then re-expands to provide sealing to a bifurcated component, if needed.

Manufacturer: Jotec, Hechingen, Germany

Platform: E-vita thoracic 3G

Stent material: nitinol

Graft material: woven polyester

Available designs: fenestrations, scallops, and branches

Application: thoracoabdominal, pararenal, and juxtarenal aneurysms

Available diameters: 24–40 mm

Delivery system diameter: 22–24 Fr

Peculiarities: E markers

Restrictions: construction time 18 days

Fenestrations are reinforced as for the Cook graft and have a diameter ranging from 6 to 12 mm, while branches have a diameter of 6–10 mm.

The anterior portion of the graft presents four "E" markers which, just like the Cook check/tick marker, provide information on anteroposterior position of the graft and its eventual rotation.

23.2.2 Off-the-Shelf Grafts

Urgent procedure seemed to be a limitation to total endovascular repair, but the introduction into the market of off-the-shelf devices has recently permitted to adopt this technique also in urgent cases.

23.2.2.1 Cook p-Branch

Intro: The p-branch was designed to manage juxtarenal aneurysms. This graft has a supraceliac fixation with a single bare steel stent, followed by one scallop for the celiac trunk, one 8-mm fenestration for the SMA, and two conical renal artery pivot fenestrations. Preloaded wires are present through both renal fenestrations. Immediately distal to the renal fenestrations, a tapered bridging stent reduces the diameter of the device to 24 mm to facilitate mating with a universal distal bifurcated body. Single diameter-reducing ties are present. Two different renal configurations are available, one with both fenestrations arising at the same height (configuration A) and one with the left renal artery (LRA) fenestration 4 mm lower than the right renal artery (RRA) fenestration (configuration B). The device is deployed through a 20-French system.

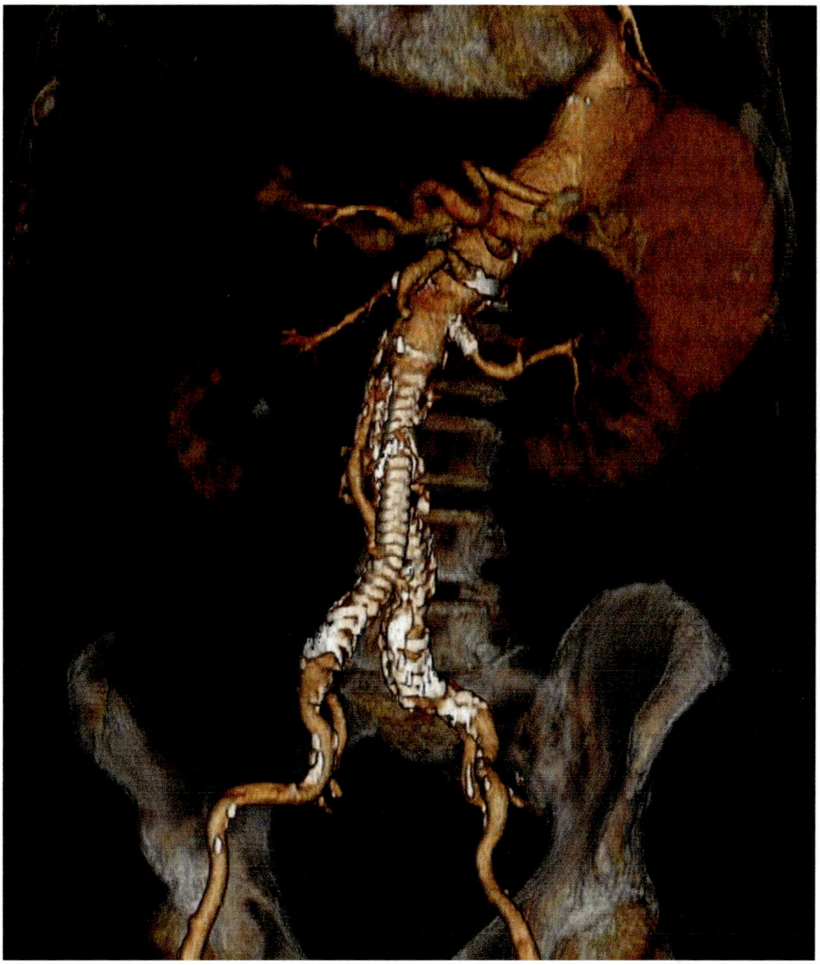

Fig. 23.3 Postoperative CTA of a patient treated with a fenestrated Anaconda stent graft

Manufacturer: Cook Medical Inc., Bloomington, IN

Platform: Zenith Fenestrated

Stent material: stainless steel uncovered barbed supraceliac stent and a series of nitinol Z-stents

Graft material: polyethylene terephthalate

Available designs: The tubular graft design provides a scallop for the celiac artery (CA) located at 12:30 and 11 mm lower 8-mm strut-free fenestration for the superior mesenteric artery (SMA), located at 12:00 o'clock. Two options for pivot fenestration of the renal arteries with respect to the SMA origin are available. *Configuration A*: the pivot fenestrations come off at the same longitudinal position of the device below the SMA. *Configuration B*: the right renal fenestration is 4 mm higher than the left renal pivot fenestration. In both configurations the 6-mm right renal and left renal fenestrations are oriented at 9:30 and 2:30.

Application: juxtarenal and pararenal aneurysms, provided a healthy neck exists below the SMA

Available diameters: 26–36 mm in diameter

Delivery system diameter: 20 Fr (internal diameter)

Peculiarities: double renal pivot fenestrations configuration, single-reducing tie, and preloaded wire in both renal fenestrations

Restrictions: Proximal sealing zone should not be shorter than 4 mm below the SMA in an aorta that is ≤32 mm in diameter. Visceral vessels have to fit within the overlay targets of the provided planning and sizing grid.

23.2.2.2 Cook t-Branch

Intro: The off-the-shelf stent graft is built on the same platform of the custom-made devices for thoracoabdominal aneurysm but differs for its fixed design; the device proximal has a proximal diameter of 34 mm and features three sealing stents (76 mm); a covered stent at the proximal end contains barbs for additional fixation of the device. The graft then tapers down to 18 mm and gives off four downward-directed branches. Total length is 202 mm. Branches to celiac trunk and superior mesenteric artery are 8 mm in diameter and 21 and 18 mm in length, respectively, and axially located at 01:00 and 12:00 o'clock positions. Right and left renal artery branches are 6 mm in diameter, 18 mm in length, and located in the 10:00 and 03:00 clock positions, respectively. Four circumferentially placed gold markers are positioned within 2 mm of the most superior aspect of the graft. Each branch features three gold markers at the proximal internal edge and two gold markers at the distal outer edge. Three markers on the third and seventh stents and an additional thick-shaped gold marker are positioned anteriorly to ease proper orientation of the graft before deployment.

Manufacturer: Cook Medical Inc., Bloomington, IN

Platform: Zenith

Stent material: stainless steel Cook Z-stents

Graft material: woven polyester

Application: thoracoabdominal aortic aneurysm even in urgent/emergent setting

Available diameters: The device features a fixed configuration with 34 mm of proximal diameter that tapers to an 18 mm distal diameter

Delivery system diameter: 22 F internal diameter

Peculiarities: four branches for visceral vessels and off-the-shelf design

Restrictions: implantation rather higher than lower to fit higher number of anatomies

23.2.2.3 Gore TAMBE

Intro: Thoracoabdominal branch endoprosthesis (TAMBE) (WL Gore, Flagstaff, AZ) is a trimodular system with a proximal multibranched aortic component, a distal bifurcated component, and iliac limb extensions. The multibranched component is now available in two different configurations. The original prototype featured a combination of antegrade and retrograde branches. The antegrade branches were dedicated to ensure direct flow to the celiac trunk (CT) and the superior mesenteric artery (SMA), while the retrograde branches were destined to the renal arteries. A second configuration that features four antegrade branches, one for each visceral vessel, is under investigation. The aortic component allows for placement of through-and-through preloaded guidewires to facilitate visceral vessel access, by eliminating the need for branch cannulation.

Manufacturer: WL Gore, Flagstaff, AZ

Platform: Gore® Excluder® AAA

Stent material: nitinol stent

Graft material: ePTFE

Available designs: combined antegrade (celiac trunk and superior mesenteric artery) and retrograde branch configuration (renal arteries) and fully antegrade branch configuration

Application: thoracoabdominal aortic aneurysm even in urgent/emergent setting

Available diameters: proximal diameters of 26, 31, and 37 mm, length of 215 mm, and distal diameter of 20 mm

Delivery system diameter: 22 Fr outer diameter

Peculiarities: The side branch components have CBAS® Heparin Surface, preloaded through-and-through guidewires, designed to be used with a dedicated covered balloon-expandable bridging stent Gore Viabahn BX or with the self-expandable Viabahn.

23.3 Bridging Stents

The choice of the correct bridging stents is crucial for the procedure's technical success and might play an important role in the short- and long-term clinical results in terms of occlusions, angulations, and stenosis. A large variety of stent grafts and bare metal stents are currently used in thoracoabdominal repair. Bare metal stents are usually used to reline distally a stent graft in order to obtain smoother curves and avoid kinks and to increase distal landing zones in visceral vessels. Their application can be particularly convenient in case of poor landing zone and side branches originating from the target vessels. The following dissertation includes the most commonly used stent grafts implanted in total endovascular thoracoabdominal repair.

A critical step in these complex procedures is the placement of bridging stent graft (BSG) in visceral vessels to connect the main stent graft with these target vessels. The commercially available BSG is either balloon-expandable or self-expandable, and none of these have been specifically approved for fenestrated or branched endovascular exclusion of TAAAs (F/BEVAR).

23.3.1 Balloon-Expandable Stents

The advantages of these stents are precision in deployment and their radial force; nevertheless, they usually lack in flexibility. Multiple balloon-expandable covered stents could be utilized for fenestrations and branches: Maquet Atrium iCAST (US market) or Advanta (EU market) stent, Bentley BeGraft, and Gore VBX stents are the three most commonly employed.

23.3.1.1 Atrium Advanta Stent

Intro: The stent structure is made up of stainless steel stent, with an open cell design, encapsulated with two layers of polytetrafluoroethylene (PTFE) (Fig. 23.4). The presence of a double layer permits on one side to avoid direct contact of the struts with the arterial wall and on the other side to reduce the shear stress with respect to the bloodstream. The balloon can be easily recognized under fluoroscopy thanks to two gold markers at the proximal and distal end. The system is 0.035" compatible and is mounted on a noncompliant balloon and is advanced under the protection of a long introducer sheath, with a profile (6–7 Fr) depending on the balloon's diameter and length. Stent's diameter ranges from 5 to 12 mm and length ranges from 22 to 59 mm.

Manufacturer: Maquet, Getinge group, Rastatt, Germany

Stent material: stainless steel

Graft material: double layer of PTFE

Available diameters: 5–12 mm

Delivery system diameter: varies according to stent diameter from 6 to 7 Fr

23.3.1.2 Bentley BeGraft Stent

Intro: The Bentley BeGraft stent has been recently introduced in the market for fenestrated and branched endografts. The single stent structure is made of chromium-cobalt and is covered with a microporous ePTFE fabric. The device is 0.035" compatible, with stent diameters of 5–10 mm and lengths of 18–58 mm. The stent is introduced using a 6 Fr (up to 8 × 58 mm) or 7 Fr delivery sheath depending on its nominal diameter.

Manufacturer: Bentley, Hechingen, Germany

Stent material: chromium-cobalt

Graft material: ePTFE

Available diameters: 5–10 mm and lengths of 18–58 mm

Delivery system diameter: 6 Fr up to 8 × 58 mm and 7 Fr for larger stents

23.3.2 Self-Expandable Stent Grafts

The main feature of these endografts is their flexibility that renders their use ideal in tortuous vessels. Their limitation is the impossibility to be

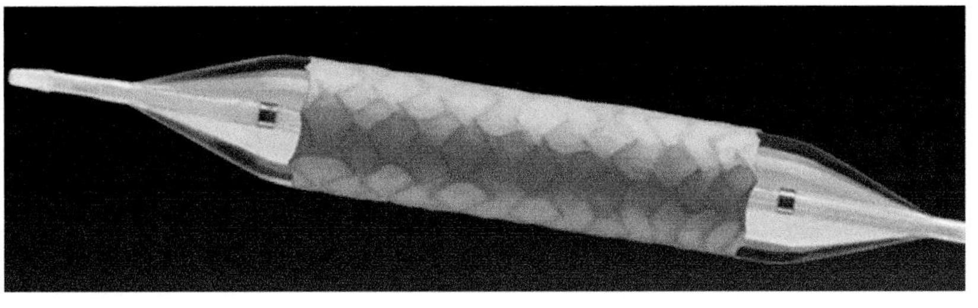

Fig. 23.4 The Atrium Advanta balloon-expandable stent graft

flared to increase seal within the fenestrations. There are multiple self-expandable stent grafts available for peripheral vascular procedures: WL Gore Viabahn and Bard Fluency being the most used.

23.3.2.1 Gore Viabahn Stent Graft

Intro: The Gore Viabahn self-expandable stent graft (WL Gore, Flagstaff, AZ) is made up of an external nitinol stent structure and an expanded PTFE fabric (ePTFE) (Fig. 23.5), with an extremely flexible structure. A balloon-expandable version of the stent is now under development and not for clinical use yet. Both 0.018" compatible and 0.035" compatible systems are available. Stent diameters range from 5 to 13 mm while available lengths 25 to 250 mm. Its profile, depending on stent diameter, ranges from 6 to 12 Fr.

Manufacturer: WL Gore, Flagstaff, AZ
Stent material: nitinol stent
Graft material: ePTFE
Available diameters: from 5 to 13 mm
Delivery system diameter: from 6 to 12 Fr

23.3.2.2 Bard Fluency Plus

Intro: The Bard Fluency Plus (Bard Peripheral Vascular, Tempe, AZ) is a self-expanding vascular ePTFE-covered stent with a nitinol structure (2 mm uncovered at each end) and inner carbon impregnation (Fig. 23.6). It is compatible with 0.035″ system. Minimum stent length is 40 and maximum is 120 mm with diameters ranging from 6 to 13.5 mm. Recommended sheath diameters are 8 to 10 Fr. It is not as flexible as the Viabahn stent graft, but its advantages are a wide spectrum of lengths and diameters and the pullback deployment system with low risk of malpositioning.

Manufacturer: Bard Peripheral Vascular, Tempe, AZ
Stent material: nitinol
Graft material: ePTFE
Available diameters: from 6 to 13.5 mm
Delivery system diameter: 8 to 10 Fr

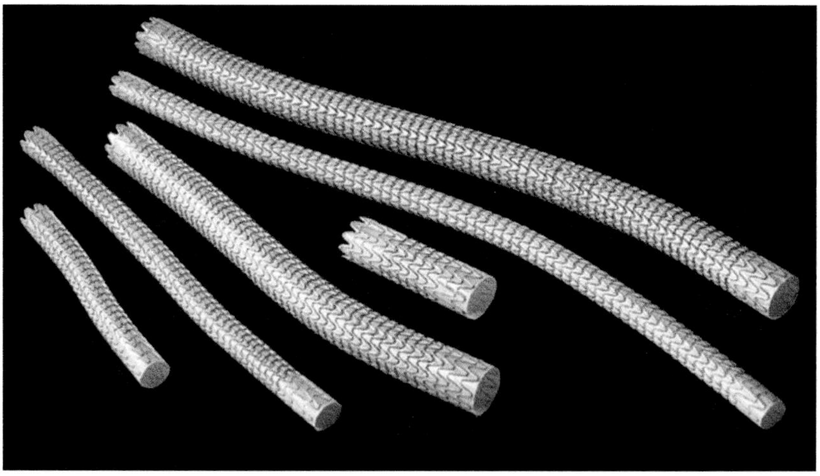

Fig. 23.5 The Gore Viabahn self-expandable stents grafts in different diameters and lengths

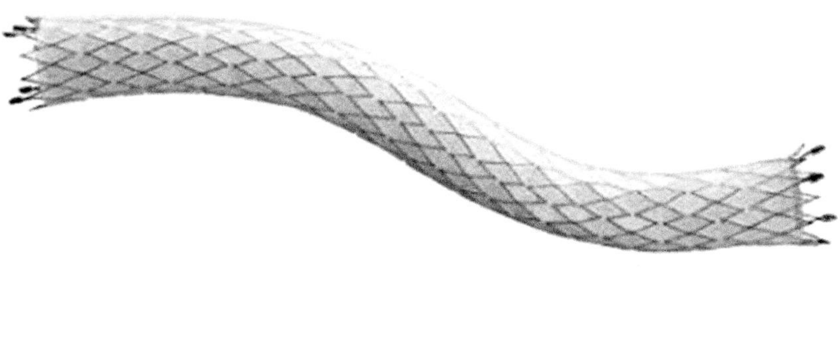

Fig. 23.6 The Bard Fluency stent graft

23.4 Lessons Learnt

23.4.1 Custom-Made Design According to Aneurysm Morphology

23.4.1.1 Branches in Large Sac

When considering custom-made graft design, a widely accepted rule is to opt for a branch to revascularize the vessel when the distance between the wall of aneurysm and that of the opening on the endograft is >10 mm.

This is the outcome of both intraoperative and postoperative considerations. If this distance is >10 mm, it means that, at that level, we most probably have a large aneurysm with little to no thrombotic apposition, and this allows an eventual branch to expand and leaves enough room to the operator to manipulate guidewires and catheters. Furthermore, deployment of endograft in large sacs can alter the desired clock orientation of the graft, thus making a fenestrated design less ideal.

In the postoperative period, we can assume that any endograft is more mobile at the level of a large sac than at the level of close apposition to the vessel wall or parietal thrombus; this mobility in a fenestrated design could eventually translate to a superior peri-fenestration stress on the bridging stent with consequent impairment on its patency and/or sealing.

23.4.1.2 Fenestrations in Dissection

Conversely in subacute and chronic dissections, the residual true lumen is usually smaller than the lumen in an atherosclerotic aneurysm. Therefore, fenestrated design is more commonly used whenever there is not enough room for a side branch to expand and allow target vessel bridging [5].

23.4.1.3 Fenestrated Previous Thoracic or Thoracoabdominal Open Surgery

The same issue with branch expansion arises whenever the patient had been previously treated for proximal aortic pathology. If the patient had undergone open thoracic aorta repair with distal anastomosis close (<5 cm) to the origin of the celiac trunk, there would be no room for branch expansion within the surgical graft (reminder: branches are 18–21 mm and need to be deployed 20–50 mm above the ostium of the vessel). The same problem arises in visceral aortic patch aneurysms, in which the graft ends exactly at the level of the CT and with previous endovascular management of proximal TAA, if the graft had been deployed just above the origin of the CT in a healthy portion of the aorta (e.g., 20 mm Ø).

23.4.2 Management of Hostile Visceral Vessels

23.4.2.1 Fenestrations in Upward Vessels

The optimal design for visceral vessels originating with an upward angle had been shown to be a fenestration [6]. Classic downward branches are intuitively suboptimal, both because they require the target vessel to be catheterized from an upper extremity access, making it technically more difficult, and because of the angle at which the bridging stent will bend, most likely affecting long-term patency. The idea of upward branches has been explored and offered both by Cook custom-made grafts and Gore off-the-shelf TAMBE, although the main concern of patency is still present regarding this design.

23.4.2.2 Distal Bare Stent Reinforcement

In extremely angulated visceral vessels, expert operators sometime employ distal reinforcement of the bridging stents with bare self-expanding stents to better accommodate vessel curvature. Nonetheless no data is yet available on the impact of such approach on short- and long-term patency of the bridging stents [7].

23.4.2.3 Occlusion of Small Vessels

Mastracci et al. highlighted the inferior long-term patency of renal arteries when compared to the celiac trunk or superior mesenteric artery [8]. One of the factors deemed responsible could be the smaller diameter of renal arteries which, together with the high resistance of the target organ, might explain the high occlusion rate. Furthermore, the smallest bridging stents available on the market are 5 mm in diameter.

23.4.2.4 No Long Bridging Stents

The relationship between bridging stent length and their patency rates has already been addressed [9]. While branched designs benefit of increased flexibility of application, both in terms of clock rotation and in terms of proximal/distal positioning, any graft should not be deployed too proximally just to fit the anatomy as longer bridging stents can both occlude and disconnect. Instead the distance between the bottom of the directional branch and the ostium of the target vessel should be between 20 and 50 mm as recommended by Cook IFU.

References

1. Park JH, Chung JW, Choo IW, et al. Fenestrated stent-grafts for preserving visceral arterial branches in the treatment of abdominal aortic aneurysms: preliminary experience. J Vasc Interv Radiol. 1996;7:819–23.
2. Anderson JL, Berce M, Hartley DE. Endoluminal aortic grafting with renal and superior mesenteric artery incorporation by graft fenestration. J Endovasc Ther. 2001;8(1):3–15.
3. Chuter TAM, Gordon RL, Reilly LM, et al. An endovascular system for thoracoabdominal aortic aneurysm repair. J Endovasc Ther. 2001;8(1):25–33.
4. Verhoeven EL, Prins TR, Tielliu IF, et al. Treatment of short-necked infrarenal aortic aneurysms with fenestrated stent-grafts: short-term results. Eur J Vasc Endovasc Surg. 2004;27(5):477–83.
5. Oikonomou K, Kopp R, Katsargyris A, Pfister K, Verhoeven EL, Kasprzak P. Outcomes of fenestrated/branched endografting in post-dissection thoracoabdominal aortic aneurysms. Eur J Vasc Endovasc Surg. 2014;48(6):641–8.
6. Martin-Gonzalez T, Pinçon C, Maurel B, Hertault A, Sobocinski J, Spear R, Le Roux M, Azzaoui R, Mastracci TM, Haulon S. Renal outcomes following fenestrated and branched endografting. Eur J Vasc Endovasc Surg. 2015;50(4):420–30.
7. Panuccio G, Bisdas T, Berekoven B, Torsello G, Austermann M. Performance of bridging stent grafts in fenestrated and branched aortic endografting. Eur J Vasc Endovasc Surg. 2015;50(1):60–70.
8. Mastracci TM, Carrell T, Constantinou J, Dias N, Martin-Gonzalez T, Katsargyris A, Modarai B, Resch T, Verhoeven EL, Burnell M, Haulon S. Editor's choice - effect of branch stent choice on branch-related outcomes in complex aortic repair. Eur J Vasc Endovasc Surg. 2016;51(4):536–42.
9. Hertault A, Haulon S. Part one: for the motion. Branched/fenestrated EVAR procedures are better than snorkels, chimneys, or periscopes in the treatment of most thoracoabdominal and juxtarenal aneurysms. Eur J Vasc Endovasc Surg. 2015;50(5):551–7.

Recurrent Thoracoabdominal Aortic Aneurysm with Visceral Artery Involvement: Treatment Options

24

Luca Bertoglio, Alessandro Grandi, Tommaso Cambiaghi, Andrea Melloni, and Simone Salvati

24.1 Introduction

Revascularization of splanchnic and renal arteries is one of the critical steps in open repair of thoracoabdominal aortic aneurysm (TAAA). Several techniques are currently employed, but the most represented is the inclusion technique proposed by Stanley Crawford in the early 1970s: it consists in a side-to-end anastomosis aimed at reimplanting, on a side opening in the synthetic Dacron graft, an island of aortic wall from which the visceral arteries arise [1].

The main drawback of this technique is that the retained portion of the diseased aorta might be prone to further dilatation, thus giving rise to a visceral aortic patch (VAP) aneurysm. The prevalence of this late complication is currently underreported, although the rate of VAP aneurysm (>5 cm) ranges from 1.1% to 7.7% after a median time interval from the index procedure ranging from 7 months to 16 years [2–5].

Different authors [2, 3, 6–21] published small series regarding both redo-open or hybrid TAAA repair with high mortality and morbidity rate, and only two authors proposed a fenestrated or branched approach for two single cases [22, 23].

L. Bertoglio (✉) · A. Grandi · T. Cambiaghi
A. Melloni · S. Salvati
Division of Vascular Surgery, "Vita—Salute" University, Scientific Institute H. San Raffaele, Milan, Italy
e-mail: bertoglio.luca@hsr.it

The real prevalence and incidence of VAP aneurysm are hard to define because long-term follow-up protocols are often lacking and a relevant proportion of TAAA patients have brief postoperative survival due to associated morbidities. However, everlasting follow-up imaging is warranted. Two clear risk factors have been associated with VAP aneurysm formation: the size of the aortic patch used to include the reimplanted visceral vessels and connective tissue disorders [24, 25].

Reimplantation of visceral vessels with the standard inclusion technique in open TAAA can be performed either with side-to-end anastomosis of an aortic patch including all vessels or including only three out of four vessels with separate reimplantation on the graft of the remaining vessel, usually the left renal artery. Obviously, the size of a four-vessel patch is going to be larger than that of a three-vessel patch, with a consequent increase in the surface of the diseased aortic wall kept exposed to the stress of systemic blood pressure. Notably, no VAP dilatation or aneurysm of a three-vessel patch was recorded in an old San Raffaele series despite the fact that in 23% of the patients of the cohort, an inclusion technique was employed to reattach the celiac trunk, the superior mesenteric, and the right renal artery [3]. Nowadays, the 3 + 1 configuration is preferred for splanchnic and renal revascularization [26].

Interestingly, the data emerging from Johns Hopkins series demonstrated that the incidence

© Springer Nature Switzerland AG 2019
Y. Tshomba et al. (eds.), *Visceral Vessels and Aortic Repair*,
https://doi.org/10.1007/978-3-319-94761-7_24

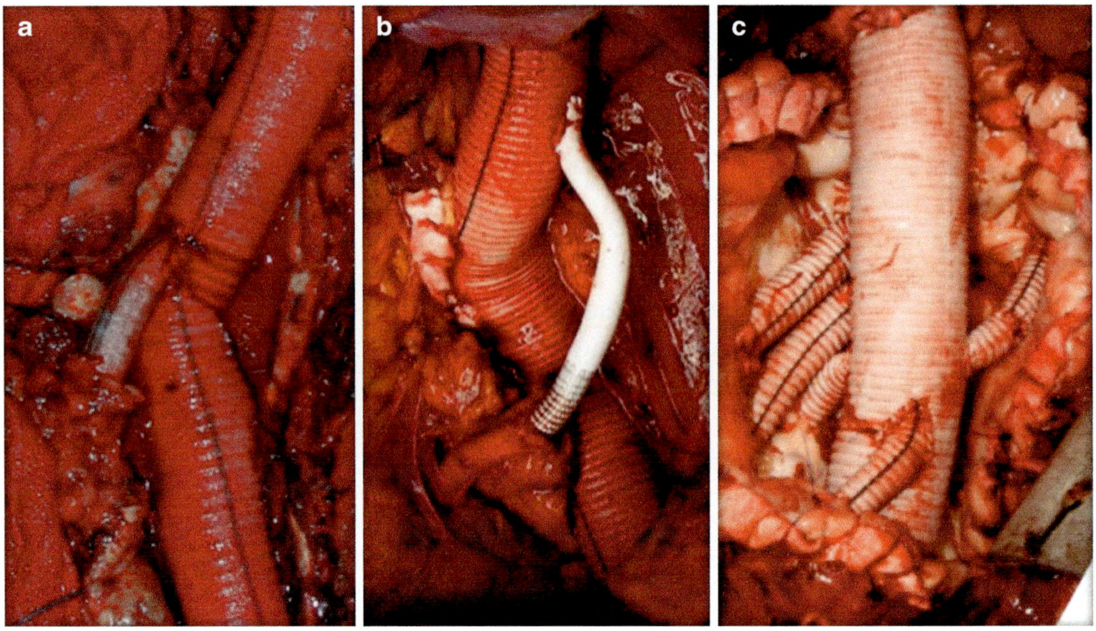

Fig. 24.1 Different types of revascularization of splanchnic and renal arteries during open repair. (**a**) Three-vessel visceral aortic patch (VAP) with separate surgical bypass to the left renal artery. (**b**) Three-vessel patch with sutureless reimplantation of the left renal artery. (**c**) Separate reimplantation of renal and splanchnic arteries with quadrifurcated branched presewn Dacron graft

of VAP aneurysm was much higher in patients affected by collagenopathy 17.6%, with respect to atherosclerotic patients 5.6% ($p = 0.034$) [2]. For those reasons, in order to ensure a durable repair, in young or connective disease patients, we employ a presewn four-branch Dacron graft to revascularize the visceral vessels during open TAAA repair, thus minimizing the amount of residual diseased aorta, thereby preventing future development of VAP aneurysms [15]. The branched graft also provides an alternate repair option in patients whose visceral and renal arteries are too far apart to obtain a reasonably sized aortic patch [27] (Fig. 24.1).

24.2 Surgical Management

Surgical management consists in an open repair with re-inclusion technique via a thoraco-phreno-laparotomy access. All the visceral vessels were separately reimplanted with quadrifurcated branched Dacron graft (Vascutek Ltd., Renfrewshire, Scotland, UK) in the most recent seven cases (50%), and in the other cases, a combination of undersized VAP and separated bypasses was used [12]. No extracorporeal circulation was used and an intraoperative hypothermic selective perfusion through 9F Pruitt-Inahara occlusion/perfusion catheters (LeMaitre Vascular, Inc., Burlington, MA) of the splanchnic vessels with cold crystalloid (lactate ringer at 4 °C) and of the renal arteries with cold enriched crystalloid solution (Custodiol 4 °C; Dr. Franz Kohler Chemie 95 GmbH, Bensheim, Germany) [28] was performed (Table 24.1, 96 Fig. 24.2).

24.3 Hybrid Management

Hybrid management, instead, consists in a single-staged repair with retrograde splanchnic and renal debranching with Dacron graft (6–8 mm in diameter) from the previous infrarenal graft or from the common iliac artery and VAP aneurysm exclusion using commercially available endograft [12]. The abdominal aorta, common iliac arteries, and the first 2 cm from the origin of

Table 24.1 Thirty-day outcome and midterm outcome

	Open ($n = 14$)	Hybrid ($n = 10$)	Endovascular ($n = 5$)	Overall ($n = 29$)	p-values
In-hospital outcomes					
Operative time (min)	220 (IQR 190–260)	255 (IQR 193–340)	320 (IQR 315–540)	250 (IQR 93–320)	Ns
Operative time >250 min	6 (43%)	5 (50%)	4 (80%)	15 (52%)	Ns
Estimated blood loss (mL)	1475 (IQR 1000–3400)	550 (IQR 380–1450)	400 (IQR 300–450)	1000 (IQR 450–1700)	Ns
Blood loss >1000 mL	11 (79%)	4 (40%)	0	15 (52%)	0.007
Number of PRBC transfusion	7.5 (IQR 4–12)	4 (IQR 3–5)	2 (IQR 2–3)	4 (IQR 3–7)	Ns
PRBC transfusion >3	14 (100%)	9 (90%)	2 (40%)	25 (86%)	0.003
Median ICU stay (days)	2 (IQR 1–3)	3 (IQR 1–5)	0 (IQR 0–1)	2 (IQR 1–4)	Ns
Need for an ICU stay >1 day	10 (71%)	7 (70%)	0	17 (58.6%)	0.014
Length of hospital stay (days)	8.5 (IQR 8–10)	8 (IQR 7–10)	5 (IQR 4–6)	8 (IQR 6–10)	Ns
Length of hospital stay >7 days	11 (79%)	8 (80%)	1 (20%)	20 (69%)	0.034
30-day outcomes					
30-day mortality	2 (14%)	2 (20%)	0	4 (14%)	Ns
Renal complications (Grade >2)	4 (29%)	1 (10%)	0	5 (17%)	Ns
Cardiac complications (Grade >2)	3 (21%)	1 (10%)	0	4 (14%)	Ns
Pulmonary complications (Grade >2)	7 (50%)	4 (40%)	0	11 (38%)	Ns
Spinal cord ischemia (Grade >2)	0	0	0	0	Ns
Any major adverse event (Grade >2)	11 (79%)	6 (50%)	0	17 (59%)	0.009
Any spinal cord ischemia	0	1 (10%)	1 (20%)	2 (7%)	Ns
Any surgical perioperative revision	3 (21%)	2 (20%)	0	5 (17%)	Ns
Midterm outcomes					
Median follow-up (months)	70 (IQR 21–84)	25 (IQR 1–38)	13 (IQR 11–14)	28 (IQR 11–74)	
Overall survival	10 (71%)	4 (40%)	5 (100%)	16 (55%)	Ns
Related mortality	0	2	0	2	Ns
Unrelated mortality	2	2	0	4	Ns

the common hepatic artery, superior mesenteric artery, and renal arteries were exposed through a transperitoneal midline approach with the patient in a supine position. Separate bypass should be used for each recipient vessel, customized "Y" grafts, customized trifurcated grafts, or single bypass with sequential graft technique related to the specific anatomy of every case. For celiac trunk revascularization, the graft was routed in front of the renal vein behind the pancreas, an arteriotomy was made in the common hepatic artery, and an end-to-side anastomosis was made. An end-to-end anastomosis was usually preferred for the superior mesenteric artery, and this type of anastomosis was always used for the renal arteries. A radiopaque marker was placed at the origin of the more proximal visceral graft when originating from native or grafted abdominal aorta. The stent graft is inserted from the common femoral artery surgically exposed, and the ballooning was performed according to the instructions for use of the device (Table 24.1, Fig. 24.3).

24.4 Endovascular Management

The experience on visceral aortic patch aneurysm management published in the literature highlights morbidity and mortality rates unfavorable with both redo-open TAAA repair and with hybrid approach [2, 3, 6–21]. These results are the rationale for an attempt of total endovascular repair

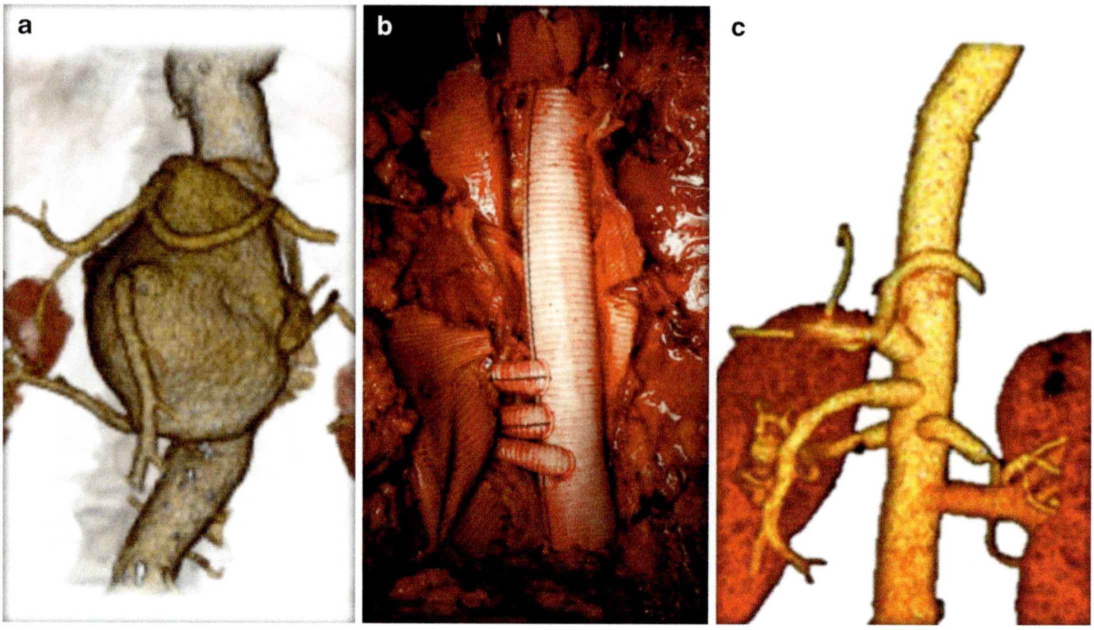

Fig. 24.2 (**a**) Preoperative three-dimensional reconstruction of a visceral aortic patch (VAP). (**b**) Treatment was by means of separate reimplantation of renal and splanchnic arteries with quadrifurcated branched presewn Dacron graft (Vascutek Ltd., Renfrewshire, Scotland, UK). (**c**) The postoperative computed tomography scan demonstrates patency of all vessels reimplanted

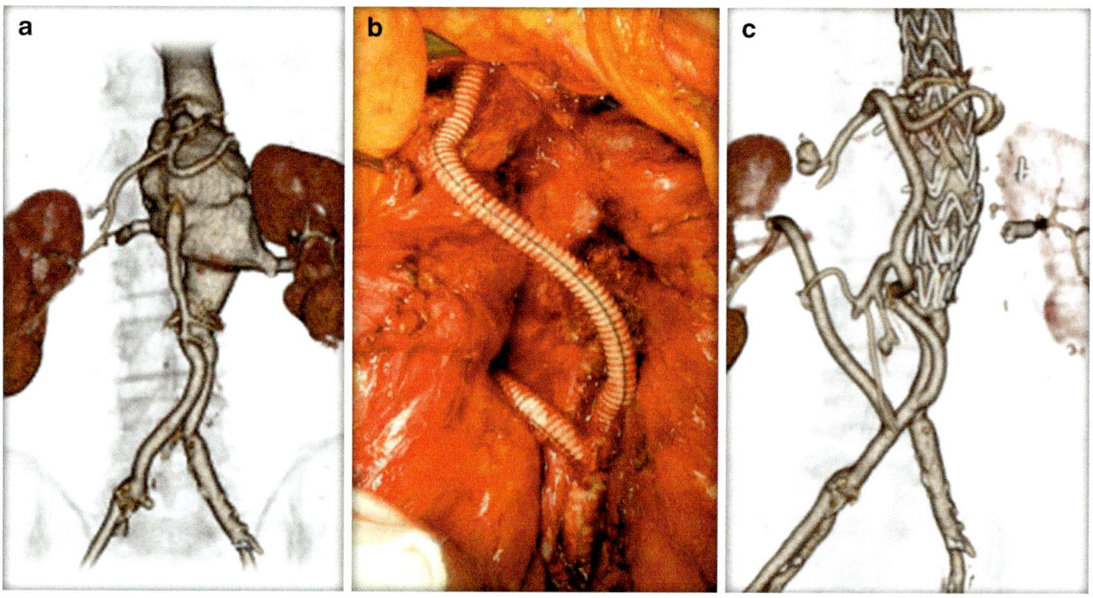

Fig. 24.3 (**a**) Preoperative three-dimensional reconstruction of a visceral aortic patch (VAP). (**b**) Treatment with a hybrid repair. A retrograde visceral and renal bypass from the right iliac artery to revascularize the right renal artery, superior mesenteric artery, and celiac trunk was performed, followed by endovascular exclusion of the aneurysm. The left renal artery revascularization was unsuccessful because of intraoperative adhesions. (**c**) The postoperative computed tomography scan demonstrates complete exclusion of the aneurysm and patency of target vessels

of VAP aneurysms. Adam et al. reported the first endovascular treatment of a VAP aneurysm with a fenestrated custom-made device in 2007 [22]. Worldwide, three other single cases were treated by means of endovascular approach with octopus graft, surgeon-modified graft, or fenestrated graft [22–25].

The latter was used in elective cases and the first two options in emergent or symptomatic cases.

The advantages of this endovascular approach compared to either open or hybrid surgery are evident: it avoids a redo thoracotomy and/or laparotomy, thus reducing the risk of blood loss, respiratory complications, and organ injuries due to severe perivisceral adhesions, leading to prolonged ICU and in-hospital stay. Moreover, the visceral reconstruction might be jeopardized by such adhesions as well as by concomitant steno-occlusive disease of target vessels with the subsequent increase in risk of end-organ ischemia and related deaths (Table 24.1, Figs. 24.4 and 24.5) [6].

24.5 Discussion

According to our experience, endovascular treatment of VAP aneurysm with custom-made devices brings along several technical challenges.

24.5.1 Graft Design

Firstly, the graft should be carefully designed, taking into consideration the reduced compliance of the Dacron graft (maximum 4 mm of oversizing instead of 20%), the limited room for guidewires and catheters maneuverability, and the alteration in visceral vessel anatomy induced by the aneurysmal degeneration of the patch. The presence of the previous surgical graft, as well as the reported [29, 30] access limitations, might worsen the navigation of the endograft and the ability to orientate the fenestrations in the desired position. For these reasons, it is of vital importance that the initial careful and correct opening of the custom-made device with double-diameter-reducing wires is of paramount importance.

24.5.2 Branch or Fenestration?

Secondly, when choosing graft designs, some adjustments are necessary in the treatment of this pathology: branches, despite being easier to manage in a more complex anatomy, are not an option for celiac trunk (CT) revascularization as its ostium is too close to the apex of suture line of the VAP, and no room for branch expansion within the previous surgical graft is left. Moreover, the splanchnic vessel course is distorted by the aneurysm itself, and, as the VAP dilates, both the CT and the superior mesenteric artery (SMA) tend to take a more and more upward direction. This typical upward direction mandates again a fenestrated design to facilitate target vessel catheterization and avoid kinking of bridging stents. The right renal artery (RRA)-bearing component is typically designed with a fenestration because of its proximity to the bottom of VAP suture line which brings it close to the surgical graft wall. Due to the likelihood of surgical modifications during initial open TAAA repair, the CT and the left renal artery (LRA) are the most complex vessels. When they are selectively anastomosed to the graft, the remaining vessel portion without branches is usually shortened, thus providing a decreased distal sealing zone for the bridging stent; while if the initial revascularization of the left renal artery had instead required graft interposition or direct stenting of the ostium, target vessel catheterization could be more difficult. In these cases, a branch design with a preloaded indwelling catheter can be considered to deal with these challenging vessel characteristics. Furthermore, in cases in which we anticipated the possible failure of targeting a vessel, the branch design allows, in the event of missed cannulation, the option of plugging it, in a second stage, after having performed revascularization of the missing vessel with an extra-anatomic bypass (i.e., iliac to renal bypass) [29].

24.5.3 Spinal Cord Ischemia

The last critical point to consider in the management of this pathology is the prevention of spinal cord ischemia. The eventual presence of

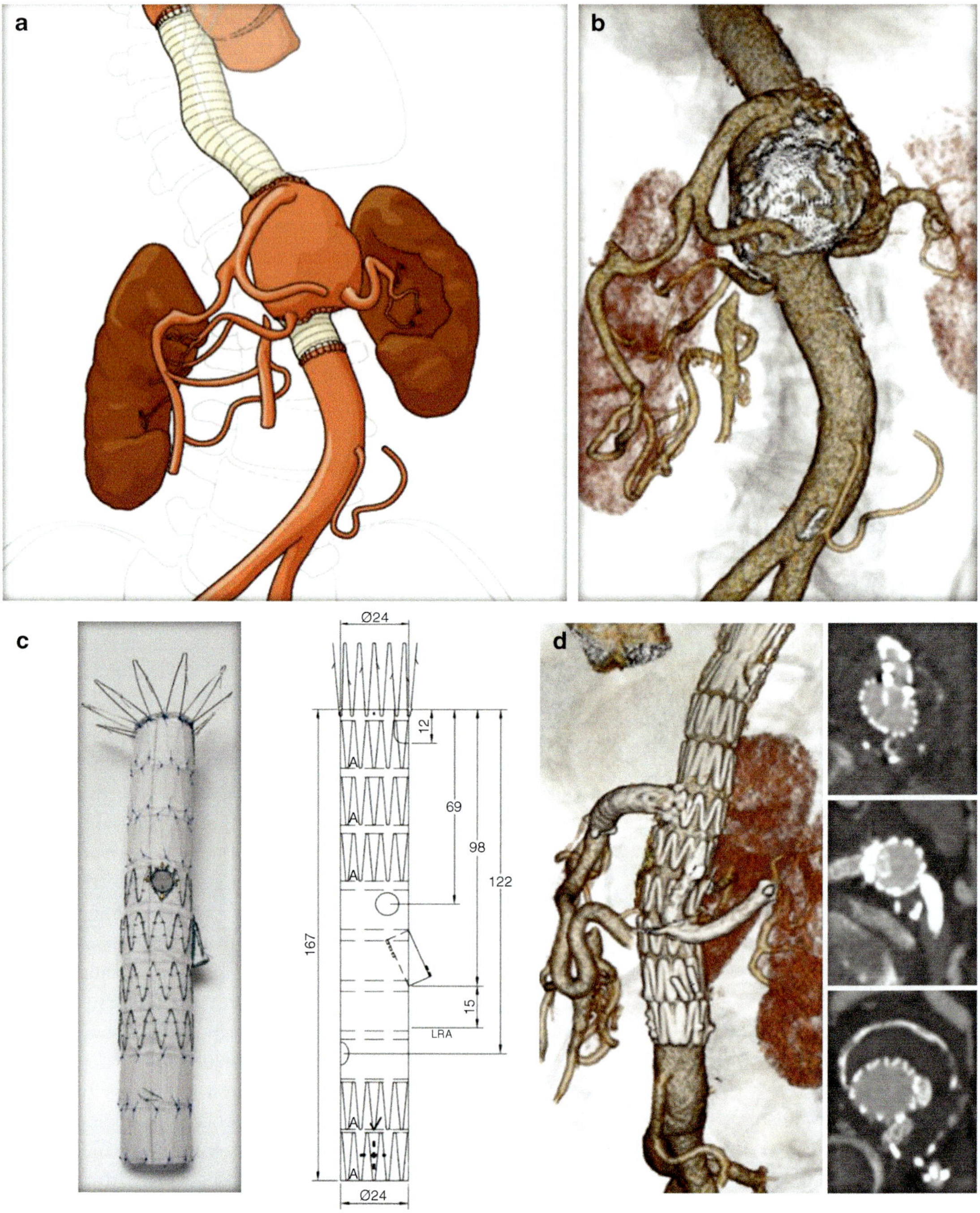

Fig. 24.4 Schematic drawing (**a**) and preoperative three-dimensional reconstruction (**b**) demonstrate a visceral aortic patch (VAP) aneurysm; the celiac trunk and the renal arteries were patent. The superior mesenteric artery was occluded at the origin, with distal revascularization from anastomotic collaterals arising from both the celiac trunk and a patent inferior mesenteric artery (**a**). A two-fenestration and one-branch custom-made device was designed to seal the aneurysm: the branch was targeted to the left renal artery (LRA) with an indwelling catheter (**c**). The postoperative scan (**d**) demonstrates successful exclusion of the aneurysm with patency of all target vessels

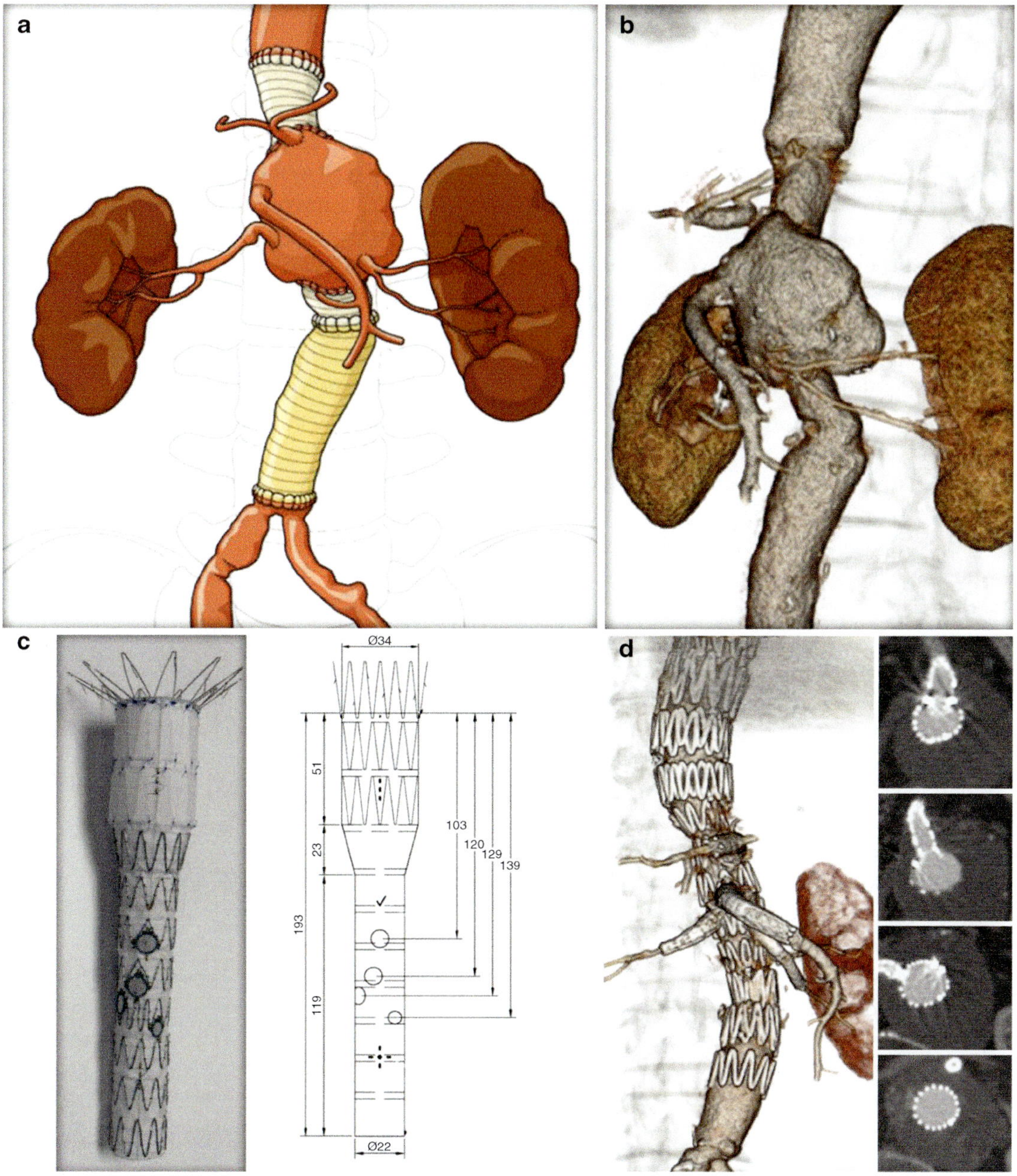

Fig. 24.5 Schematic drawing (**a**) and preoperative three-dimensional reconstruction (**b**) demonstrate a visceral aortic patch (VAP) aneurysm with all the visceral vessel patents. However, the celiac trunk presented with a tight stenosis near the patch suture line, and the left renal artery common trunk was shortened by the previous reimplantation. There was caliber mismatch between the native aorta and the surgical graft, so the planned strategy was a two-step repair. The first step was aimed at fixing the dilation at the level of the proximal anastomosis with a custom-made short-tapered thoracic component to create a proximal fixation site for the four fenestrations of the custom-made endograft (**c**) to be deployed in the second step. (**d**) Postoperative scan confirms complete exclusion of the VAP aneurysm with patency of all target vessels

intercostal artery patches or selective reimplantations on the surgical graft at the level of the proximal sealing zone should be evaluated, and while planning the custom-made graft, any attempt of not covering the intercostal patch with either the fabric or the proximal bare stent must be made. If sparing of this area is unachievable, a careful evaluation of risks/benefits needs to be carried on, staging should be considered, and preoperative cerebrospinal fluid drainage is strongly recommended. Such staging can be performed with an initial thoracic stent grafting in order to create a proximal sealing zone with covering the intercostal patch, if present, or a portion of the native thoracic aorta proximal to the open repair. Even if no adjunctive native aorta coverage is required, other factors might determine spinal cord ischemia such as hypotension, anemia, and intraoperative temporary hypogastric artery occlusion by the delivery system. Indeed, the whole planning procedure should be aimed at early removal of large femoral sheaths in order to reduce the pelvic and lower limb ischemia time [30]. However, in our experience, the procedural time was longer than expected because of increased difficulties during catheterization, and, in these patients with a "compulsory" fenestrated design, two possible solutions have been adopted to obtain early pelvic reperfusion: keeping the main large introducer below the hypogastric artery during the transfemoral bridging maneuvers and targeting at least one vessel from above through a brachial or axillary access so as to limit the size of the required contralateral femoral sheath.

24.6 Conclusion

In the last two decades, we managed different VAP aneurysms by means of open and hybrid repairs [3, 12], and although the results were acceptable for such complex operations, the mortality and morbidity rates were not negligible.

It is the authors' opinion that endovascular option, whenever applicable, should be strongly recommended in patients unfit for open surgery, while hybrid surgery should be limited to single-vessel revascularization in the cases of endovascular failure of bridging stent placement or in very selected cases due to the poorer outcomes reported in our experience. Although concerns remain for young patients or patients with connective tissue disease, in whom the long-term patency and sealing of target vessels still need to be proven, a proximal and distal aortic neck within a previous surgical graft seems a safe landing zone even in cases with connective tissue disorders. In the future, in order to answer these questions, we would need an analysis of a larger series collected from a retrospective registry gathering the few cases treated in large-volume centers dealing with endovascular TAAA treatment.

References

1. Crawford ES. Thoraco-abdominal and abdominal aortic aneurysms involving renal, superior mesenteric, celiac arteries. Ann Surg. 1974;179:763–72.
2. Dardik A, Perler BA, Roseborough GS, Williams GM. Aneurysmal expansion of the visceral patch after thoracoabdominal aortic replacement: an argument for limiting patch size? J Vasc Surg. 2001;34:405–9.
3. Tshomba Y, Melissano G, Civilini E, Setacci F, Chiesa R. Fate of the visceral aortic patch after thoracoabdominal aortic repair. Eur J Vasc Endovasc Surg. 2005;29:383–9.
4. Schepens MA, Kelder JC, Morshuis WJ, Heijmen RH, van Dongen EP, ter Beek HT. Long-term follow-up after thoracoabdominal aortic aneurysm repair. Ann Thorac Surg. 2007;83:S851–5.
5. Coselli JS, LeMaire SA, Preventza O, de la Cruz KI, Cooley DA, Price MD, et al. Outcomes of 3309 thoracoabdominal aortic aneurysm repairs. J Thorac Cardiovasc Surg. 2016;151:1323–37.
6. Quiñones-Baldrich WJ, Nene SM, Gelabert HA, Moore WS. Rupture of the perivisceral aorta: atherosclerotic versus mycotic aneurysm. Ann Vasc Surg. 1997;11:331–41.
7. Carrel TP, Signer C. Separate revascularization of the visceral arteries in thoracoabdominal aneurysm repair. Ann Thorac Surg. 1999;68:573–5.
8. Gasparis AP, Da Silva MS, Semel L. Visceral patch rupture after repair of thoracoabdominal aortic aneurysm—a case report. Vasc Surg. 2001;35:491–4.
9. Clouse WD, Marone LK, Davison JK, Dorer DJ, Brewster DC, LaMuraglia GM, et al. Late aortic and graft-related events after thoracoabdominal aneurysm repair. J Vasc Surg. 2003;37:254–61.
10. Dias RR, Coselli JS, Stolf NA, Dias AR, Mady C, Oliveira SA. Aneurysmal dilation of the reimplant segment of the visceral vessels after thoracoab-

dominal aneurysm correction. Arq Bras Cardiol. 2003;81:273–8.
11. Lombardi JV, Carpenter JP, Pochettino A, Sonnad SS, Bavaria JE. Thoracoabdominal aortic aneurysm repair after prior aortic surgery. J Vasc Surg. 2003;38:1185–90.
12. Tshomba Y, Bertoglio L, Marone EM, Melissano G, Chiesa R. Visceral aortic patch aneurysm after thoracoabdominal aortic repair: conventional vs hybrid treatment. J Vasc Surg. 2008;48:1083–91.
13. Suzuki K, Kazui T, Ohno T, Sugiki K, Doi H, Ohkawa Y. Re-reconstruction of visceral arteries with thoracoabdominal aortic replacement using a branched graft. Jpn J Thorac Cardiovasc Surg. 2005;53:217–9.
14. LeMaire SA, Carter SA, Volguina IV, Laux AT, Milewicz DM, Borsato GW, et al. Spectrum of aortic operations in 300 patients with confirmed or suspected Marfan syndrome. Ann Thorac Surg. 2006;81:2063–78.
15. Cochennec F, Kobeiter H, Gohel M, Leopardi M, Raux M, Majewski M, et al. Early results of physician modified fenestrated stent grafts for the treatment of thoraco-abdominal aortic aneurysms. Eur J Vasc Endovasc Surg. 2015;50:583–92.
16. van de Mortel RH, Vahl AC, Balm R, Buth J, Hamming JF, Schurink GW, et al. Collective experience with hybrid procedures for suprarenal and thoracoabdominal aneurysms. Vascular. 2008;16:140–6.
17. Kasirajan K. Branched grafts for thoracoabdominal aneurysms: off-label use of FDA-approved devices. J Endovasc Ther. 2011;18:471–6.
18. Juvonen T, Biancari F, Ylönen K, Perälä J, Rimpiläinen J, Lepojärvi M. Combined surgical and endovascular treatment of pseudoaneurysms of the visceral arteries and of the left iliac arteries after thoracoabdominal aortic surgery. Eur J Vasc Endovasc Surg. 2001;22:275–7.
19. Flye MW, Choi ET, Sanchez LA, Curci JA, Thompson RW, Rubin BG, et al. Retrograde visceral vessel revascularization followed by endovascular aneurysm exclusion as an alternative to open surgical repair of thoracoabdominal aortic aneurysm. J Vasc Surg. 2004;39:454–8.
20. Bakken AM, Protack CD, Waldman DL, Davies MG. Hybrid debranching-endovascular repair of visceral patch aneurysm after thoracoabdominal aneurysm repair. Vasc Endovasc Surg. 2007;41:249–53.
21. O'Connor DJ, Vouyouka A, Ellozy SH, Sundick SA, Lemasters P, Marin ML, et al. Stent graft repair of paraanastomotic aneurysms after open descending thoracic and thoracoabdominal aortic aneurysm repair. Ann Vasc Surg. 2013;27:693–8.
22. Adam DJ, Berce M, Hartley DE, Robinson DA, Anderson JL. Repair of recurrent visceral aortic patch aneurysm after thoracoabdominal aortic aneurysm repair with a branched endovascular stent graft. J Vasc Surg. 2007;45:183–5.
23. Gargiulo M, Gallitto E, Freyrie A, Stella A. Fenestrated endograft for recurrent paravisceral aortic pseudoaneurysm after thoracoabdominal aortic aneurysm open repair. J Vasc Surg. 2013;58:790–3.
24. Bertoglio L, Mascia D, Cambiaghi T, Kahlberg A, Melissano G, Chiesa R. Fenestrated and branched endovascular treatment of recurrent visceral aortic patch aneurysm after open thoracoabdominal repair. J Vasc Interv Radiol. 2018;29:72–7.
25. Bertoglio L, Mascia D, Cambiaghi T, Kahlberg A, Tshomba Y, Gomez JS, et al. Management of visceral aortic patch aneurysms after thoracoabdominal repair: open, hybrid and endovascular approach. J Vasc Surg. 2018;67:1358–69.
26. Chiesa R, Kahlberg A, Mascia D, Tshomba Y, Civilini E, Melissano G. Use of a novel hybrid vascular graft for sutureless revascularization of the renal arteries during open thoracoabdominal aortic aneurysm repair. J Vasc Surg. 2014;60:622–30.
27. de la Cruz KI, LeMaire SA, Weldon SA, Coselli JS. Thoracoabdominal aortic aneurysm repair with a branched graft. Ann Cardiothorac Surg. 2012;1:381–93.
28. Tshomba Y, Kahlberg A, Melissano G, Coppi G, Marone E, Ferrari D, et al. Comparison of renal perfusion solutions during thoracoabdominal aortic aneurysm repair. J Vasc Surg. 2014;59:623–33.
29. Verhoeven EL, Katsargyris A, Bekkema F, Oikonomou K, Zeebregts CJ, Ritter W, et al. Ten-year experience with endovascular repair of thoracoabdominal aortic aneurysms: results from 166 consecutive patients. Eur J Vasc Endovasc Surg. 2015;49:524–31.
30. Maurel B, Delclaux N, Sobocinski J, Hertault A, Martin-Gonzalez T, Moussa M, et al. The impact of early pelvic and lower limb reperfusion and attentive peri-operative management on the incidence of spinal cord ischemia during thoracoabdominal aortic aneurysm endovascular repair. Eur J Vasc Endovasc Surg. 2015;49:248–54.

Preoperative Assessment of the Spinal Cord Vasculature

25

Alexandre Campos Moraes Amato and Noedir Antonio Groppo Stolf

25.1 Introduction

Spinal cord ischemia is a rare and devastating complication of aortic aneurysm repair that has a great impact on quality of life and surgical success. Given the difficulty in predicting paraplegia in patients with aortic pathologies, new strategies are being studied to prevent spinal cord injury after aortic surgery.

Surgical repair of thoracoabdominal aneurysms was first described in 1955, and, despite improvements, the risk of spinal cord ischemia remained substantial, between 4% and 11%, with a mortality risk ranging from 3% to 17%, even at centers with extensive experience [1–3]. Therefore, the search for a better treatment option is still ongoing. One such improvement was the development of thoracic endovascular aortic repair (TEVAR). Because the technique does not require aortic cross-clamping, has shorter surgery times, and involves less invasive procedures, it lowered the incidence of spinal cord ischemia to 1–5% [4–7], a rate that is nevertheless high.

Understanding the spinal cord (SC) vascular supply is key when treating patients with aortic diseases; however, the SC vasculature is complex and difficult to study because it consists of very small vessels running in intricate, three-dimensional planes with highly variable anatomy [8]. Current noninvasive imaging techniques can identify the artery of Adamkiewicz (AKA, also known as arteria radicularis magna) and show spinal cord vasculature; however, their sensitivity and specificity are insufficient, with several factors affecting their detection capability [9, 10]. Conversely, angiography, formerly considered the gold standard method, is too invasive for current clinical routine use, hence the need for post-processing of images using three-dimensional multiplanar reconstruction to enhance detection of critical closure sites.

25.2 Anatomy

Blood supply to the medulla comes from the intercostal and lumbar arteries, which split three times before reaching the spinal cord, and from the subclavian and hypogastric branches. Except for the hypogastric arteries, which originate from the iliac arteries, the others arise from the aorta. After the first branch, the spinal branch, which

A. C. M. Amato (✉)
Vascular Surgery, Santo Amaro University, São Paulo, SP, Brazil

Amato—Instituto de Medicina Avançada, São Paulo, SP, Brazil
e-mail: alexandre@amato.com.br

N. A. G. Stolf
Thoracic and Cardiovascular Surgery, School of Medicine, University of São Paulo, São Paulo, SP, Brazil
e-mail: stolf@incor.usp.br

© Springer Nature Switzerland AG 2019
Y. Tshomba et al. (eds.), *Visceral Vessels and Aortic Repair*, https://doi.org/10.1007/978-3-319-94761-7_25

divides into anterior and posterior radicular arteries, the intercostal artery bifurcates into the dorsal and vertebral branches. Only at some spinal levels do the anterior and posterior radicular arteries penetrate the dura mater, reaching the spinal cord. Only some of the original segmental branches persist into adulthood (2–14, mean = 6). The anterior spinal artery (ASA), which is a key component of the vascularization of the spinal cord and anterior and lateral funiculi, is basically an anastomotic channel between the ascending and descending branches of neighboring anterior radicular arteries (Fig. 25.1) [11]. The last bifurcation of the spinal branch provides a constant supply of oxygenated blood to the anterior and posterior spinal cord, nerve roots, and dura mater.

Generally, the largest of the anterior radicular arteries, with its characteristic "hairpin" shape, is referred to as the great anterior radicular artery or artery of Adamkiewicz (AKA) (Fig. 25.2) [11].

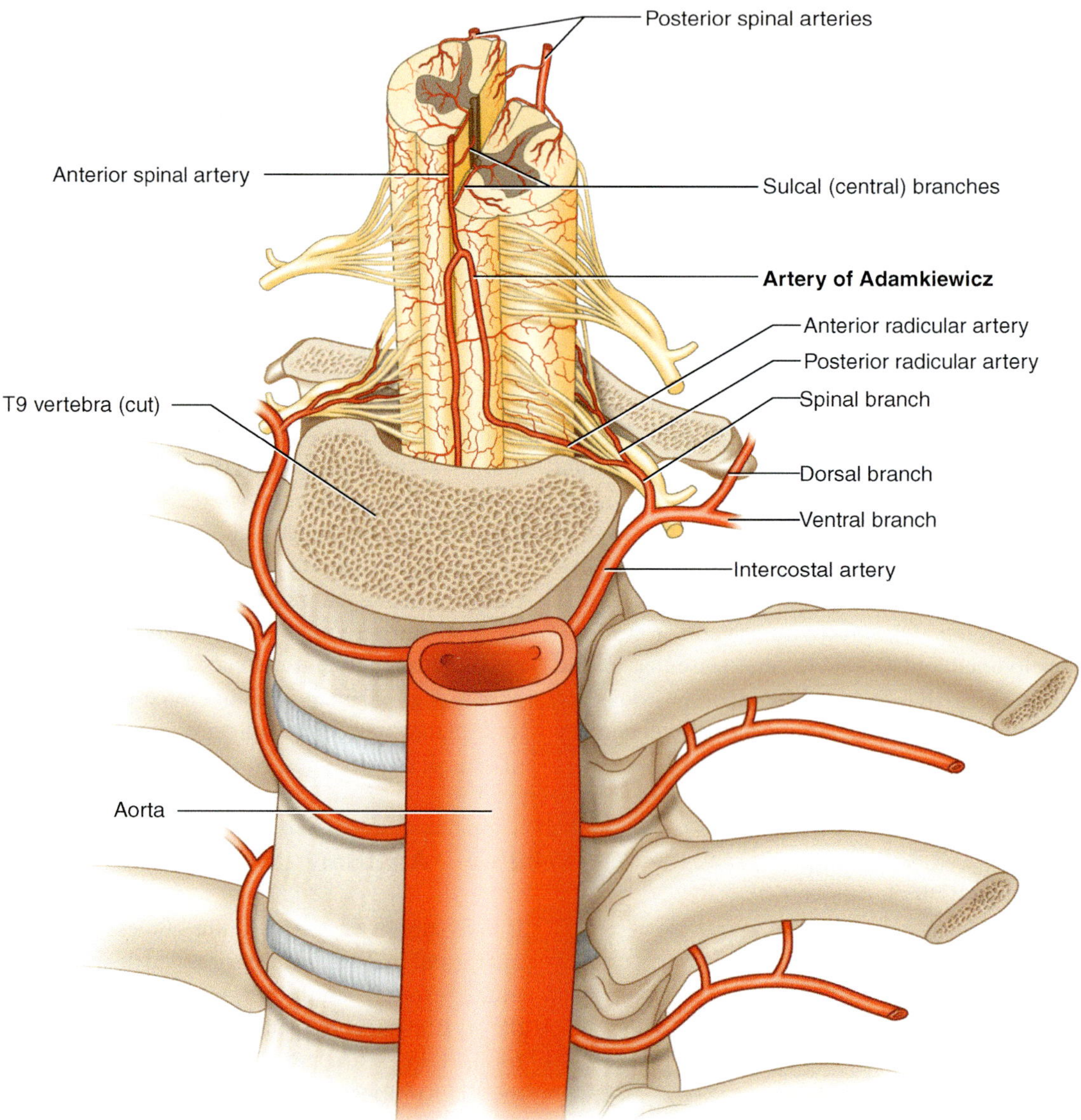

Fig. 25.1 Schematic drawing of the blood supply to the spinal cord [11]

The posterior radicular artery follows a pattern similar to the anterior radicular artery but gives rise to two longitudinal anastomotic channels, the posterolateral spinal arteries. Arteries that supply the spinal cord are divided into a central system supplied by the sulcal arteries and a peripheral system, the pial plexus, from which the perforating branches originate (Fig. 25.2) [8, 12–14]. The AKA usually originates from a left posterior intercostal artery at the levels of T9–T12 (Fig. 25.6) [9].

The venous drainage of the spinal cord is no less controversial and characterized mainly by the great posterior radicular vein, identified by its "coat hook" appearance, the posterior spinal vein, and the anterior spinal vein [27]. The anatomic significance of venous drainage preoperative planning of aortic surgery lies in its differentiation, in the image exams, from the arterial system (Fig. 25.3). Posteriorly, there is just one posterior spinal vein, as opposed to two posterolateral arteries, which is often larger than the anterior median vein [28].

Even though there is a single identifiable artery supplying the spinal cord at the thoracic level, it is not the only source of medullary blood supply. Griepp et al. refined the anatomic conceptualization of the collateral circulation network for spinal cord blood supply [29] (Fig. 25.4), providing details of its vascular redundancy. There is an axial network of small arteries in the spinal canal, paravertebral tissues, and paraspinal muscles that anastomose with each other and with the nutrient arteries of the spinal cord. Inputs

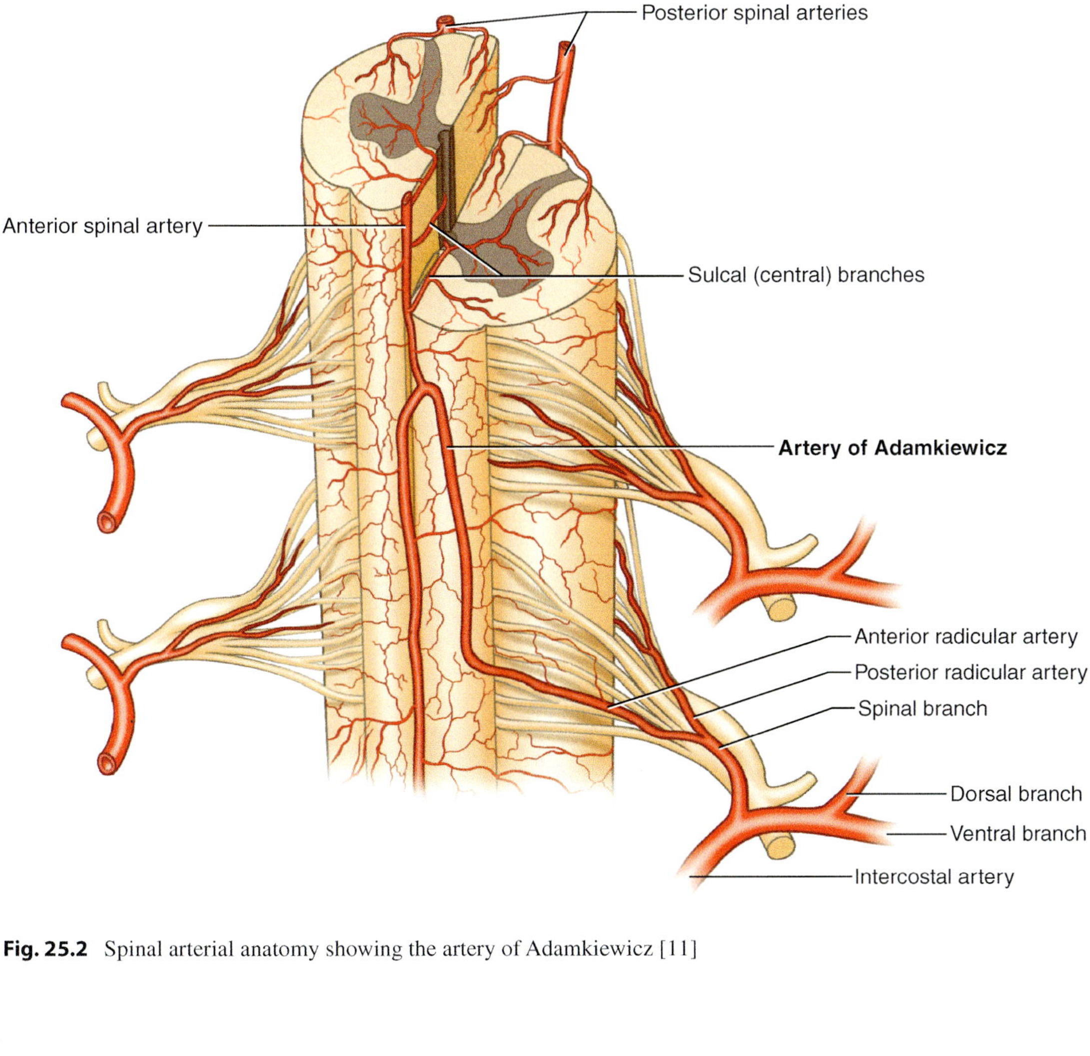

Fig. 25.2 Spinal arterial anatomy showing the artery of Adamkiewicz [11]

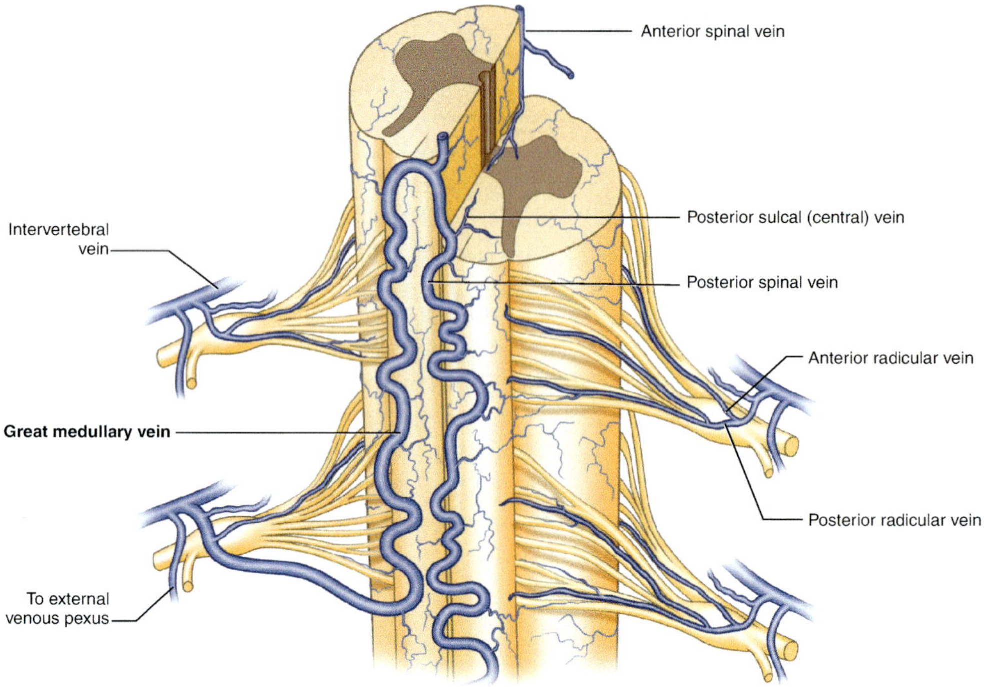

Fig. 25.3 Spinal venous anatomy [11]

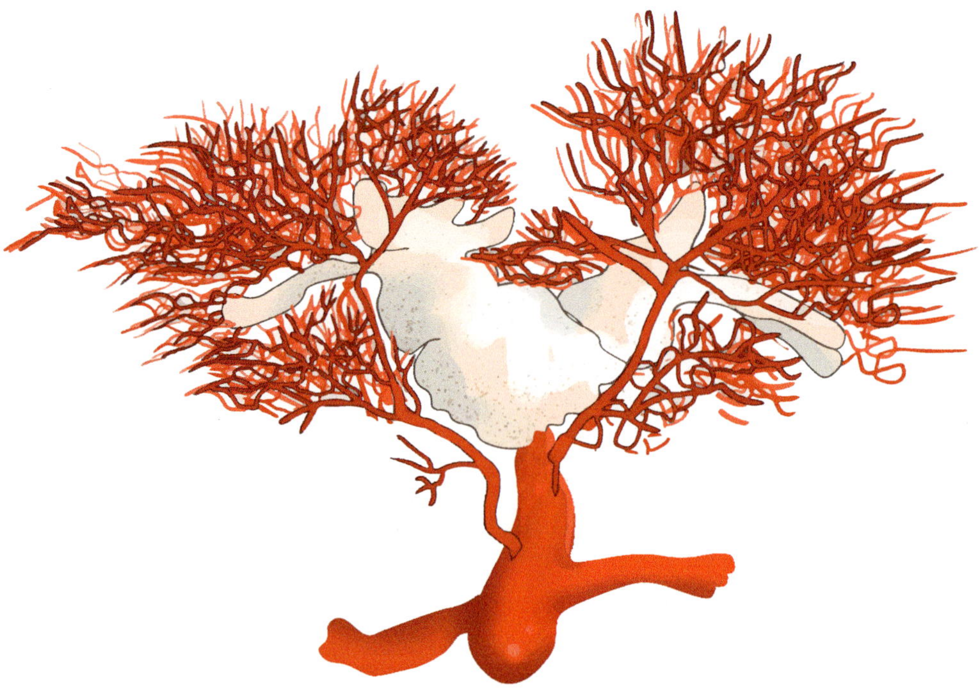

Fig. 25.4 The aorta is seen giving off segmental arteries which course around the vertebral body to supply the paraspinal muscles and, in the midline, the anterior spinal artery. The image shows the extensive anastomotic network for spinal cord blood supply

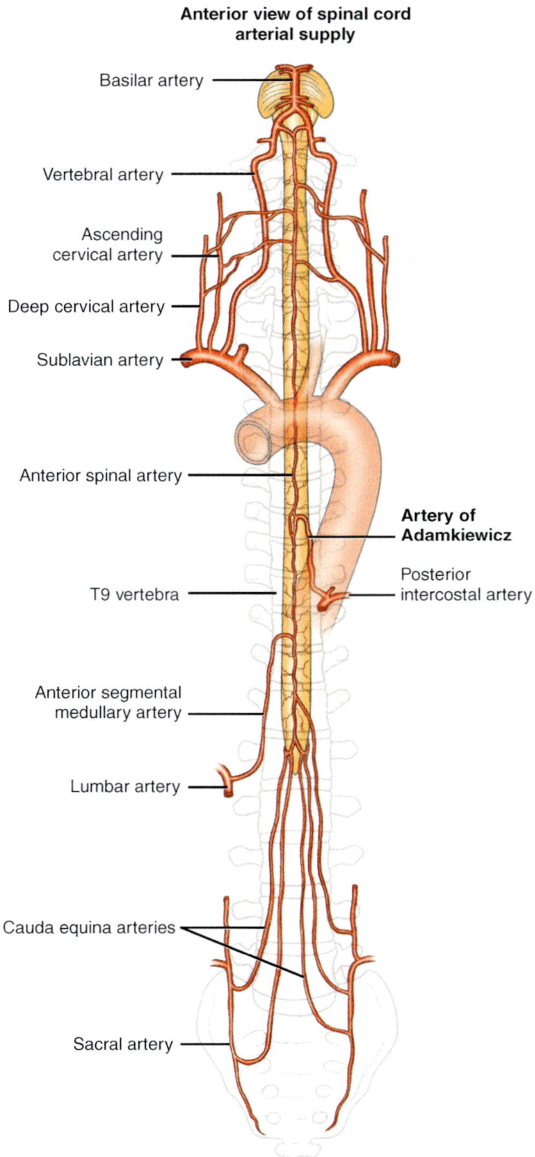

Fig. 25.5 Network of collateral vessels: subclavian, hypogastric, intercostal, and lumbar arteries

into this network include the segmental vessels (intercostal and lumbar arteries), subclavian arteries, hypogastric arteries, and their branches (Fig. 25.5) [30, 31]. In addition to these multiple inputs, there is also an extensive network of epidural arterial and small vessels that supply the paraspinal musculature (Fig. 25.4). All these vessels are interconnected and have anastomoses with the subclavian arteries, cranially, and the hypogastric arteries, caudally [31].

This network of collateral vessels can provide compensatory flow to the spinal cord in the event of occlusion of large caliber vessels [31] and increase cord nutrient flow from one source when another is reduced. Conversely, flow can be decreased if an alternate low resistance pathway is opened, such as when arterial steal occurs [29]. According to Adamkiewicz's partial flow theory, the bloodstreams of the radicular arteries reach the medullary surface in two streams, one running cranially and one caudally [13].

25.3 Imaging Acquisition Techniques

The importance of identifying and localizing the artery of Adamkiewicz prior to thoracic and thoracoabdominal surgery to prevent spinal cord injury was demonstrated by Kieffer et al. in the 1980s [32] using angiography. Arterial and posterior radicular arteries and spinal artery branches with calibers greater than 200–400 μm have been demonstrated angiographically [13]; however, this procedure is invasive, and its risks, including the risk of embolization [33], are currently considered unacceptable [34].

Computed tomography angiography (CTA) and magnetic resonance angiography (MRA) are minimally invasive imaging techniques currently used to assess spinal cord blood supply [28]. There is growing evidence that the artery of Adamkiewicz can be identified by these noninvasive techniques [15–21, 33, 35–40]. AKA detection rates range from 67% to 100% with MRA [28]; however, this imaging technique is not routinely used for the preoperative assessment of patients with aortic diseases. Conversely, CTA is performed routinely, but AKA detection rates vary widely from 18% to 100% [28] depending on post-processing technique, type of scanner, and operator experience. In addition, atherosclerotic disease and atherosclerotic risk factors may hinder SC blood supply visualization [9]. AKA identification rates are higher in studies using multiple detection techniques [18, 19, 41] (Fig. 25.6).

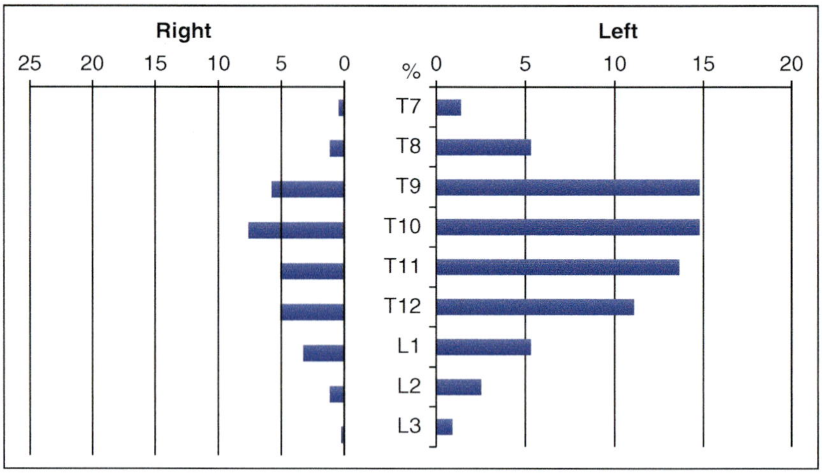

Fig. 25.6 Frequency distribution of the side of origin in studies that used computed tomography angiography for AKA identification [9, 15–26]

Even though magnetic resonance does not involve exposure to ionizing radiation and has a small risk for complications [28], it is not tolerated by all patients due to the long scan times [42]. The ability to discriminate between arterial supply and venous drainage is a clear advantage of MRA, while the proximity to skeletal structures is irrelevant, but special acquisition protocols, particularly fast acquisition techniques that use a strong bolus, in addition to good skill and dedication in image post-processing, are required for optimal results [28].

25.4 Influence of Artery Detection or Presence of Artery on Postoperative Spinal Cord Ischemia

A retrospective study using a risk model for the analysis of a database with 2235 patients from 19 European centers revealed 38 (1.7%) cases of symptomatic spinal cord ischemia. This study indicated that endovascular closure of intercostal arteries combined with occlusion of collateral vessels supplying the spinal cord is a risk factor for symptomatic spinal cord ischemia. The mathematical algorithm employed identified that intraoperative hypotension and simultaneous closure of at least two spinal cord vascular territories were relevant in the development of ischemia and that extensive coverage of intercostal arteries alone is not associated with symptomatic spinal cord ischemia [30]. Also, Murakami et al. suggested that the AKA is not the only source of SC blood supply [43]. Nevertheless, retrospective analysis of 457 patients and their in-hospital complications revealed that paraplegia and paraparesis were significantly associated with a length of the covered aorta >20 cm [44], which supports the importance of segmental arteries for SC blood supply. Yingbin et al. demonstrated the importance of identifying the AKA for selecting long endografts in cases of thoracic aortic dissection [45].

The mechanism of spinal cord ischemia after thoracic endovascular aortic repair (TEVAR) has not been fully clarified and appears to be multifactorial [3, 33]. Spinal cord perfusion depends on the gradient between arterial pressure and cerebrospinal fluid pressure [33].

25.5 Spinal Cord Visualization Technique

For AKA visualization [9, 21, 46], axial images are scrolled over at a large magnification and examined for the presence of two enhanced spots in the spinal cord, corresponding to the ASA and AKA, while tracing their cranial-caudal trajectory. Next, three-dimensional multiplanar reconstruction is used, enabling the simultaneous visualization, in three windows,

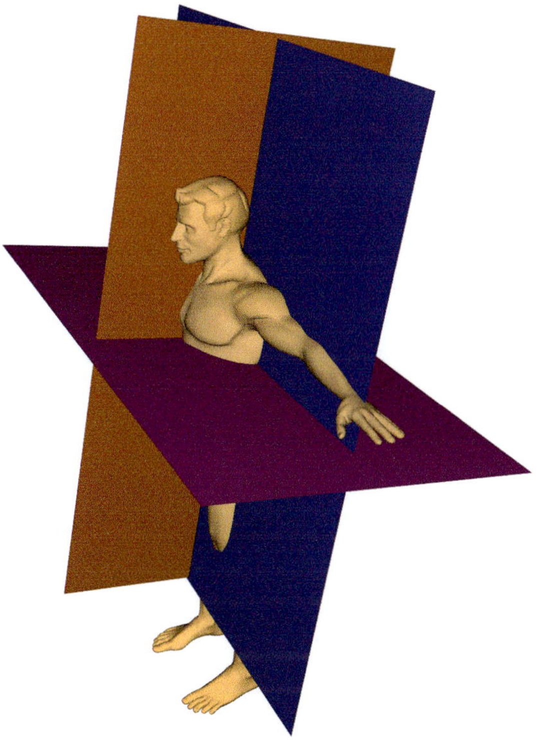

Fig. 25.7 Oblique planes used for AKA localization on three-dimensional multiplanar reconstruction

of three oblique planes at 90° in relation to each other (Fig. 25.7). The entire spinal cord can be visualized by moving the crosshair. A video illustrating the technique is available at http://vascular.cc/aka.html, and an AKA identification prediction model can be seen here https://vascular.pro/aka-model.

The crosshair is placed on the spinal cord at the level of the last thoracic vertebrae, and a sagittal view is displayed in the upper left window. By adjusting the position and angle of the crosshair to cover most of the spinal cord longitudinally in the upper left window and adjusting slice thickness using the maximum intensity projection (MIP) algorithm and "windowing" (apparent Hounsfield scale), an oblique coronal or paracoronal view of the spinal cord is produced in the large window. Tilting the crosshair and scrolling over the images along the anteroposterior direction allows a quick exploration of the entire spinal cord (Fig. 25.9) [21].

The ASA is identified, in the anterior aspect of the spinal cord, as a thin longitudinal vessel (Fig. 25.8a), whereas the AKA is readily identified by its "hairpin" appearance, supplying the

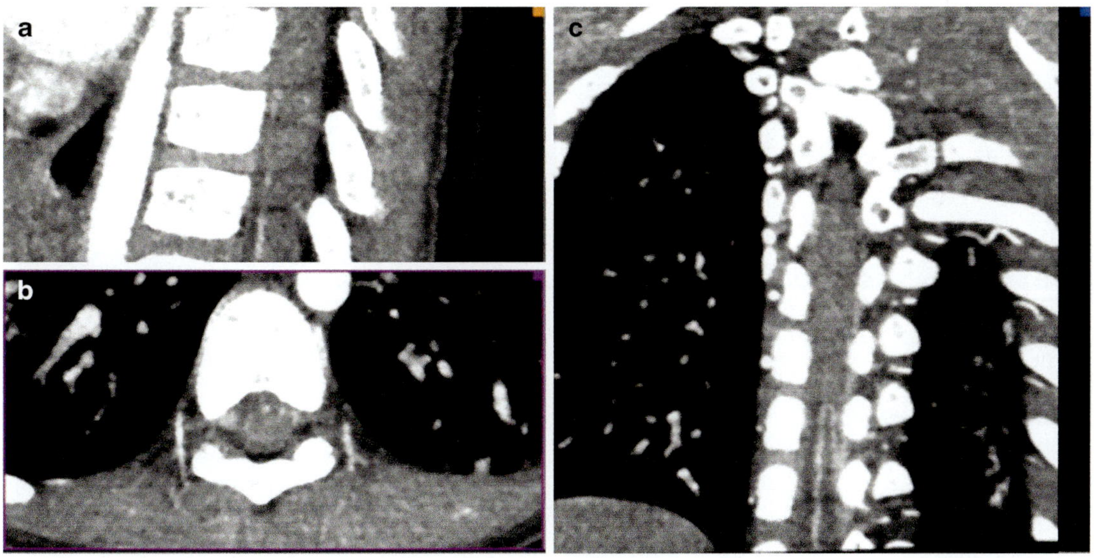

Fig. 25.8 *OsiriX* software window. The green arrow shows the ASA, and the red arrow shows the AKA. (**a**) Sagittal view. (**b**) Axial view. (**c**) Coronal oblique view

anterior spinal artery, in a paracoronal view using two-dimensional multiplanar reconstruction (MPR) (Figs. 25.8c and 25.9).

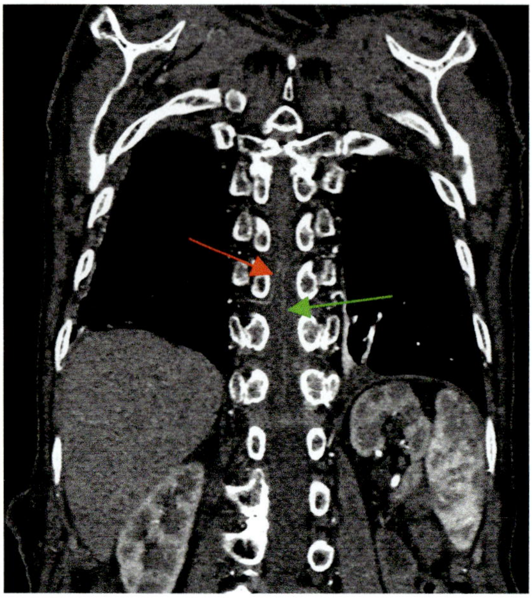

Fig. 25.9 Three-dimensional MPR oblique view showing the AKA (red arrow) with its typical "hairpin" appearance and the ASA (green arrow)

The identification of the AKA and ASA is based on the following criteria:

- Continuity of the AKA traceable to vessels of known arterial nature such as the intercostal artery or aorta (Fig. 25.10) [16, 19, 20, 36]. Continuity with arteries is certainly a highly relevant factor; however, this is not always achieved and other criteria are needed [16, 19, 20, 28, 36].
- Simultaneous identification of the AKA and ASA as two enhanced spots in the ventral aspect of the spinal cord on consecutive axial scans [19, 20, 28].
- Characteristic anatomic relationship of the two vessels, i.e., "hairpin" shape (Fig. 25.3) [19].
- Failure of venous enhancement and visualization of the posterior spinal vein and other veins surrounding the spinal column (intercostal, lumbar, and azygos veins) [28].

The AKA can be identified with computed tomography angiography in approximately 70% of cases [9, 17–20, 26, 27, 38, 41, 47–50], and this imaging modality is routinely used in the

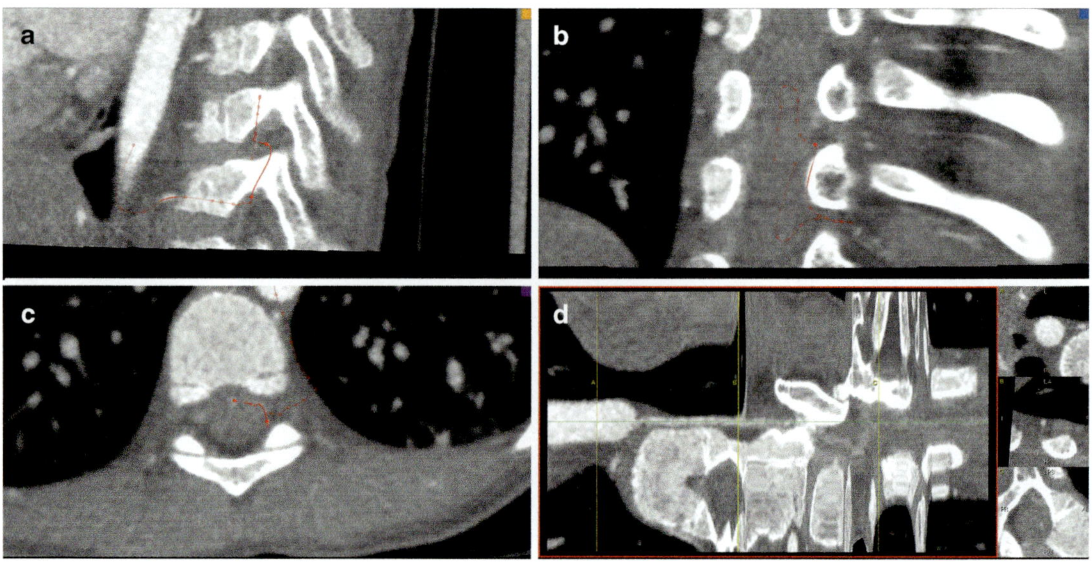

Fig. 25.10 (**a**–**c**) Oblique views showing the three-dimensional path of the AKA. (**d**) Continuity of the AKA (red arrow) from the aorta (yellow arrow) through the intercostal artery (blue arrow) and ASA (green arrow) on three-dimensional curved multiplanar reconstruction, which reconstructs the course of the vessel from its origin in the aorta through the spinal cord

preoperative assessment of thoracoabdominal aortic aneurysms. The imaging acquisition protocol for SC blood supply visualization is similar to standard angio-CT protocols used in most centers.

25.6 Conclusion

When the risk of intraoperative closure of two vascular territories supplying the spinal cord [30] is identified in the presurgical planning of aortic aneurysm repair, AKA disruption—or at least that of collateral vessels—can be prevented with prior knowledge of its location using the method described here.

If the AKA identification method proposed cannot be applied to a patient, the surgical team should then rely on anatomic studies [9] that show the existence of a critical area of great importance for SC circulation between the levels of T9 and T12. This area requires special attention from the surgeon to preserve the AKA as well as if possible the other spinal cord blood supply sources.

References

1. Greenberg RK, Lytle B. Endovascular repair of thoracoabdominal aneurysms. Circulation. 2008;117(17):2288–96.
2. Svensson LG, Crawford ES, Hess KR, Coselli JS, Safi HJ. Experience with 1509 patients undergoing thoracoabdominal aortic operations. J Vasc Surg. 1993;17(2):357–68.
3. Chiesa R, Melissano G, Bertoglio L, Amato ACM, Tshomba Y, Civilini E, et al. The risk of spinal cord ischemia during thoracic aorta endografting. Acta Chir Belg. 2008;108:492–502.
4. Gottardi R, Dumfarth J, Holfeld J, Schoder M, Funovics M, Laufer G, et al. Symptomatic spinal cord malperfusion after stent-graft coverage of the entire descending aorta. Eur J Cardiothorac Surg. 2010;37(5):1081–5.
5. Eggebrecht H, Nienaber CA, Neuhäuser M, Baumgart D, Kische S, Schmermund A, et al. Endovascular stent-graft placement in aortic dissection: a meta-analysis. Eur Heart J. 2006;27(4):489–98.
6. Czerny M, Funovics M, Sodeck G, Dumfarth J, Schoder M, Juraszek A, et al. Long-term results of thoracic endovascular aortic repair in atherosclerotic aneurysms involving the descending aorta. J Thorac Cardiovasc Surg. 2010;140(6 Suppl):S179–84.
7. Buth J, Harris PL, Hobo R, van Eps R, Cuypers P, Duijm L, Tielbeek X. Neurologic complications associated with endovascular repair of thoracic aortic pathology: incidence and risk factors. A study from the european collaborators on stent/graft techniques for aortic aneurysm repair (EUROSTAR) registry. J Vasc Surg. 2007;46(6):1103–10.
8. Melissano G, Civilini E, Bertoglio L, Calliari F, Campos Moraes Amato A, Chiesa R. Angio-CT imaging of the spinal cord vascularisation: a pictorial essay. Eur J Vasc Endovasc Surg. 2010;39(4):436–40.
9. Amato ACM, Parga Filho JR, Stolf NAG. Influential factors on the evaluation of Adamkiewicz artery using a 320-detector row computed tomography device. Ann Vasc Surg. 2017;44:136–45.
10. Amato ACM, Parga Filho JR, Stolf NAG. Predictors of Adamkiewicz artery and anterior spinal artery detection through computerized tomographic angiography. SAGE Open Med. 2017;5:2050312117711599.
11. Amato ACM, Stolf NAG. Anatomy of spinal blood supply. J Vasc Bras. 2015;14(3):248–52.
12. Thron AK. Vascular anatomy of the spine. Oxford: Oxford University Press; 2002.
13. Thron AK, Rossberg C. Vascular anatomy of the spinal cord: neuroradiological investigations and clinical syndromes. New York: Springer; 1988.
14. Thron AK. Vascular anatomy of the spinal cord: neuroradiological investigations and clinical syndromes. New York: Springer-Verlag; 1989.
15. Kudo K, Terae S, Asano T, Oka M, Kaneko K, Ushikoshi S, Miyasaka K. Anterior spinal artery and artery of Adamkiewicz detected by using multi-detector row CT. AJNR Am J Neuroradiol. 2003;24(1):13–7.
16. Uotani K, Yamada N, Kono AK, Taniguchi T, Sugimoto K, Fujii M, et al. Preoperative visualization of the artery of Adamkiewicz by intra-arterial CT angiography. AJNR Am J Neuroradiol. 2008;29(2):314–8.
17. Nojiri J, Matsumoto K, Kato A, Miho T, Furukawa K, Ohtsubo S, et al. The Adamkiewicz artery: demonstration by intra-arterial computed tomographic angiography. Eur J Cardiothorac Surg. 2007;31(2):249–55.
18. Yoshioka K, Niinuma H, Ohira A, Nasu K, Kawakami T, Sasaki M, Kawazoe K. MR angiography and CT angiography of the artery of Adamkiewicz: noninvasive preoperative assessment of thoracoabdominal aortic aneurysm. Radiographics. 2003;23(5):1215–25.
19. Yoshioka K, Niinuma H, Ehara S, Nakajima T, Nakamura M, Kawazoe K. MR angiography and CT angiography of the artery of Adamkiewicz: state of the art. Radiographics. 2006;26(Suppl 1):S63–73.
20. Takase K, Sawamura Y, Igarashi K, Chiba Y, Haga K, Saito H, Takahashi S. Demonstration of the artery of Adamkiewicz at multi- detector row helical CT. Radiology. 2002;223(1):39–45.
21. Melissano G, Amato ACM, Bertoglio L, Civilini E, Civelli V, Coppi G, et al. Demonstration of the

Adamkiewicz artery by multidetector computed tomography angiography analysed with open-source software OsiriX. Eur J Vasc Endovasc Surg. 2009;37(4):395–400.
22. Nishimura J, Lee J, Koike S, Kurihara H, Ozawa Y, Abe A, et al. Identification of the segmental artery feeding the anterior spinal artery: correlation between helical CT and angiography. Radiat Med. 2005;23(4):271–6.
23. von Tengg-Kobligk H, Böckler D, Jose TM, Ganten M, Kotelis D, Nagel S, et al. Feeding arteries of the spinal cord at CT angiography before and after thoracic aortic endografting. J Endovasc Ther. 2007;14(5):639–49.
24. Nakayama Y, Awai K, Yanaga Y, Nakaura T, Funama Y, Hirai T, Yamashita Y. Optimal contrast medium injection protocols for the depiction of the Adamkiewicz artery using 64-detector CT angiography. Clin Radiol. 2008;63(8):880–7.
25. Zhao S, Logan L, Schraedley P, Rubin GD. Multidetector CT angiography for the assessment of anterior spinal artery and artery of Adamkiewicz patency in patients suspected of having thoracic aortic pathology. J Geriatr Cardiol. 2006;3(1):52–6.
26. Ou P, Schmit P, Layouss W, Sidi D, Bonnet D, Brunelle F. CT angiography of the artery of Adamkiewicz with 64-section technology: first experience in children. AJNR Am J Neuroradiol. 2007;28(2):216–9.
27. Takase K, Akasaka J, Sawamura Y, Ota H, Sato A, Yamada T, et al. Preoperative MDCT evaluation of the artery of Adamkiewicz and its origin. J Comput Assist Tomogr. 2006;30(5):716–22.
28. Melissano G, Chiesa R. Advances in imaging of the spinal cord vascular supply and its relationship with paraplegia after aortic interventions. A review. Eur J Vasc Endovasc Surg. 2009;38(5):567–77.
29. Griepp RB, Griepp EB. Spinal cord perfusion and protection during descending thoracic and thoracoabdominal aortic surgery: the collateral network concept. Ann Thorac Surg. 2007;83(2):S865–9.
30. Czerny M, Eggebrecht H, Sodeck G, Verzini F, Cao P, Maritati G, et al. Mechanisms of symptomatic spinal cord ischemia after TEVAR: insights from the european registry of endovascular aortic repair complications (eurec). J Endovasc Ther. 2012;19(1):37–43.
31. Griepp R, Luozzo GD, Schray D, Stefanovic A, Geisbüsch S, Randall BRB. The anatomy of the spinal cord collateral circulation. Ann Cardiothorac Surg. 2012;1(3):350–7.
32. Kieffer E, Richard T, Chiras J, Godet G, Cormier E. Preoperative spinal cord arteriography in aneurysmal disease of the descending thoracic and thoracoabdominal aorta: preliminary results in 45 patients. Ann Vasc Surg. 1989;3(1):34–46.
33. Chiesa R, Melissano G, Marrocco-Trischitta MM, Civilini E, Setacci F. Spinal cord ischemia after elective stent-graft repair of the thoracic aorta. J Vasc Surg. 2005;42(1):11–7.
34. Forbes G, Nichols DA, Jack CR, Ilstrup DM, Kispert DB, Piepgras DG, et al. Complications of spinal cord arteriography: prospective assessment of risk for diagnostic procedures. Radiology. 1988;169(2):479–84.
35. Schurink GW, Nijenhuis RJ, Backes WH, Mess W, de Haan MW, Mochtar B, Jacobs MJ. Assessment of spinal cord circulation and function in endovascular treatment of thoracic aortic aneurysms. Ann Thorac Surg. 2007;83(2):S877–81.
36. Yamada N, Okita Y, Minatoya K, Tagusari O, Ando M, Takamiya M, Kitamura S. Preoperative demonstration of the Adamkiewicz artery by magnetic resonance angiography in patients with descending or thoracoabdominal aortic aneurysms. Eur J Cardiothorac Surg. 2000;18(1):104–11.
37. Kawaharada N, Morishita K, Fukada J, Yamada A, Muraki S, Hyodoh H, Abe T. Thoracoabdominal or descending aortic aneurysm repair after preoperative demonstration of the Adamkiewicz artery by magnetic resonance angiography. Eur J Cardiothorac Surg. 2002;21(6):970–4.
38. Nijenhuis RJ, Gerretsen S, Leiner T, Jacobs MJ, van Engelshoven JM, Backes WH. Comparison of 0.5-M gd-dtpa with 1.0-M gadobutrol for magnetic resonance angiography of the supplying arteries of the spinal cord in thoracoabdominal aortic aneurysm patients. J Magn Reson Imaging. 2005;22(1):136–44.
39. Hyodoh H, Shirase R, Akiba H, Tamakawa M, Hyodoh K, Yama N, et al. Double-subtraction maximum intensity projection MR angiography for detecting the artery of Adamkiewicz and differentiating it from the drainage vein. J Magn Reson Imaging. 2007;26(2):359–65.
40. Hyodoh H, Kawaharada N, Akiba H, Tamakawa M, Hyodoh K, Fukada J, et al. Usefulness of preoperative detection of artery of Adamkiewicz with dynamic contrast-enhanced MR angiography. Radiology. 2005;236(3):1004–9.
41. Nijenhuis RJ, Jacobs MJ, Schurink GW, Kessels AG, van Engelshoven JM, Backes WH. Magnetic resonance angiography and neuromonitoring to assess spinal cord blood supply in thoracic and thoracoabdominal aortic aneurysm surgery. J Vasc Surg. 2007;45(1):71–7.
42. Katz RC, Wilson L, Frazer N. Anxiety and its determinants in patients undergoing magnetic resonance imaging. J Behav Ther Exp Psychiatry. 1994;25(2):131–4.
43. Murakami H, Kawahara N, Tomita K, Demura S, Kato S, Yoshioka K. Does interruption of the artery of Adamkiewicz during total en bloc spondylectomy affect neurologic function? Spine (Phila Pa 1976). 2010;35(22):E1187–92.
44. Fattori R, Nienaber CA, Rousseau H, Beregi JP, Heijmen R, Grabenwöger M, et al. Results of endovascular repair of the thoracic aorta with the talent thoracic stent graft: the talent thoracic retrospective registry. J Thorac Cardiovasc Surg. 2006;132(2):332–9.
45. Yingbin J, Jiefei M, Jian L, Yonghui S, Haiyan P, Baimeng Z, Weigoo F. Evaluation of the thoracic aortic dissection treated by endografts covering a longer distance of aorta according to the location of

the Adamkiewicz artery. Thorac Cardiovasc Surg. 2013;61(07):569–74.
46. Amato ACM, Melissano G, Giovanni C, Civilini E, Civelli V, Calori G, et al. Available from: http://vascular.cc/aka.html. Accessed 18 Dec 2012.
47. Nijenhuis RJ, Jacobs MJ, Jaspers K, Reinders M, Reijnders M, van Engelshoven JM, et al. Comparison of magnetic resonance with computed tomography angiography for preoperative localization of the Adamkiewicz artery in thoracoabdominal aortic aneurysm patients. J Vasc Surg. 2007;45(4):677–85.
48. Boll DT, Bulow H, Blackham KA, Aschoff AJ, Schmitz BL. MDCT angiography of the spinal vasculature and the artery of Adamkiewicz. AJR Am J Roentgenol. 2006;187(4):1054–60.
49. Nijenhuis RJ, Mull M, Wilmink JT, Thron AK, Backes WH. MR angiography of the great anterior radiculomedullary artery (Adamkiewicz artery) validated by digital subtraction angiography. AJNR Am J Neuroradiol. 2006;27(7):1565–72.
50. Nijenhuis RJ, Jacobs MJ, van Engelshoven JM, Backes WH. MR angiography of the Adamkiewicz artery and anterior radiculomedullary vein: postmortem validation. AJNR Am J Neuroradiol. 2006;27(7):1573–5.

Intercostal Artery Reattachment Guided by Intraoperative Neurophysiologic Monitoring During Open Thoracoabdominal Aortic Repair: Basic Principles and Clinical Experience

26

Ubaldo Del Carro, Francesca Bianchi, Marco Cursi, and Heike Caravati

Spinal cord ischemia (SCI) is one of the most important complications during thoracoabdominal aortic aneurysm (TAAA) repair. In an effort to reduce this risk, over the last few years, operative strategies have evolved from the traditional clamp-and-sew technique with epidural cooling to one applying distal aortic perfusion with a variety of additional strategies to protect the spinal cord [1]. Among these strategies, intraoperative neuromonitoring (IOM) allows for a real-time assessment of spinal cord functional integrity and early detection of SCI, providing the team with the opportunity to promptly trigger interventions for maximizing spinal perfusion and potentially reverse spinal injury [2–4]. Type I to III TAAAs are often repaired with distal perfusion techniques and neuromonitoring, while the use of such adjuncts is irregularly applied in the repair of type IV TAAA [5–7]. Literature data support the use of IOM as a strategy to detect SCI and to guide hemodynamic optimization and/or reimplantation of intercostal arteries to prevent or treat SCI, providing a level B of evidence [8]. The neuromonitoring modalities used during TAAA surgery are the somatosensory evoked potentials (SSEPs) and the motor evoked potentials (MEPs) because their neural pathways pass through the spinal cord and their sensitivity to ischemia [9]. These techniques are safe, do not interfere with surgical procedures, or modify the clamping time. SSEPs provide information about the somatosensory pathway in the spinal dorsal columns. Furthermore, their peripheral response (i.e., popliteal potential) is useful to monitor the impending peripheral nerve injury and therefore differentiates SCI from peripheral ischemia. Nielsen and Kardel studied the peripheral nerve conduction during ischemia and found that sensory conduction velocity exhibits a temporospatial slowing along the ischemic nerve segment, determining that conduction time increases and amplitude decreases rectilinearly with the squared duration of ischemia and proportionally to segment length [10]. Because TAAA surgery is more likely to compromise blood flow in the anterior spinal artery territory, the presence of synapses in the anterior horn gray matter makes MEPs more sensitive than SSEPs in detecting SCI. Furthermore, MEP monitoring has a better

U. Del Carro (✉)
Department of Neurology and INSPE, Vita-Salute University, San Raffaele Scientific Institute, Milan, Italy
e-mail: delcarro.ubaldo@hsr.it

F. Bianchi · M. Cursi · H. Caravati
Department of Neurology and INSPE, San Raffaele Scientific Institute, Milan, Italy
e-mail: bianchi.francesca@hsr.it; cursi.marco@hsr.it; caravati.heike@hsr.it

© Springer Nature Switzerland AG 2019
Y. Tshomba et al. (eds.), *Visceral Vessels and Aortic Repair*,
https://doi.org/10.1007/978-3-319-94761-7_26

correlation with motor outcome because it monitors the corticospinal tract [9]. However, SSEPs can provide a neurophysiologic "background" on which to interpret MEP changes, and the use of both these techniques may offer a better vigilance on neurological complication [9]. MEPs are elicited by transcranial electrical stimulation applied through corkscrew electrodes placed at FC3 and FC4 scalp sites and recorded from limb muscles. The electrical stimulation consisted in a train-of-five monophasic or biphasic stimuli of 500 μs duration, intensity ranging from 200 to 400 V (avoiding to exceed 600 V), and interstimulus interval of 4 ms. MEPs are recorded by needle electrodes placed into limb muscles and monitored bilaterally in lower limbs. Responses from the upper limb are frequently used as internal control to rule out the effects of systemic factors. There is no literature agreement on the MEP warning criteria, and even if different percentages of amplitude reduction compared to the baseline value have been proposed, a recent meta-analysis showed that the "all-or-none" cutoff may be the best criterion [11]. SSEPs are obtained by electric stimulation of the posterior tibial nerve at the ankle and usually recorded from the popliteal fossa and the scalp. The right and left posterior tibial nerves are alternatively stimulated at the internal malleolus. The stimulus consists in a single current pulse, with intensity high enough to obtain motor twitch, duration of 200 μs, and repetition rate of 4.6 Hz. Cortical potentials are recorded by means of corkscrew electrodes using a multichannel montage that includes Fz–CPz and CP3–CP4 derivations. Peripheral potentials are recorded bilaterally by needle electrodes placed in the popliteal fossa. A range of 300–500 repetitions are averaged to produce reproducible SSEPs. The traditional 10/50 rule is considered to define SSEP abnormalities (Fig. 26.1). A baseline MEP

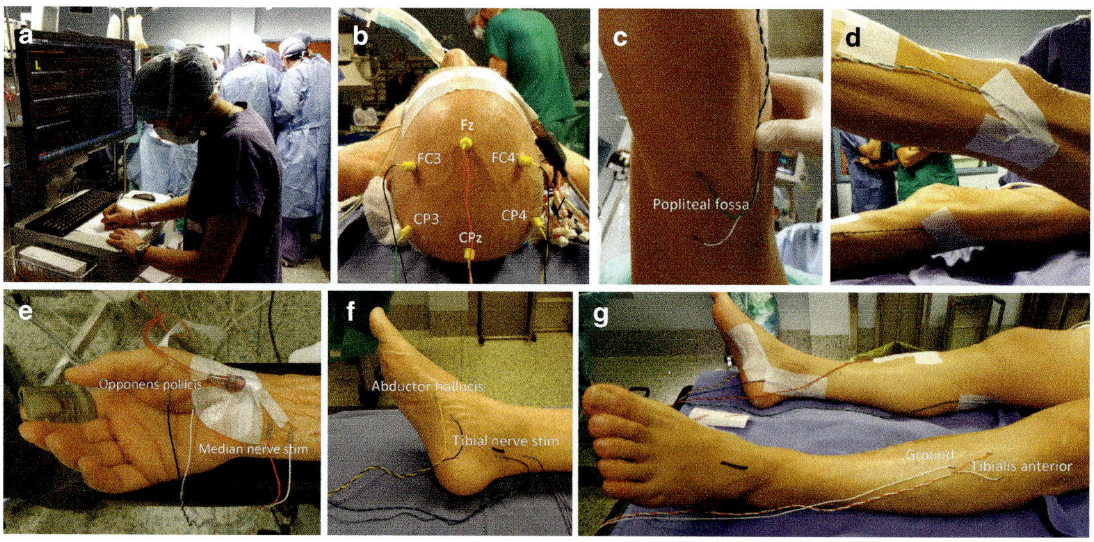

Fig. 26.1 Neurophysiological intraoperative monitoring during TAAA repair. The neurophysiological monitoring system is located in the operating room near the surgical table (**a**). Corkscrew electrodes are used to record SSEPs and to deliver the transcranial electrical stimulation for MEPs (**b**). Cortical SSEPs are recorded from two channels: Fz–CPz and CP3–CP4. The transcranial electrical stimulus for MEPs is applied between FC3 and FC4. Twisted pair needle electrodes are placed at the left (**c**) and right popliteal fossa to record SAPs. Needle electrodes are secured to the patient skin with Hypafix non-woven fabric adhesive patch (**d**, **g**). Twisted pair needle electrodes are placed on the right opponens pollicis muscle for recording three different responses: the MEP, the MAP, and the TOF. Another couple of needle electrodes is placed at the wrist to stimulate the median nerve for obtaining TOF and MAP responses (**e**). Twisted pairs needle electrodes are positioned bilaterally on the abductor hallucis (**f**) and tibialis anterior (**g**) for recording lower limb MEPs. Two couples of twisted needle electrodes are placed bilaterally at the ankle (**f**, **g**) to stimulate the tibial nerve for obtaining MAPs and SSEPs. The ground electrode is placed on the left leg (**g**)

and SSEP recording is suggested after anesthetic induction and intubation maneuvers, in order to guarantee the measurements when a steady anesthetic state has been reached and the effect of the initial dose of muscle relaxant has disappeared. All subsequent measurements are compared with the baseline recordings. MEPs are checked intermittently until the aorta is cross-clamped and more regularly during and after the cross-clamping (e.g., every 5 min). SSEPs are monitored continuously. A critical aspect of this neurophysiologic monitoring is the interpretation of the MEP and SSEP changes occurring after aortic cross-clamping, specifically the distinction between those changes due to SCI and false-positive results. There is a clear need to better interpret these changes in order to guide more precisely the choice of appropriate surgical strategies for each patient, increasing the speed and safety of the procedures and avoiding unnecessary time-consuming maneuvers. Intraoperative evoked potential (EP) changes may result from ischemia of their specific neural pathway or may be due to nonspecific systemic factors. When systemic factors take place, there is a concomitant reduction of both upper and lower limb EPs. Hence, the simultaneous use of an upper limb recording represents an important internal control to detect unspecific EP changes. Among systemic causes that may influence EPs, there are physiologic factors (e.g., blood pressure, temperature) and pharmacologic agents (i.e., anesthetic drugs, neuromuscular blocking agents). The use of inhalation anesthetic agents has an inhibitory effect on neurotransmission, and total intravenous anesthesia is widely recommended when neurophysiological monitoring is needed. Deepening anesthesia and administering boluses decrease EP responses, and the maintenance of a stable concentration of anesthetics is advisable. Several different methods of EEG processing have been developed to evaluate the intraoperative anesthetic depth, and among these the bispectral index (BIS) provides a quantitative measure easy to interpret. Neuromuscular blockade can influence IOM results, especially decreasing MEP signals. For this reason, it is often omitted after intubation or controlled by means of different methods throughout the surgery. Among these, the train-of-four (TOF) test is based on four supramaximal stimulation of peripheral nerve resulting in four twitches: T1, T2, T3, and T4. The assessment of the neuromuscular blockade is performed by measurement of the amplitude of the compound muscle action potential (CMAP) and calculation of percentage of CMAP decrement from T1 to T4. Hypothermia decreases the reliability of EP monitoring, even if a stable temperature above 32 °C seems to be sufficient enough to record the signal. Once excluding systemic factors, the role of hypoperfusion must be considered. Hypoperfusion can be due to both surgical maneuvers and arterial hypotension and can involve the spinal cord and/or lower limbs. In both of these cases, an alteration of lower limb EPs with preserved upper limb response should be expected. Lower limb ischemia may occur when the surgeon performs distal aortic or iliac anastomosis and suspends retrograde perfusion, or it happens frequently in the left leg used for femoral artery cannulation. To overcome this limitation, several studies proposed monitoring only the right leg, others the use of a left femoral side graft rather than a second cannula to maintain the left leg perfused and available for monitoring cord functions. SSEPs could be useful to identify limb ischemia, showing a concomitant alteration of popliteal and cortical potentials. Another method consists in the study of CMAP is obtained by stimulating a peripheral nerve (i.e., tibial nerve at the ankle) and recording the motor response from the muscle (i.e., abductor hallucis). CMAP provides a further intraoperative measure of the peripheral nerve functional integrity and could be useful to differentiate SCI from limb ischemia. When CMAPs and MEPs are both reduced at the lower limbs, the surgeon can suspect that EP changes are due to peripheral rather than spinal ischemia. In such scenario, more complexed maneuvers, such as selective perfusion or reimplantation of intercostal arteries, may be unnecessary. On the other hand, when MEPs are altered and CMAPs remain unchanged, the surgeon is sufficiently confident that an ischemic injury to the spinal cord is ongoing.

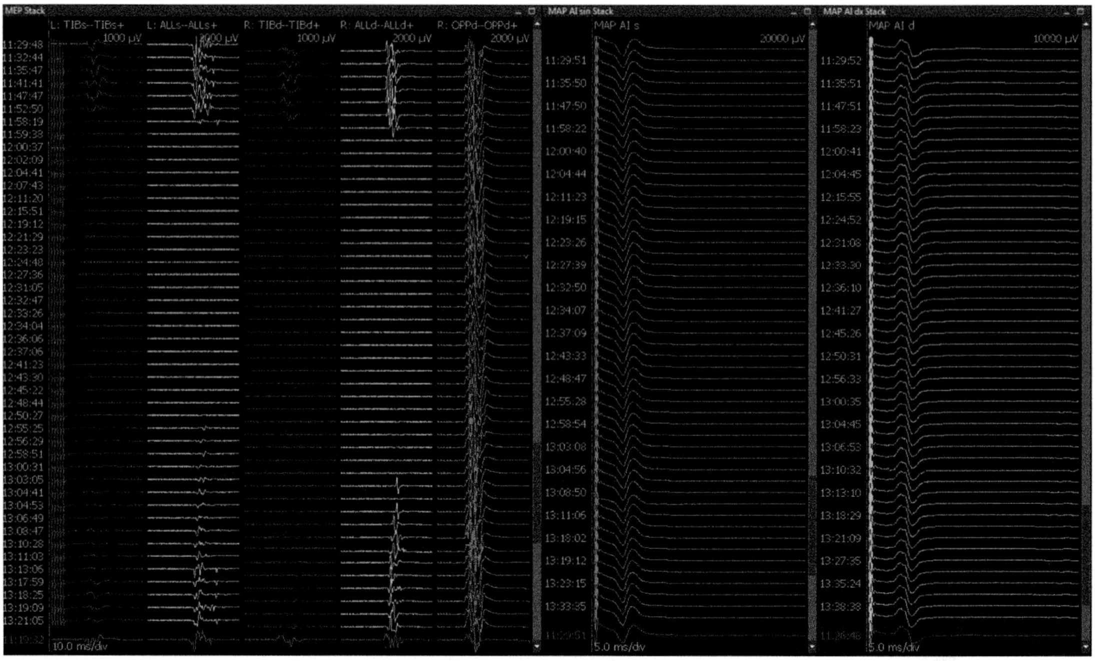

Fig. 26.2 Case 1: spinal cord ischemia after aorta cross-clamping. In the figure MEP and CMAP time courses are reported for patient (AM) with TAAA type II. From left to right: MEPs recorded from the left tibialis anterior (first column), left abductor hallucis (second column), right tibialis anterior (third column), right abductor hallucis (fourth column), and right opponens pollicis (fifth column) and CMAPs recorded from left and right abductor hallucis (sixth and seventh columns). Baseline tracings (represented by the red line) are shown at the bottom of the stack. Aorta cross-clamping occurred at 11:32. At 11:58 MEPs were abruptly lost in the left lower limb and, 1 min later, also in the right lower limb. No changes were observed in upper limb MEPs and in lower limb CMAPS. Distal aortic clamp was removed, and anterograde lower extremity perfusion restored at 12:22 but MEPs did not recover. Six intercostal arteries were identified and reattached to the graft, determining a slow restoration of MEPs to the baseline levels

A selection of clinical cases is reported in Figs. 26.2, 26.3, 26.4, 26.5, 26.6, and 26.7. In order to verify the sensitivity of CMAP amplitude in peripheral ischemia and the usefulness of this method combined with MEP and SSEP monitoring in differentiating spinal versus peripheral ischemia, we draw a prospective open-label study on patients with TAAA undergoing surgical repair. The study has been approved by local ethics committee on 8 October 2015 and registered on ClinicalTrials.gov website (ID: NCT02644681), and it is still ongoing. The segmental artery reimplantation represents a strategy to reduce the risk of SCI based on specific pathophysiologic prerequisite, especially when the other strategies are not able to restore MEP changes. The pathophysiology of spinal cord injury in TAAA surgery is essentially based on ischemia-infarction model. Thoracic aortic clamping reduces arterial blood supply to the spinal cord, increases spinal fluid pressure, and produces inadequate oxygen delivery and ischemia [12–14]. Infarction occurs when the ischemic tolerance of the spinal cord is exceeded or when aortic replacement permanently interrupts critical radicular arteries supplying the anterior spinal artery. To reduce the risk of spinal infarction during TAAA surgery, it is necessary to increase the ischemic tolerance of the spinal cord and maximize spinal cord perfusion. Typically, the anterior spinal artery is fed by several anterior radiculomedullary arteries, and, among these, the intercostal arteries arising from the thoracic and lumbar aorta are considered critical to spinal cord blood supply [15]. This is the rationale for the importance of critical segmental artery reimplantation in TAAA surgery. However, only a few of the segmental arteries supply radicular arteries contributing to

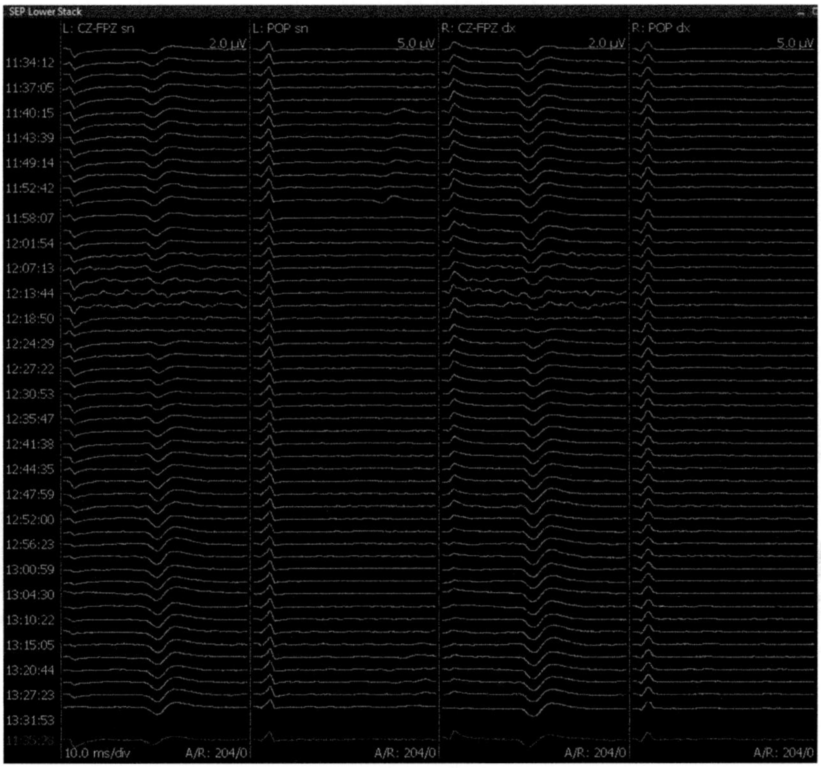

Fig. 26.3 Case 1: spinal cord ischemia after aorta cross-clamping. In the figure, same patient (AM), of Fig. 26.2, SSEP time course is reported. From left to right: CPz–Fpz derivation (first columns), popliteal fossa (second column) for left stimulation, CPz–Fpz and popliteal fossa for right stimulation (third and fourth columns). Baseline tracings (represented by the red line) are shown at the bottom of the stack. A brief amplitude decrease of cortical SSEPs was observed between 12:13 and 12:24, while no changes occurred in peripheral responses. However, the concomitant persistence of MEP changes motivated the intercostal arteries reimplantation

the anterior spinal artery [16], and their identification could be difficult [17]. Furthermore, reimplanting intercostal arteries is technically challenging because open intercostals are often small and atherosclerotic in patients with TAAA [18]. The spinal cord has also a complex collateral circulation fed by other thoracic arteries that contribute significantly to anterior spinal cord blood flow [16, 19]. The concept of collateral circulation explains how maintaining high arterial blood pressure reduces spinal cord ischemia and infarction in TAAA surgery.

Although majority of surgeons consider reimplantation of critical segmental arteries, controversies still exist about the clinical benefits [20, 21]. Several studies sought to prevent ischemia by reimplanting segmental arteries with particular focus on those arising between T7 and L1, believing that paraplegia is the consequence of hypoperfusion after the sacrifice of critical spinal cord arteries [5, 22]. Because these reports combine intercostal reimplantation with other protective strategies, it is impossible to determine how much intercostal reattachment itself contributes to improve results. How many and which arteries have to be reimplanted is not completely clarified. This dilemma could be elucidated with preoperative radiological studies [23, 24], intraoperative neurophysiological monitoring [25, 26], or both [27, 28]. SSEPs do not seem suitable for determination of critical segmental arteries because of a relative high false-positive rate [29]. More often the selective reconstruction of segmental arteries is guided by MEP monitoring [30, 31]. According to this method, when the exclusion of an aortic segment results in ischemic

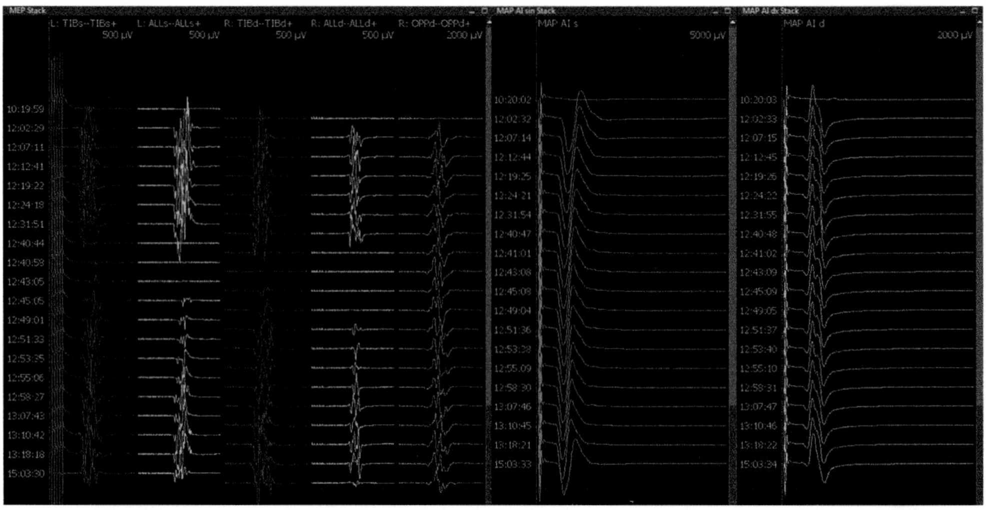

Fig. 26.4 Case 2: spinal cord ischemia related to intercostal artery blood reflux. MEP and CMAP time courses are reported for a patient suffering of TAAA type I (CA). From left to right: MEPs from the left tibialis anterior (first column), left abductor hallucis (second column), right tibialis anterior (third column), right abductor hallucis (fourth column), and right opponens pollicis (fifth column) and CMAPs from left and right abductor hallucis (sixth and seventh columns). Aorta cross-clamping occurs at 12:10. At 12:40 an amplitude reduction in MEPs is observed for muscles of the left and right inferior limb. No modification is observed for the upper limb, used as control. No modification is present for CMAPs. This situation, suggesting a central involvement, appears strictly related to a sudden, massive, blood reflux from intercostal arteries, occurring at 12:35. After intercostal sewing, MEPs rapidly come back to the baseline condition. No SSEP changes were observed: as known, the presence of synapses in the anterior horn gray matter makes MEPs more sensitive than SSEPs in detecting SCI

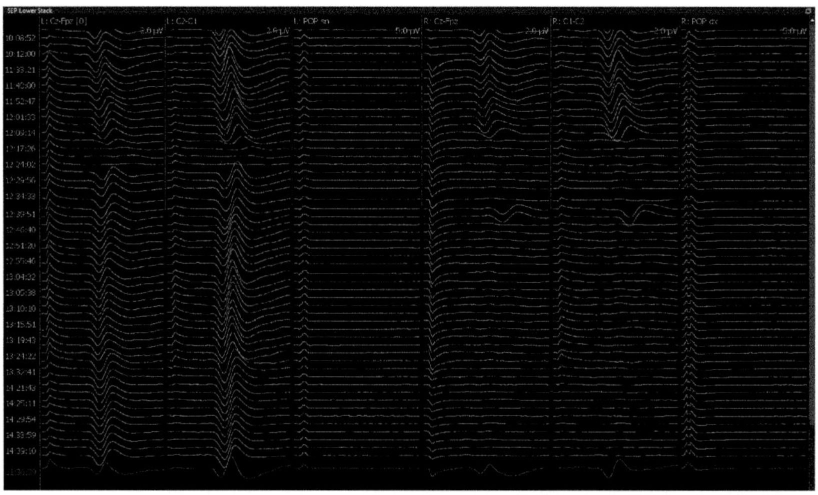

Fig. 26.5 Case 3: left hemispheric ischemic stroke. In the figure SSEP time courses for a patient suffering of TAAA type II (TV) are reported. From left to right: CPz–Fpz derivation (first columns) and C2–C1 (second column), popliteal fossa (third column) for left stimulation and CPz–Fpz, C1–C2, and popliteal fossa for right stimulation (fourth, fifth, and sixth columns). Baseline tracings (represented by the red line) are shown at the bottom of the stack. Aorta cross-clamping occurs between 11:19 and 12:23. No MEP changes were observed throughout the surgery. A temporary amplitude decrease of cortical SSEPs and SAPs was observed between 12:09 and 12:29 in the left side and between 12:09 and 12:39 in the right side. After an initial recovery for left and right SSEPs, a sudden disappearance of right stimulus-related cortical SSEP derivation is observed, maintained until the end of the surgery. A CT scan after intervention showed a left hemispheric ischemic stroke. An involvement of the cortical territory of the middle cerebral artery (MCA) can explain a sudden disappearance of the cortical SSEP and the initial persistence of MEP response, because the transcranial electrical stimulation can depolarize pyramidal axons deeper in the cerebral hemisphere

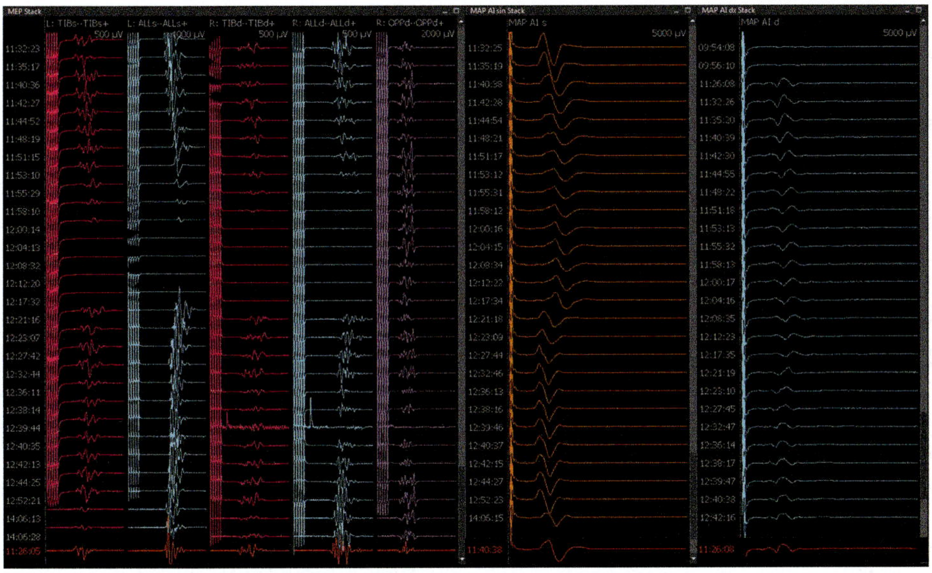

Fig. 26.6 Case 4: lower limb ischemia. MEP and CMAP time courses, for a patient (FL) suffering of TAAA type IV, are reported. No perfusion assistance is used during surgery. From left to right: MEPs from the left tibialis anterior (first column), left abductor hallucis (second column), right tibialis anterior (third column), right abductor hallucis (fourth column), and right opponens pollicis (fifth column) and CMAPs from the left and right abductor hallucis (sixth and seventh columns). Aorta cross-clamping occurs at 11:26. At 11:53 an amplitude reduction in MEPs is observed for muscles of the left and right inferior limbs. No modification is observed for the upper limb, used as control. A concomitant amplitude reduction and temporal spreading are shown by left and right CMAPs. This last modification is suggesting for a peripheral suffering. After aorta declamp, at 12:18, a quite rapid return to the baseline condition is achieved for both peripheral and central responses

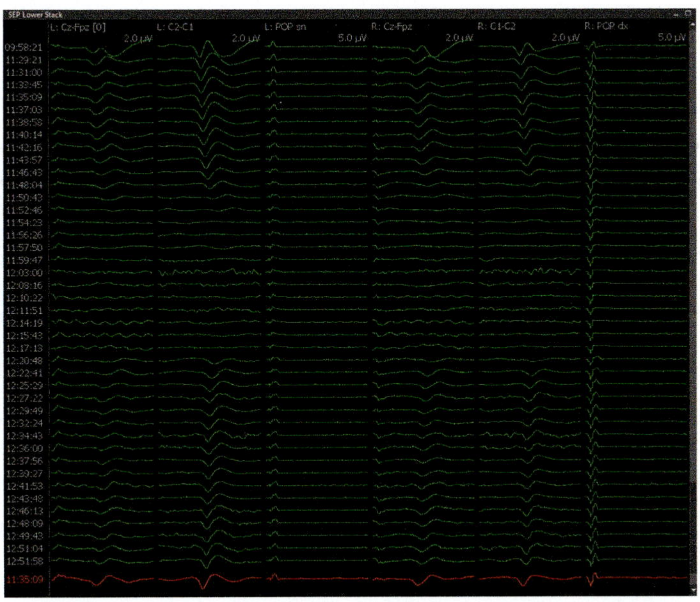

Fig. 26.7 Case 4: lower limb ischemia. For the same patient of Fig. 26.6 (FL), SSEP time course is reported. From left to right: CPz–Fpz derivation (first columns), C2–C1 (second column), and popliteal fossa (third column) for left stimulation and CPz–Fpz, C1–C2, and popliteal fossa for right stimulation (fourth, fifth, and sixth columns). An amplitude decrease for scalp and peripheral derivations is observed between 11:46 and 12:25. Also in this case, a peripheral suffering is testified by an amplitude reduction, and temporal spreading of sensory action potential (SAP) registered at popliteal fossa as shown in columns 3 and 6

MEP changes, the intercostal or lumbar arteries in that segment are considered critical to spinal cord blood supply and reimplanted.

The concept of selective reconstruction of critical arteries was developed by Svensson [32] in an attempt to avoid injury resulting from failure to restore spinal blood flow and to shorten the time required for implantation of the vessels, since reconstruction of the noncritical arteries is shown to be associated with increased risk of injury [33].

Other authors argue that reimplantation of the critical segmental arteries is unnecessary or not critical at least [20, 21]. This idea is supported by the anatomic evidence that the Adamkiewicz artery (AKA) is not the single source of perfusion to the distal spinal cord [34, 35]. Some of them reported a reduced paralysis risk without any intercostal reimplantation [15, 18, 21], using other strategies to increase ischemic tolerance and maximize collateral circulation. However, other authors suggested that nonselective reimplantation of segmental arteries may be protective by increasing perfusion to the collateral network even if they are not the direct origin of the AKA [20, 36]. Animal experiments show that when one intercostal artery is ligated, spinal cord blood flow arising from the preserved intercostals increases [37]. This suggests that any intercostal artery can supply blood to the spinal cord and become collateral circulation to the anterior spinal artery. In patients with reduced collateral circulation, reimplanting any intercostal in the critical zone from T8 to L1 may permanently increase perfusion pressure in the collateral network, and this may be the important factor in preventing spinal cord infarction. The advantages are the minimization of procedural time and the length of anastomotic line that carries a risk of bleeding. However, if the incidence of immediate neurological deficits is significantly reduced using both selective and empirical reimplantations, the incidence of delayed spinal cord ischemia is not completely clarified [15, 20, 36].

Therefore, if MEP changes represent a warning toward the reimplantation of intercostal arteries, on the contrary, stable MEPs throughout the surgery could indicate that segmental artery reattachment could not be necessary [38].

In conclusion, literature data suggest that MEP monitoring is reliable in detecting SCI, allowing the determination of critical segmental arteries and the assessment of the effects of protective techniques. A multimodal IOM can be useful to assess the various factors that may contribute to SCI, to help guiding specific measures to reduce neural risk and minimize the overall ischemic time by focusing efforts only on the necessary maneuvers.

References

1. Melissano G, Bertoglio L, Mascia D, Rinaldi E, Del Carro U, Nardelli P, et al. Spinal cord ischemia is multifactorial: what is the best protocol? J Cardiovasc Surg. 2016;57(2):191–201.
2. Kahn RA, Stone ME, Moskowitz DM. Anesthetic consideration for descending thoracic aortic aneurysm repair. Semin Cardiothorac Vasc Anesth. 2007;11(3):205–23.
3. Greenberg RK, Lytle B. Endovascular repair of thoracoabdominal aneurysms. Circulation. 2008;117(17):2288–96.
4. Cambria RP, Davison JK, Carter C, Brewster DC, Chang Y, Clark KA, et al. Epidural cooling for spinal cord protection during thoracoabdominal aneurysm repair: a five-year experience. J Vasc Surg. 2000;31(6):1093–102.
5. Coselli JS, Bozinovski J, LeMaire SA. Open surgical repair of 2286 thoracoabdominal aortic aneurysms. Ann Thorac Surg. 2007;83(2):S862–4. discussion S890–892
6. Kieffer E, Chiche L, Godet G, Koskas F, Bahnini A, Bertrand M, et al. Type IV thoracoabdominal aneurysm repair: predictors of postoperative mortality, spinal cord injury, and acute intestinal ischemia. Ann Vasc Surg. 2008;22(6):822–8.
7. Bicknell CD, Cowan AR, Kerle MI, Mansfield AO, Cheshire NJW, Wolfe JHN. Renal dysfunction and prolonged visceral ischaemia increase mortality rate after suprarenal aneurysm repair. Br J Surg. 2003;90(9):1142–6.
8. Hiratzka LF, Bakris GL, Beckman JA, Bersin RM, Carr VF, Casey DE, et al. 2010 ACCF/AHA/AATS/ACR/ASA/SCA/SCAI/SIR/STS/SVM guidelines for the diagnosis and management of patients with thoracic aortic disease: executive summary. A report of the American College of Cardiology Foundation/American Heart Association Task Force on Practice Guidelines, American Association for Thoracic Surgery, American College of Radiology, American Stroke Association, Society of Cardiovascular Anesthesiologists, Society for Cardiovascular Angiography and Interventions, Society of Interventional Radiology, Society of

Thoracic Surgeons, and Society for Vascular Medicine. Catheter Cardiovasc Interv Off J Soc Card Angiogr Interv. 2010;76(2):E43–86.
9. Sloan TB, Edmonds HL, Koht A. Intraoperative electrophysiologic monitoring in aortic surgery. J Cardiothorac Vasc Anesth. 2013;27(6):1364–73.
10. Nielsen VK, Kardel T. Temporospatial effects on orthodromic sensory potential propagation during ischemia. Ann Neurol. 1981;9(6):597–604.
11. Tanaka Y, Kawaguchi M, Noguchi Y, Yoshitani K, Kawamata M, Masui K, et al. Systematic review of motor evoked potentials monitoring during thoracic and thoracoabdominal aortic aneurysm open repair surgery: a diagnostic meta-analysis. J Anesth. 2016;30(6):1037–50.
12. Svensson LG, Rickards E, Coull A, Rogers G, Fimmel CJ, Hinder RA. Relationship of spinal cord blood flow to vascular anatomy during thoracic aortic cross-clamping and shunting. J Thorac Cardiovasc Surg. 1986;91(1):71–8.
13. Marini CP, Levison J, Caliendo F, Nathan IM, Cohen JR. Control of proximal hypertension during aortic cross-clamping: its effect on cerebrospinal fluid dynamics and spinal cord perfusion pressure. Semin Thorac Cardiovasc Surg. 1998;10(1):51–6.
14. Marsala M, Sorkin LS, Yaksh TL. Transient spinal ischemia in rat: characterization of spinal cord blood flow, extracellular amino acid release, and concurrent histopathological damage. J Cereb Blood Flow Metab Off J Int Soc Cereb Blood Flow Metab. 1994;14(4):604–14.
15. Acher CW, Wynn MM, Hoch JR, Popic P, Archibald J, Turnipseed WD. Combined use of cerebral spinal fluid drainage and naloxone reduces the risk of paraplegia in thoracoabdominal aneurysm repair. J Vasc Surg. 1994;19(2):236–46. discussion 247–248
16. Christiansson L, Ulus AT, Hellberg A, Bergqvist D, Wiklund L, Karacagil S. Aspects of the spinal cord circulation as assessed by intrathecal oxygen tension monitoring during various arterial interruptions in the pig. J Thorac Cardiovasc Surg. 2001;121(4):762–72.
17. Williams GM, Roseborough GS, Webb TH, Perler BA, Krosnick T. Preoperative selective intercostal angiography in patients undergoing thoracoabdominal aneurysm repair. J Vasc Surg. 2004;39(2):314–21.
18. Griepp RB, Ergin MA, Galla JD, Lansman S, Khan N, Quintana C, et al. Looking for the artery of Adamkiewicz: a quest to minimize paraplegia after operations for aneurysms of the descending thoracic and thoracoabdominal aorta. J Thorac Cardiovasc Surg. 1996;112(5):1202–13. discussion 1213–1215
19. Lazorthes G, Gouaze A, Zadeh JO, Santini JJ, Lazorthes Y, Burdin P. Arterial vascularization of the spinal cord. Recent studies of the anastomotic substitution pathways. J Neurosurg. 1971;35(3):253–62.
20. Acher CW, Wynn MM, Mell MW, Tefera G, Hoch JR. A quantitative assessment of the impact of intercostal artery reimplantation on paralysis risk in thoracoabdominal aortic aneurysm repair. Ann Surg. 2008;248(4):529–40.
21. Etz CD, Halstead JC, Spielvogel D, Shahani R, Lazala R, Homann TM, et al. Thoracic and thoracoabdominal aneurysm repair: is reimplantation of spinal cord arteries a waste of time? Ann Thorac Surg. 2006;82(5):1670–7.
22. Cambria RP, Clouse WD, Davison JK, Dunn PF, Corey M, Dorer D. Thoracoabdominal aneurysm repair: results with 337 operations performed over a 15-year interval. Ann Surg. 2002;236(4):471–9. discussion 479
23. Yamada N, Takamiya M, Kuribayashi S, Okita Y, Minatoya K, Tanaka R. MRA of the Adamkiewicz artery: a preoperative study for thoracic aortic aneurysm. J Comput Assist Tomogr. 2000;24(3):362–8.
24. Kawaharada N, Morishita K, Fukada J, Yamada A, Muraki S, Hyodoh H, et al. Thoracoabdominal or descending aortic aneurysm repair after preoperative demonstration of the Adamkiewicz artery by magnetic resonance angiography. Eur J Cardio-Thorac Surg Off J Eur Assoc Cardio-Thorac Surg. 2002;21(6):970–4.
25. Jacobs MJ, de Mol BA, Elenbaas T, Mess WH, Kalkman CJ, Schurink GW, et al. Spinal cord blood supply in patients with thoracoabdominal aortic aneurysms. J Vasc Surg. 2002;35(1):30–7.
26. van Dongen EP, Schepens MA, Morshuis WJ, ter Beek HT, Aarts LP, de Boer A, et al. Thoracic and thoracoabdominal aortic aneurysm repair: use of evoked potential monitoring in 118 patients. J Vasc Surg. 2001;34(6):1035–40.
27. Ogino H, Sasaki H, Minatoya K, Matsuda H, Yamada N, Kitamura S. Combined use of adamkiewicz artery demonstration and motor-evoked potentials in descending and thoracoabdominal repair. Ann Thorac Surg. 2006;82(2):592–6.
28. Takahashi S, Orihashi K, Imai K, Mizukami T, Takasaki T, Sueda T. Cold blood spinoplegia under motor-evoked potential monitoring during thoracic aortic surgery. J Thorac Cardiovasc Surg. 2011;141(3):755–61.
29. Crawford ES, Mizrahi EM, Hess KR, Coselli JS, Safi HJ, Patel VM. The impact of distal aortic perfusion and somatosensory evoked potential monitoring on prevention of paraplegia after aortic aneurysm operation. J Thorac Cardiovasc Surg. 1988;95(3):357–67.
30. Shiiya N, Yasuda K, Matsui Y, Sakuma M, Sasaki S. Spinal cord protection during thoracoabdominal aortic aneurysm repair: results of selective reconstruction of the critical segmental arteries guided by evoked spinal cord potential monitoring. J Vasc Surg. 1995;21(6):970–5.
31. Jacobs MJ, Meylaerts SA, de Haan P, de Mol BA, Kalkman CJ. Strategies to prevent neurologic deficit based on motor-evoked potentials in type I and II thoracoabdominal aortic aneurysm repair. J Vasc Surg. 1999;29(1):48–57. discussion 57–59
32. Svensson LG, Patel V, Robinson MF, Ueda T, Roehm JO, Crawford ES. Influence of preservation or perfusion of intraoperatively identified spinal cord blood supply on spinal motor evoked potentials

and paraplegia after aortic surgery. J Vasc Surg. 1991;13(3):355–65.
33. Svensson LG, Hess KR, Coselli JS, Safi HJ. Influence of segmental arteries, extent, and atriofemoral bypass on postoperative paraplegia after thoracoabdominal aortic operations. J Vasc Surg. 1994;20(2): 255–62.
34. Etz CD, Kari FA, Mueller CS, Silovitz D, Brenner RM, Lin H-M, et al. The collateral network concept: a reassessment of the anatomy of spinal cord perfusion. J Thorac Cardiovasc Surg. 2011;141(4):1020–8.
35. Biglioli P, Roberto M, Cannata A, Parolari A, Fumero A, Grillo F, et al. Upper and lower spinal cord blood supply: the continuity of the anterior spinal artery and the relevance of the lumbar arteries. J Thorac Cardiovasc Surg. 2004;127(4):1188–92.
36. Park KH, Lim C, Kim TH, Park I, Jung Y. Outcome of extensive descending aorta repair adopting present concepts of spinal cord preservation. J Cardiovasc Surg. 2016;57(1):58–65.
37. Uezu T, Koja K, Kuniyoshi Y, Miyagi K, Shimoji M, Arakaki K, et al. Blood distribution to the anterior spinal artery from each segment of intercostal and lumbar arteries. J Cardiovasc Surg. 2003;44(5):637–45.
38. Conrad MF, Ergul EA, Patel VI, Cambria MR, Lamuraglia GM, Simon M, et al. Evolution of operative strategies in open thoracoabdominal aneurysm repair. J Vasc Surg. 2011;53(5):1195–1201.e1.

Spinal Cord Protection During Open and Endovascular Aortic Repair: State of the Art

27

Carlo Setacci, Marco Tadiello, Matteo Tozzi, Giancarlo Palasciano, Domenico Benevento, Gianmarco de Donato, and Francesco Setacci

27.1 Introduction

Spinal cord protection during aortic surgery has spelled trouble since the beginning of aortic surgery.

As reported by Clopton in 1911 [1], A. Carrel said: "The main danger of the aortic operation does not come from the heart or from the aorta itself, but from the central nervous system. Spastic paralysis develops when the descending aorta has been clamped for more than ten or fifteen minutes due to a degeneration of the cells in the anterior horn".

A hundred years later, spinal cord protection during aortic repair still remains a topic of major debate.

The incidence of paraplegia was reported to be as high as 20% in the early 1990s [2], and current scientific literature describes spinal cord ischaemia (SCI) as the most dreaded complication of both open and endovascular repair of thoracoabdominal aortic disease, with reported rates between 5 and 31% [3–7].

27.1.1 Anatomy of the Spinal Cord Blood Supply

Understanding the spinal cord (SC) blood supply is a cornerstone when treating patients requiring thoracic and thoracoabdominal aortic repair. The SC vessel network is complex and difficult to study because it consists of very small and intricate vessels with substantial regional and interindividual variability. Most of our anatomical knowledge about SC circulation derives from microinjections of different staining fluids and micro-radiological studies in postmortem specimens [8].

The extrinsic arterial system, supplying inflow vessels to the SC, is constituted by the subclavian artery through the vertebral artery, the thyrocervical trunk and the costocervical trunk, several segmental feeders from the intercostal and lumbar arteries and the hypogastric artery through the lateral sacral and iliolumbar arteries [9].

C. Setacci (✉) · M. Tadiello · G. Palasciano
D. Benevento · G. de Donato
Vascular and Endovascular Surgery Unit, Department of Medicine, Surgery and Neurological Sciences, University of Siena, Siena, Italy
e-mail: carlo.setacci@unisi.it; marco.tadiello@student.unisi.it; giancarlo.palasciano@unisi.it; d.benevento@ao-siena.toscana.it; gianmarco.dedonato@unisi.it

M. Tozzi
Vascular Surgery, Department of Medicine and Surgery, Circolo University Teaching Hospital, University of Insubria School of Medicine, Varese, Italy
e-mail: matteo.tozzi@uninsubria.it

F. Setacci
Vascular Surgery Unit, Multimedica Institute for Scientific Research, Milan, Italy
e-mail: francesco.setacci@multimedica.it

© Springer Nature Switzerland AG 2019
Y. Tshomba et al. (eds.), *Visceral Vessels and Aortic Repair*,
https://doi.org/10.1007/978-3-319-94761-7_27

The intrinsic arterial system, directly supplying the SC, is divided into a central system (supplying blood to the spinal grey matter) fed by the sulcal arteries, arising from the anterior spinal artery (ASA), and a peripheral system, the pial plexus (or pial network), which gives rise to perforating branches. The pial plexus covers the entire length of the SC and forms an elaborate secondary anastomotic system between the anterior and posterolateral longitudinal vessels that may only be important for slower circulatory adjustments. Intraparenchymal anastomoses have rarely been demonstrated.

The intercostal arteries divide three times before reaching the ASA: the first branch of the intercostal artery is the nervomedullary artery, the latter divides into an anterior and a posterior radicular artery, and the anterior radicular artery divides into a descending and an ascending branch.

The ASA is essentially an anastomotic channel between ascending and descending branches of neighbouring anterior radicular arteries.

In the thoracolumbar region, one (occasionally two or three) anterior radicular artery (the artery of Adamkiewicz) is always distinctly dominant in calibre and is therefore called the great radicular artery or ARM [10].

The importance of the ARM was early described by A. Adamkiewicz in 1881–1882 [11]. Adamkiewicz demonstrated that blood from the radicular arteries flows upwards in the ascending branches and downwards in the descending ones. He also pointed out that the ARM is characterized by the most stable morphology and course. In 60% of the population it branches off at the level of the ninth to twelfth thoracic segment; in 15%, at the level of the fifth to eighth segment; and in approximately 25%, at the first lumbar segment [12].

The majority of Adamkiewicz's observations are fully confirmed by today's knowledge of the variability of the spinal cord vascular system and origin of the ARM.

Some peculiar anatomical variant types can hide the highest risk of paraplegia. Fortunately, in most rare anatomical variants with poor development of the ARM or a lack of continuity of the anterior spinal artery (i.e. it is interrupted in the majority of cases in its thoracic segment), clamping the thoracic aorta in the course of surgery, or covering a certain region with endografts, is associated with the highest risk of paraplegia [13].

27.1.2 Imaging for Spinal Cord Protection

The importance of preoperative knowledge of the location of the artery of Adamkiewicz (arteria radicularis magna, ARM) before thoracic and thoracoabdominal aortic surgery was demonstrated by Kieffer and co-workers back in the 1980s [14], and its clinical importance in both open and in endovascular aortic repair has been widely confirmed in more recent times for the prevention of spinal ischaemia [2, 15, 16].

In open surgery, the precise preoperative location of ARM contributes to the reduction of the incidence of spinal cord ischaemia in thoracic aortic disease, shortening clamp time by identifying intercostal arteries that need to be reimplanted [17]. In endovascular aortic repair, it may define the most appropriate landing zone, avoiding unnecessary coverage of important intercostal arteries [18].

The rapid evolution of digital imaging techniques and the increasing number of multidimensional and multimodality studies constitute a challenge for picture archiving and communication system (PACS) workstations and image display programs. Traditional 2D image viewers and image display programs have become inadequate for interpretation of large sets of images. The large sets of images acquired by multidetector CT scanners require additional image processing and reformatting to make them suitable for efficient and rapid image navigation and interpretation. In most cases, this can only be achieved on high-end dedicated workstations that provide multiplanar/centre line reconstruction and 3D volume surface. Access to these techniques is usually limited to high-end users in a radiology

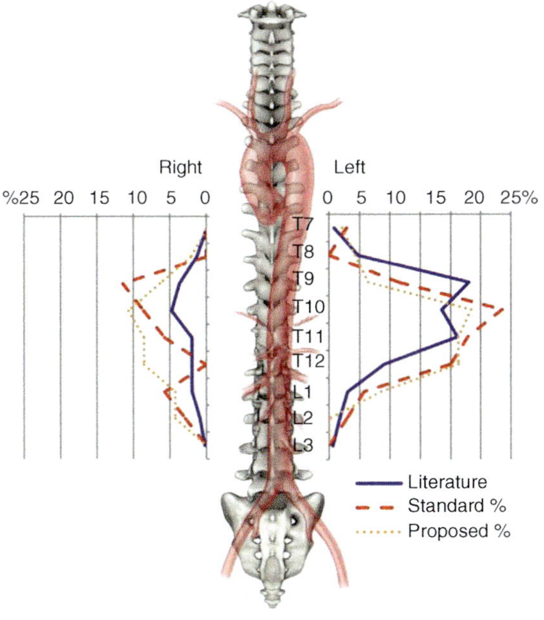

Fig. 27.1 Percentage of ARM origin level in relation to the intercostal artery, its location and method used. Note the higher left T9–T12 prevalence (G. Melissano, L. Bertoglio, V. Civelli, A.C. Moraes Amato, G. Coppi, E. Civilini, G. Calori, F. De Cobelli, A. Del Maschio, R. Chiesa, Demonstration of the Adamkiewicz Artery by Multidetector Computed Tomography Angiography Analysed with the Open-Source Software OsiriX. Eur J Vasc Endovasc Surg (2009) 37, 395e400)

department, but since the last decade, many attractive alternatives to dedicated workstations have been made available. The most popular and easy to use is the software OsiriX, developed 8 years ago by Ratib and Rosset at the Department of Medical Imaging and Information Sciences at the University Hospital of Geneva, Switzerland [19].

A recent study by Melissano et al. [20] proposed a method for the demonstration of the ARM using OsiriX software.

In this study, the proposed method for ARM identification, using OsiriX software, had a substantial recognition consensus of 85.07% compared to the standard method, using a dedicated workstation and when applied to the same patients. The proposed method presents a higher prevalence of left (T9–T12) ARM arteries (Fig. 27.1) that is consistent with the standard method and the analysis of the literature.

In employing this versatile tool, they realized that identification of the ARM could be quite simple from a standard set of contrast-enhanced CT scans, showing the feasibility of ARM location by using low-cost hardware and software, with standard contrast protocol [20] (Fig. 27.2).

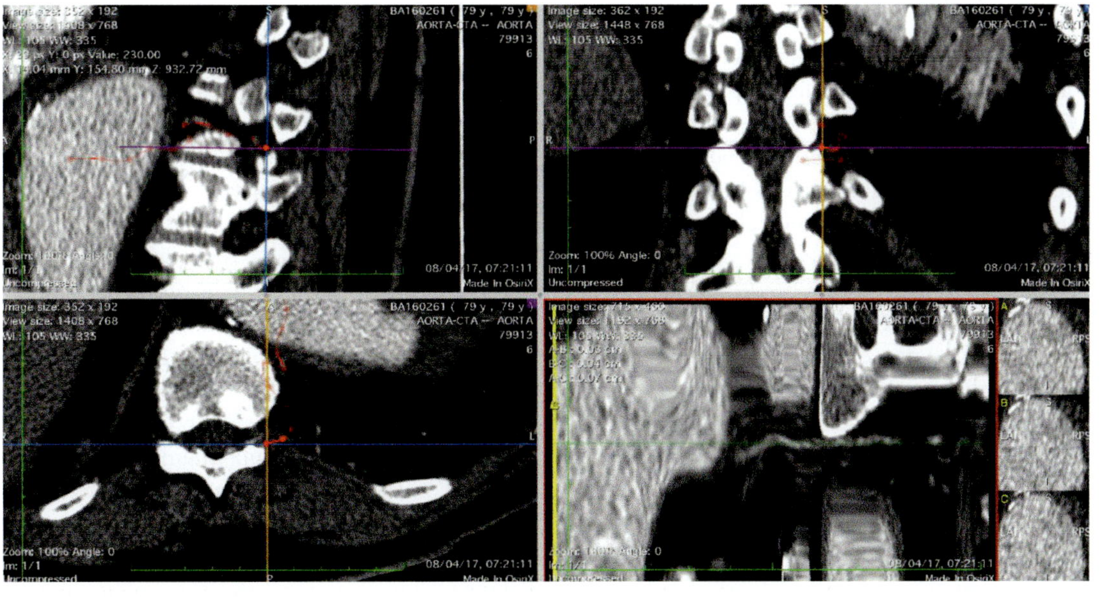

Fig. 27.2 Spinal artery multiplanar rendering using OsiriX software (Courtesy of M. Bossi, MD, HSR, Milan)

27.2 Mechanism of Spinal Cord Ischaemia

Spinal cord ischaemia can develop basically after coverage/exclusion of intercostal arteries or after small thrombus fragment embolization.

Data from the EuREC (European Registry of Endovascular Aortic Repair Complications) suggest that extensive coverage of intercostal arteries by a thoracic stent graft alone is not associated with symptomatic spinal cord ischaemia, as the sacrifice of one vascular territory supplying the spinal cord is irrelevant. Simultaneous closure of at least two vascular territories instead is highly relevant, especially in combination with prolonged intraoperative hypotension.

By regarding all four vascular territories supplying the spinal cord—left subclavian, intercostal, lumbar and hypogastric arteries—as equally important, risk modelling found strong associations between simultaneous coverage of two of these independent vascular territories, intraoperative prolonged hypotension and the occurrence of symptomatic spinal cord injury.

It is well known how the preservation of the left subclavian artery, not because of left upper extremity perfusion, as this is always well maintained by collateral circulation, but to maintain the important perfusion pathway for the spinal cord, results in a low rate of paraplegia after TEVAR.

Interestingly, occlusion of one hypogastric artery during vascular access surgery was of equal importance as was the occlusion of the left subclavian artery [21].

The same notable remark derives from M. Eagleton's work (Cleveland Clinic, OH) with the observation that extensive coverage of intercostal arteries by TEVAR alone was not associated with symptomatic SCI, as the sacrifice of one collateral bed was irrelevant. In particular, he also suggested that efforts to reduce the untoward effects of spinal cord malperfusion may be achieved by preserving flow (or restoring flow) to occluded subclavian and hypogastric collaterals prior to extensive endovascular aortic coverage [22].

27.3 Spinal Cord Monitoring

The assessment of spinal cord vascularization during surgery is a difficult goal to achieve due to the anatomical position of the spine and its extremely complex vessel net. Indirect techniques can however assess the SC vitality and can lead the surgeon's decisions during either open or endovascular procedures and in the immediate postoperative period.

27.3.1 Cerebrospinal Fluid Drainage

The choroid plexus and walls of the ventricles produce cerebrospinal fluid at a rate that varies in a diurnal rhythm from 0.2 to 0.7 mL/min, producing 400–600 mL of fluid every 24 h. Cerebrospinal fluid circulates from the brain to the spinal canal and back to the brain where it is reabsorbed in the venous sinuses. The total volume of spinal circulating fluid is approximately 140 mL in an adult, and the ventricles hold an additional 25 mL. Spinal cord perfusion pressure derives from the difference between arterial blood pressure and SCF pressure. When SCF pressure exceeds spinal arterial pressure, a critical closing pressure is achieved [23].

The relationship between cerebrospinal fluid pressure and the development of paraplegia during repairs of the thoracic aorta was first suggested by Sugie and colleagues in 1957 [24].

Almost three decades later, experimental work by McCullough and colleagues [25] and Bower and colleagues [26] at the Mayo clinic led to reports on the benefit of perioperative cerebrospinal fluid drainage (CSFD) and renewed interest in the use of CSFD for thoracic aortic repairs.

Nowadays, hundreds of clinical studies focus on CSFD, and the protocol for its management is quite different from one team to another: intraoperative or both intra- and postoperative, at 24–72 h postoperatively, maintaining cerebrospinal fluid pressure at 5 or 10 mmHg (or cm H2O) and systematic drainage of 50 mL or more.

An example of the current policies is the one of King's College London, UK. Their protocol is to place a spinal drain prior to surgery for all Crawford type I, II, III and V TAAAs and to begin prophylactic CSF drainage intraoperatively. Passive drainage of CSF is done at 10 cm H2O until postoperative day 2, during which time all patients are monitored hourly for the presence of lower limb neurology. If any signs or symptoms of spinal cord ischaemia develop, the MAP is raised to >90 to 100 mmHg using inotropic support and the CSF drain initially lowered to 5 cm H2O, maintaining drainage for up to 5 days [6].

In order to avoid many practical disadvantages of the current gravity-based drip chamber system, some automatic drainage systems are appearing. The most remarkable drawbacks of the current systems are the impossibility of a simultaneous drainage and pressure measurement and possible handling mistakes that are related to concerns of safety, sterility and human error, leading to potentially dangerous over-/underdrainage and catheter contamination.

The San Raffaele group (Y. Tshomba et al.) recently utilized an automatic drainage system (the LiquoGuard (Möller Medical GmbH, Fulda, Germany)). This device allows CSF drainage according to CSF pressure changes. The pressure sensor, along the tubing, continuously measures the pressure in the CSF catheter, and the volume of CSF pumped out is also continuously measured. The CSF automatic drainage system has the advantage that the CSF is drained not simply on the basis of the excess pressure but is actively pumped out in a controlled manner, with the possibility of controlling hourly drainage speed, maximum and minimum CSF pressure and maximum amount to be drained per hour.

Apart from the previously mentioned advantages, they observed a reduced post-dural puncture headache with earlier patient mobilization and better compliance [27].

27.3.2 Neuromonitoring

Since the early work of Coles and colleagues [28] and Cunnigam and colleagues [29, 30] in 1982, demonstrating that it was possible to detect spinal cord ischaemia intraoperatively by monitoring somatosensory evoked potential (SSEPs), growing interest has spread among vascular surgeons in applying this technique to TAAA surgery.

Nowadays, motor evoked potentials (MEPs) enable the surgeon to better understand the ischaemic damage of the spinal cord.

From a physio-anatomical point of view, SSEPs are the expression of the spinal grey matter dorsal column vitality, while MEPs are the expression of the anterolateral ones.

In brief, electrical charges sent to the motor cortex through C3/C4 scalp electrodes evoke MEPs through the motor pathway, and values are recorded down the cord over multiple muscles in the upper and lower extremities. An upper extremity muscle is recorded to help differentiate neurogenic impairment from nonspecific changes. Bilateral lower extremity muscles are recorded using subdermal electroencephalographic (EEG) electrodes generally placed in the hamstring, tibialis anterior and abductor hallucis muscles. In addition, SSEPs, consisting of electrical stimulus generated at the ulnar or tibial nerve that travels from the distal extremity, are recorded over the neck and scalp. A ≥75% consistent reduction from baseline evoked potential amplitude is generally considered to be significant (Fig. 27.3).

The main goal of neuromonitoring is to help identify ischaemia of the anterior and lateral spinal columns, which are sensitive to a decrease in oxygen supply. Because signal changes can result from dysfunction in any of the recorded pathways, including the brain, peripheral nerves, receptors or muscles, as well as technical issues, interpretation requires correlation with the clinical scenario.

During endovascular procedures, early detection of these changes allows the surgical team to put in place manoeuvres designed to optimize spinal cord perfusion pressure (augmentation of MAP, reduction of CSF pressure, early restoration of pelvis and lower limb flow) in order to reduce the risk of spinal cord injury.

During open TAAA repair, this technique has helped guide selective intercostal artery reimplantation and the aforementioned intraoperative manoeuvres designed to improve spinal cord perfusion [31].

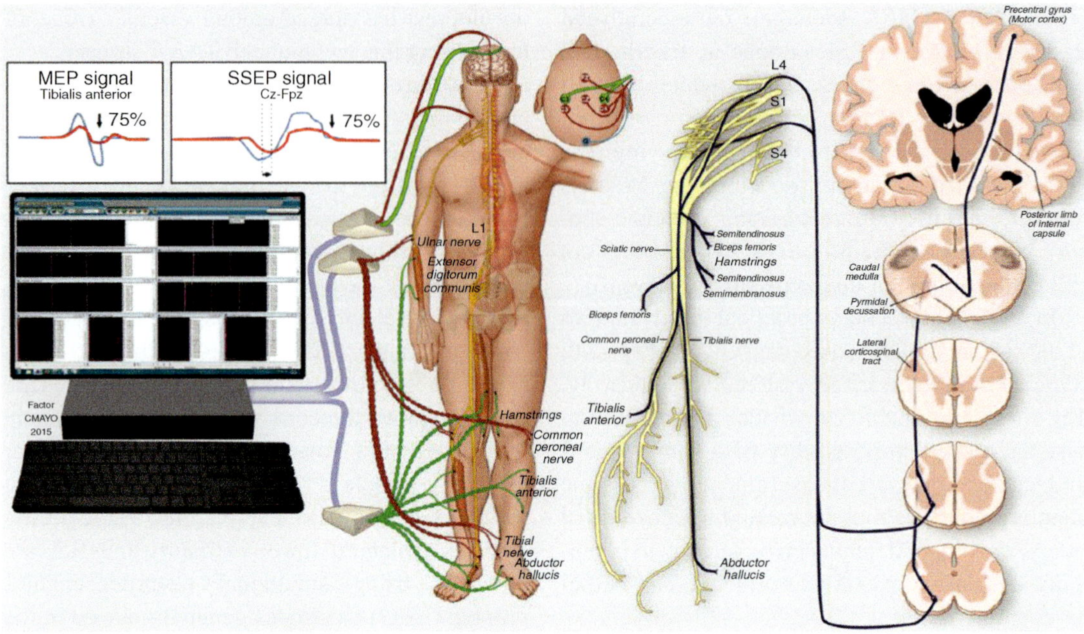

Fig. 27.3 Illustration depicting the placement of electrodes for monitoring of motor evoked potentials (MEPs) and somatosensory evoked potentials (SSEPs) during complex endovascular aortic repair. A significant change is defined by >75% decline in amplitude in MEPs or SSEPs (Peter V. Banga, Gustavo S. Oderich, Leonardo Reis de Souza, Jan Hofer, Meaghan L. Cazares Gonzalez, Juan N. Pulido, Stephen Cha, Peter Gloviczki, Neuromonitoring, Cerebrospinal Fluid Drainage, and Selective Use of Iliofemoral Conduits to Minimize Risk of Spinal Cord Injury During Complex Endovascular Aortic Repair, Journal of Endovascular Therapy 2016, Vol. 23(1) 139–149)

27.4 Operative Strategies for Preventing SCI in Endovascular Aortic Repair

Following endovascular aortic procedures, SCI can occur from a combination of reduced spinal cord perfusion, because of hypotension, coverage of lumbar and intercostal arteries and/or embolization of atheroma/thrombus into the aforementioned.

If the risk of thrombus mobilization and embolization during endovascular manoeuvers remains a less predictable inconvenience, the "haemodynamic" causes of SC ischaemia are a foreseeable one. Careful management of the arterial pressure during the intervention is mandatory. The preservation of the left subclavian/hypogastric arteries, in cases of favourable anatomy, in order to maintain the collateral extrinsic SC vasculature is at present a solid knowledge; in addition, the early removal of large sheets and the selective use of iliofemoral conduit are proved to be solid adjuncts in order to prevent SC ischaemia.

The deepest consciousness of the spinal cord vasculature acquired with the aforementioned diagnostic tools and the so-derived collateral network concept allows the clinician to put in place several methods to stimulate the spinal cord collateral network in order to avoid the onset of ischaemia.

27.4.1 Staged Endovascular Repair and Temporary Aneurysm Sac Perfusion

Early reports of successful thoracoabdominal aneurysm repair suggested that postoperative neurologic dysfunction occurred in proportion to the extent of aortic replacement [2]. The endovascular approach to the aorta allows minimal surgical injury and the absence of organ ischaemia, but it does require the coverage of any patent intercostals and/or lumbar vessels that may contribute to spinal cord blood flow suffering from the inability to maintain their direct perfusion. Aortic coverage is identified as a variable that has a fundamental role in the development of SC ischaemia. Some authors identified a precise cut-off length (205 mm [32]), above which the aortic coverage length was showed to be an independent predictor of SCI. Almost the same covering length of 20 cm emerges from EUROSTAR data [5] as a threshold for other protocols that express the same aortic length. In these cases, a CSF drain should be placed between 12 and 20 cm.

Some attempts to overstep the limit imposed by the endovascular approach have been made, from the successful creation of a type Ib endoleak to perfuse the lumbar vessels following the development of paraplegia (Reilly et al. [33]) to the less successful incorporation of spinal perfusion branches in the endograft design (Ivanchev et al. [34]).

In recent years, in light of the "collateral network concept" (Furthermore, Etz et al. [35]), the staged repair is becoming a solid practice in the Crawford type II procedures, in an effort to maximize collateralization after the loss of elements of the collateral supply (Fig. 27.4).

O' Callaghan and Eagleton et al. (Cleveland Clinic, OH) analysed their experience comparing single and staged Crawford type II TAAA procedures, with the result of a significantly lower overall rate of spinal injury (37.5% vs 11%) and mortality (Fig. 27.5). No optimal time interval between stages is described with certainty at present. The interval proposed in their analysis is determined by the 6- to 12-week delay in constructing a custom device, resulting in the median of 5 months. Two patients had rup-

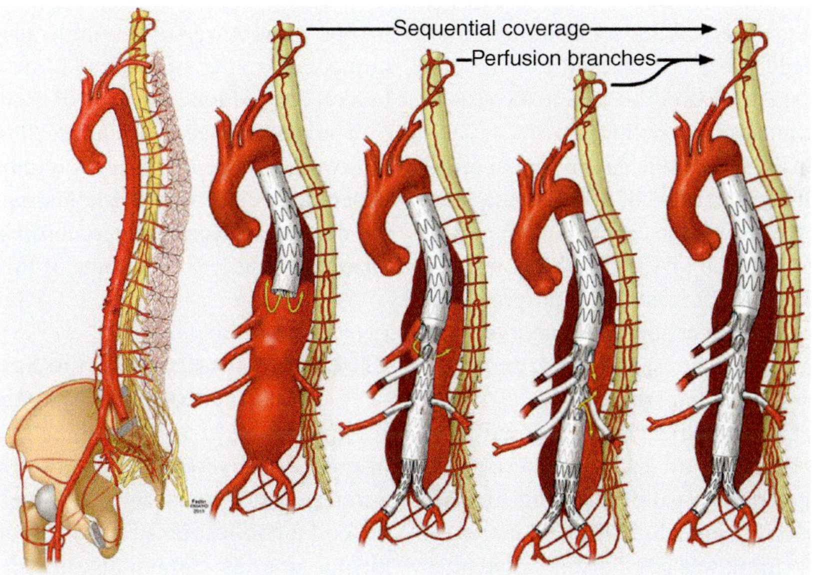

Fig. 27.4 Optimization of the extensive spine collateral network, including vertebral, intercostal, lumbar and hypogastric arteries, forms the basis for staged endovascular repair of complex aneurysms. Strategies include coverage of the proximal thoracic aorta up to the celiac axis, followed by visceral branch stenting in the second stage. Alternatively the sac can be perfused via perfusion branches or unstented celiac axis or contralateral iliac limb. The addition of two perfusion branches is favoured by some to improve haemodynamics and avoid hyperpressurization of the sac by single branches (Peter V. Banga, Gustavo S. Oderich, Leonardo Reis de Souza, Jan Hofer, Meaghan L. Cazares Gonzalez, Juan N. Pulido, Stephen Cha, Peter Gloviczki, Neuromonitoring, Cerebrospinal Fluid Drainage, and Selective Use of Iliofemoral Conduits to Minimize Risk of Spinal Cord Injury During Complex Endovascular Aortic Repair, Journal of Endovascular Therapy 2016, Vol. 23(1) 139–149)

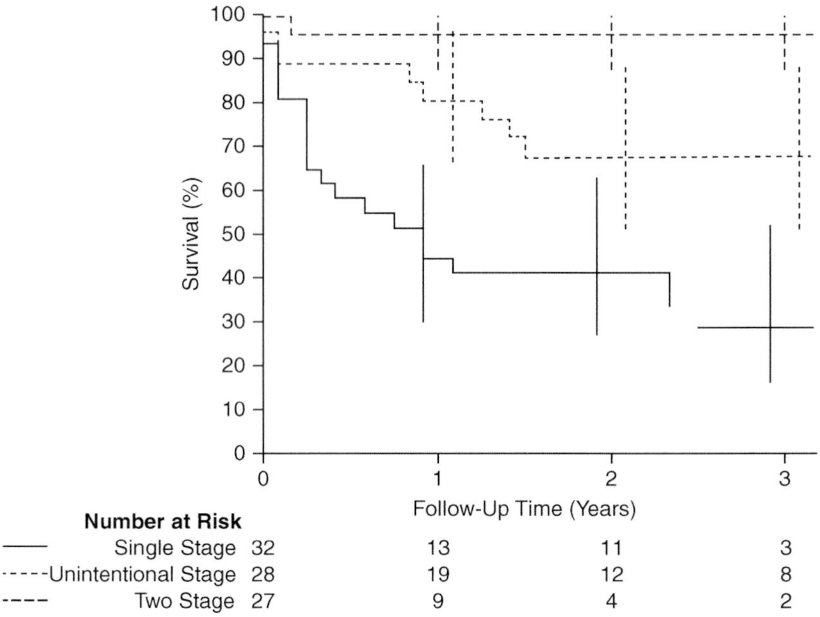

Fig. 27.5 Kaplan-Meier showing how the two-stage procedure affects patient survival

ture while they were waiting for completion of the second stage, so it is desirable to limit the time between stages in order to reduce the risk of rupture in the intervening period [36].

To maintain the intercostal and/or lumbar arteries patent after the first stage of endovascular aortic repair is at the base of the concept of temporary aneurysm sac perfusion (TASP). TASP consist of the noncompletion of at least one stent-graft side branch in order to prevent complete aneurysm sac thrombosis and maintain spinal cord perfusion through intercostal-lumbar arteries.

Kasprzak et al. studied the feasibility and early perioperative outcome of TAAAs treated with bEVAR compared with patients having bEVAR with immediate side branch. For TASP preferentially the celiac trunk was left noncompleted after uncomplicated superior mesenteric artery (SMA) and renal artery stent-graft implantation. Second-stage branch completion was recommended within 4 weeks of the initial bEVAR, and all patients with symptomatic TAAA had primary side branch completion. As a result they observed severe SCI in the non-TASP group immediately after the intervention in six patients and delayed in one patient versus a single paraplegia case immediately after bEVAR and one after the side branch completion in the TASP group.

The risk of aneurysm rupture during the TASP interval has to be considered, and based on their experience, early side branch completion within 4 weeks is recommended according to the presence or absence of symptoms of SCI [37].

27.4.2 Minimally Invasive Segmental Artery Coil Embolization

In order to overcome the need for staged procedures in the endovascular treatment of TAAA, the coil embolization strategy for intercostal segmental arteries (minimally invasive segmental artery coil embolization—MISACE) has been proposed.

As a result of the animal model studies [38], this technique, carried out through a percutaneous femoral approach, may allow extensive aortic repair in a single surgical time, increasing the resilience of spinal cord perfusion prior to definite aortic repair.

Tilo Kolbel's group described the first-in-man (two patients) clinical application of endovascular coil embolization to precondition the spinal cord collateral network before open and totally endovascular extensive TAAA repair. After the identification of target spinal arteries (SAs), the first stage of the treatment consists of embolization of the SAs of the thoracic or abdominal level under local anaesthesia, aiming to occlude the vessels in their ostial segment to preserve the ability of the collateral network to compensate to a maximum extent (2.7 F microcatheter and 0.018 microcoils). Endovascular coil embolization did not result in any neurologic impairment, and both patients were discharged after 72 h of clinical surveillance.

The interval between the MISACE and the second stage was 4–8 weeks, although probably a shorter time may be sufficient to trigger the collateral network response, and the second procedures had a successful outcome [39].

Although minimally invasive segmental coil embolization seems feasible, risks and limitations need to be addressed to further optimize this technique.

27.5 Operative Strategies for Preventing SCI in Open Repair

During the clamp and sew era, aortic cross-clamp time was the principal predictor of neurologic impairment during thoracic and thoracoabdominal aortic repair. In Crawford's experience with 1509 patients, aortic cross-clamp time of more than 60 min was associated with a 27% incidence of paraplegia overall and 50% for the extent II TAAA [2].

A decade of study definitely refined a series of adjuncts, which includes distal aortic perfusion, selective intercostal artery reimplantation, cerebrospinal fluid drainage and neuromonitoring, that led to the separation of clamp time from ischaemic time when a multimodal SC prevention protocol is used.

In order to preserve the SC cord supply, solid preoperative planning with the study of "critical" intercostal arteries must precede the surgical act; in addition to surgery, anaesthesiologic adjuncts can aim to increase SC tolerance to ischaemia, such as mild systemic hypothermia or deep hypothermic circulatory arrest, pharmacologic neuroprotection and controlled hypertension.

During open surgical aortic repair, three periods when the spinal cord is vulnerable to ischaemia are described: during aortic cross-clamping, after the clamp is removed if crucial spinal arteries are not perfused and, in some patients, for several days or weeks postoperatively [23].

27.5.1 Intercostal Artery Reimplant

While in the past authors advocated expeditious aortic repair with systemic sacrifice of intercostal arteries [40], with "the clamp and sew technique", being confident in the SC collateral network, at present, the role of preservation of spinal flow in reducing the risk of paraplegia/paraparesis is well known. The importance of the reattachment of critical intercostal arteries (T8–L2 zone) is widely demonstrated [41], and the procedure can be performed either systematically or selectively. The routine reimplant of all patent intercostal arteries in T7–L2 segment proved to reduce paraplegia rate below 10% in some series [42], but it can be time-consuming, and large "Carrel" patches may be susceptible to further dilatation. Therefore, it is questionable whether a large number of reimplanted intercostal arteries justify the effort and the risk for every patient; in particular it would probably be better to avoid unnecessary reimplantations especially in patients with connective tissue disorders. Interestingly, recent advances in CT and MR imaging technology may play a role in planning a selective reimplantation of the principal SC feeders [43].

The goal of selective reimplantation of the intercostal arteries is to overcome the disadvantages of systematic reimplantation, reducing the clamping time as well as the time of the entire procedure.

ARM or some peculiar intercostal arteries that had potentially emerged at the preoperative imaging are certainly prone to selective reimplantation. Otherwise, intercostal arteries may be temporarily occluded during the procedure, and MEP/SSEP modification can guide intraoperative decisions. Only intercostal/lumbar arteries that lead to instrumental modification could potentially be reimplanted, preventing unnecessary intercostal artery reimplantation [44]. Otherwise intercostal arteries may even be sacrificed if MEP-SSEP monitoring remains unchanged.

Other authors advocate expeditious aortic repair with the systemic sacrifice of the intercostal arteries [40], "the clamp and sew technique", where the rationale is to avoid "the steal" phenomenon, sacrificing intercostal arteries and being confident in the spinal cord collateral network.

27.5.2 Distal Aortic Perfusion

The basic premise for distal aortic perfusion has been that increasing the distal aortic perfusion pressure will result in improved blood flow to the spinal cord and result in the benefit of decreased spinal cord ischaemic injury.

Retrograde distal aortic perfusion was imposed as a necessary prevention of spinal and visceral ischaemia when aortic clamping lasts longer than 30 min. A number of approaches have been attempted for distal aortic perfusion and have included passive shunts, roller pumps, centrifugal pumps or total cardiopulmonary bypass. Passive pump shunts cannot regulate flow, while cardiopulmonary bypass needs significant systemic heparinization with the possibility of excessive bleeding. It has been our preference to use centrifugal pumps that have the advantage of avoiding or at least reducing heparinization, as well as the ability to control distal flow.

Coselli et al. reported a protective effect of the left heart bypass combined with sequential clamping compared with the simple "clamp and sew" technique. In his experience, patients treated with this adjunct had an incidence of SC ischaemia of 4.5% versus 11.2% in those with simple clamping technique, concluding that left heart bypass may play a crucial role in cases of unexpected complications or extensive repair [45].

27.6 Postoperative SCI Prevention

In the immediate postoperative period, it is mandatory to focus on a close neurological monitoring in order to put potential manoeuvers in place to minimize the risk of paraplegia at a very first sign of spinal cord ischaemia. Various protocols suggest different evaluation time and scales. One way to standardize the evaluation involves the use of muscle strength grading scale, for example, in assessing hip flexion and flexion and dorsiflexion of the foot.

The score is made as follows: 0, no muscle contraction; 1, contraction but no muscle shortening; 2, with shortening but unable to overcome gravity; 3, shortening able to overcome gravity, but no ability to gain additional strength; 4, shortening, able to gain a small additional force; 5, normal.

Different options have been explored for the management of CSF drainage: one option is to maintain or decrease the intraoperative target of drainage postoperatively for about 24–36 h and then clamp the drain following its removal at 48 h, maintaining a MAP of 75–85 mmHg. Another approach is to suspend drainage postoperatively as soon as the patient is able to demonstrate normal force in the lower limbs, keeping MAP at 90–100 mmHg. If the patient develops symptoms, a neurological evaluation is recommended followed by haemodynamic optimization and CSF drainage increase (if it has been decreased in the meantime) [46].

Permissive hypertension (mean MAP of 90) is recommended, keeping haemoglobin >9 mg/dL for the first 5 days post-op, and if the patient develops SCI, haemoglobin should be raised by >10 mg/dL [3].

27.7 Conclusions

Spinal cord protection during open and endovascular aortic repair is still a major challenge. It is multifactorial and this underlines the need for a multimodal approach in the attempt to prevent it. The "aortic team" must involve surgeons, anaesthesiologists and intensive care specialists in order to put in place the best knowledge with the strongest efforts.

Spinal cord ischaemia is also time-dependent, forcing the team to act fast and resolutely. Focusing on that aspect, it may be auspicable to have bundled protocols with the rationale to facilitate guideline application by identifying key interventions from evidence-based guidelines or best clinical practices.

Even if recent studies and innovation have provided the surgeon with instruments for detecting early spinal cord injuries, an affordable and precise diagnostic tool does not yet exist. Further effort has to be made in that field.

At present, the state of the art in spinal cord protection can be resumed in an apparent contradictory sentence: try to implement multimodal bundled protocol in order to standardize surgical and rescue procedures, but at the same time remember to apply tailored techniques and procedures in order to fit each patient peculiarity.

References

1. Clopton MB. Surgery of the heart and blood vessels. A review of recent literature. 211 Clopton: Surgery of the heart. St. Louis Interstate Medical Journal Co, 1911.
2. Svensson LG, Crawford ES, Hess KR, Coselli JS, Safi HJ. Experience with 1509 patients undergoing thoracoabdominal aortic operations. J Vasc Surg. 1993;17:357–70.
3. Scali ST, Kim M, Kubilis P, Feezor RJ, Giles KA, Miller B, Fatima J, Huber TS, Berceli SA, Back M, Beck AW. Implementation of a bundled protocol significantly reduces risk of spinal cord ischemia after branched or fenestrated endovascular aortic repair. J Vasc Surg. 2017;67(2):409.e4–23.e4.
4. Bobadilla JL, Wynn M, Tefera G, Acher CW. Low incidence of paraplegia after thoracic endovascular aneurysm repair with proactive spinal cord protective protocols. J Vasc Surg. 2013;57:1537–42.
5. Buth J, Harris PL, Hobo R, van Eps R, Cuypers P, Duijm L, et al. Neurologic complications associated with endovascular repair of thoracic aortic pathology: incidence and risk factors. A study from the European Collaborators on Stent/Graft Techniques for Aortic Aneurysm Repair (EUROSTAR) registry. J Vasc Surg. 2007;46:1103–10. discussion: 1110–1.
6. Rossi SH, Patel A, Saha P, Gwozdz A, Salter R, Gkoutzios P, et al. Neuroprotective strategies can prevent permanent paraplegia in the majority of patients who develop spinal cord ischaemia after endovascular repair of thoracoabdominal aortic aneurysms. Eur J Vasc Endovasc Surg. 2015;50:599–607.
7. Schlosser FJ, Verhagen HJ, Lin PH, Verhoeven EL, van Herwaarden JA, Moll FL, et al. TEVAR following prior abdominal aortic aneurysm surgery: increased risk of neurological deficit. J Vasc Surg. 2009;49:308–14. discussion: 314.
8. Thron AK. Vascular anatomy of the spinal cord: neuroradiological investigations and clinical syndromes. New York: Springer; 1989.
9. Melissano G, Bertoglio L, Rinaldi E, Leopardi M, Chiesa R. An anatomical review of spinal cord blood supply. J Cardiovasc Surg. 2015;56(5):699–706.
10. Melissano G, Civilini E, Bertoglio L, Calliari F, Campos Moraes Amato A, Chiesa R. Angio-CT imaging of the spinal cord vascularisation: a pictorial essay. Eur J Vasc Endovasc Surg. 2010;39:436–40.
11. Adamkiewicz A. Die Blutgefasse des menschlichen Ruckenmarkes, I: Die Gefasse der Ruckenmarksubstanz. Sitzb Akad Wiss. 1881;84:469–598; II Die Gefasse der Ruckenmarksoberflache. Sitzb Akad Wiss. 1882;85:101–30.
12. Kirklin JW, Barrat Boyes BG. Acute traumatic aortic transection. In: Cardiac surgery. New York: Wiley; 1986. p. 1462–4.
13. Skalski JH, Zembala M. Albert Wojciech Adamkiewicz: the discoverer of the variable vascularity of the spinal cord. Ann Thorac Surg. 2005;80:1971–5.
14. Kieffer E, Richard T, Chiras J, Godet G, Cormier E. Preoperative spinal cord arteriography in aneurysmal disease of the descending thoracic and thoracoabdominal aorta: preliminary results in 45 patients. Ann Vasc Surg. 1989;3:34e46.
15. Hyodoh H, Kawaharada N, Akiba H, Tamakawa M, Hyodoh K, Fukada J, et al. Usefulness of preoperative detection of artery of Adamkiewicz with dynamic contrast-enhanced MR angiography. Radiology. 2005;236(3):1004–9.
16. Svensson LG, Hess KR, Coselli JS, Safi HJ. Influence of segmental arteries, extent, and atriofemoral bypass on postoperative paraplegia after thoracoabdominal aortic operations. J Vasc Surg. 1994;20:255–62.
17. Kawaharada N, Morishita K, Fukada J, Yamada A, Muraki S, Hyodoh H, et al. Thoracoabdominal or descending aortic aneurysm repair after preoperative demonstration of the Adamkiewicz artery by magnetic resonance angiography. Eur J Cardiothorac Surg. 2002;21(6):970–4.

18. Chiesa R, Melissano G, Marrocco-Trischitta MM, Civilini E, Setacci F. Spinal cord ischemia after elective stent-graft repair of the thoracic aorta. J Vasc Surg. 2005;42:11–7.
19. Setacci F, Sirignano P, Cappelli A, Setacci C. The wonders of a newly available post-analysis ct software in the hands of vascular surgeons. Eur J Vasc Endovasc Surg. 2012;43:404–6.
20. Melissano G, Bertoglio L, Civelli V, Moraes Amato AC, Coppi G, Civilini E, Calori G, De Cobelli F, Del Maschio A, Chiesa R. Demonstration of the Adamkiewicz artery by multidetector computed tomography angiography analysed with the open-source Software OsiriX. Eur J Vasc Endovasc Surg. 2009;37:395–400.
21. Czerny M, Eggebrecht H, Sodeck G, Verzini F, Cao P, Maritati G, Riambau V, Beyersdorf F, Rylski B, Funovics M, Loewe C, Schmidli J, Tozzi P, Weigang E, Kuratani T, Livi U, Esposito G, Trimarchi S, van den Berg JC, Weiguo F, Chiesa R, Melissano G, Bertoglio L, Lonn L, Schuster I, Grimm M. Mechanisms of symptomatic spinal cord ischemia after TEVAR: insights from the European registry of endovascular aortic repair complications (EuREC). J Endovasc Ther. 2012;19:37–43.
22. Eagleton MJ, Shah S, Petkosevek D, Mastracci TM, Greenberg RK. Hypogastric and subclavian artery patency affects onset and recovery of spinal cord ischemia associated with aortic endografting. J Vasc Surg. 2014;59:89–95.
23. Godet G, Bertrand M, Fléron M-H, Goarin J-P, Colson P, Cardon A, Koskas F, Verhoye J-P, Kieffer E. Cerebrospinal fluid drainage and thoracic endovascular aneurysm repair. Asian Cardiovasc Thorac Ann. 2017;25(9):608–17.
24. Sugie S, Nakajima M, Ueno A, et al. Studies on occlusion and replacement of the thoracic aorta. Nippon J Angiocardiol. 1957;20:120.
25. McCullough JL, Hollier LH, Nugent M. Paraplegia after thoracic aortic occlusion: influence of cerebrospinal fluid drainage. Experimental and early clinical results. J Vasc Surg. 1988;7:153–60.
26. Bower TC, Murray MJ, Gloviczki P, et al. Effects of thoracic aortic occlusion and cerebrospinal fluid drainage on regional spinal cord blood flow in dogs: correlation with neurologic outcome. J Vasc Surg. 1989;9:135–44.
27. Tshomba Y, Leopardi M, Mascia D, Kahlberg A, Carozzo A, Magrin S, Melissano G, Chiesa R. Automated pressure-controlled cerebrospinal fluid drainage during open thoracoabdominal aortic aneurysm repair. J Vasc Surg. 2017;66:37–44.
28. Coles JG, Wilson GJ, Sima AF, et al. Intraoperative detection of spinal cord ischemia using somatosensory cortical evoked potentials during thoracic aortic occlusion. Ann Thorac Surg. 1982;34(3):299–306.
29. Cunnigham JN Jr, Lashinger JC, Spencer FC. Monitoring of somatosensory evoked potentials during surgical procedures on the thoracoabdominal aorta. IV. Clinical observations and results. J Thorac Cardiovasc Surg. 1987;94(2):275–85.
30. Laschinger JC, Cunnigham JN Jr, Cooper MM, et al. Monitoring of somatosensory evoked potentials during surgical procedures on the thoracoabdominal aorta. I. Relationship of aortic cross-clamp duration, changes in somatosensory evoked potentials, and incidence of neurologic dysfunction. J Thorac Cardiovasc Surg. 1987;94(2):260–5.
31. Banga PV, Oderich GS, de Souza LR, Hofer J, Cazares Gonzalez ML, Pulido JN, Cha S, Gloviczki P. Neuromonitoring. Cerebrospinal fluid drainage, and selective use of iliofemoral conduits to minimize risk of spinal cord injury during complex endovascular aortic repair. J Endovasc Ther. 2016;23(1):139–49.
32. Amabile P, Grisoli D, Giorgi R, et al. Incidence and determinants of spinal cord ischaemia in stent-graft repair of the thoracic aorta. Eur J Vasc Endovasc Surg. 2008;35:455–61.
33. Reilly LM, Chuter TA. Reversal of fortune: induced endoleak to resolve neurological deficit after endovascular repair of thoracoabdominal aortic aneurysm. J Endovasc Ther. 2010;17:21–9.
34. Harrison SC, Agu O, Harris PL, Ivancev K. Elective sac perfusion to reduce the risk of neurologic events following endovascular repair of thoracoabdominal aneurysms. J Vasc Surg. 2012;55:1202–5.
35. Etz CD, Kari FA, Mueller CS, Brenner RM, Lin HM, Griepp RB. The collateral network concept: remodeling of the arterial collateral network after experimental segmental artery sacrifice. J Thorac Cardiovasc Surg. 2011;141:1029–36.
36. O'Callaghan A, Mastracci TM, Eagleton MJ. Staged endovascular repair of thoracoabdominal aortic aneurysms limits incidence and severity of spinal cord ischemia. J Vasc Surg. 2015;61:347–54.
37. Kasprzak PM, Gallis K, Cucuruz B, Pfister K, Janotta M, Kopp R. Editor's choice—temporary aneurysm sac perfusion as an adjunct for prevention of spinal cord ischemia after branched endovascular repair of thoracoabdominal aneurysms. Eur J Vasc Endovasc Surg. 2014;48(3):258–65.
38. Luehr M, Salameh A, Haunschild J, et al. Minimally invasive segmental artery coil embolization for preconditioning of the spinal cord collateral network before one stage descending and thoracoabdominal aneurysm repair. Innovations. 2014;9:60–5.
39. Christian D, Sebastian Debus E, Moh F-W, Kolbel T. First-in-man endovascular preconditioning of the paraspinal collateral network by segmental artery coil embolization to prevent ischemic spinal cord injury. J Thorac Cardiovasc Surg. 2015;149(4):1074–9.
40. Galla JD, Ergin MA, Lansman SL, McCullough JN, Nguyen KH, Spielvogel D, Klein JJ, Griepp RB. Use of somatosensory evoked potentials for thoracic and thoracoabdominal aortic resections. Ann Thorac Surg. 1999;67(6):1947–52. discussion 1953–8.

41. Safi HJ, Miller CC, Carr C, Iliopoulos DC, Dorsay DA, Baldwin JC. Importance of intercostal artery reattachment during thoracoabdominal aortic aneurysm repair. J Vasc Surg. 1998;27(1):58–66. discussion 66–8.
42. Jacobs MJ, de Mol BA, Elenbaas T, Mess WH, Kalkman CJ, Schurink GW, Mochtar B. Spinal cord blood supply in patients with thoracoabdominal aortic aneurysms. J Vasc Surg. 2002;35(1):30–7.
43. Melissano G, Bertoglio L, Mascia D, Rinaldi E, Del Carro U, Nardelli P, Chiesa R. Spinal cord ischemia is multifactorial: what is the best protocol? J Cardiovasc Surg. 2016;57(2):191–201.
44. Davidovic L, Ilic N. Spinal cord ischemia after aortic surgery. J Cardiovasc Surg. 2014;55(6):741–57.
45. Coselli JS. The use of left heart bypass in the repair of thoracoabdominal aortic aneurysms: current techniques and results. Semin Thorac Cardiovasc Surg. 2003;15(4):326–32.
46. Dias-Neto M, Reis PV, Rolim D, Ramos J'F, Teixeira J'F, Sampaio S. Strategies to prevent TEVAR-related spinal cord ischemia. Vascular. 2017;25(3):307–15.

28 Current Trends of Treatment Options for Complex Aortic Pathology with Visceral Artery Involvement in a Large Single-Center Experience

Nicola Mangialardi, Matteo Orrico, Sonia Ronchey, and Andrea Esposito

28.1 Introduction

Currently, there are no prospective randomized trials that compare open versus endovascular repair for thoracoabdominal aortic diseases. Open surgical repair represents the "gold standard" for the treatment of thoracoabdominal aortic aneurysm (TAAA) or dissection.

Over the last 40 years, advances in perioperative care, surgical techniques, and adjuncts for organ protection have greatly improved morbidity and mortality rates in experienced surgical centers, even in patients undergoing extensive repair [1] .The contemporary results of open surgical repair of thoracoabdominal aneurysms come from the very few centers with expertise in this area, so it is difficult to make a reliable comparison between open and endovascular repair. Furthermore, the mortality rates reported for open procedures are still high. The most encouraging results for open procedures including the repair of the visceral aorta are based on cohorts of patients aged 50 years or younger [1]. It is clear from the experience of the same centers reporting these good results that the mean age for these conditions is close to 70 years, so when speaking about complex aortic pathologies involving the visceral aorta, a less-invasive approach should be considered both for age and for comorbidities of this population [2]. The endovascular option shows an immediate advantage on the open approach, and this consideration is modifying the attitude toward such patients [3]. We herein report a retrospective analysis of patients treated for complex aortic pathologies with visceral artery involvement in the last year.

N. Mangialardi (✉) · M. Orrico
Ospedale San Camillo, Rome, Italy
e-mail: nicola.mangialardi@asl-rme.it

S. Ronchey · A. Esposito
Ospedale San Filippo Neri, Rome, Italy

28.2 Decision-Making

When a complex aortic pathology with visceral artery involvement is present, patients' age and clinical conditions usually drive the choice of the surgical approach. Young patients, and those in good clinical conditions with pararenal pathology which may not imply a thoracotomy, may benefit from open or hybrid treatment. If the patient is considered unfit for open surgery, the anatomy should be the factor determining which endovascular option between Ch-EVAR, custom

© Springer Nature Switzerland AG 2019
Y. Tshomba et al. (eds.), *Visceral Vessels and Aortic Repair*,
https://doi.org/10.1007/978-3-319-94761-7_28

FEVAR/BEVAR, and "off-the-shelf" BEVAR should be chosen, while for thoracoabdominal aneurysms which would need a thoracotomy for the open repair, the endovascular option with FEVAR and BEVAR should be considered a good alternative [3] (treatment algorithm is schematized in Fig. 28.1).

28.3 Patient Populations

A retrospective analysis of our cohort of patients from December 2016 to December 2017 showed a total of 64 patients treated for complex aortic pathologies with visceral artery involvement (the intended meaning for visceral artery involvement is a primary aortic pathology with proximal extent to reno-visceral segment or an evolution of the index pathology after an infrarenal repair for which the correction would include an extent to the reno-visceral segment). Of these, seven were treated as an urgency/emergency. Distribution of treatment options with the number of managed reno-visceral branches is shown in Figs. 28.2 and 28.3.

28.4 Open Procedures

In our cohort of patients (11 male patients), all of them were treated by an open approach. The mean age in this subgroup was 65 years. The comorbidities are reported in Table 28.1.

The primary open repairs were nine; two patients underwent open conversion of a previous EVAR, one as an emergency. In these two

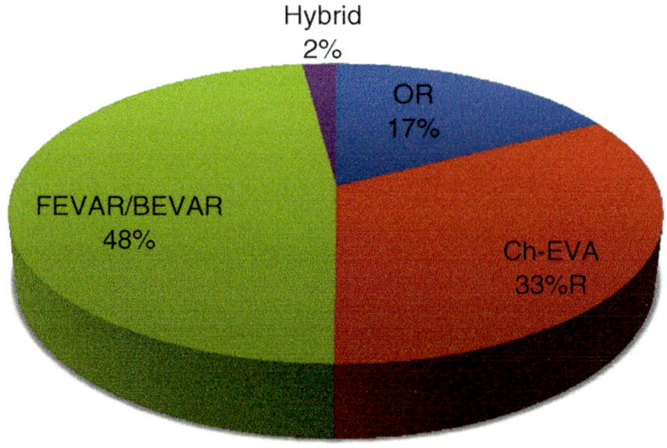

Fig. 28.2 Distribution of complex aortic procedure in 2017 at San Filippo Neri Hospital in Rome

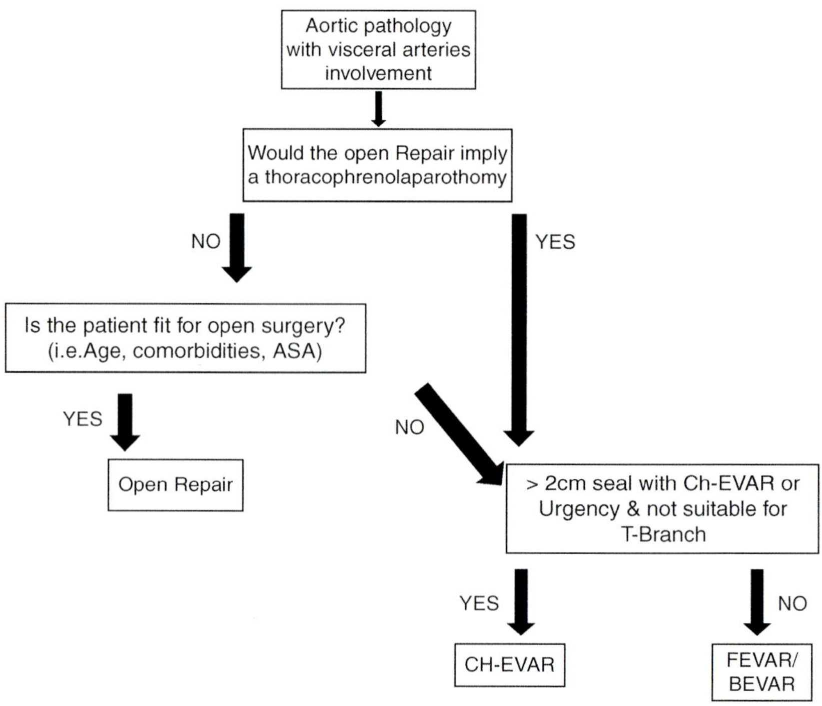

Fig. 28.1 Treatment algorithm for complex aortic aneurysms at our center

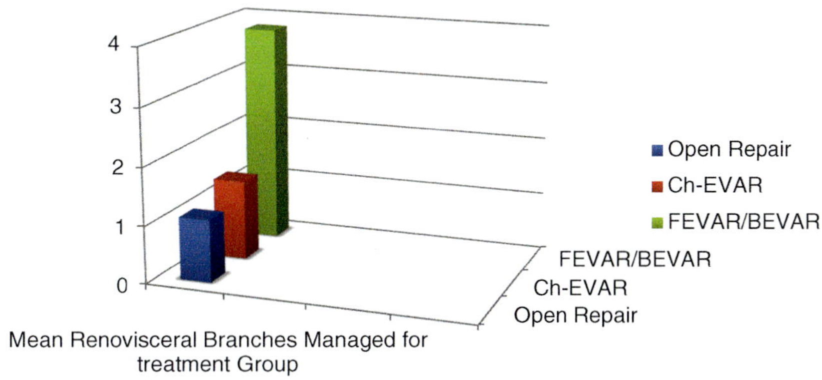

Fig. 28.3 Mean number of reno-visceral arteries managed in every treatment group. Only one patient was treated in the hybrid group with the debranching of all four reno-visceral branches

Table 28.1 Open repair group demographics

Demographic	*N* (%)
Age	65 (61–75)
Smoke	9/11 (81%)
Hypertension	9/11 (81%)
Dyslipidemia	6/11 (54%)
COPD	4/11 (36%)
Diabetes	3/11 (27%)
ASA III/IV	3/11 (27%)

patients, it was not necessary to surgically manage the reno-visceral branches. They are part of this population as the previously implanted graft was a suprarenal fixation endoprosthesis, so that the repair implied a supraceliac clamping. In both patients, the indication was a type I and II endoleak. The patient was treated as an emergency and presented with an aneurysmal sac rupture after being lost at 5 years follow-up. The index repair was performed in 2010 via a Jotec E-vita endograft, a type II endoleak was clear since the initial follow-up, and after 1 year, a 5 mm aneurysmal sac growth was evident. Unfortunately, the patient never returned for follow-up until presentation at the emergency room with abdominal pain. The CTA showed a rupture with an associated type I and II endoleak. We performed an emergent open conversion with graft explantation and aorto-bysiliac bypass. The patient died 5 days later in the ICU due to cardiopulmonary failure. The patient treated with open conversion in elective setting also had a mixed type I and II endoleak with associated aneurysmal sac growth. It had been treated with Endurant (Medtronic Vascular, Santa Rosa, California) 3 years earlier and had an overall aneurysmal sac growth of 1.5 cm. An open conversion was performed electively through a translumbar approach, with supraceliac clamping. The patient was discharged on the sixth postoperative day in a good condition. For the remaining nine patients, the open procedure was primary repair. In eight patients, the aneurysm had no infrarenal neck for EVAR, and they were in good clinical condition, so an open repair was planned with the reimplantation of one (seven) or both (one) renal arteries. One last patient had a horseshoe-shaped kidney, and so we provided the open repair of his aneurysm with reimplantation of three renal arteries (Fig. 28.4). In this cohort of patients, 30-day mortality was 0.9% (one emergent conversion), and the overall mortality was 1.8% (one death at 40 days in the ICU due to pulmonary complications). It is not possible to compare these results with the endo-cohort as the visceral artery involvement of this cohort of patients was limited in the large majority of cases to one renal artery and the patients were always in good clinical conditions.

28.5 Endovascular Procedures

28.5.1 Chimney Repair

This technique is preferred to fenestrated/branched technology, if based on the preoperative planning; a single/double chimney is enough to exclude the aneurysm with 2 cm of new sealing neck. Twenty-one patients have been treated

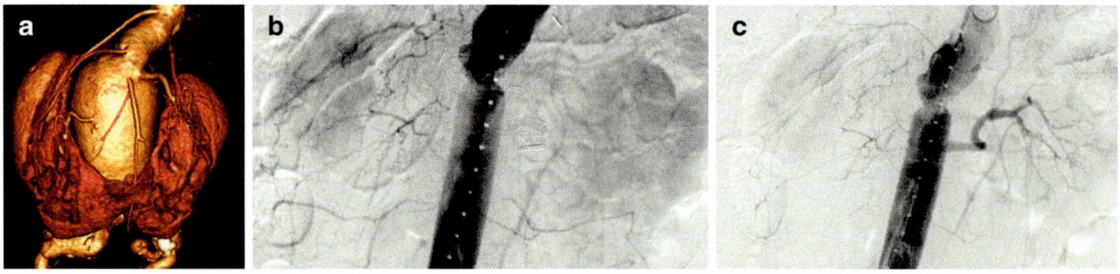

Fig. 28.4 (**a**) CTA of AAA associated with a horseshoe kidney; (**b/c**) control angiograms showing the good perfusion of the kidney after OR and renal artery reimplantation

over the last year with chimney technology (single, double, or triple), as they were all considered unfit for open surgery. Seventeen patients were treated in an elective setting, four in emergency. Out of the general population, two were treated with Nellix (Endologix, Irvine, California), plus Advanta V12 (Atrium Europe B.V., Mijdrecht, The Netherlands) as parallel graft (one single chimney on a right renal, one triple chimney on both renals and the superior mesenteric artery). Thirty-eight percent were treated by Endurant IIs plus Advanta as parallel graft (75% single chimney, 25% double, of which one case was a patient with a previous nephrectomy and in which the double chimney included a left renal and a superior mesenteric). Forty-three percent were treated by Gore C3 excluder and Viabahn (W. L. Gore & Associates, Inc., Flagstaff, Arizona) (67% single chimney, 33% double). The remaining 9.5% were treated by Cook Alpha Abdominal (Cook Medical Inc., Bloomington, Indiana) (one single chimney with Advanta and one double chimney with bare-metal stents).

We planned one case of chimney repair with bare-metal stent due to short infrarenal aortic segment, for which it was necessary to partially cover the renal ostia, which were coplanar, so since there were no sealing concerns in the infrarenal neck, chimney was necessary only to safeguard renal flow.

We prefer this technique to FEVAR technology when the repair includes one or two visceral arteries to reduce the extent of aortic repair and for compromised patients, with short life expectancy, and of course in emergency settings.

The main concern of this technique is still type I endoleak from gutters [4]. In order to reduce such complications, adequate planning is required, and the size choice of the parallel graft and the main graft is of utmost importance. We recently described our sizing method for arch chimney, which is basically the same as for an abdominal chimney. This method is described with the name of Over-SIRIX and consists in calculating the correct graft diameter with a disease-specific oversizing, based on the simulation of presumed circumferential graft length adjusted to fill the gutters between the main and the parallel grafts [5]. With the aim of reducing chimney numbers, a good adjunct in emergency situations is represented by homemade fenestrations (Fig. 28.5).

A crucial point in reducing gutters is the choice of the materials, as various reports suggest that similar materials perform better. For this reason, chimney with Gore C3 is generally made with Gore Viabahn as a parallel graft and reinforced if needed [6]. As far as Ch-EVAR with Endurant is concerned, the most often used parallel graft is the Advanta V12 stents based on the data reported by the PERICLES and PROTAGORAS registry [7, 8]: IFUs of the Endurant for the parallel graft technique do not force the use of this stent but advise the use of any balloon-expandable stent. It is now agreed that this technique should be standardized, just like the fenestrated and branched repairs. This is the reason the planning should be accurate and take consideration remove and angulate the side vessels, the need for reinforcement, and visceral landing zone, which should, when possible, be in a straight segment of the artery and not in unfavorable angulations.

It is noteworthy that favorable removal for the chimney configuration is typically a caudally

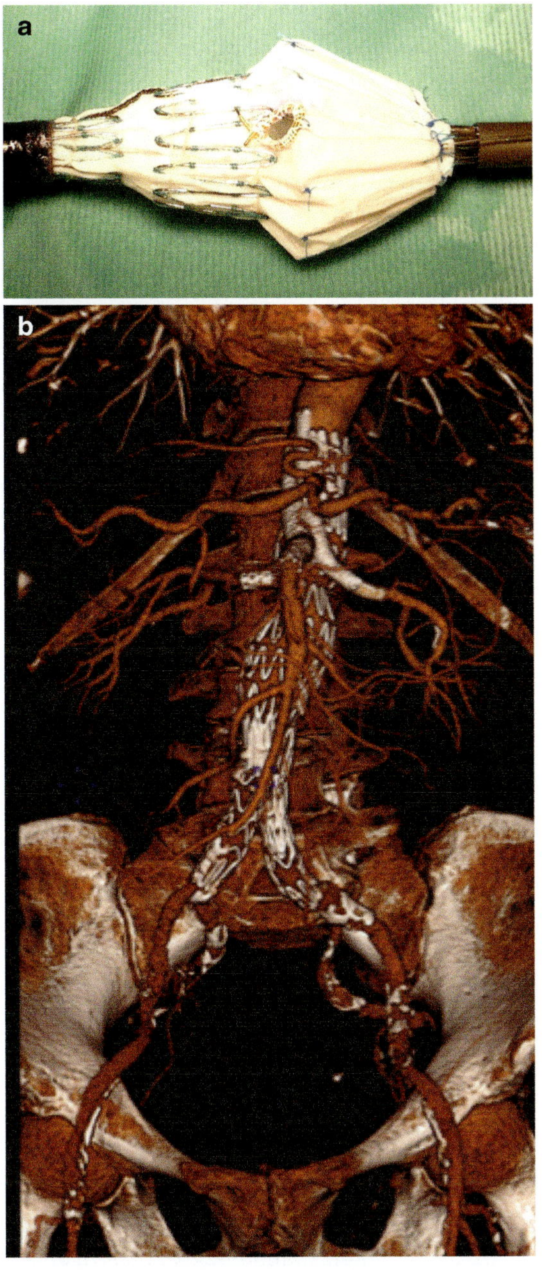

Fig. 28.5 (**a**) Homemade fenestrations; (**b**) triple chimney (SMA, CT, LRA) homemade fenestration on RRA

oriented vessel. When a cranial orientation is present, however, fenestrations or alternative parallel graft configurations should be considered.

Stroke and TIA are complications to consider in this technique and to always prevent with an accurate study of the arch since in well-experienced centers this complication still ranges around 1.9% with risk factors being bilateral upper extremity access, aneurysm rupture, and prolonged operation time [9].

Using this technique, we registered a type I endoleak rate of 4.7% in the last year, which is considered acceptable. Four cases (19%) of this subgroup of patients presented for correction of a type I endoleak. This is our technique of choice for type I endoleak with aneurysmal growth and resistance to endotherapy. Thirty-day mortality rate was 0%, with no major complications. The strength of Ch-EVAR over FEVAR for type I endoleak is the availability of the material, so that an emergency repair can easily be performed. The chimney method is easier than FEVAR in type I endoleak because no difficulties in orienting the markers which can be superimposed to the previous graft ones exist for Ch-EVAR. In FEVAR, on the other hand, this can represent a major problem. The technique is a valid alternative in cases of aortic pathology involving less than three visceral vessels and gaining a total of 2 cm sealing neck, with a new neck of at least 1 cm. This limitation comes from the results of PERICLES registry in which good early and late results, even in terms of effective aneurysmal sac exclusion, are reported for single and double chimney, because of the limited number of gutters. This technique should be indicated for pararenal rather than for thoracoabdominal aneurysm with the exception of the very few cases unfit for open surgery and/or for off-the-shelf thoracoabdominal grafts and those that cannot wait for a custom repair. Of note, very few reports have been published regarding thoracoabdominal repair with Ch-EVAR, mostly in emergency, and high rates of type I endoleak are reported [10].

28.5.2 FEVAR and BEVAR

Thirty-one patients were treated by FEVAR/BEVAR repair. This, in our opinion, should be the preferred option for aneurysm or dissections with the involvement of more than two vessels, as it is strongly standardized and has good results in the follow-up. Of our 31 patients, 7 were treated with an off-the-shelf graft, the t-Branch from Cook, and 24 by custom fenestrated and branch devices with Cook, Anaconda (Vascutek, Renfrewshire, Scotland), and Jotec (GmbH, Hechingen, Germany) endografts. In cases of visceral artery involvement, with more than two vessels, we always check for feasibility of an off-the-shelf complex solution. t-Branch from Cook is indicated for aneurysms with important proximal extension, and one of the most frequent reasons for unsuitability is generally the diameter of the aorta which should at least be 30 mm at the visceral segment [11]. In cases of unsuitability, we then look for a custom solution. Our preference is to actively participate in the planning of our custom graft and, when possible, plan our own graft. One concern about this technique is the risk of spinal cord ischemia related to extensive aortic coverage. Whenever possible, even in post-dissected aneurysm, we try to obtain a graft with at least one branch. The reason for this is that in cases of extensive aortic coverage, more than 4 cm above the celiac trunk, the repair is always performed in two stages, supported by literature findings [12]: in the first one, the main graft is deployed every branch, and fenestration is completed but one branch, usually the celiac trunk, which is connected to the main graft only with a bare-metal stent; in the second step, under local anesthesia and from a brachial access, this branch is re-catheterized and a balloon is kept inflated for 20 min to simulate aneurysmal sac exclusion [13]. If there are no neurological alterations, the repair is completed with the reliance of a bare stent (Fig. 28.6). So far, in the subgroup of patients treated with this approach, we had one transient paraparesis noted at 4/5 but it was transient and fully recovered so that we have a rate of permanent deficit of 0%.

Beside the total aortic coverage, which should be minimized to avoid paraplegia, the planning of the custom graft should always take into consideration the removal of visceral branches to decide whether a fenestration or a branch is more convenient. The general rule is that upward vessels are better managed with fenestrations and downward vessels are ideal for branches. It is also very important to check for early branches: a visceral neck of at least 10 mm should always exist so that if there is a bifurcation before 10 mm, the larger branch should always be considered, and the smaller should be sacrificed. In cases of similar dimensions, a selective angiography is performed in order to visualize the amount of parenchyma supplied by every branch. In our cohort of patients, 29 (93%) were treated in an elective setting and 2 (7%) in emergency for symptomatic aneurysm or rupture. An iliac conduit was necessary in three cases, always planned, for both external iliac arteries <than 8.1 mm. Fourteen were type III TAAA (45%), seven (22.5%) type II, five type I, and five type II (32.5%) according to the Crawford classification. The total mean aortic coverage was 402 mm (210–570 mm), while the mean coverage above the celiac trunk was 285 mm (110–406 mm). We routinely use a preventive CSF drainage for supraceliac coverage of more than 4 cm.

In this subgroup of patients, 26 repairs included all four reno-visceral branches (1 case

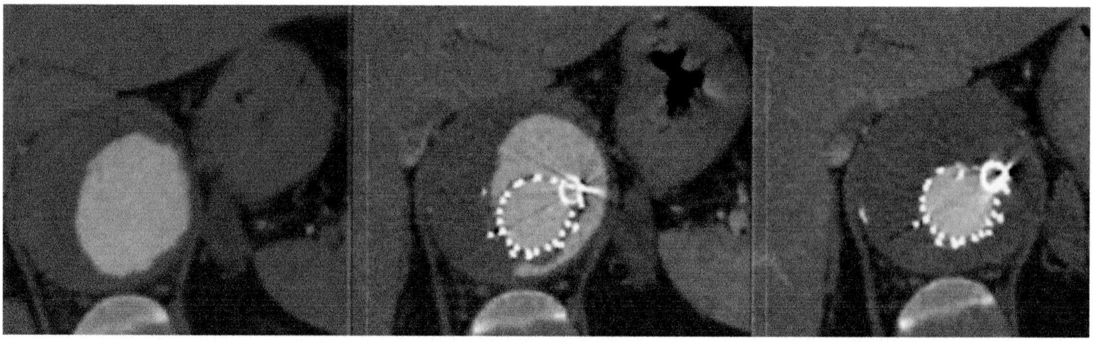

Fig. 28.6 Temporary perfusion of the aneurysmal sac in a "t-Branch" type III thoracoabdominal patient

of proximal evolution after infrarenal open repair and 1 of proximal evolution after EVAR), 4 included three (2 cases of previous nephrectomy, 2 cases of occluded celiac trunk), 1 case had only 2 fenestrations (SMA and CT) because the patient was already in dialysis, and so we did not manage the renal arteries for a total of 118 visceral arteries to target. Four repairs were for a post-dissective aneurysm.

In the last 31 TAAAs of our experience, we used BeGraft (Bentley GmbH, Hechingen, Germany) balloon-expandable stents, mainly because of their low profile. We usually reinforce them with bare-metal stent only if needed (i.e., landing in angulated segment with post-stenting kinking).

In this series, we registered a technical success of 96.7% with a successful revascularization rate of target vessels of 98.3%: in one case of type B aortic dissection, despite the correct alignment of the markers, it was not possible to catheterize CT and SMA, and they were rescued by periscope (Fig. 28.7). This accounts for an assisted patency rate of 100%. The SCI rate was 9.6%: one case of fully recovered paraparesis after a staged procedure and two regressive paraparesis in "four fens" one-stage repair, of which one had a partial recovery. The mean procedural length was 160 min (140–300 min), and the mean hospital stay was 8.9 days (4–10). The second stages were performed at a mean time of 7.5 weeks after the first stage (6–10 weeks) and were always performed under local anesthesia. We had a morbidity rate of 9.6% (three supracited cases of SCI), and minor complication rate was 6.4% (with two cases of brachial hematoma). In this cohort of patients, the type I endoleak rate is 0%, to note that we re-intervened on a t-Branch case with an endoleak from the CT stent which we misdiagnosed as a type III endoleak, but that was actually due to a fracture of the BeGraft which we treated with relining with a covered stent.

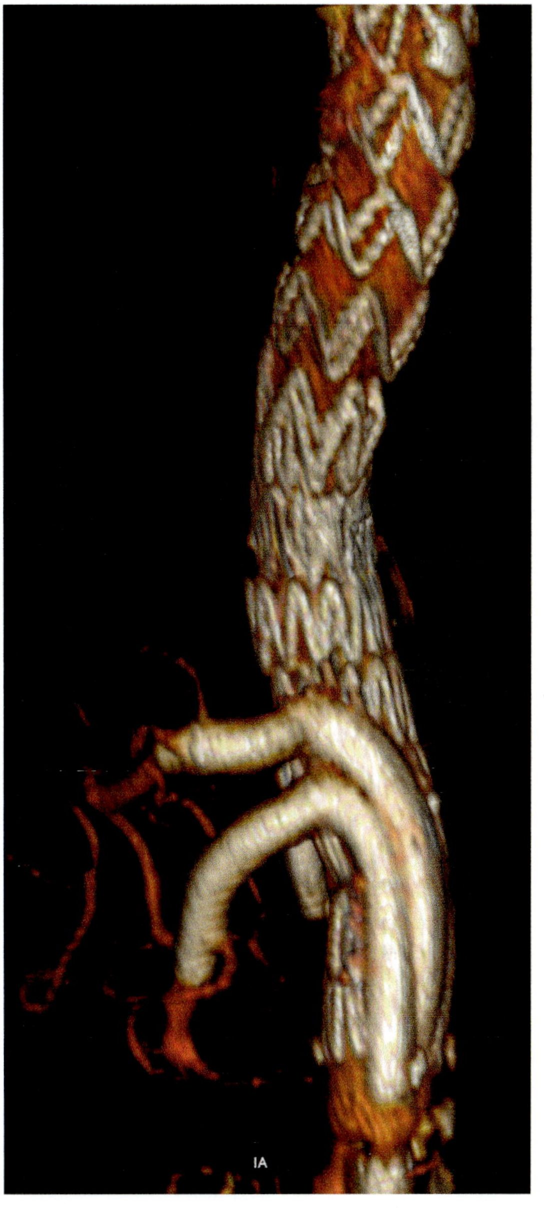

Fig. 28.7 Periscope for rescue of a CT and SMA in a FEVAR procedure for dissection

28.6 Hybrid Procedures

Hybrid repair can be a valid alternative and is more often considered since the VORTEC technique was first described [14]. In the examined amount of time, we only used this technique once. In our opinion, this has to be considered a major intervention because it implies an extensive dissection of the aorta and selection of the population is of utmost importance. There are no well-defined criteria for such a technique, but in our opinion, it should be reserved to the very few patients in good conditions but cannot undergo a thoracotomy.

28.7 Final Considerations

The approach to such pathologies should be tailored to the patient: knowing that the open repair is still the gold standard, patients unfit for open surgery may be sent to the endovascular repair which has demonstrated an early advantage over the open repair. The choice between chimney and FEVAR/BEVAR technology should always be based on the amount of the aorta to cover and on the life expectancy of the patient. Confidence with the technique and accurate preoperative planning are of paramount importance to achieve the technical success.

References

1. Coselli JS, Amarasekara HS, Green SY, et al. Open repair of thoracoabdominal aortic aneurysm in patients 50 years old and younger. Ann Thorac Surg. 2017;103(6):1849–57.
2. LeMaire SA, Price MD, Green SY, et al. Results of open thoracoabdominal aortic aneurysm repair. Ann Cardiothorac Surg. 2012;1(3):286–92.
3. Ferrer C, Cao P, De Rango P, et al. A propensity-matched comparison for endovascular and open repair of thoracoabdominal aortic aneurysms. J Vasc Surg. 2016;63(5):1201–7.
4. Adovasio R, Chiarandini S, Calvagna C, et al. Treatment of complex abdominal aortic aneurysms with parallel graft-endovascular aneurysm repair. Retrospective analysis of a single center experience and midterm results. Ann Vasc Surg. 2018;47:260.
5. Fazzini S, Ronchey S, Orrico M. "Over-SIRIX": a new method for sizing aortic endografts in combination with the chimney grafts: early experience with aortic arch disease. Ann Vasc Surg. 2018;46:285.
6. Montelione N, Pecoraro F, Puippe G. A 12-year experience with chimney and periscope grafts for treatment of type I endoleaks. J Endovasc Ther. 2015;22(4):568–74.
7. Donas KP, Lee JT, Lachat M. Collected world experience about the performance of the snorkel/chimney endovascular technique in the treatment of complex aortic pathologies: the PERICLES registry. Ann Surg. 2015;262(3):546–53.
8. Donas KP, Torsello GB, Piccoli G. The PROTAGORAS study to evaluate the performance of the Endurant stent graft for patients with pararenal pathologic processes treated by the chimney/snorkel endovascular technique. J Vasc Surg. 2016;63(1):1–7.
9. Bosiers MJ, Tran K, Lee JT, et al. Incidence and prognostic factors related to major adverse cerebrovascular events in patients with complex aortic diseases treated by the chimney technique. J Vasc Surg. 2018;67:1372.
10. Pecoraro F, Pfammatter T, Mayer D, et al. Multiple periscope and chimney grafts to treat ruptured thoracoabdominal and pararenal aortic aneurysms. J Endovasc Ther. 2011;18(5):642–9.
11. Silingardi R, Gennai S, Leone N. Standard "off-the-shelf" multibranched thoracoabdominal endograft in urgent and elective patients with single and staged procedures in a multicenter experience. J Vasc Surg. 2018;67:1005.
12. Kasprzak PM, Gallis K, Cucuruz B. Temporary aneurysm sac perfusion as an adjunct for prevention of spinal cord ischemia after branched endovascular repair of thoracoabdominal aneurysms. Eur J Vasc Endovasc Surg. 2014;48(3):258–65.
13. Mangialardi N, Lachat M, Esposito A. The "open branch" technique: a new way to prevent paraplegia after total endovascular repair of thoracoabdominal aneurysm. Catheter Cardiovasc Interv. 2016;87(4):773–80.
14. Setacci F, Pecoraro F, Chaykovska L. The gore hybrid vascular graft in renovisceral debranching for complex aortic aneurysm repair. J Vasc Surg. 2016;64(1):33–8.

Visceral Ischemia During Type B Dissection: Incidence, Prognostic Value, Diagnosis, and Operative Management

29

Domenico Spinelli, Hector W. L. de Beaufort, and Santi Trimarchi

29.1 Introduction

Organ malperfusion is a possible complication of acute Type B aortic dissection (AD). Theoretically each branch arising from dissected aorta or downstream may be affected, resulting in end-organ ischemia. Obstruction of the celiac and/or mesenteric arteries may lead to visceral ischemia, which is one of the most lethal complications of AD. A timely diagnosis and treatment are crucial to increase the chances of survival. Nowadays, the endovascular approach is the most frequently adopted in order to restore blood flow to the bowel, while open surgery is usually reserved for the cases of failure of endovascular treatment. In this chapter, the incidence, prognostic value, diagnosis, and operative management of this dreaded complication of AD will be described.

D. Spinelli
Thoracic Aortic Research Center, IRCCS Policlinico San Donato, San Donato Milanese, Italy

Department of Biomedical and Dental Sciences and Morphofunctional Imaging, Policlinico G. Martino, University of Messina, Messina, Italy

H. W. L. de Beaufort
Thoracic Aortic Research Center, IRCCS Policlinico San Donato, San Donato Milanese, Italy

S. Trimarchi (✉)
Thoracic Aortic Research Center, IRCCS Policlinico San Donato, San Donato Milanese, Italy

Department of Scienze Biomediche per la Salute, University of Milan, Milan, Italy
e-mail: santi.trimarchi@unimi.it

29.2 Incidence and Prognostic Value

Two different mechanisms can lead to branch vessel obstruction: dynamic obstruction and static obstruction. The most common, occurring in about 80% of cases, is the dynamic obstruction. The incidence of malperfusion syndrome in acute Type B AD is about 20% [1], with mesenteric ischemia accounting for about one third of cases. Among complicated ATBAD, contemporary series report an incidence of visceral ischemia ranging from 14 to 25% [2]. Overall, in-hospital mortality directly related to the visceral ischemia ranges from 2 to 11% [2]. In the IRAD registry, visceral ischemia of TBAD patients was 7%, and it heavily affected in-hospital mortality, which was more than triplicated compared to patients without visceral ischemia (31% versus 9%) [3]. In this cohort, patients with visceral ischemia were slightly but significantly younger than patients without visceral ischemia (59 vs 64 years) and often had malperfusion of other organs associated. On average, Type B AD patients with visceral ischemia are younger than patients without visceral ischemia [3, 4].

© Springer Nature Switzerland AG 2019
Y. Tshomba et al. (eds.), *Visceral Vessels and Aortic Repair*,
https://doi.org/10.1007/978-3-319-94761-7_29

29.3 Diagnosis

In AD, malperfusion syndrome may become evident through onset of end-organ specific signs of ischemia. It is usually more severe in case of static malperfusion, while it may be intermittent and of varying intensity in case of dynamic obstruction. In this case, care must be taken not to overlook the signs of ischemia, which can lead to a delay in diagnosis. Abdominal pain is present in the majority of cases of visceral ischemia. Nonetheless it is not an exclusive sign of malperfusion syndrome in AD, as it was reported to be present in 40% of patients without visceral ischemia [3]. Vomiting, diarrhea, and bloody defecation are more specific but later signs. Malperfusion of visceral organs may be associated with malperfusion of other districts. Kidney malperfusion with acute renal failure was reported in 40% of cases with celiac-mesenteric ischemia and only in 14% without. Femoral pulse deficit may be present, and a 28% rate of lower limb ischemia has been reported in patients with visceral malperfusion, while in patients without visceral malperfusion, it was 13%. Also spinal cord ischemia has been reported more often in association with visceral malperfusion (5% versus 2%). The suspicion of visceral malperfusion should increase in case of positivization of blood markers of ischemia. Levels of D-dimer, lactate, ammonia, transaminase, creatine phosphokinase, and leukocytes may be elevated. Recently, other markers of mesenteric ischemia have been tested. The intestinal fatty acid-binding protein (I-FABP) was reported to have a sensitivity of 79% and a specificity of 91% [5]. However many markers of ischemia increase only after the intestine has become necrotic. Therefore, negative biochemical markers should not delay intervention if there is a strong suspicion of visceral malperfusion. In presence of clear peritoneal signs, the patient should be treated without hesitation. Imaging evidence of visceral malperfusion syndrome includes true lumen compression, branch vessel dissection and thrombosis, and reduced late-phase visceral enhancement on computed tomography angiography (CTA) (Fig. 29.1). Doppler ultrasonography can show arterial thrombosis, dissection, or patterns of altered flow, but the sensitivity is not high.

29.4 Operative Management

Thoracic endovascular aortic repair (TEVAR) is currently the first-line treatment in acute complicated Type B AD patients [6, 7]. The treatment consists in the coverage of the proximal entry tear in order to achieve expansion of the true lumen and decompression of the false lumen. Thus, celiac or mesenteric artery obstruction are reversed in most cases. Otherwise, additional branch vessel stenting may be necessary in up to 20% of the cases [8–10]. TEVAR is therefore effective in treating mesenteric malperfusion in the setting of dynamic obstruction [8]. However, in-hospital mortality rates are still considerable, ranging from 20 to 40% [9–11].

Furthermore, TEVAR-related complications may also occur in a small percentage of cases. Retrograde Type A AD and stent graft-induced new entry tears have been described, in particular in relation to the use of stent grafts provided of proximal bare spring [12, 13] or in case of excessive oversizing [14]. In order to prevent such complications, the stent graft oversizing in Type B AD should not exceed 10%, and the proximal edge of the stent graft should be deployed in a non-dissected zone. The use of a distal aortic bare metal stent in combination with the standard TEVAR (PETTICOAT—Provisional Extension To Induce Complete ATtachment—technique) [15] has been proposed both for the treatment of persistence of malperfusion after TEVAR and for the prevention of late complications. In the long run, complications may occur in patients treated with TEVAR, and in particular an aneurysmal evolution should be expected. In these cases, an endovascular treatment with branched stent graft is feasible, but additional difficulties should be anticipated, especially if the visceral vessels originate from different lumina [16, 17].

Endovascular fenestration of the dissection flap is a valid treatment option in case of persistence of false lumen pressurization and dynamic obstruction. It can be performed also as

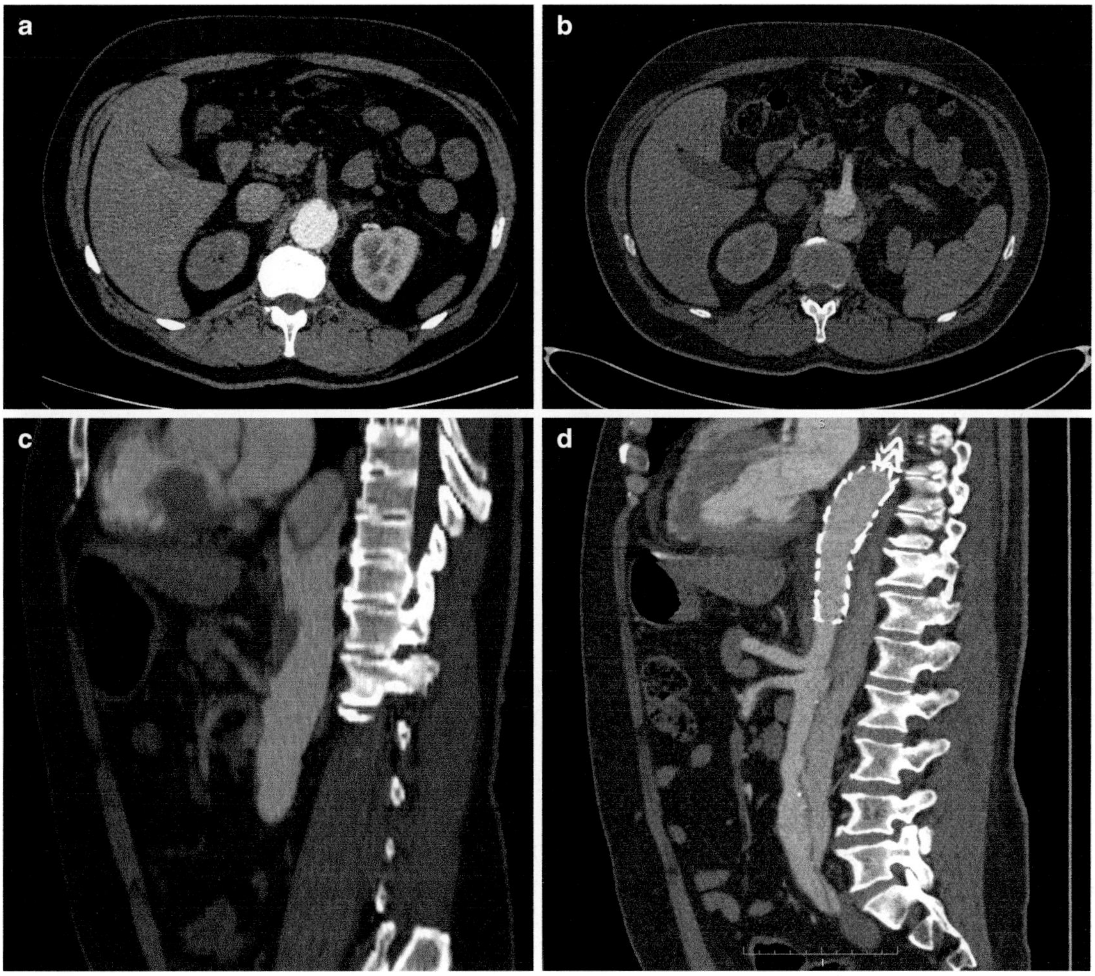

Fig. 29.1 Dynamic obstruction of visceral arteries (**a** axial view, **c** sagittal view), resolved after TEVAR (**b** axial view, **d** sagittal view)

an alternative to TEVAR. If necessary, it can be accompanied by branch vessel stenting if static obstruction of a branch vessel is present.

A 17% early mortality rate was reported after endovascular fenestration in a cohort of 69 Type B AD patients with malperfusion performed in an experienced center. Mortality was due to aortic rupture in 7% of cases and malperfusion complications in 10% [18]. Following endovascular fenestration, even more than after TEVAR, the risk of late aortic dilatation should be taken into account. Freedom from aortic rupture or aortic repair rates at 1, 5, and 8 years of 80%, 68%, and 54% have been reported [18]. The technique of endovascular flap fenestration entails gaining access to both lumina as a first step. In this phase, intravascular or intraesophageal ultrasonography may be of great help to distinguish the two lumina and identify the tears. It also helps reduce the use of iodinated contrast medium, which is particularly important in case of renal malperfusion to lower the risk of renal failure [15]. Pressure measurements allow to detect a pressure gradient between the two lumina, as well as between the proximal aorta and the branch vessels, providing an objective assessment of malperfusion. It is important to document the patency status of all branches before and after the procedure, as the resolution of obstruction in one branch vessel may lead to unpredictable changes in mobility of the dissection flap and potentially cause dynamic obstruction of other branch vessels. If static obstruction of a branch vessel is found, this should be treated by stenting prior to the fenestration procedure. In order to perform fenestration, the dissection flap needs to be crossed through a reentry tear, which is usually present at the level of branch vessels. Because the true lumen is smaller, it is usually easier to cross from the true lumen to the false lumen. If no reentry tears are found, it is possible to pierce the dissection flap using a catheter and a stiff guidewire at the level of the obstructed artery. Then a guidewire is advanced through the fenestration, and serial balloon angioplasty is performed until the pressure differential between the two lumina is abolished. If necessary, a bare metal stent may be placed in the true lumen to preserve patency of the fenestration. Other fenestration techniques have been described, such as the scissor technique and the cheese wire fenestration technique. In the latter, the guidewire, after crossing the septum, is captured with a snare device and pulled out through the contralateral groin access. Then the guidewire is pulled inferiorly with a sawing motion to shear the dissection flap, stopping before the aortic bifurcation. However, pulling the flap downward carries a risk of circumferential detachment of the intimal layer, which can result in aortic intussusception and obstruction [15]. TEVAR is currently considered the first-line treatment in most cases [7]. Fenestration may be more appropriate than TEVAR in patients with increased risk of spinal cord ischemia such as those with history of previous abdominal aortic repair and occlusion of hypogastric, subclavian, or vertebral artery. On the contrary, TEVAR is particularly indicated in elderly patients, in case of aortic dilatation, and for intermediate-risk patients (i.e., patients with refractory/recurrent pain or hypertension). Overall, the endovascular approach was used in almost 70% of patients with visceral ischemia enrolled in the IRAD in recent years [3]. In case of suspicion of intestinal infarction, an explorative laparoscopy or laparotomy is indicated. Acute abdomen, refractory lactic acidosis, and hemodynamic instability due to ongoing intestinal malperfusion warrant immediate laparotomy and resection of necrotic intestinal tracts. A temporary closure technique such as Bogota bag or VAC closure system can be used to allow later inspection of the abdominal organs. In case endovascular techniques fail to restore vascularization to the visceral arteries, open surgery is necessary [3]. Surgical vascular reconstruction should also be considered in case of anatomical contraindication for TEVAR, such as unsuitable iliac accesses and insufficient proximal landing zones [6]. Furthermore, for patients with connective tissue disorders, TEVAR can be used as a bridge treatment, while open surgical aortic replacement is the treatment of choice. Open surgery should be considered also in younger patients, since long-term durability of TEVAR is still unclear.

Open surgical options to treat visceral malperfusion include open fenestration and aortic graft replacement. Open fenestration requires exposure of the visceral segment of the aorta and clamping in supraceliac position. A longitudinal aortotomy is then carried out on the left anterolateral aortic wall, and the dissection flap is widely resected to maximize the size of the single aortic lumen. The restoration of flow in the branch vessels may be assessed through intraoperative Doppler ultrasound.

Although open surgical fenestration appears to be effective at relieving malperfusion, it is still burdened by rates of in-hospital mortality of 20% [19]. There are concerns about late aneurysmal evolution after surgical fenestration. However positive results have been reported in this regard when reduction of aortic diameter at the closure of aortotomy was carried out. In fact, according to the law of Laplace, the tension on the aortic wall decreases by reducing the radius [19].

Graft replacement of thoracic or thoracoabdominal aorta is a more definitive option [3]. However, in the acute setting, in AD patients, it is associated with about 30% mortality [20] and a relevant risk of spinal cord ischemia in case of extensive distal thoracoabdominal resection [3]. Although the visceral malperfusion is an absolute indication for invasive treatment, the rate of patients with visceral ischemia who only receive medical management is around 20% in IRAD [3].

The reason for this discrepancy may be partially due to the presence in multicenter registries of patients with radiological or angiographic signs suggestive of mesenteric obstruction without matching clinical signs [21]. More often, these patients are in such a poor clinical condition that are deemed unsuitable for endovascular or surgical intervention, and an attempt of operative management is denied. In this class of patients, the mortality rate reaches 50%. Indeed, in these patients the conservative treatment independently predicted in-hospital mortality [3]. Conversely, mortality rates after surgical and endovascular management of visceral ischemia were comparable (25.8% and 25.5%). However, the endovascular approach is considered the first-line treatment [6, 7].

29.5 Conclusion

Visceral ischemia is a life-threatening complication of acute Type B AD that mandates prompt intervention. Timeliness of diagnosis and treatment is crucial in order to successfully reverse end-organ ischemia. TEVAR is the first-line treatment. Endovascular fenestration can be used either as an alternative to TEVAR in selected patients or after TEVAR when it was not effective in restoring perfusion to the affected branch vessels. Open surgery should be limited to cases in which endovascular techniques are contraindicated or unsuccessful.

References

1. Suzuki T, Mehta RH, Ince H, et al. Clinical profiles and outcomes of acute type B aortic dissection in the current era: lessons from the International Registry of Aortic Dissection (IRAD). Circulation. 2003;108:II312–7.
2. Kamman AV, Yang B, Kim KM, Williams DM, Deeb GM, Patel HJ. Visceral malperfusion in aortic dissection: the Michigan experience. In: Seminars in thoracic and cardiovascular surgery. Philadelphia: W. B. Saunders; 2016.
3. Jonker FH, Patel HJ, Upchurch GR, et al. Acute type B aortic dissection complicated by visceral ischemia. J Thorac Cardiovasc Surg. 2015;149(4):1081–6.e1.
4. Jonker FH, Trimarchi S, Muhs BE, et al. The role of age in complicated acute type B aortic dissection. Ann Thorac Surg. 2013;96(6):2129–34.
5. Treskes N, Persoon AM, van Zanten AR. Diagnostic accuracy of novel serological biomarkers to detect acute mesenteric ischemia: a systematic review and meta-analysis. Intern Emerg Med. 2017;12(6):1–6.
6. Fattori R, Cao P, De Rango P, et al. Interdisciplinary expert consensus document on management of type B aortic dissection. J Am Coll Cardiol. 2013;61(16):1661–78.
7. Riambau V, Böckler D, Brunkwall J, Cao P, Chiesa R, Coppi G, Czerny M, Fraedrich G, Haulon S, Jacobs MJ, Lachat ML. Editor's choice–management of descending thoracic aorta diseases. Eur J Vasc Endovasc Surg. 2017;53(1):4–52.
8. Szeto WY, McGarvey M, Pochettino A, et al. Results of a new surgical paradigm: endovascular repair for acute complicated type B aortic dissection. Ann Thorac Surg. 2008;86(1):87–93; discussion 93-4.
9. Sfyroeras GS, Rubio V, Pagan P, Diethrich EB, Rodriguez JA. Endovascular management of malperfusion in acute type B aortic dissections. J Endovasc Ther. 2011;18(1):78–86.
10. Ryan C, Vargas L, Mastracci T, et al. Progress in management of malperfusion syndrome from type B dissections. J Vasc Surg. 2013;57(5):1283–90; discussion 90.
11. Khoynezhad A, Donayre CE, Omari BO, Kopchok GE, Walot I, White RA. Midterm results of endovascular treatment of complicated acute type B aortic dissection. J Thorac Cardiovasc Surg. 2009;138(3):625–31.
12. Dong ZH, Fu WG, Wang YQ, da Guo Q, Xu X, Ji Y, et al. Retrograde type A aortic dissection after endovascular stent graft placement for treatment of type B dissection. Circulation. 2009;119:735–41.
13. Eggebrecht H, Thompson M, Rousseau H, Czerny M, Lönn L, Mehta RH, et al. Retrograde ascending aortic dissection during or after thoracic aortic stent graft placement: insight from the European registry on endovascular aortic repair complications. Circulation. 2009;120(11 Suppl):S276–81.
14. Canaud L, Ozdemir BA, Patterson BO, Holt PJ, Loftus IM, Thompson MM. Retrograde aortic dissection after thoracic endovascular aortic repair. Ann Surg. 2014;260:389–95.
15. Canaud L, Faure EM, Ozdemir BA, Alric P, Thompson M. Systematic review of outcomes of combined proximal stent-grafting with distal bare stenting for management of aortic dissection. Ann Cardiothorac Surg. 2014;3(3):223–33.
16. Oikonomou K, Kopp R, Katsargyris A, Pfister K, Verhoeven EL, Kasprzak P. Outcomes of fenestrated/branched endografting in post-dissection thoracoabdominal aortic aneurysms. Eur J Vasc Endovasc Surg. 2014;48(6):641–8.
17. Oikonomou K, Katsargyris A, Ritter W, Spinelli D, Seto Y, Verhoeven EL. Endovascular management of

chronic post-dissection aneurysms. Ann Cardiothorac Surg. 2014;3(3):307.
18. Patel HJ, Williams DM, Meerkov M, Dasika NL, Upchurch GR Jr, Deeb GM. Long-term results of percutaneous management of malperfusion in acute type B aortic dissection: implications for thoracic aortic endovascular repair. J Thorac Cardiovasc Surg. 2009;138(2):300–8.
19. Trimarchi S, Segreti S, Grassi V, et al. Open fenestration for complicated acute aortic B dissection. Ann Cardiothorac Surg. 2014;3(4):418–22.
20. Conrad M, Cambria R. Aortic dissection. In: Cronenwett J, Johnston KW, editors. Rutherford's vascular surgery. 8th ed. Philadelphia: Elsevier Saunders; 2014. p. 2179–85.
21. Lauterbach SR, Cambria RP, Brewster DC, et al. Contemporary management of aortic branch compromise resulting from acute aortic dissection. J Vasc Surg. 2001;33(6):1185–92.

30 Understanding Visceral Ischaemia in Acute Type B Dissection: State of the Art, Challenges and Future Perspectives

T. Donati, A. Patel, and M. Sallam

30.1 Visceral Malperfusion

30.1.1 Definition

Visceral malperfusion is an ill-defined entity; in the available literature, it is variably used to refer to mesenteric and renal malperfusion or to mesenteric malperfusion alone with or without end-organ ischaemia. This distinction is crucial to allow clarity of discussion and avoid misinterpretation or misuse of available data from the literature.

It is our opinion that when referring to visceral malperfusion in the context of aortic dissection, this has to refer to the clinical scenario related to malperfusion of the visceral branches of the aorta.

According to Henry Gray's textbook of anatomy [1], the visceral branches of the abdominal aorta include the coeliac axis, the superior mesenteric, the inferior mesenteric, the middle suprarenals, the renals, the internal spermatic and the ovarian arteries.

Within the limits of our knowledge, only involvement of the superior mesenteric and renal arteries (with the occasional exception of the coeliac axis) is related to relevant clinical scenarios in the clinical setting and therefore can be the object of a meaningful discussion; however other entities like MP and ischaemia of the adrenal gland might be clinically relevant and wrongly overlooked.

T. Donati (✉) · A. Patel · M. Sallam
Guy's and St Thomas' NHS Foundation Trust, London, UK
e-mail: tommaso.donati@gstt.nhs.uk

30.1.2 The Relevance of VMP in the Setting of Type A and B Dissection and Why We Cannot Ignore Type A Dissections

The incidence of visceral malperfusion differs between type A and type B reflecting somehow the different populations of patients affected by these very closely related but at the same time different conditions [2–4].

Distal extension of a type A dissection to the aorta and its branches is an independent marker of a severity [5, 6]. In-hospital mortality for patients included in the IRAD registry presenting with type A dissections complicated by mesenteric malperfusion undergoing surgical or hybrid treatment has been reported to be 41.7% [7, 8].

Although strictly speaking beyond the aim of this chapter, we believe it is also important to highlight the relevance of visceral malperfusion in setting of acute type A dissection.

There are multiple reasons for it:

– Visceral malperfusion (with particular mention to mesenteric malperfusion) in the setting

© Springer Nature Switzerland AG 2019
Y. Tshomba et al. (eds.), *Visceral Vessels and Aortic Repair*,
https://doi.org/10.1007/978-3-319-94761-7_30

of acute type A dissection is a leading cause and independent predictor factor for in-hospital mortality; distal extension of a type A dissection to the aorta and its branches is an independent marker of a severity [5, 6, 9]. In-hospital mortality for patients included in the IRAD registry presenting with type A dissections complicated by mesenteric malperfusion undergoing surgical or hybrid treatment has been reported to be as high as 41.7% [7, 8].

- Recognition of this complication is often delayed as a consequence of the predominant role given to emergency repair of the ascending aorta and the difficult assessment of signs and symptoms in the immediate postoperative period.
- There is increasing interest for a staged approach for acute type A dissection complicated by visceral malperfusion advocating treatment of the malperfusion first followed by surgical repair of the ascending aorta (hence in a certain way questioning the dogma of the neat separation between type A and type B in terms of timing and strategy of treatment) [2, 10, 11].
- Even after successful repair of the ascending aorta, type A dissection with distal progression to the descending thoracic and visceral aorta can present exactly the same challenges of a type B dissection and in the long term can result in chronic "type B" dissection.
- Given the current strategies for treatment of VMP, a better communication and a better integration between different teams (cardiothoracic, vascular and endovascular interventionist) is likely beneficial for patients for a multidisciplinary approach aiming at early detection and treatment of reversible cause of a clinically relevant VMP.

30.1.3 Mechanisms of Obstruction Reviewed

Williams and his collaborators in a paper published in 1997 have described the mechanisms involved in the obstruction of the visceral branches of the aorta for the first time. They described two main mechanisms that are still accepted today, one "dynamic" and one "static" [12].

Although further mechanisms have been proposed [13] mainly as a combination of dynamic and static components, ultimately the main—and most relevant—difference between the two mechanisms is the direct involvement or not of the ostia of the aortic branch in consideration.

A *dynamic obstruction* refers mainly to the reduction of flow to a given artery due to a haemodynamic conflict between the true and the false lumen in the aorta. Dynamic obstructions can be responsible of clinical pictures of intermittent malperfusion; however it is also important to clarify that "dynamic" does not necessarily translate with "intermittent" (Fig. 30.1).

Static obstructions on the other hand are characterised by a direct involvement of the ostia of the aortic branch with possible progression of the dissection into the branch and a possible conflict between the true and the false lumen within the aortic branch.

The involvement of a branch can result in different scenarios of which the most common are:

- Progression of the false lumen into a branch with distal re-entry and maintained perfusion of vessel through the false, or both the true and false, lumen (Fig. 30.2)

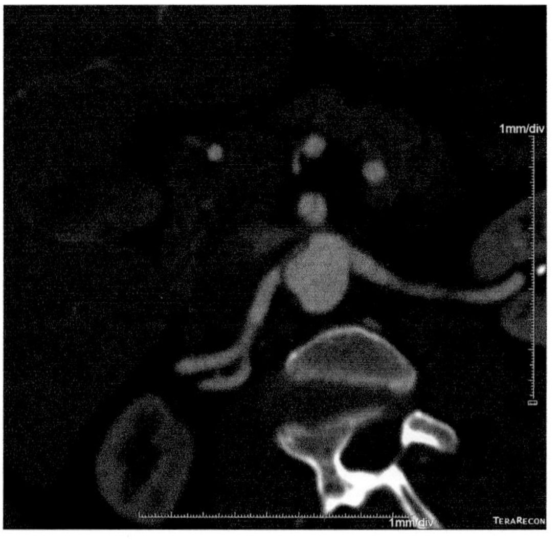

Fig. 30.1 Dynamic obstruction of the right renal artery with delayed perfusion but no obvious malperfusion

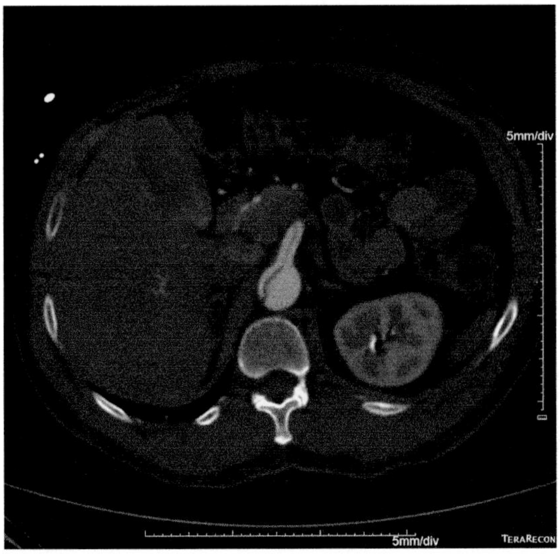

Fig. 30.2 Progression of the false lumen into the superior mesenteric artery with distal outflow and maintained perfusion of both true and false lumen

- Progression of the false lumen into a branch (eccentric or circumferential) without distal re-entry resulting in an extrinsic compression of the true lumen and various degrees of malperfusion (from flow reduction to complete obstruction of both lumina) (Fig. 30.3a–c)
- Ostial disconnection with or without flow-limiting intimal tears

The understanding of these mechanisms is crucial to identify the right strategy to resolve a possible malperfusion, hence the importance of imaging modalities and their interpretation.

30.2 The Role of Imaging

The term malperfusion—as opposed to hypoperfusion—suggests a lack of adequate blood supply; however it is commonly used both in the context of hypoperfusion with and without end-organ ischaemia. This distinction is relevant both in terms of terminology and for clinical decision-making as the end-organ ischaemia and not the malperfusion alone (usually based on radiological findings) that defines the need for intervention.

Imaging plays a critical role in suggesting a visceral malperfusion and in defining the mechanism of the malperfusion; it has however significant limitations when it comes to differentiating between hypoperfusion and end-organ ischaemia.

CT tomography, MR and ultrasound imaging all play an important role in the imaging of aortic dissection [9, 14–16].

30.2.1 Computed Tomography

In the acute setting, computed tomography remains the imaging of choice for the diagnosis and characterisation of aortic dissection.

CT angiography is widely available in the emergency setting and combines a high spatial resolution with a rapid acquisition time. Sequences in the arterial phase and venous phase can allow a reasonably good description of both the true and the false lumen and their relative perfusion. Several factors however can influence the quality of the imaging and the enhancement of both lumina and the aortic branches. Those factors include heart rate, ejection fraction, blood pressure and movement artefacts. All these factors are particularly relevant in the diagnosis of visceral malperfusion (in setting of an acute aortic dissection). The right timing of the acquisition can be difficult to predict, and this can influence significantly the enhancement of true and false lumen. In most cases CT angiography is accurate in demonstrating the involvement of the ostia of the main visceral arteries and in differentiation between different mechanisms of obstruction. Triple-phase CT has improved our ability to assess flow and thrombosis in the true and false lumen and should be considered the protocol of choice in most instances. ECG-gated protocols have proven to be useful to reduce misinterpretations due to motion artefact and more importantly to characterise intimal flap motion although its use is somehow limited by the reduced field of acquisition and their role in the diagnosis of visceral branch malperfusion still has to be demonstrated [16–18].

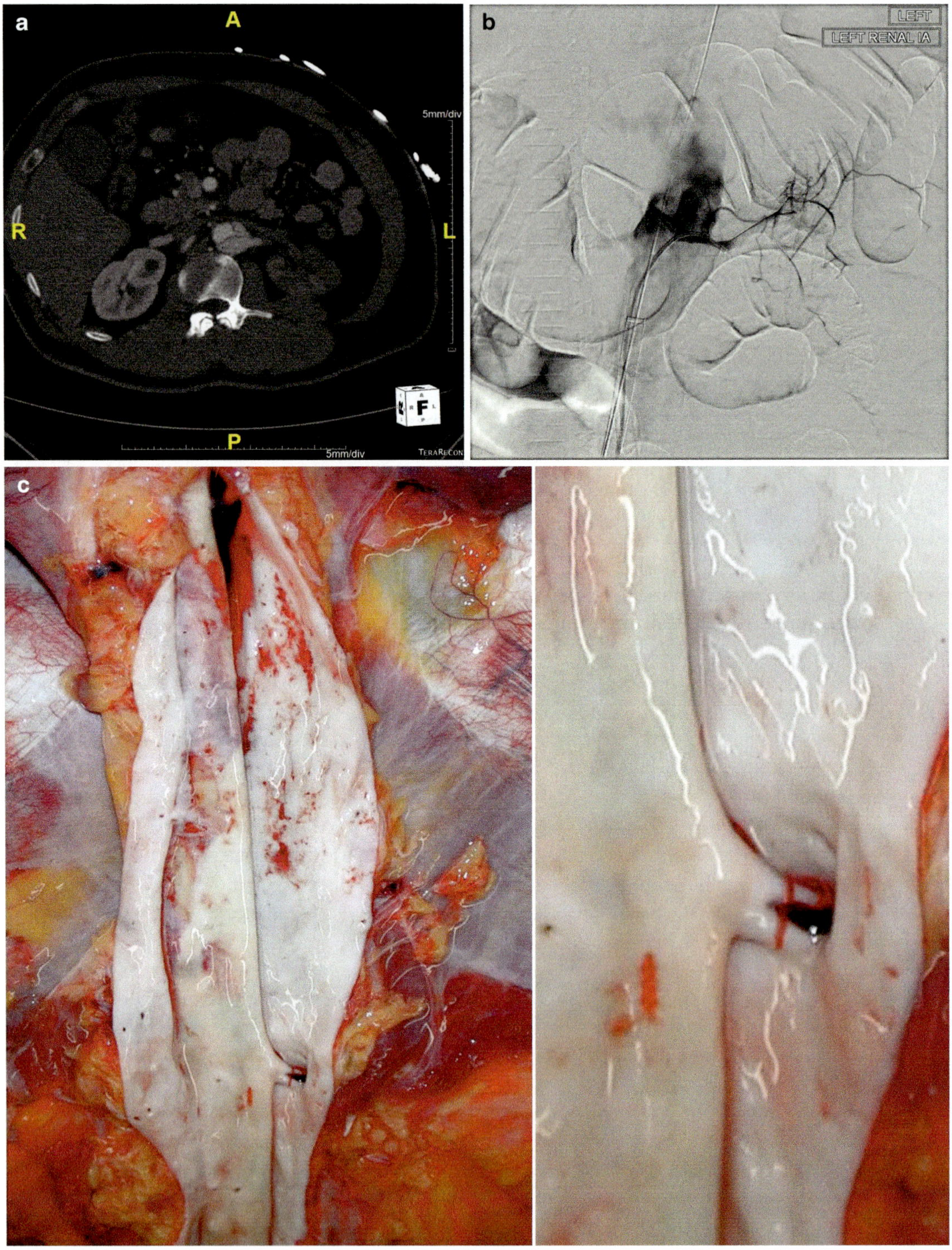

Fig. 30.3 (**a**, **b**) Progression of false lumen into the left renal artery with no distal re-entry with compression of the true lumen and organ malperfusion. (**c**) Autoptic findings of progression of the false lumen into the left renal artery (Courtesy of Chiesa/Tshomba et al., San Raffaele Hospital, Milan)

30.2.2 MR Imaging

MR has an increasingly important role, both in the acute and in the chronic phase, for its potential of providing simultaneously morphological and functional information and for the absence of ionising radiations [14]. In the acute setting the main limitations remain availability and acquisition time. The most commonly used modality is MR angiogram. First-pass MRI is commonly used to identify false lumen thrombosis. However it is important to remember that both CT angiography and first-pass MRI have been shown to overestimate the amount of false lumen thrombosis by up to sixfold when compared to more advanced although not commonly available MRI protocols [19], hence the need for a high degree of circumspection when interpreting those investigations [16]. MR is a fast-evolving technology, and it will certainly play an increasingly important role in acute aortic syndromes [20].

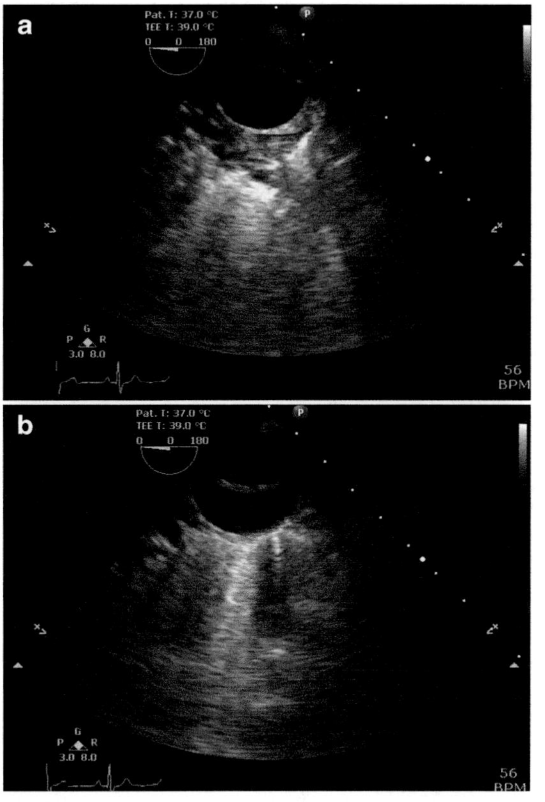

Fig. 30.4 (**a**) Dynamic compression of the true lumen during the systolic phase on TEE. (**b**) Distension of the true lumen during the diastolic phase on TEE

30.2.3 Ultrasound Modalities

Ultrasound modalities have a somehow limited but important role in the diagnosis of aortic dissections complicated by visceral malperfusion.

Colour Doppler ultrasonography can be extremely helpful to evaluate a haemodynamic compromise at the level of the renal and superior mesenteric artery [9, 21–23]. Limitations intrinsic to the technique are represented by the availability of experienced operators in an urgent setting, the morphology and the clinical and haemodynamic status of the patient. Intravascular ultrasound (IVUS) is mainly used intraoperatively to define the anatomy and the interaction between true and false lumen and to guide precise treatment both at the level of the aorta and its branches [24].

Transoesophageal ultrasound can demonstrate the haemodynamic conflict between true and false lumen helping to rule out dynamic, intermittent compressions of the true lumen at the level of the descending thoracic aorta (Fig. 30.4a, b).

30.2.4 Limitations and Perspective in Imaging of Renal Malperfusion

In case of involvement of the renal arteries, it is a common finding to observe a defect or delay of enhancement of one or—rarely—both kidneys. Given the above-mentioned limitation and the rapid acquisition, it is somehow difficult to give a functional interpretation to these findings as the organ can still be well perfused despite a poor enhancement. While renal perfusion scintigraphy might have a role in the subacute and chronic phase, interesting perspectives are suggested by preliminary studies investigating the use of CT perfusion scanning for renal malperfusion [25]. In a report from Johns Hopkins Hospital on 38 patients, renal malperfusion could be accurately predicted by end-diastolic velocity (EDV) measurements on duplex ultrasound imaging [26]. IVUS and selective pressure measurements have been used successfully to define and guide treatment for renal malperfusion; however, there is no clear description on the technique to measure pressure gradients (whether, e.g. it is measured in the aorta or in the target vessel), and specific advantages with the use of IVUS assessment as opposed to standard imaging with CTA and intraoperative angiography still have to be demonstrated [27].

30.2.5 Limitations and Perspectives in Imaging of Mesenteric Malperfusion

Radiological diagnosis of mesenteric malperfusion is still extremely difficult.

Multiphase CT (usually biphasic is recommended, but in the context of an acute dissection, a triple-phase CT should be considered the gold standard) remains the imaging of choice. CT findings have been associated with advanced and in most cases irreversible mesenteric ischaemia and include intestinal dilatation and thickness, reduction or absence of visceral enhancement, pneumatosis intestinalis and portal venous gas and free intraperitoneal air [28]. On the other hand, improvement in CT protocols and interpretation are showing promising results for the diagnosis of intermediate grades of ischaemia [29]. Of note no other imaging modalities are currently recommended by international guideline on management of acute mesenteric ischaemia [30, 31]; nevertheless there is evidence and hope that different imaging modalities, namely, MRI, will be in the future validated and will become an additional tool in the diagnosis of mesenteric ischaemia [32, 33].

30.3 Recognition and Management of Visceral Malperfusion

Distinction between hypoperfusion and malperfusion is often difficult as malperfusion does not automatically translate in end-organ ischaemia. Signs and symptoms can be difficult to interpret; however, clinical assessment of the patient remains key for the diagnosis and for decision-making particular when there is discrepancy between clinical and radiological findings.

Operative treatments whether this translates in open or endovascular interventions carry significant risks and should be justified on clinical ground.

Although surgical aortic replacement remains the gold standard in management of type A aortic dissections [9], there is increasing interest and awareness regarding the potential role of *malperfusion first* strategies that combine endovascular and open surgical techniques to improve outcomes in patient presenting with visceral malperfusion and stable type A dissections [2].

Endovascular stent grafting is widely recognised as the treatment of choice in acute complicated type B dissections, and endovascular techniques should be favoured as the first choice in the management of visceral malperfusion in most cases [34–37]. Open surgical repair for visceral malperfusion in aortic dissection requires experience and can be considered in selected patients and high-volume centres for this kind of surgery [37].

Understanding the mechanism of obstruction plays an important role for the choice of the most appropriate from of intervention. Dynamic obstruction will almost invariably need a central aortic treatment aiming at covering the proximal entry tear and re-equilibrate the perfusion pressure between true and false lumen, while static obstructions of the visceral branches might benefit of more focused treatment that can include selective stenting and fenestration techniques, and combined mechanisms of dynamic and static obstructions conversely need a combined approach.

There are however not large series or high-quality literature reporting combined approaches and strategies detailing the suspected mechanisms of malperfusion; aortic treatment has been adopted as the first-line strategy in a large centre, while on the other hand, there are relatively small series reporting fenestration techniques as the main treatment for visceral malperfusion [27, 34, 38, 39].

It is of extreme interest to notice that multiple reports failed to show an advantage in survival for patients who underwent branch vessel stenting or any intervention for malperfusion with particular regard to renal malperfusion raising the question whether renal malperfusion alone (particularly when it comes to a single kidney malperfusion) should be an indication at all for any kind of treatment [26, 38].

30.3.1 A Note on Blood Pressure Management in Acute Aortic Dissections Complicated by Visceral Malperfusion: Is There a Role for Permissive Hypertension in the Presence of Malperfusion?

Aggressive blood pressure management has an established role in the treatment of acute aortic dissections for prevention of progression of the dissection and rupture of the aorta [39, 40].

However there is some evidence that higher blood perfusion pressure might be beneficial in patients with visceral malperfusion [38]. High mean arterial pressures (MAP) are also often adopted as a standard practice in the management of acute dissections complicated pre- or postoperatively by spinal cord ischaemia. Despite convincing data supporting this practice [41], it is interesting to highlight that in traumatic spinal cord injuries, no advantages have been demonstrated with arbitrarily set high MAP goals [42], and overall there is limited evidence to support it.

Overall there is certainly scope to further investigate the role of permissive hypertension in the acute setting of aortic dissections complicated by malperfusion.

30.4 Challenges of Renal Malperfusion

A degree of renal failure is very common in the setting of acute aortic dissections. The aetiology of possible acute kidney injury in this context is most of the times the results of a multifactorial insult to the kidney [9]. Regardless of concomitant findings of delayed perfusion of the kidney with evidence of dynamic or static compression (usually this inflects in a picture of true lumen compression causing haemodynamic compression and flow reduction associated or less to extension of the dissection into the lumen of the artery), a state of shock, possible dehydration, aggressive intravenous blood pressure control and multiple imaging with contrast can all contribute to an acute kidney injury even in an otherwise well-perused organ. In most cases a reduced enhancement on CT imaging of a kidney will be interpreted as a sign of malperfusion of the organ. However the distinction between delayed perfusion, malperfusion and end-organ ischaemia is not only an academic exercise as it affects the decision-making and possibly the prognosis of the patient. CT findings however are known to be unreliable as they depend on the haemodynamic in and between the two lumina, and even with multiple-phase CT or gated imaging, they should be interpreted with caution [16, 19]. More subtle interpretation of the CT (as kidney size or presence of contrast in a delayed phase) can still give testimony of the perfusion of the kidney despite poor enhancement.

When it comes to indications to treatment, renal failure is a well-known predictor of poor prognosis in cardiovascular interventions as well as in acute aortic dissections [9]. This usually leads to the somehow logical temptation of aggressively correcting any reversible cause of it. Different considerations though seem to be necessary when it comes to chronic kidney disease (CKD) and acute kidney injuries in the setting of aortic dissection with or without underlying CKD.

Chronic kidney disease can be a marker of a more advanced form of atheromasic disease and/or underlying comorbidities (diabetes) as this can often explain its importance as a prognostic factor. Similarly in the setting of acute aortic dissection, a renal malperfusion could be the marker of a more severe form of dissection, hence its relationship with poorer outcomes.

Overall aggressive revascularisation strategies based on the presence of kidney malperfusion and a biochemical picture of renal failure could be a complete inappropriate approach, and it should be carefully weighted with the complexity of the required/proposed treatment.

On the other hand, a possible rationale for treatment even in the case of a single renal malperfusion could be a refractory hypertension [as mentioned before though that there is some evidence that hypertension might be linked to better outcome in the presence of a malperfusion syndrome [38]].

30.5 Challenges of Mesenteric Malperfusion

Mesenteric malperfusion is the more insidious and serious form of malperfusion, and overall it is associated with a poor prognosis in the setting of acute aortic dissection [4, 7].

As discussed previously the instrumental diagnosis is often difficult, and often only irreversible ischaemia is clearly demonstrated on imaging.

On the other hand, available biomarkers have failed to demonstrate high sensitivity and specificity. As stated in the guidelines of the World Society of Emergency Surgery, "There are no laboratory studies that are sufficiently accurate to identify the presence or absence of ischemic or necrotic bowel, although elevated L-lactate, and D-dimer may assist," and this statement is supported by most of the available literature [30, 43, 44]. According to the European Society of Trauma and Emergency Surgery (ESTES), "Normal serum lactate level does not exclude acute mesenteric ischemia (AMI) and should not be used for diagnosis" [31].

Once mesenteric ischaemia has been demonstrated on clinical ground and with ominous signs on CT imaging, it will require in most of the cases immediate laparotomy and bowel resection more than any form of revascularisation.

As a result clinical diagnosis together with a suspicion of malperfusion on CT imaging should guide clinical practice. This is of course made even more difficult by confusing factor as could be sedation, analgesia and concomitant malperfusion of different aortic branches. Feasibility and safety of laparoscopy for early detection of bowel ischaemia has been demonstrated [45]; however there is insufficient evidence to support the routine use of laparoscopy in AMI [31].

Overall the early diagnosis of mesenteric malperfusion remains an unresolved challenge. In the next paragraph, we will expand further on emerging biomarkers that might radically change our practice in the future.

30.6 Future Perspectives: Biomarkers and Early Diagnosis of Visceral Malperfusion

Early recognition and diagnosis remain the greatest challenge and play a crucial role in improving our understanding and ultimately our management of acute aortic dissection complicated by visceral malperfusion.

The use of biomarkers, in combination with advanced imaging techniques and conventional biochemistry analysis, may provide a better way of assessing ongoing VMP following aortic dissection. A good biomarker should be easy to measure, have an earlier detectability than conventional assays (such as creatinine/lactate), be organ-specific identity type and preferably be able to predict the severity of malperfusion as well as allow for monitoring of any pharmacological/surgical responses to therapy. Theoretically, these biomarkers can be measured at the gene, RNA and protein (including cell surface, intracellular and circulating) level. It is generally the circulating proteins that are easier to measure, although techniques such a flow cytometry and polymerase chain reaction are now utilised relatively routinely in the clinic.

During the period of organ ischaemia, the function of the endothelial cell barrier is impaired [46], resulting in an increase in vascular permeability and leakage [47]. During this period, a range of changes occurs in the transcriptional control of gene expression. For example, oxygen-sensing prolyl hydroxylase (PHD) enzymes, which require oxygen as a cofactor, are inhibited which leads to the activation of hypoxia and inflammatory signalling cascades that control the stability of the transcription factors hypoxia-inducible factor (HIF) and nuclear factor-κB (NF-κB), respectively [48]. Reactive oxygen species (ROS) increased ischaemia and reperfusion [49] and are implicated in the tissue damage that occurs during this period by altering cellular ribonucleic acids (RNAs), lipids and proteins. Measurement of the redox state of patients may provide a way of assessing for VMR as well as predicting clinical outcome [50].

Tissue ischaemia also results in acute changes in cellular infiltrate within the circulation and organ itself. Studies have shown that T cell lymphocytes accumulate during organ ischaemia and reperfusion [51] and measurement of changes in T cell subsets and phenotype using flow cytometry may provide evidence of ongoing organ ischaemia. For example, further, IL-17 is produced by γδ T cells during ischaemia and reperfusion injury [52]. This sterile inflammation during ischaemia is also characterised by the recruitment of specific subsets of monocytes from the bone marrow and splenic reservoir to participate in healing [53, 54]. One disadvantage of these assays is that changes in cellular phenotype are not usually organ specific and further work is needed to determine specific changes in mononuclear cell populations during, for example, bowel, liver and renal ischaemia.

Despite its poor sensitivity and specificity, serum creatinine is still utilised as the indicator for renal injury/ischaemia. Cystatin C may be a more reliable biomarker of renal malperfusion, and more novel markers such as urinary *N*-acetyl-β-D-glucosaminidase (NAG), kidney injury molecule-1 (KIM-1) and neutrophil gelatinase-associated lipocalin (NGAL) have recently been shown to be sensitive, early markers of tubular damage in renal ischaemia [55]. There is increasing interest in the use of microRNAs (miRNAs), noncoding RNAs that post-transcriptionally regulate gene expression, for detecting organ-specific changes. These biomarkers are stable, have low interindividual variability and can be measured in samples of serum and plasma. For example, miR-30a, miR-30e and miR-188 are upregulated between two- and threefold [56] during kidney injury. Further research is needed into evaluating changes that occur in circulating miRNAs during aortic dissection and then correlating these with organ ischaemia.

The emerging use of "omics" in the discovery of biomarkers with the aid of mass spectrometry and bioinformatics has also recently provided new avenues in the monitoring of visceral malperfusion. Proteomic studies investigate the pool of full-length, truncated and post-transductionally modified proteins and peptides, whereas metabolomics explores the metabolic process of peptides, saccharides and lipids. Studies have utilised the omics approach for the assessment of biomarkers of gut malperfusion. The mature enterocyte expresses intestinal FABP (I-FABP), and urinary I-FABP has been shown to be a biomarker with high specificity and sensitivity for the diagnosis of acute intestinal ischaemia [57, 58]. I-FABP is considered to be one of the most promising biomarkers for intestinal ischaemia along with D-dimer and a-GST [59]. The advantage of I-FABP above a-GST and D-dimer is, of course, its tissue specificity [60].

During liver ischaemia, activated Kupffer cells, liver tissue and distant organs secrete TNF-α [61] which can be measured in serum. Matrix metalloproteinases (MMPs), such as MMP-9, are detected in the serum of patients following liver ischaemia/reperfusion, and a range of MMPs, including MMP-2, MMP-3, MMP-8, MMP-10, MMP-12 and MMP-13, are upregulated during hepatic ischaemia [62]. However, neither TNF-α nor MMPs are liver specific as they can be increased during systemic inflammation, and further work is needed in biomarkers that can detect VMP due to reduced flow in the coeliac axis.

References

1. Gray H. Anatomy of the human body. 23rd ed. Philadelphia: Lea & Febiger; 1936.
2. Kamman AV, Yang B, Kim KM, Williams DM, Michael Deeb G, Patel HJ. Visceral malperfusion in aortic dissection: the Michigan experience. Semin Thorac Cardiovasc Surg. 2017;29(2):173–8.

3. Tanaka A, Estrera AL. Mesenteric malperfusion: the insidious, dreadful enemy. Semin Thorac Cardiovasc Surg. 2017;29(2):179–80.
4. Jonker FH, Patel HJ, Upchurch GR, Williams DM, Montgomery DG, Gleason TG, et al. Acute type B aortic dissection complicated by visceral ischemia. J Thorac Cardiovasc Surg. 2015;149(4):1081–6.e1.
5. Rampoldi V, Trimarchi S, Eagle KA, Nienaber CA, Oh JK, Bossone E, et al. Simple risk models to predict surgical mortality in acute type A aortic dissection: the International Registry of Acute Aortic Dissection score. Ann Thorac Surg. 2007;83(1):55–61.
6. Geirsson A, Szeto WY, Pochettino A, McGarvey ML, Keane MG, Woo YJ, et al. Significance of malperfusion syndromes prior to contemporary surgical repair for acute type A dissection: outcomes and need for additional revascularizations. Eur J Cardiothorac Surg. 2007;32(2):255–62.
7. Berretta P, Patel HJ, Gleason TG, Sundt TM, Myrmel T, Desai N, et al. IRAD experience on surgical type A acute dissection patients: results and predictors of mortality. Ann Cardiothorac Surg. 2016;5(4):346–51.
8. Di Eusanio M, Trimarchi S, Patel HJ, Hutchison S, Suzuki T, Peterson MD, et al. Clinical presentation, management, and short-term outcome of patients with type A acute dissection complicated by mesenteric malperfusion: observations from the International Registry of Acute Aortic Dissection. J Thorac Cardiovasc Surg. 2013;145(2):385–90.e1.
9. Crawford TC, Beaulieu RJ, Ehlert BA, Ratchford EV, Black JH 3rd. Malperfusion syndromes in aortic dissections. Vasc Med. 2016;21(3):264–73.
10. Goldberg JB, Lansman SL, Kai M, Tang GHL, Malekan R, Spielvogel D. Malperfusion in type A dissection: consider reperfusion first. Semin Thorac Cardiovasc Surg. 2017;29(2):181–5.
11. Tanaka K, Chikazawa G, Sakaguchi T, Totsugawa T, Tamura K, Yoshitaka H. Hybrid treatment for type A acute aortic dissection with multiorgan malperfusion. Ann Thorac Surg. 2014;98(3):1118–20.
12. Williams DM, Lee DY, Hamilton BH, Marx MV, Narasimham DL, Kazanjian SN, et al. The dissected aorta: part III. Anatomy and radiologic diagnosis of branch-vessel compromise. Radiology. 1997;203(1):37–44.
13. Midulla M, Fattori R, Beregi JP, Dake M, Rousseau H. Aortic dissection and malperfusion syndrome: a when, what and how-to guide. Radiol Med. 2013;118(1):74–88.
14. Moore AG, Eagle KA, Bruckman D, Moon BS, Malouf JF, Fattori R, et al. Choice of computed tomography, transesophageal echocardiography, magnetic resonance imaging, and aortography in acute aortic dissection: International Registry of Acute Aortic Dissection (IRAD). Am J Cardiol. 2002;89(10):1235–8.
15. Baliga RR, Nienaber CA, Bossone E, Oh JK, Isselbacher EM, Sechtem U, et al. The role of imaging in aortic dissection and related syndromes. JACC Cardiovasc Imaging. 2014;7(4):406–24.
16. Donati T, Wilson J, Kolbel T, Clough RE. Modern diagnostics for type B aortic dissection. Gefässchirurgie. 2015;20(6):420–7.
17. Yang S, Li X, Chao B, Wu L, Cheng Z, Duan Y, et al. Abdominal aortic intimal flap motion characterization in acute aortic dissection: assessed with retrospective ECG-gated thoracoabdominal aorta dual-source CT angiography. PLoS One. 2014;9(2):e87664.
18. Ganten MK, Weber TF, von Tengg-Kobligk H, Bockler D, Stiller W, Geisbusch P, et al. Motion characterization of aortic wall and intimal flap by ECG-gated CT in patients with chronic B-dissection. Eur J Radiol. 2009;72(1):146–53.
19. Clough RE, Hussain T, Uribe S, Greil GF, Razavi R, Taylor PR, et al. A new method for quantification of false lumen thrombosis in aortic dissection using magnetic resonance imaging and a blood pool contrast agent. J Vasc Surg. 2011;54(5):1251–8.
20. Wang GX, Hedgire SS, Le TQ, Sonis JD, Yun BJ, Lev MH, et al. MR angiography can guide ED management of suspected acute aortic dissection. Am J Emerg Med. 2017;35(4):527–30.
21. Catalini R, Alborino S, Giovagnoli A, Zingaretti O. Color Duplex evaluation of the mesenteric artery (). J Ultrasound. 2010;13(3):118–22.
22. Perko MJ. Duplex ultrasound for assessment of superior mesenteric artery blood flow. Eur J Vasc Endovasc Surg. 2001;21(2):106–17.
23. AbuRahma AF, Stone PA, Srivastava M, Dean LS, Keiffer T, Hass SM, et al. Mesenteric/celiac duplex ultrasound interpretation criteria revisited. J Vasc Surg. 2012;55(2):428–36.e6; discussion 35-6.
24. Koschyk DH, Meinertz T, Hofmann T, Kodolitsch YV, Dieckmann C, Wolf W, et al. Value of intravascular ultrasound for endovascular stent-graft placement in aortic dissection and aneurysm. J Card Surg. 2003;18(5):471–7.
25. Liu D, Liu J, Wen Z, Li Y, Sun Z, Xu Q, et al. 320-row CT renal perfusion imaging in patients with aortic dissection: a preliminary study. PLoS One. 2017;12(2):e0171235.
26. Osgood MJ, Grimm J, Abularrage CJ, Lum YW, Call D, Black JH III. VESS24. Duplex ultrasound assessment and outcomes of renal malperfusion syndromes after acute aortic dissection. J Vasc Surg. 2017;65(6):29S.
27. Barnes DM, Williams DM, Dasika NL, Patel HJ, Weder AB, Stanley JC, et al. A single-center experience treating renal malperfusion after aortic dissection with central aortic fenestration and renal artery stenting. J Vasc Surg. 2008;47(5):903–10; discussion 10-1.
28. Kirkpatrick ID, Kroeker MA, Greenberg HM. Biphasic CT with mesenteric CT angiography in the evaluation of acute mesenteric ischemia: initial experience. Radiology. 2003;229(1):91–8.
29. Moschetta M, Telegrafo M, Rella L, Stabile Ianora AA, Angelelli G. Multi-detector CT features of acute intestinal ischemia and their prognostic correlations. World J Radiol. 2014;6(5):130–8.

30. Bala M, Kashuk J, Moore EE, Kluger Y, Biffl W, Gomes CA, et al. Acute mesenteric ischemia: guidelines of the World Society of Emergency Surgery. World J Emerg Surg. 2017;12:38.
31. Tilsed JVT, Casamassima A, Kurihara H, Mariani D, Martinez I, Pereira J, et al. ESTES guidelines: acute mesenteric ischaemia. Eur J Trauma Emerg Surg. 2016;42:253–70.
32. Mazzei MA, Guerrini S, Cioffi Squitieri N, Imbriaco G, Chieca R, Civitelli S, et al. Magnetic resonance imaging: is there a role in clinical management for acute ischemic colitis? World J Gastroenterol. 2013;19(8):1256–63.
33. Saba L, Berritto D, Iacobellis F, Scaglione M, Castaldo S, Cozzolino S, et al. Acute arterial mesenteric ischemia and reperfusion: macroscopic and MRI findings, preliminary report. World J Gastroenterol. 2013;19(40):6825–33.
34. Lauterbach SR, Cambria RP, Brewster DC, Gertler JP, Lamuraglia GM, Isselbacher EM, et al. Contemporary management of aortic branch compromise resulting from acute aortic dissection. J Vasc Surg. 2001;33(6):1185–92.
35. White RA, Miller DC, Criado FJ, Dake MD, Diethrich EB, Greenberg RK, et al. Report on the results of thoracic endovascular aortic repair for acute, complicated, type B aortic dissection at 30 days and 1 year from a multidisciplinary subcommittee of the Society for Vascular Surgery Outcomes Committee. J Vasc Surg. 2011;53(4):1082–90.
36. Nienaber CA, Fattori R, Lund G, Dieckmann C, Wolf W, von Kodolitsch Y, et al. Nonsurgical reconstruction of thoracic aortic dissection by stent-graft placement. N Engl J Med. 1999;340(20):1539–45.
37. Szeberin Z, Dosa E, Fehervari M, Csobay-Novak C, Pinter N, Entz L. Early and long-term outcome after open surgical suprarenal aortic fenestration in patients with complicated acute type B aortic dissection. Eur J Vasc Endovasc Surg. 2015;50(1):44–50.
38. Ryan C, Vargas L, Mastracci T, Srivastava S, Eagleton M, Kelso R, et al. Progress in management of malperfusion syndrome from type B dissections. J Vasc Surg. 2013;57(5):1283–90; discussion 90.
39. Mokashi SA, Svensson LG. Guidelines for the management of thoracic aortic disease in 2017. Gen Thorac Cardiovasc Surg. 2017.
40. Writing C, Riambau V, Bockler D, Brunkwall J, Cao P, Chiesa R, et al. Editor's choice—Management of descending thoracic aorta diseases: clinical practice guidelines of the European Society for Vascular Surgery (ESVS). Eur J Vasc Endovasc Surg. 2017;53(1):4–52.
41. Kise Y, Kuniyoshi Y, Inafuku H, Nagano T, Hirayasu T, Yamashiro S. Directly measuring spinal cord blood flow and spinal cord perfusion pressure via the collateral network: correlations with changes in systemic blood pressure. J Thorac Cardiovasc Surg. 2015;149(1):360–6.
42. Martin ND, Kepler C, Zubair M, Sayadipour A, Cohen M, Weinstein M. Increased mean arterial pressure goals after spinal cord injury and functional outcome. J Emerg Trauma Shock. 2015;8(2):94–8.
43. Acosta S, Nilsson T. Current status on plasma biomarkers for acute mesenteric ischemia. J Thromb Thrombolysis. 2012;33(4):355–61.
44. Ambe PC, Kang K, Papadakis M, Zirngibl H. Can the preoperative serum lactate level predict the extent of bowel ischemia in patients presenting to the emergency department with acute mesenteric ischemia? Biomed Res Int. 2017;2017:8038796.
45. Tshomba Y, Coppi G, Marone EM, Bertoglio L, Kahlberg A, Carlucci M, et al. Diagnostic laparoscopy for early detection of acute mesenteric ischaemia in patients with aortic dissection. Eur J Vasc Endovasc Surg. 2012;43(6):690–7.
46. Ogawa S, Gerlach H, Esposito C, Pasagian-Macaulay A, Brett J, Stern D. Hypoxia modulates the barrier and coagulant function of cultured bovine endothelium. Increased monolayer permeability and induction of procoagulant properties. J Clin Invest. 1990;85(4):1090–8.
47. Ogawa S, Koga S, Kuwabara K, Brett J, Morrow B, Morris SA, et al. Hypoxia-induced increased permeability of endothelial monolayers occurs through lowering of cellular cAMP levels. Am J Phys. 1992;262(3 Pt 1):C546–54.
48. Eltzschig HK, Carmeliet P. Hypoxia and inflammation. N Engl J Med. 2011;364(7):656–65.
49. Iadecola C, Anrather J. The immunology of stroke: from mechanisms to translation. Nat Med. 2011;17(7):796–808.
50. Paspalj D, Nikic P, Savic M, Djuric D, Simanic I, Zivkovic V, et al. Redox status in acute ischemic stroke: correlation with clinical outcome. Mol Cell Biochem. 2015;406(1-2):75–81.
51. Schroeter M, Jander S, Witte OW, Stoll G. Local immune responses in the rat cerebral cortex after middle cerebral artery occlusion. J Neuroimmunol. 1994;55(2):195–203.
52. Shichita T, Sugiyama Y, Ooboshi H, Sugimori H, Nakagawa R, Takada I, et al. Pivotal role of cerebral interleukin-17-producing gammadeltaT cells in the delayed phase of ischemic brain injury. Nat Med. 2009;15(8):946–50.
53. Swirski FK, Nahrendorf M, Etzrodt M, Wildgruber M, Cortez-Retamozo V, Panizzi P, et al. Identification of splenic reservoir monocytes and their deployment to inflammatory sites. Science. 2009;325(5940):612–6.
54. Patel AS, Smith A, Nucera S, Biziato D, Saha P, Attia RQ, et al. TIE2-expressing monocytes/macrophages regulate revascularization of the ischemic limb. EMBO Mol Med. 2013;5(6):858–69.
55. Andreucci M, Faga T, Pisani A, Perticone M, Michael A. The ischemic/nephrotoxic acute kidney injury and the use of renal biomarkers in clinical practice. Eur J Intern Med. 2017;39:1–8.
56. Sun SQ, Zhang T, Ding D, Zhang WF, Wang XL, Sun Z, et al. Circulating microRNA-188, -30a, and -30e as early biomarkers for contrast-induced acute kidney injury. J Am Heart Assoc. 2016;5(8):e004138.

57. Salim SY, Young PY, Churchill TA, Khadaroo RG. Urine intestinal fatty acid-binding protein predicts acute mesenteric ischemia in patients. J Surg Res. 2017;209:258–65.
58. Sun DL, Cen YY, Li SM, Li WM, Lu QP, Xu PY. Accuracy of the serum intestinal fatty-acid-binding protein for diagnosis of acute intestinal ischemia: a meta-analysis. Sci Rep. 2016;6:34371.
59. Derikx JP, Schellekens DH, Acosta S. Serological markers for human intestinal ischemia: a systematic review. Best Pract Res Clin Gastroenterol. 2017;31(1):69–74.
60. Pelsers MM, Namiot Z, Kisielewski W, Namiot A, Januszkiewicz M, Hermens WT, et al. Intestinal-type and liver-type fatty acid-binding protein in the intestine. Tissue distribution and clinical utility. Clin Biochem. 2003;36(7):529–35.
61. Peralta C, Fernandez L, Panes J, Prats N, Sans M, Pique JM, et al. Preconditioning protects against systemic disorders associated with hepatic ischemia-reperfusion through blockade of tumor necrosis factor-induced P-selectin up-regulation in the rat. Hepatology. 2001;33(1):100–13.
62. Hamada T, Duarte S, Tsuchihashi S, Busuttil RW, Coito AJ. Inducible nitric oxide synthase deficiency impairs matrix metalloproteinase-9 activity and disrupts leukocyte migration in hepatic ischemia/reperfusion injury. Am J Pathol. 2009;174(6):2265–77.

Part IV

Visceral Vessels Management in Oncologic, Infectious and Inflammatory Diseases

31 Vascular Reconstruction in Oncologic Patients with Aortic and Visceral Artery Involvement

Domenico Palombo and Simone Mambrini

31.1 Introduction

Vascular surgeons play an important role in surgical oncology due to their familiarity with the preparation of vessels; their routine use of reconstructive techniques, be they vascular replacement or arterial and venous repair; their knowledge of surgical anatomy related to their experience with surgical access to the neck, chest, abdomen and limbs; and the knowledge they have of anaesthesiological and extracorporeal methods of circulation support.

While respecting oncology guidelines, it is conceivable that mixed surgical teams made up of vascular surgeons and general or thoracic surgeons could deal with locally advanced tumour lesions that would otherwise not be eligible for surgical treatment. Vascular surgery could, therefore, improve the outcomes of surgical oncology by increasing the radicality and safety of surgical procedures and in selected cases by broadening the range of surgical indications.

Clearly, both the patient's survival profile with regard to the neoplasm and the rationalization of resources must be respected. Therefore, once the oncology disease management team (DMT) has discussed and accepted the indications for surgery, high-volume surgical oncology centres could identify the surgically excisable tumours, and multispecialist teams, including vascular surgeons, would perform the surgery.

The role of the DMT in oncology is of paramount importance. It represents an opportunity for the oncologist and the surgeon to compare and discuss their specific surgical and oncological knowledge and experience with regard to a given case: the former must indicate what the most appropriate step is, while the latter must state whether surgery is indicated, i.e. whether surgery is feasible for the patient. In other words, the role of the oncology DMT consists in evaluating the best therapeutic strategy for the patient with respect to the tumour, its features and its developmental stage. The team must identify which patients should be sent directly to surgery, which should undergo alternative treatments (adjuvant or neoadjuvant radio-chemotherapy) prior to carrying out a safer surgical approach and which patients are still inoperable. This can be done thanks to our ever-increasing knowledge of oncology, as defined in terms of prognosis related to localization of the primary tumour lesion, its size and the presence and type of metastasis. It is also possible, thanks to the new perspectives provided by pharmacological and physical therapies (i.e. chemotherapy with new-generation drugs, radiation therapy with more powerful instruments), to obtain curative or palliative value. In particular, invasion of the vascular, arterial and/or

D. Palombo (✉) · S. Mambrini
Vascular and Endovascular Surgery Unit, University Hospital Policlinic San Martino of Genoa, University of Genoa, Genoa, Italy
e-mail: domenico.palombo@unige.it

© Springer Nature Switzerland AG 2019
Y. Tshomba et al. (eds.), *Visceral Vessels and Aortic Repair*,
https://doi.org/10.1007/978-3-319-94761-7_31

venous structures by the neoplasm is often considered a condition that excludes surgery. In fact, even tumours that are typically considered inoperable, such as pancreatic carcinoma with invasion of the mesenteric arterial axis or infiltrating lung neoplasms, can be eradicated by expert hands by combining the excision of the tumour mass, the necessary manoeuvres of cleavage from the vessels or resection and vascular reconstruction, often leading to surprisingly good results. Switching the various teams intraoperatively depends on the type of cancer being treated, the technical skills of the various surgeons and the teamwork that is created between them. Since the frequency of this type of surgery is rather limited (even in high-volume centres), to improve the degree of knowledge and mutual trust between the teams, as well as the technical skills and quality of work, it is important for a small number of vascular surgeon to be designated for this type of surgery.

For example, Fig. 31.1 shows the imaging of a typical case where a collegial discussion among the various specialists is needed to define the most appropriate therapeutic approach.

Although it is difficult to talk about rules in surgery, the experience gained in the field of surgical oncology over the years (averaging 12 interventions/year for locally advanced tumours involving the neck, chest, abdomen and limbs) has allowed us to reflect on what should or should not be done in this context.

Very few cases of arterial infiltration by neoplasms without coexistent venous involvement have been seen. Therefore, we must also consider the venous aspects of vascular treatment of locally advanced tumours. Moreover, extensive aortic infiltration continues to represent a contraindication to surgical oncology in most cases.

Our experience has led us to elaborate a number of general and specific standards or recommendations. Here we report the salient data of our experience.

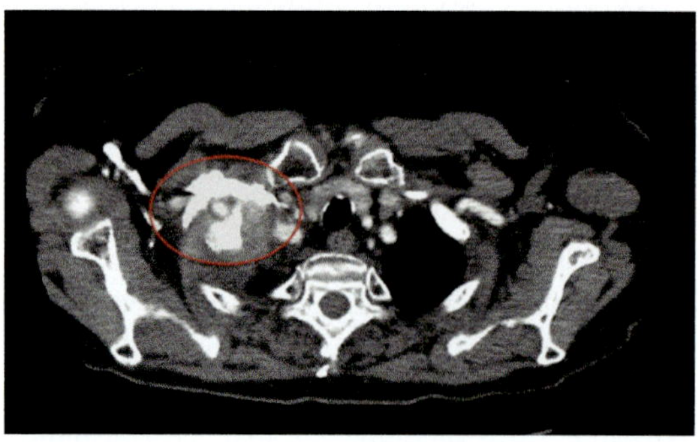

Fig. 31.1 A Pancoast tumour involving the right pulmonary apex and nearby vascular and neural structures

31.2 General Standards

It is important to plan the operative strategy and to share the surgical approach accurately, especially with regard to the need for vascular control upstream and downstream of the tumour mass. For example, Fig. 31.1 shows an angio-CT picture of a massive Pancoast tumour. It is evident that thoracotomy would not provide adequate vascular control given the presence of the first rib and clavicle and the apical site of the lesion. We prefer to approach similar cases using cervical-ministerno-thoracotomy and disconnecting the clavicle from the sternal manubrium in order to obtain adequate arterial and venous vascular control upstream and downstream of the lesion (brachiocephalic trunk, subclavian artery and its collaterals for the arterial part and the innominate, internal jugular and subclavian veins for the venous slope). Figure 31.2 shows the surgical preparation of a tumour mass infiltrating the superior vena cava which could force surgeons to broaden the surgical preparation given that such manoeuvers are time-consuming. This should be done prior to dealing with the tumour mass and certainly not only when intraoperative emergency situations occur, such as the rupture of a large vessel which makes every manoeuver more complex. In other words, whenever possible, calling the vascular surgeon must be avoided in emergency settings, such as during surgery following unexpected intraoperative findings which differ from preoperative imaging or, worse, that were underestimated a priori. For example, we were forced to perform surgery on the descending thoracic aorta through a right thoracotomy access. Thus, it is important to evaluate the option of a

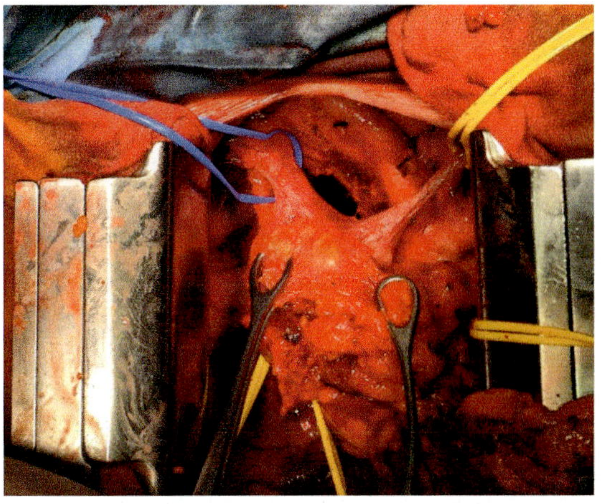

Fig. 31.2 Surgical preparation of a tumour mass infiltrating the superior vena cava; you can see that the innominate-caval system has been prepared above and below the tumour mass; two yellow silastic bands located below the mass surround the azygos vein (on the left) and the atrial outlet of the superior vena cava (on the right). In the background are the aortic arch and the supra-aortic vessels that have been cluttered by the tumour mass

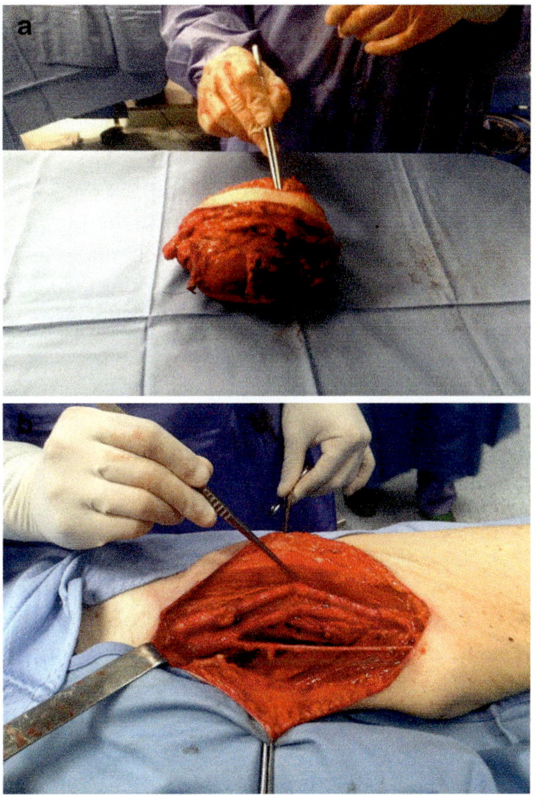

Fig. 31.3 Sarcoma of the thigh in which the tumour mass was removed with complete vascular arterial and venous preservation. (**a**) Tumour mass. (**b**) Intraoperative feature after sarcoma removal

vascular approach through other routes than the ones that are traditionally employed to treat the tumour lesion.

With regard to the type and site of the involved vessel, the possibility of saving the vessel, or the most reasonable reconstructive solutions, must be evaluated in advance, taking into account the high degree of invasiveness of cancer surgery in these cases. Figure 31.3 shows a case of sarcoma of the thigh in which the tumour mass is excised with complete vascular preservation.

It is imperative to preserve the integrity of the tumour mass in order to avoid coarse dissemination of neoplastic cells in the operative field which could be the cause of a local recurrence or distant metastases. This is the concept of "no-touch dissection".

Preserving the main vascular axis is a definite advantage in terms of both immediate and future outcome. The decision regarding the option of preservation or resection depends on the degree of adhesion of the tumour to the vessel and the presence of clear vascular infiltration. For example, Fig. 31.4 is a case of clear infiltration of the innominate-caval confluence and of the superior vena cava by a mediastinal tumour.

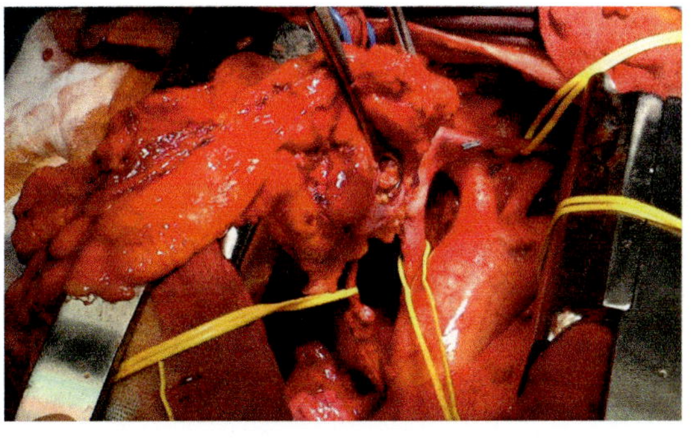

Fig. 31.4 Case of a clear infiltration of the innominate-caval confluence and of the superior vena cava by a mediastinal tumour. It should be noted that even the vagus and phrenic nerves are embedded in the cancerous mass

Once vascular control has been achieved upstream and downstream of the tumour, careful preparation of the vessels is required along their adventitial or sub-adventitial layer. The manoeuver is carried out in both directions, from the centre towards the distal end and from the distal end towards the centre along the vascular axis with respect to the greatest adhesion portion between the vessels and the tumour. This must be done taking into account the possible presence of structures (e.g. the thoracic duct, the phrenic nerve, the vagus nerve in Pancoast lesions) which are increasingly incorporated in the tumour mass and thus require arterial and venous interruption.

When the tumour does not infiltrate the vessel, as is often observed in the presence of sarcomas, various branches of the main vessel enter into the cancerous mass. These branches should be interrupted to allow removal of the tumour without injuring the main vessel. It is preferable to interrupt the vascular branches by affixing sutures on the main vascular trunk (polypropylene 5/0 or 6/0, depending on their size) and clipping the branches on the side which penetrates the tumour mass.

Once the cleavage of the neoplastic lesion along the vessel makes the media easily recognizable in the arteries by the change in colour and consistency of the vessel, there are two options, (a) dissection and (b) "en bloc" resection. In the former case, the vascular wall must be reinforced by the use of banding techniques in order to prevent secondary fractures or pseudoaneurysm. In the latter case, reconstruction by termino-terminal grafts is necessary. An example is shown in Fig. 31.5.

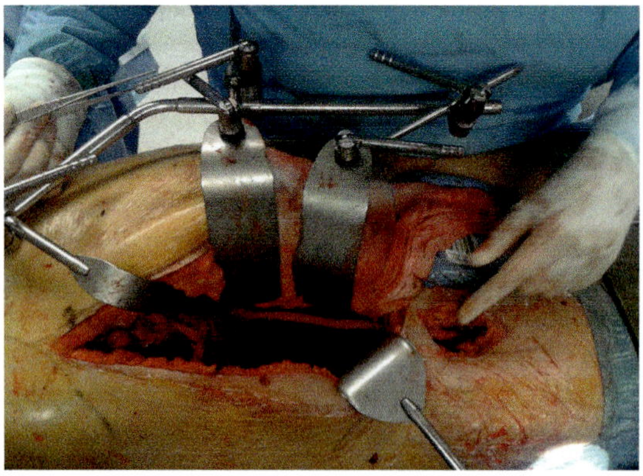

Fig. 31.5 Iliofemoral saphenous bypass graft after wide excision of endo- and retro-peritoneal metastatic carcinoma

31.3 Specific Standards

31.3.1 Large Vessel Involvement

In the presence of large vessel involvement (the aorta or abdominal veins), a rapid infusion system (RIS) is mandatory, while if lesions of the superior vena cava with atrial infiltration or an involvement of the suprahepatic segment of the inferior vena cava are suspected, it is appropriate to plan the use of extracorporeal circulation (ECC).

When the need for resection of the large vessels is expected, it is also important to have a suitable graft for reconstruction, including tubular segments of reinforced large calibre ePTFE (from 14 mm to 20 mm) or thoracic arterial homografts for the venae cavae, Dacron or Dacron Silver for arterial reconstruction and suitable saphenous segments or superficial autologous femoral veins (the validity of which will obviously have been studied preoperatively). For example, Fig. 31.6 shows a reconstruction of the superior vena cava carried out by the interposition of a tubular

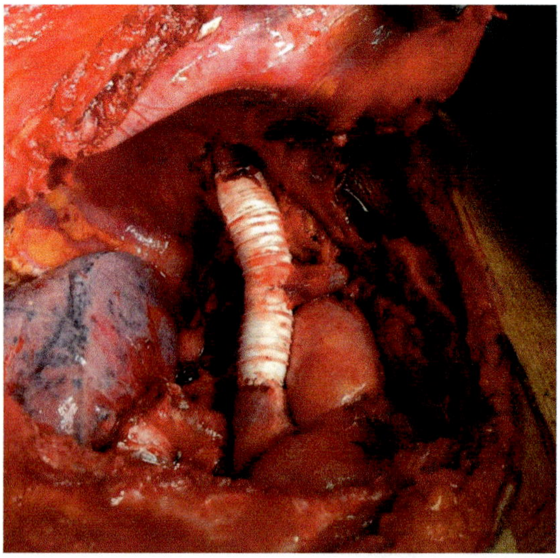

Fig. 31.6 Reconstruction of the superior vena cava carried out by interposition of a tubular ring-reinforced ePTFE (14 mm), placed between the right innominate vein and the inferior portion of the superior vena cava to which the left innominate vein was attached. Note the sterno-thoracic access with disengagement of the first rib from the sternum bar

ring-reinforced ePTFE placed between the right innominate vein and the inferior portion of the native vena cava to which the left innominate vein was attached.

31.3.2 Involvement of the Aorta

In the presence of aortic lesions (arch, thoracic or abdominal aorta), reconstruction significantly affects the outcome for obvious reasons. In these cases, our experience suggests the use of the most conservative techniques possible such as banding the aorta with Teflon or, better yet, with an autologous pericardial patch or, in the presence of accidental iatrogenic lesions, by directly suturing the aorta using Teflon pledgets. An example of an autologous pericardial patch for aortic banding is depicted in Fig. 31.7. All the aortic reconstructions by tubular substitution that we have carried out involve cases where the intraoperative picture was different from what was assumed by preoperative imaging or due to iatrogenic lesions that could not be repaired using a different conservative technique. In fact, we believe that lesions that extensively infiltrate the thoracic or abdominal aorta, in which oncological radicality depends on resection with tubular reconstruction, are contraindications to surgery. Regardless of perioperative outcomes, the prognosis of these patients remains burdened by very high short-term mortality. Therefore, the prerequisite for dealing with surgery on cancerous lesions that touch or infiltrate the aorta is the possibility to cleave the tumour or to limit the excision to a cuneiform resection.

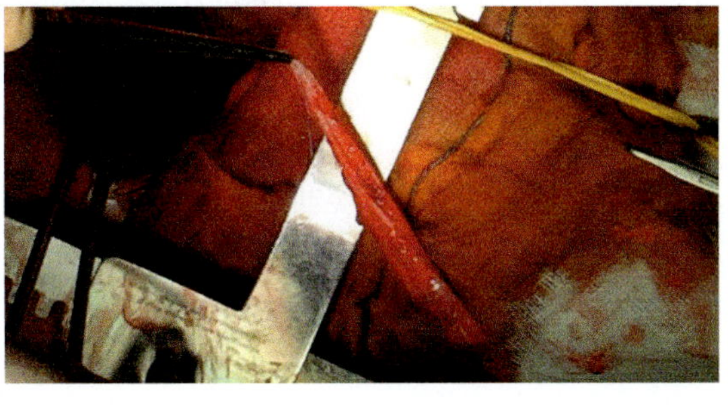

Fig. 31.7 Autologous pericardial patch for aortic banding

The access route depends on the aortic segment that is involved and on the nature and extent of the original neoplasm.

With regard to the ascending aorta and arch, the pathways we most frequently travelled included median sternotomy, sterno-cervicotomy and sterno-thoracotomy with possible detachment of the clavicle from the sternal manubrium.

One patient required descending thoracic aorta repair due to a recurrence of stromal carcinoma of the posterior mediastinum, which we carried out by right thoracotomy. The case in question is purely anecdotal and involved aortic clamping with retro-cardio-esophageal banding to reinforce the vessel. Unfortunately, traditional access to the thoracic aorta by left thoracotomy is not the most convenient way to excise tumour lesions of the posterior mediastinum, while it is optimal in the presence of aortic infiltration by tumours of the main bronchus or of the left lung.

31.3.3 Involvement of Large Veins

When the affected vessel is a vein, resection is more frequent because of the weaker structure of the vessel as compared to that of an artery. If in doubt, which is frequent when dealing with patients undergoing adjuvant radiotherapy due to the intense fibrotic reaction between the tumour and the vessel, the choice of the most appropriate dissection plane for cancer lesions may require an impromptu histological evaluation. The presence of neoplastic cellularity in the tested fragment often leads to resection. Figure 31.8 shows the dissection of an irradiated Pancoast tumour.

We limit vein reconstruction to the caval system and to the innominate trunk. In other cases, the solution may involve suturing the venous stump, possibly in the vicinity of side vessels or venous confluences in order to avoid a "cul-de-sac" effect, using an allez-retour polypropylene 4/0 or 5/0 on the vascular stumps. If a segmental resection of the vein wall can be performed, reconstruction with an autologous venous or pericardial patch sutured with polypropylene 5/0 or 6/0 or direct suture with the same procedures can be carried out. For example, in Fig. 31.9, a

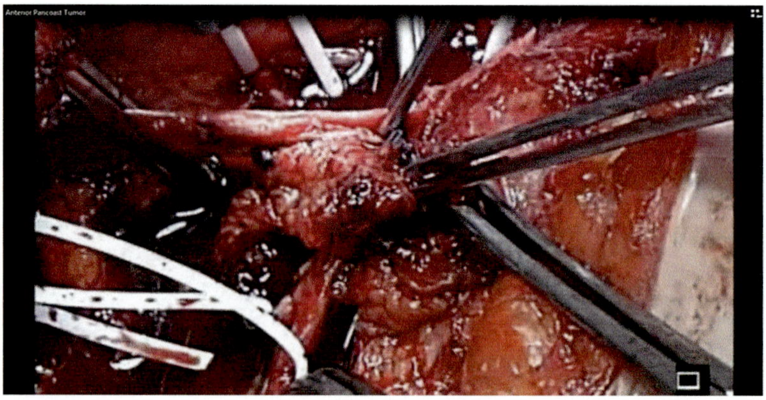

Fig. 31.8 Dissection of the irradiated Pancoast tumour

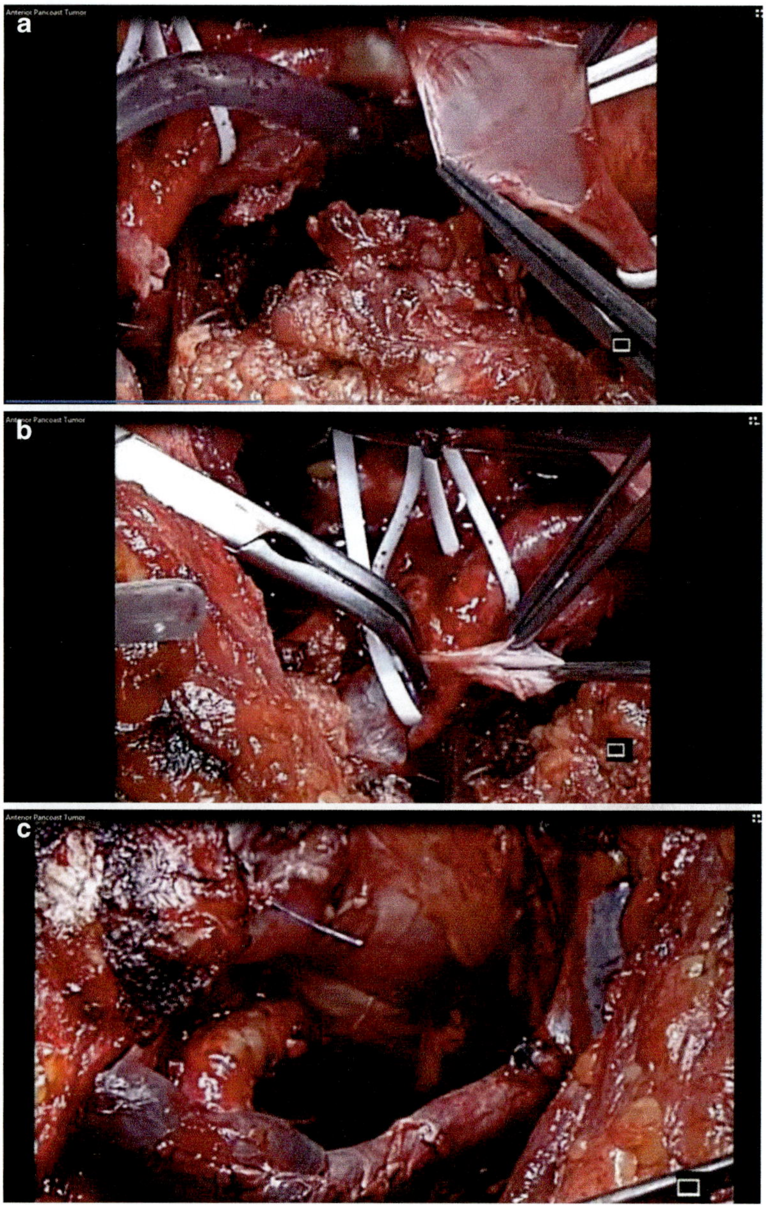

Fig. 31.9 Partial resection of the innominate vein and superior vena cava (**a** + **b**) with reconstruction and transposition (**c**)

partial resection of the innominate vein and superior vena cava reconstruction with transposition are shown, while Fig. 31.10 depicts a similar case in which we preferred reconstruction using an autologous pericardial patch.

Innominate or caval reconstruction may be done by end-to-end anastomosis of the venous stumps using polypropylene sutures 4/0 or 5/0 in the presence of limited resections or by using saphenous duplications, transpositions of the femoral vein and substitutes such as suitable calibre-reinforced ePTFE or homografts. In Fig. 31.11, a ringed ePTFE reconstruction of the left innominate vein is reported.

In the presence of neoplastic thrombosis of a venous trunk, and if it is not the cause of severe symptoms (such as mediastinal syndrome, Budd-Chiari syndrome or massive oedema of a limb), the fastest and most effective solution consists in resection without reconstruction of the venous trunk. On the contrary, cancerous lesions of the retro- or suprahepatic vena cava, secondary to the intraluminal extension of a renal adenocarcinoma or primary malignant disease of the vessel wall (angiosarcoma or leiomyosarcoma), warrant special treatment with regard to the preparation of surgical procedures and to the support that is sometimes needed for the circulation. In these cases, we emphasize the importance of careful haemodynamic monitoring using echo-transesophageal cardiography; the availability of RIS and ECC in the operating room is equally important. In these cases, full mobilization of the liver is imperative. This manoeuvre requires a rooftop incision or a Mercedes incision, preparation of the vascular pedicle, sectioning of all hepatic ligaments including the hepato-caval ligament, interruption of the Spigelian veins which should be clipped and sutured on both sides (vena cava and hepatic parenchyma), preparation of the suprahepatic veins (left, right and common trunk of the respective branches) and the preparation of the caval hiatus of the diaphragm which must be sectioned by the lateral-right phrenic approach

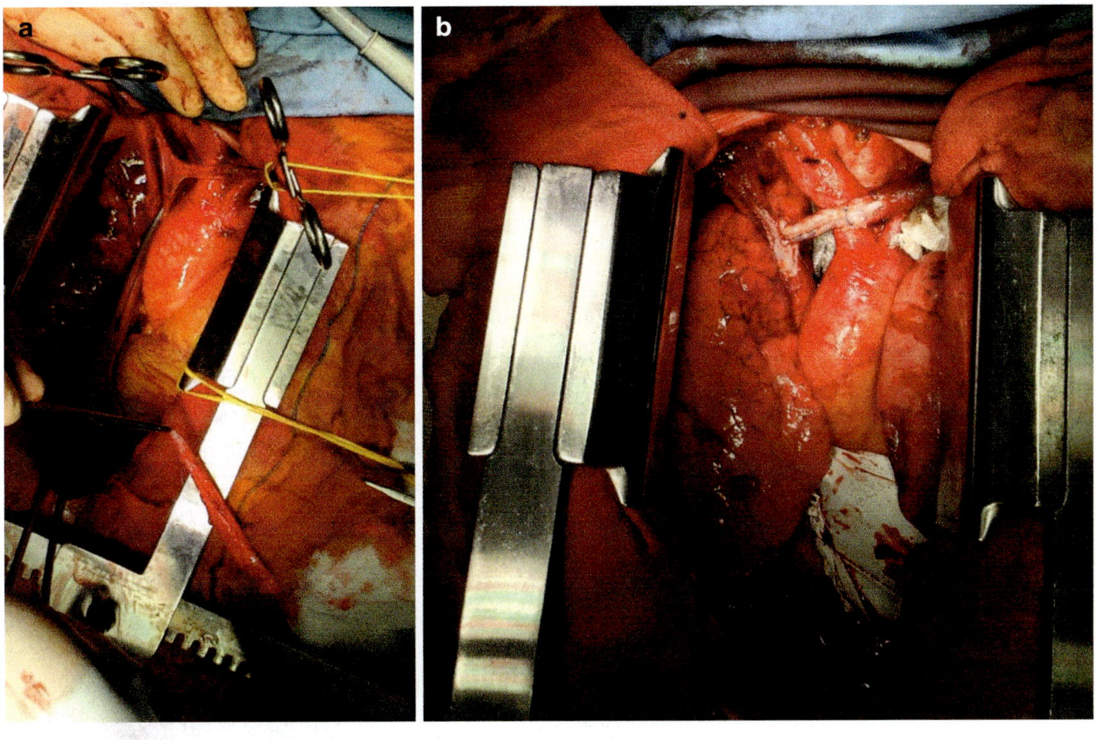

Fig. 31.10 Partial resection of the innominate vein and superior vena cava (**a**) with reconstruction using an autologous pericardial patch (**b**). In (**b**) note the presence of an ePTFE patch used to reconstruct the pericardium in order to avoid the twist of the heart in the perioperative

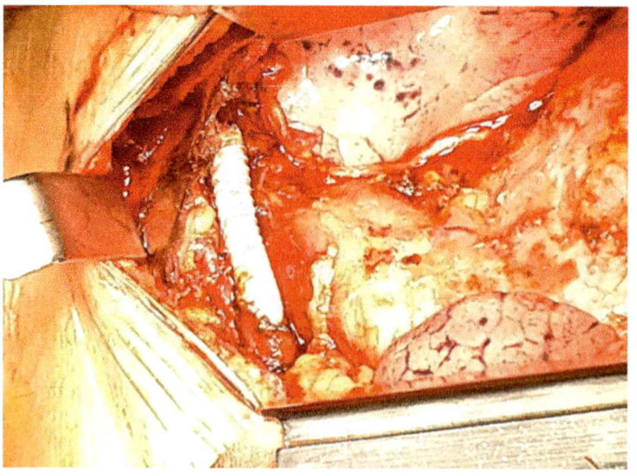

Fig. 31.11 Ringed ePTFE reconstruction of the left innominate vein after resection of a thymic carcinoma

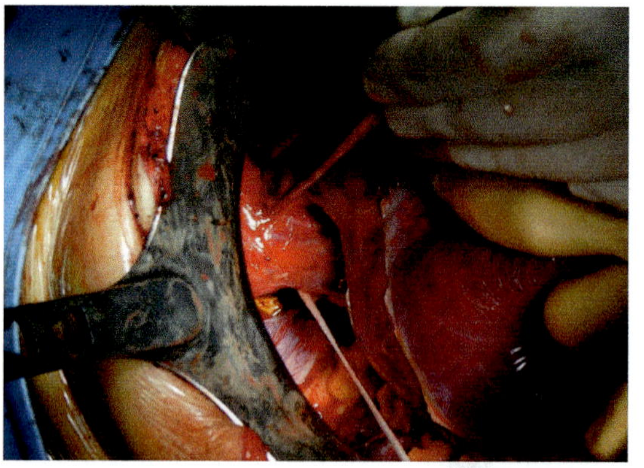

Fig. 31.12 Preparation of the suprahepatic segment of the inferior vena cava

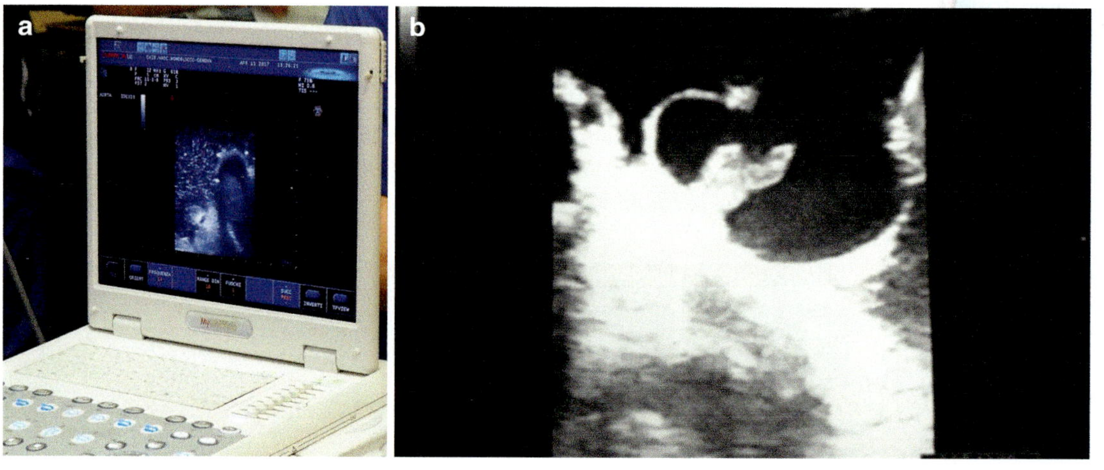

Fig. 31.13 Precise localization of the tumour along the vascular axis using intraoperative colour duplex scan (**a** + **b**)

in order to gain control of the intra-pericardial segment of the vessel. Figure 31.12 depicts the preparation of the suprahepatic segment of the lower vena cava.

If inferior vena cava cross-clamping is necessary, we prefer to test the caval cross-clamping tolerance before performing the cavotomy. In case of haemodynamic instability that cannot be anaesthesiologically controlled, it is imperative to guarantee adequate venous return to the right atrium by means of veno-venous splanchnic and somatic extracorporeal circulation (femoral vein + superior mesenteric vein to axillary vein) using a centrifugal pump. Furthermore, we prefer to perform an intraoperative colour duplex scan to evaluate the points of clamping which must be upstream and downstream to the longitudinal extension of the tumour, as shown in Fig. 31.13.

In cases of renal adenocarcinoma with invasion of the renal and inferior caval veins, the tumour does not adhere to the caval wall, except in the presence of superimposed paraneoplastic thrombosis. This results in very short infrarenal and above-the-liver (extra- or intra-pericardial) caval clamping time with contralateral renal vein clamping. The caval ostium of the renal vein that is attached to the neoplasm is used as the access site for the complete removal of the tumour. This is followed by caval side clamping, excluding the incision, and venous unclamping that restores physiological venous return. The surgical steps involved in these cases are described in Fig. 31.14.

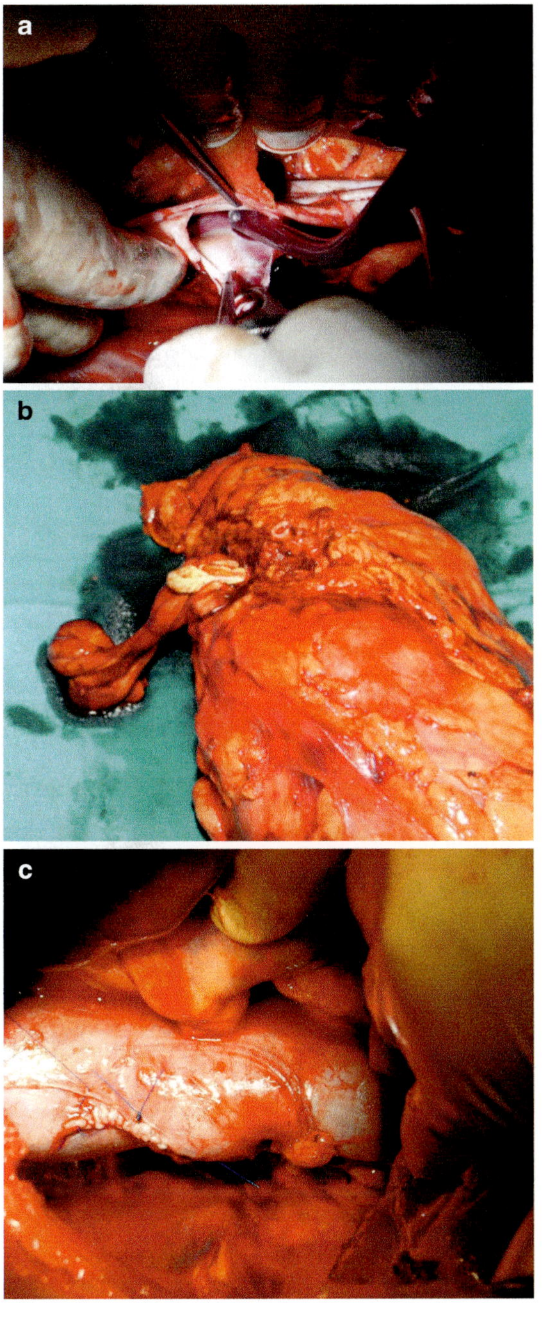

Fig. 31.14 Renal adenocarcinoma with invasion of the renal and inferior caval veins. (**a**) The caval ostium of the renal vein attached to the neoplasm is used as the access site for total removal of the tumour. (**b**) Surgical specimen coming from the kidney, deformed by adenocarcinoma and the neoplastic reno-caval thrombus. (**c**) Caval suture with the impression of the tangential clamping that was just made

The homografts we used were made up of descending thoracic aorta segments that had been cryopreserved and then grafted end to end between the caval stumps using polypropylene suture 3/0 or 4/0. The choice of the most suitable-sized homograft requires preoperative assessment of the patient's CT scan (on a workstation) in order to evaluate the minimum length and diameter of the segment to be replaced.

In cases of caval infiltration by adjacent neoplastic structures, such as lymph node packages or adrenal glands, segmental resection of the infiltrated portion of the cava is possible. During caval cross-clamping, we perform a longitudinal caval incision followed by a segmental transcaval excision of the infiltrated portion of vessel and by a direct suture of caval margins of the resection; then, suture of the first cavotomy is performed during caval side clamping. The surgical steps involved in these cases are described in Fig. 31.15.

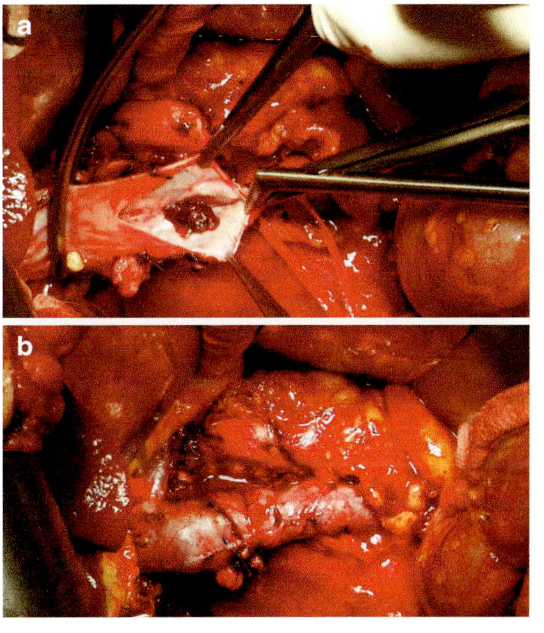

Fig. 31.15 Caval infiltration by adjacent neoplastic structures. (**a**) Segmental resection of the infiltrated portion of the cava using a trans-caval approach with direct longitudinal caval incision with total caval clamping. (**b**) Direct suture of the inferior vena cava after caval side clamping

31.3.4 Vascular Preparation to Myocutaneous Flap

In cases of wide resection of the chest or abdominal wall that has been infiltrated by cancer, it is important to evaluate the anatomic requirements for the possible reconstruction with a myocutaneous flap. Indeed, in the presence of extensive venous demolition, it is sometimes necessary to resort to autologous bridging to lengthen the vascular pedicles of the reconstruction flap.

31.4 Conclusions

The role of the vascular surgeon is of great importance in the treatment of locally advanced cancer cases.

A detailed collegial discussion of the individual case during oncological DMT meetings is equally important in order to accurately plan the surgery.

Cooperation among the various specialists is the only way to broaden indications and improve outcomes.

Despite the appealing possibility of dealing with injuries of almost any kind, oncological and surgical common sense is the main criterion when establishing indications to surgery.

Oncovascular Surgery; Surgery of the Vena Cava-Related Tumors

32

Kareem Sallam

One really wonders whether surgery is a branch of medicine or is it a branch of construction engineering

32.1 Introduction

The inferior vena cava, one of the most dreaded organs in abdominal surgery, is always blamed for killing subjects and more often is held the responsibility of the inoperability and irresectability of malignant disease.

Lying silently in the very depth of the abdominal cavity with many organs on its top, remaining patent despite its low pressure and unenforced wall.

The case for vena cava's implication in irresectability of tumors is similar to the usual scenario of living with human beings, the more you take responsibilities and commitments on your shoulder, the more you will be involved in issues of different kinds. The more you do, the more you will be blamed. This is the case with the vena cava, an organ with a very major role and numerous responsibilities and commitments to other organs with which it is connected to with tributaries many of which are critical.

As surgeons we commonly respond to this condition by abandoning or at least inconsistently doing surgery for tumors around the cava. While in fact all what it takes to perform surgery on an organ with multiple commitments is to be patient enough in the preparatory phase of surgery to repeat multiply the same step should the organ have had a single commitment.

If one would invest time to free the vena cava from its commitments and tributaries, he would find a very cooperative organ that would stand to his side and the side of the patient I assure.

So here comes the question: can all the vena cava-related tumors be resected?

With the use of current surgical and anesthesia facilities, perhaps the answer will be yes.

32.2 Types and Different Views for Classifying Vena Cava-Related Tumors

Vena cava-related tumors can have three different classifications (Table 32.1):

First is anatomical, i.e., according to the organ of origin.

Second is pathological, i.e., according to the histopathology of the tumor.

Third is technical (see later).

When you add the anatomy to the pathology, you can get numerous possibilities and combinations of anatomies-pathologies complexes.

The surprise carried by this chapter is that it is not about listing the vena cava-related tumors and then running through them to describe different operations for different tumors. Not at all.

K. Sallam (✉)
Surgical Oncology Unit, Helwan University Hospitals, Cairo, Egypt
e-mail: kareem.sallam@med.helwan.edu.eg.

© Springer Nature Switzerland AG 2019
Y. Tshomba et al. (eds.), *Visceral Vessels and Aortic Repair*,
https://doi.org/10.1007/978-3-319-94761-7_32

Table 32.1 Different ways to classify vena cava-related tumors

1. Anatomical, according to organ of origin:
Posterior segment rt.lobe liver
Caudate lobe liver
Suprarenal gland
Kidney
Soft tissue of retroperitoneum
2. Histopathological:
Different types of carcinomas and sarcomas according to the organ
Some benign and low-grade tumors of retroperitoneal tissues and organs
3. Technical:
1. Tumors adjacent to the cava or encasing without infiltration
2. Tumors infiltrating the full thickness of the wall
3. Tumors inside the caval lumen

Table 32.2 The four main phases for resection of vena cava-related tumor

Look at the scans and define the circle of interest, i.e., field of surgery (see text for description)
Phase 1: Mobilization of organs from in front of the circle of interest
Phase 2: Control of "ins and outs" to and from the circle of interest defined and now cleared from superficial structures by virtue of phase one
Phase 3: Complete (lateral and posterior) mobilization of the tumor-cava complex
Phase 4: Three options
1. Subadventitial dissection of the cava
2. Resection of cava with the tumor and replacement as appropriate
3. Opening the cava to excise a tumor from within the lumen

This article is about introducing, as the title described, the concept of vena cava-related tumors all in one and encompassed as a single entity. The chapter's purpose is to describe the basic principles and the logic behind a *single unified approach* for what the author sees as a single entity from the technical standpoint unifying a variety of anatomies and pathologies when it comes to resection, an approach that enables getting to terms with the vena cava and may be with every retroperitoneal resection surgery.

Technically speaking, IVC-related tumors can be looked at as of three types:

Tumors adjacent to the cava without infiltration
Tumors infiltrating the caval wall
Tumors inside the cava

32.2.1 General strategy of resection (the 4 phases of the surgery)

The approach entails four main phases. The titles of which are given in Table 32.2 and the description follows.

There will be no surgery for any retroperitoneal structure (which is the case for the cava) without the more superficial organs regardless their name, size, and relevance being moved out of the way. This is basic and final. The problem is that sometimes the size of the tumor overshadows the organs and attracts the surgeons' attention as soon as the abdomen is open, and therefore the surgeon goes straight to the visible and palpable part of the tumor disregarding the invisible part and disregarding the fact that he is only palpating the tumor through the full thickness of other organ, for instance, a thinned out mesentery of small bowl and colon. The anatomy will stay a fact; no matter how big the tumor is, this will never get the organs and their attachments to disappear. They might just be overshadowed or change the very usual position, but they will indeed remain in the abdomen.

The general configuration of organs in the abdomen is that we have two central structures which offer blood supply—namely, IVC and aorta—while the rest of the organs are on either sides of such central structures or on top of it. Whether on the sides or on top, they need to connect to the central structures by branches which will run in an axial plane for organs on the sides and in a sagittal plane for organs on top (superficial).

The organs in the abdomen lie in specific locations. Two categories of attachments keep them in position. First is their "ins and outs," namely, blood vessels and ducts, if any. These are unnegotiable; there interruption entails either resection of the organ or the need for a restorative surgery in most of the occasions.

What is dispensable in almost all abdominal organs is the second category which is the ligamentous attachments which in fact are nothing but perfectly dispensable peritoneal folds.

One would be amazed how much mobility that the organs acquire as a consequence to the *complete* division of these almost bloodless and routinely accessible peritoneal reflections. A degree of mobility that makes the need to divide any of the first category attachments unnecessary in almost all surgeries of the abdomen. When these cuts are made as complete as they can get, every organ on the right-hand side can go to the extreme left and vice versa and sometimes can be even flipped cranially or caudally. In a sense the blood supply will act as a fulcrum with the organ at its distal end having a 3D mobility in different directions and hence exposing the central structures in the retroperitoneum.

The ability and the will for mobilizing whatever necessary of the abdominal organs is the key to accessing the vena cava.

Access solves almost all problems in surgery because otherwise one would do nothing but making a cut or placing a stitch or multiples of the two. Making a cut and placing a stitch is something that all surgeons do with reasonable ease and efficiency on the skin level. The only difference between skin and retroperitoneal surgery (including the vena cava-related tumors) is the access.

Here comes the list of organs that is on the way to the vena cava if the full length of the vena cava is to be exposed (Fig. 32.1):

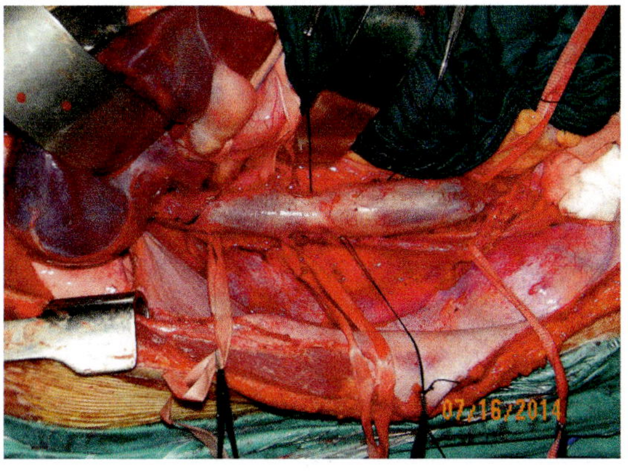

Fig. 32.1 The full length of vena cava exposed from diaphragm down to iliac bifurcation. Note the clearance of *left* side of the intrahepatic vena cava off the caudate lobe of liver. The free space here allows the passage of a big side clamp that controls the confluence of hepatic veins to cava as shown in Fig. 32.2a

- From top to bottom: Liver, Rt. colon, duodenum- head of pancreas and small bowel. (The last 3 are in a sense a complex since the fulcrum of the tree is the Superior mesenteric vessel).

Mobilizing the liver entails cutting the falciform (and round ligament), rt. triangular ligament, coronary ligament (and rt. triangular ligament)

The tricky part of freeing the cava from the liver is in freeing the short hepatic veins and clearing the left side of the upper cava from its intimate relation to the caudate lobe in particular. This maneuver is seriously important as it (1) prevents back bleeds from these veins, (2) enables placing a clamp on the joint venture of the hepatic veins preventing back bleeding even if the cava is opened straight away to the atrium as is required in some surgeries (Fig. 32.2), and (3) gives the cava this desired complete freedom and mobility facilitating opening, repairs, and resection and replacement should this be chosen for any reason.

During mobilization of the cava at this segment, it is to be appreciated and taken advantage of that the cava in its retrohepatic and intrahepatic segments is completely devoid of tributaries to its posterior surface. All what is to be handled with care and patience is the anterior and anterolaterally placed tributaries (short hepatic veins). Otherwise posterior mobilization can be done strictly by *blunt finger* dissection passed with relative impunity underneath the cava between it and the crus of the diaphragm. It is to be noted however that blunt finger dissection is not a careless forceful dissection. It is still to be done with gentleness. To the maximum, this can be upgraded to "conscious firmness" concentrating on the tactile feedback and stopping as resistance is encountered. When this resistance is met, the surgeon can retract the part that has been mobilized, sit on a stool to have a look behind the cava to see, and handle whatever is stopping the blunt dissection. Figure 32.2 shows options for hepatic veins control. Table 32.3 contains notes on hepatic veins control.

On mobilizing the rt. colon-small bowel complex, the surgeon needs to pay attention to cut the root of the mesentery of the small bowel and not to settle only to evisceration of the bowl. The root of the mesentery crosses obliquely in

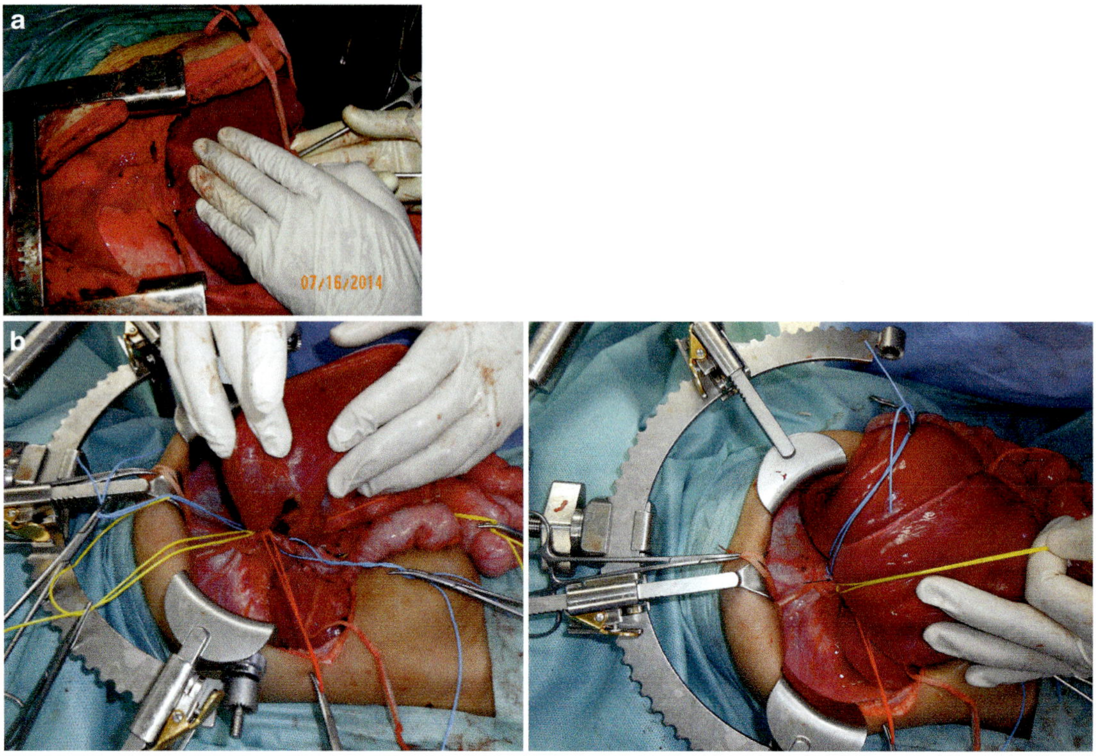

Fig. 32.2 Options for hepatic veins control. (**a**) Common control; A Satinsky clamp controlling the hepatic veins entry to cava in totality. (**b**) Selective control; Selective control by rubber slings. Please see text for description

Table 32.3 Notes on hepatic veins control

Notes on hepatic veins control
1. In either A or B, hepatic veins control is not to be attempted before complete freedom of intrahepatic cava is achieved by ligation of short hepatic veins from all directions. The hepatic vein stumps gain much length when this is done combined by outward traction on the liver. Care is to be taken not to misidentify the main hepatic veins as a large short hepatic vein
2. Main hepatic veins are wide based, and therefore standard looping using a right angled forceps is usually not possible if not hazardous; the rt. angled forceps' blade is never long enough to cover the whole width of them. The technique used by the author is as follows:
–Complete freeing of the cava from short hepatic veins
–An artery forceps has its back lying flat on the midline of the cava (i.e., the tip is toward the ceiling) from the caudal side and from the cranial side alternatively until it shows up from the other direction. This necessitates observing a characteristic notch that appears on the caval wall at the central tendon side demarcating the boundary between the rt. and the middle hepatic vein marked by an arrow in Fig. 32.2b lt. This notch guides the placement and direction of the aforementioned artery forceps. As the artery forceps aims at coming out from the other side, its tip should stay directed to the ceiling till showing up again after traversing the full length of the hepatic vein entry to cava. This avoids faulty outwarding through the hepatic vein wall itself which is thin and compressible and might give the operator an impression that it is a connective tissue band specially when flattened against the artery forceps or indeed the rt. angled forceps (Fig. 32.3)
3. Lt. hepatic vein isolation requires working from the left-hand side and division of the lesser omentum in order to gain access to the area of concern (Fig. 32.4). It might require as well clearing off hepatic parenchyma that usually covers part of the lt. hepatic vein entry to cava

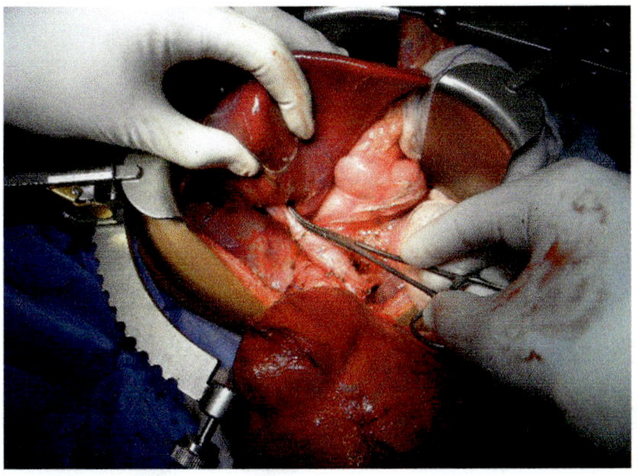

Fig. 32.3 Slinging the rt. hepatic vein: the use of an artery forceps and the direction of its introduction

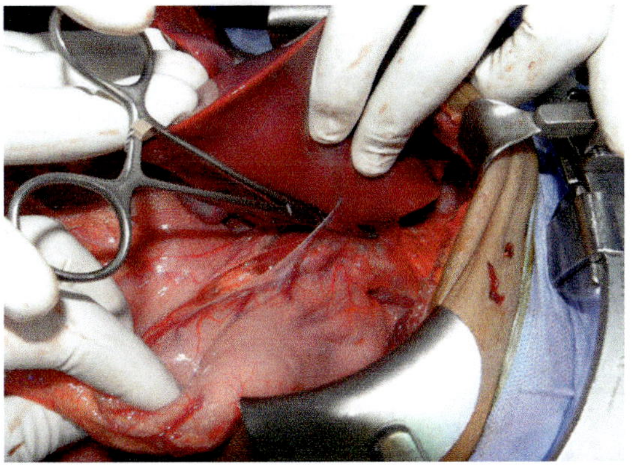

Fig. 32.4 Exposure of lt. hepatic vein from lt. side: division of the lesser omentum gives access to cava from lt. side

front of the retroperitoneal central structures (Fig. 32.5). Cutting this flimsy attachment maximizes exposure and enables flipping of the bowel cranially toward the patient's chest. A maneuver helps much in access and in freeing the hands of the assistants (Fig. 32.6).

Cranial as opposed to lateral flipping of small bowel is to be used when exposure of the aorta and cava is required to take place at the same time and in the same field. In these occasions, cranial flipping might be better (Fig. 32.6).

Table 32.4 describes the different options for small bowel mobilization according to the required magnitude of exposure of the retroperitoneum.

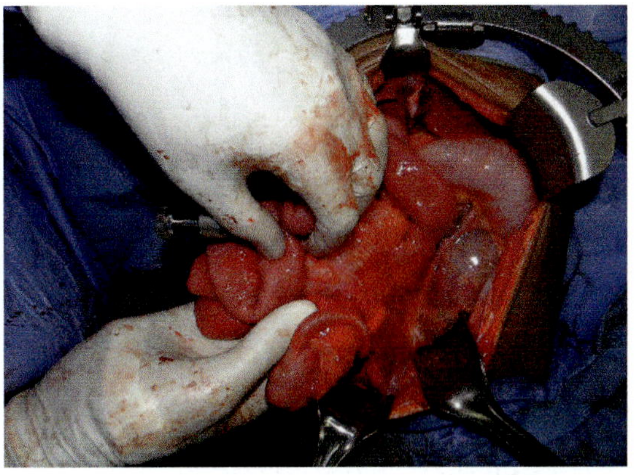

Fig. 32.5 The root of the small bowel mesentery; note that the small bowel is already eviscerated and mobilized laterally. Releasing the root of the small bowel mesentery enables flipping the bowel cranially and not only laterally maximizing the exposure of the vena cava and its tributaries and indeed the related tumor as shown in Fig. 32.1

Though mobilizing the organs is the first manual step, it is preceded by a mental one, a step that the author describes as step zero. This step is done on the scans in which the surgeon, with eye on the scans, defines the circle of interest which is the field of surgery, the field that needs to be cleared to start dissection of the tumor. This circle will be the surgeon's world for the surgery of resection, but one has to define it in the first place, and the advice here is to delineate a circle that encompasses the tumor range and a "bit more" in every direction.

This "bit more" is a rim of anatomical field all around the tumor in which the surgeon will patrol looking for blood vessels and ducts getting in and out of the field of the tumor to identify and sling. On top of which undoubtedly is the proximal and distal control of the vena cava. This step of patrolling and slinging comes as the second phase of the surgery after the organ mobilization phase. When completed, and only when it is, the surgeon can now "recall" that he is here to resect a tumor and pay attention to the tumor-vena cava complex.

Now the surgeon has the cava adherent to the tumor and the tumor adherent to the retroperitoneal structures and posterior abdominal wall, so where to start?

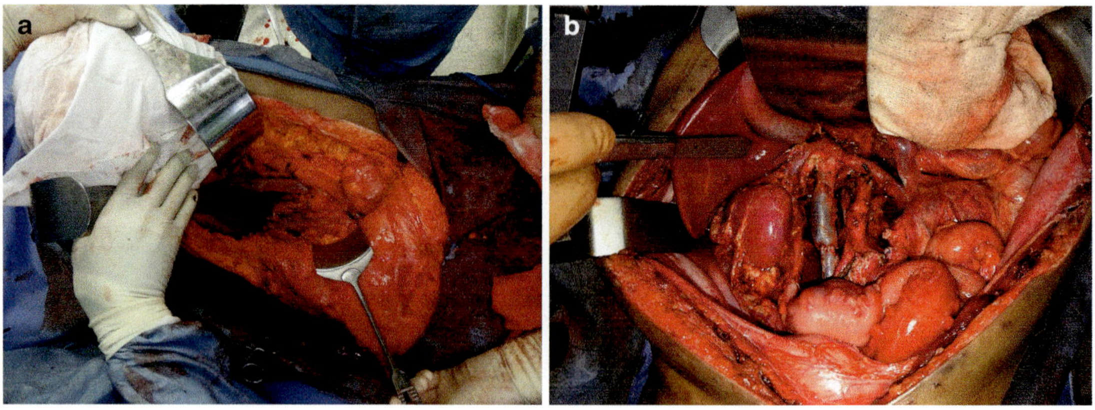

Fig. 32.6 (**a**) Cranial flipping of small bowel. (**b**) Another example of cranial flipping of small bowel wrapped in white towels. This maneuver exposes both cava and aorta in the same field

Table 32.4 Options for small bowel

Options for small bowel
This is a ladder of options according to degree of exposure required
1. Packing
2. Evisceration
3. Tenting: In which root of mesentery released yet coecum stays in right iliac fossa, and the surgery takes place underneath the small bowel and rt. colon mesentery (Fig. 32.7)
4. Complete mobilization: Root of mesentery released and coecum released completely as well leading to "mobile evisceration" of whole small bowel and rt. colon (Figs. 32.5 and 32.6)

It is usually tempting to many surgeons to go straight to the cava to take off the tumor and breathe the sigh of relief and as well decide "resectability," for some will abandon the procedure if the vena cava is inseparable from the lesion.

The answer to the question "where to start?" is fairly similar to the situation of examining the abdomen in clinical rounds. You ask where the pain is and you start at the farthest point palpating the abdomen leaving the quadrant of pain till the end.

The tumor is to be mobilized laterally first with complete disregard to the cava. Only when the tumor and cava are mobilized as one complex one can start handling the cava, and this marks the fourth and final phase of the surgery, the phase of handling the cava.

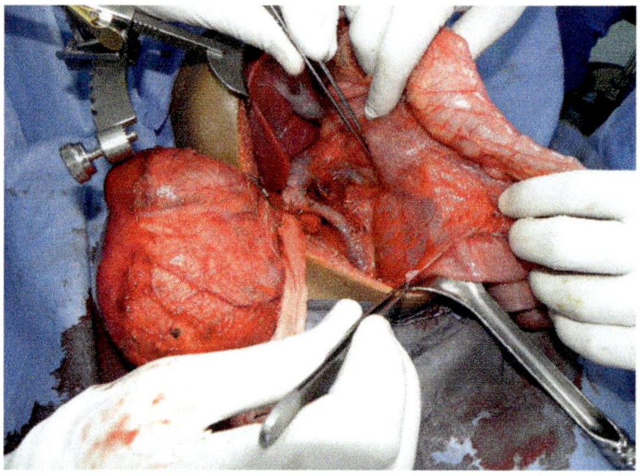

Fig. 32.7 Tenting of the small bowl mesentery and working from underneath. The coecum can stay in place in the rt. iliac fossa or acquire partial mobilization

This is the variable step of the procedure and the options are (Fig. 32.8):

1. Subadventitial dissection of the cava off the tumor
2. Resection of the tumor-cava complex and replacement by a graft
3. Opening the cava to excise a tumor thrombus

Even for surgeons who are making a decision to abandon the procedure if the cava is inseparable from the tumor, the author would recommend leaving the cava till the end. One will be amazed how friendly is this badly reputed organ will be when the procedure is done in this order. The surgical

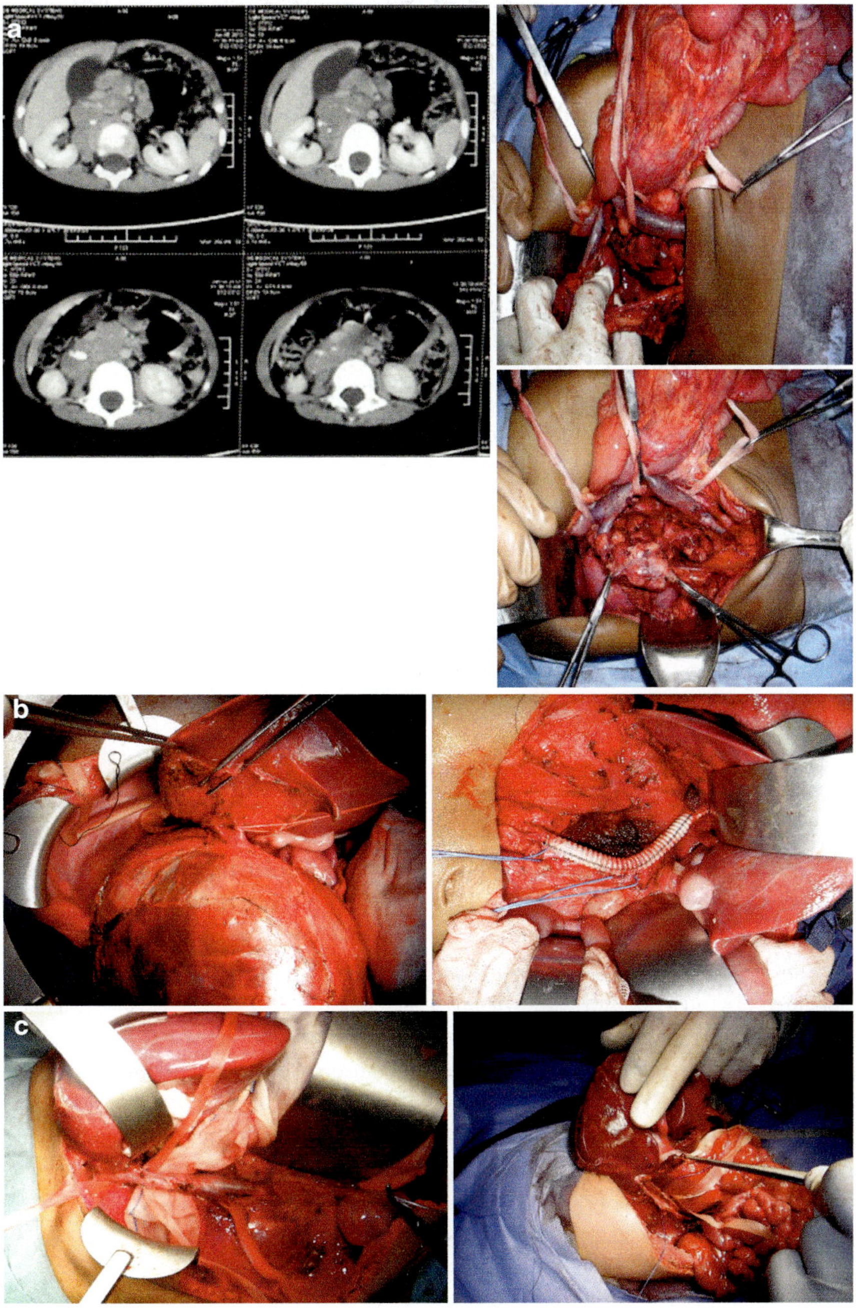

Fig. 32.8 The three options of phase 4 in surgery of vena cava-related tumors; (**a**) Subadventitial dissection, a patient with centrally located neuroblastoma: demonstration of the use of slings to retract the cava in different directions and perform subadventitial dissection. (**b**) Resection and replacement: a patient with retroperitoneal recurrent soft tissue sarcoma status post-resection and rt. nephrectomy. Now with recurrence encasing and infiltrating the IVC and part of the lt. renal vein caudal surface. Resection was performed with replacement of the IVC by Dacron graft and patch graft on the renal vein with internal jugular vein graft. The patient underwent uneventful recovery and discharged on therapeutic anticoagulation. (**c**) Extraction of a tumor from within the caval lumen. Lt.: complete exposure of cava by mobilization of bowel and liver, proximal and distal control as well as control of tributaries. Complete freeing of the cava as demonstrated by the small swab passing freely round the cava. Rt.: now the cava can be opened and the thrombus dissected off the wall by a variety of instruments including endarterectomy dissector. Note the en bloc excision of the thrombus

team will find a cooperative organ tolerating much traction, dissection, and repairs when needed, all enabling dissection of the cava that would, in other wise order, have seemed inseparable from the tumor.

The technique of dissection of the vena cava off the tumor entails using No. 15 blade lying flat. As soon as a window can be opened anywhere along the caval segment in question, a sling is to be passed round the cava and pulled in different directions including upward. This sling retraction enables maneuvering the cava here and there giving access to its different facets including the posterior one, and hence dissection can proceed and the short-stumped tributaries viewed and get a bit of length for control and division.

The sling belongs to the main operator's dominant hand with a dissection tool in the other being it a blade, a scissors, a dissection forceps, a sponge on a stick, or a Poole Suction Tip with the shield removed. Poole Suction Tips with holes very close to the tip are favored when suction tips are used for dissection. The proximity of holes to the tip makes them suck minute amount of blood rapidly and hence clearing the field for dissection. For scissors, a standard Metzenbaum is one friendly instrument. It is of value to add to the set a round-tipped Reynolds scissors of variable lengths.

An experienced assistant would have forceps in his non-dominant hand and suction tip in the other if the main operator is not holding it. Otherwise another forceps or counter traction by a small swab should be the case. The suction in whoever's hand is not only for sucking but also for teasing the tissues trying to open up the plane.

The case for vena cava dissection is the same for the dissection of any vessel; the more you go close to its wall, the easier is and the safer is the plane and not otherwise. That is why it is called subadventitial dissection. The cava lies within a sheath. The first step in dissection is opening up this sheath longitudinally along the vena caval segment in question. It is as if the cava is putting on a shirt with buttons on the front. Desheathing the cava is like taking off a shirt off a man's body, you release the buttons from the front surface and the rest of the sheath will then retract to either side (Fig. 32.9).

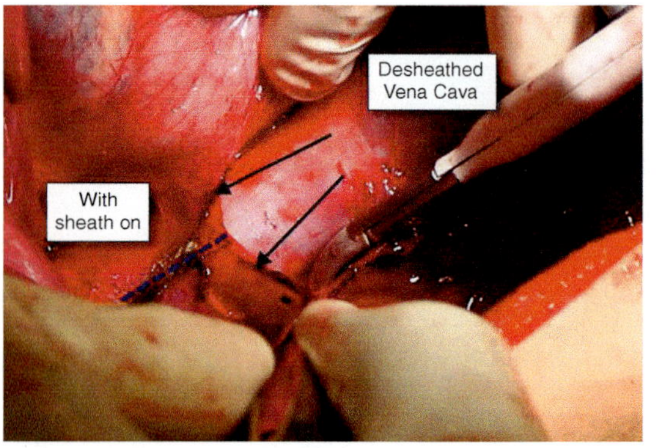

Fig. 32.9 Desheathing of the cava in progress. The view obtained in figure one with all tributaries looped around is facilitated by desheathing of the cava (see text for description). The cut edge of the sheath is pointed to with black arrows with a vena caval segment. When the sheath is cut on the strict front side of the cava longitudinally, this allows the side sheath to retract laterally; with the aid of a blunt instrument, the desheathing is completed in the opened plan. In this photograph a bipolar biclamp cautery instrument (LigaSure, precise handle by Covidien) is being in use. The dotted line represents the presumed direction of initial cut to be made by the cautery instrument

32.3 Remarks, Adjunctive Techniques, and Special Situations

32.3.1 Remarks

This section draws some light on specific points in the approach abovementioned. The points chosen are presented in a chronological sequence as they happen in surgery.

- Tumor embolism and the use of preoperative IVC filters
- Positioning of the patient
- Incision
- Role of table-mounted retraction and magnification
- The difference between lateral dissection and posterior dissection
- Vena cava clamping
- Vena cava grafting
- Inviting an old technique: vena cava compartmentalization

32.3.1.1 Tumor Embolism and the Use of Preoperative IVC Filters

Particularly for the case of intraluminal tumor thrombi, the risk of embolism is of concern. Early proximal clamp is always advisable. The use of preoperative IVC filters is another option. These are better to be retrievable, and there needs to be a space of at least 4 cm before the cavo-atrial junction to enable deployment of the filter. Transfemoral access routes are strictly prohibited for the risk of embolism as a result of manipulation of the thrombus by the passing endovascular tools.

The authors have dealt with four types of intraluminal tumors in the cava and some other veins, namely, Wilm's tumor, sarcomas of different kinds, renal cell carcinomas, and thyroid carcinoma.

Out of the four, the renal cell carcinoma has been found to be very liable to detachment, and hence early proximal *clamping* is mandatory. The other three has been found friendlier. Particularly with Wilm's tumor, thrombi tend to be adherent to the wall by synechia which probably arise after chemotherapy. Sarcomas have been found to be firm and compact and rubbery. The initial touch of the thrombus informs about its firmness, attachment to the wall, and coherence. This should indicate the need for early proximal clamping.

32.3.1.2 Positioning of the Patient

A roll underneath the site of surgery is the standard for abdominal surgery. When surgery includes resection of a tumor, surgeons tend to put the roll underneath the equator of the tumor. The recommendation here is, again, to ignore the main bulk of the tumor and its equator. The roll is best put underneath the part of surgery that is farthest or critical in access. In the case of vena cava-related tumors, this is usually the upper pole of the field of surgery rather than the equator of the tumor. This is the point of proximal control.

32.3.1.3 Incision (Fig. 32.10)

Options are:

Bilateral Transverse with Supraumbilical Midline Extension

It gives very good vertical access as well as horizontal one where the surgeon can approach the cava from top view or from sides with side rotation of the operating table and the surgeon sitting on an operating room stool. This helps much in lateral and posterior dissection of tumors, a note on which will be given later.

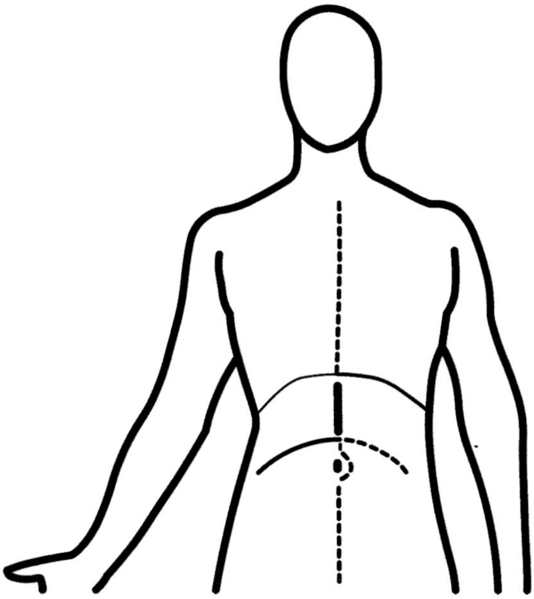

Fig. 32.10 Incision options. See text for description

Midline With or Without Transverse Extension

Obese patients whom their fat is extra-abdominal are far friendlier than what one would expect. The weight of the abdominal wall fat seems to make it to fall off to the sides offering an unexpected access from the midline incision only.

Any of the Above 2 with a Median Sternotomy

Any of the above 2 can have a median sternotomy (partial or complete) as an extension according to ease of access to suprahepatic cava keeping a low threshold to do so. Its merits supersede morbidities. Patients with narrow subcostal angle or those with a decubitus characterized by big anteroposterior diameters at the level of epigastrium will probably require it for suprahepatic control. Should one be in a position to do a suprahepatic cava control for other reason than a large neoplasm, he would find this readily accessible without a sternotomy. And probably he will judge the recommendation of sternotomy as unnecessary or overdoing. This does not apply when a big tumor is inside especially for rt.-sided upper quadrant tumors which pushes the liver cephalad preventing downward pull on the liver even when mobilized. This downward pull is pivotal in the access. In addition, the process of liver mobilization itself can be very difficult, time consuming, and bloody when tumors in these locations are accessed without a thoracoabdominal incision. The authors choose the sternotomy out of the thoracoabdominal incisions options for its more suitability for the task and its lower morbidity including pain control and lesser respiratory complications.

In conclusion, the midline supraumbilical component of the wound and the rt. transverse component are the most mandatory and extendable. Therefore, one of them is favored for initial exploration. Should more access be needed for exploration the other is to be added. At this point one can decide—according to the lower limit of tumor—whether to extend the midline downward or do a left transverse extension. The median sternotomy is the same in either case.

One should not extend the rt. transverse to the lt. side until the lower limit is settled because this lt. side extension is a giveaway of the chance to extend the midline caudally.

32.3.1.4 Role of Table-Mounted Retraction and Magnification

There has to be a serious reason to start this type of surgery without the presence of a table-mounted retractor of any form, at least present in the operating room. The commercially available ones are many. These include the Bookwalter, the Omni-Tract, and the Iron Intern. They can all serve the task. It just takes some exercise to get to know how to maximize the benefit from any of them in a particular surgery with a particular incision. The author believes that surgeons need to know how to literally exploit such instruments (Fig. 32.11).

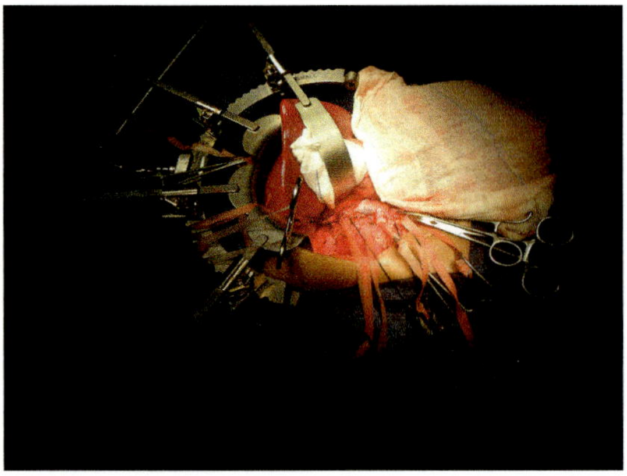

Fig. 32.11 The Bookwalter retractor in exposure of a vena cava harboring a tumor thrombus. From down the renal veins up to the intrahepatic vena cava, the field of surgery is exposed without a single hand of a human yet introduced. This frees the hands of the surgical team yet to come for some other tasks

There might be an exception for the above-mentioned near mandation of the use of table-mounted retractors which in case of huge tumors stretch the abdominal wall. The latter falls off the tumor as soon as the abdomen is opened facilitating retraction. The choice of the table-mounted retractor and its positioning need to take into account the possible need for a sternotomy. They need to be placed from the beginning of surgery to allow this to happen swiftly when needed without disturbing the whole setup. One does not have to place them all away from the whole chest field though, for one will not be operating in the cephalic part of the chest. What is required is just a draping and positioning that allows the passage of the sternal saw to make the cut.

Combining the usage of two different table-mounted retraction systems might be some surgeon's choice, for example, a combination of a cable winch retractor for the costal margin and a Bookwalter or Omni-Tract for sides, caudal and visceral retraction. The cable winch retractor has a supreme performance in costal margin. As well, it offers ample space underneath to open the chest when needed. The Bookwalter and the Omni-Tract take on the side and caudal retraction as mentioned. It is therefore up to the surgeon and the availability of equipment.

One method for side retraction of abdominal wall is the use of the Finochietto chest wall retractor. This can be used instead of the standard

Balfour retractor designed for the purpose. The Finochietto has a wider span and therefore suitable for midline incisions in subjects with big decubitus. The ones with fenestrated blades are favored as these fenestrations enable passing a stitch through them that anchors the blades to the abdominal wall to prevent its slippage from the abdominal wall edge.

As for magnification, though the cava is a gross structure and so is every structure in the field of vena cava-related tumors including the tumor itself, though this is the case, yet the author recommends the use of 2.5× magnifying loupe for most of the length of the surgery. Though structures are gross, yet it is not structures that one is after while using the loupes; one is after the tissue plans. The use of magnification helps much in defining tissue plans to desheath the cava and loop around the tributaries in proper planes with right angled forceps. During this looping one does not see the whole length of process of looping. The reliance here is on that the instrument has started in the *proper subadventitial plan* and therefore it is assumed that it will continue in it till the tip shows up again from the other side. This makes this *proper* start very important. Magnification is an important adjunct to this proper start.

32.3.1.5 The Difference Between Lateral Dissection and Posterior Dissection

Posterior dissection is complete when the tumor-cava complex is mobile over the vertebral column. The only way to do this is through opening of the inter-aortocaval plane with complete exposure of the aorta and ligation of lumbar arteries as necessary. It is complete only when a finger can be insinuated easily between the "tumor-cava complex" and the *vertebral column* all through the length of the tumor (Fig. 32.12).

When both aorta and cava are encased or in considerable contact with the tumor, it might be difficult to attain this step preserving both structures. For this "a cut to flip" technique can be introduced while handling the cava in which it is divided distally and flipped cranially to be taken out of the field allowing a safer dissection lateral to and *underneath* the aorta (Fig. 32.13).

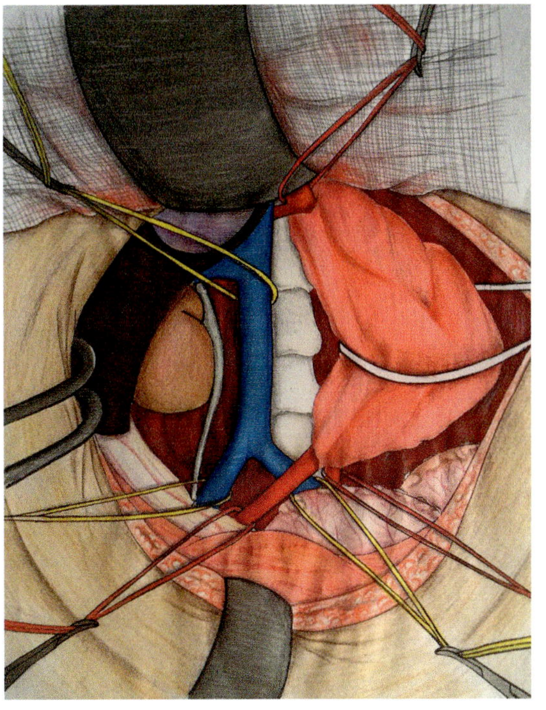

Fig. 32.12 Neuroblastoma encasing the aorta; demonstration of the so called completed posterior dissection as the aorta encased within a neuroblastoma is lifted over from the vertebral column completely

The aforementioned technique should be done with no hesitation. Merits far supersede cost in the given situations. Attempts to preserve both structures are a waste of time, blood, and effort of the patient and the team.

For tumors with adequate tissue planes, lateral dissection progresses seamlessly to the posterior dissection as the surgeon pulls on the tumor. Tumors with extensive desmoplastic reaction do not follow this. The lateral dissection is difficult and so is the posterior dissection. The lateral dissection does not take the surgeon seamlessly to the posterior one. In addition, they both will require too much sharp dissection and cautery. Tissues turn to sort of a "multilayered clothing" blending in with surroundings, and hence they require handling and cutting more or less like a parenchymatous organ harboring a tumor inside it that you cannot avoid cutting through it.

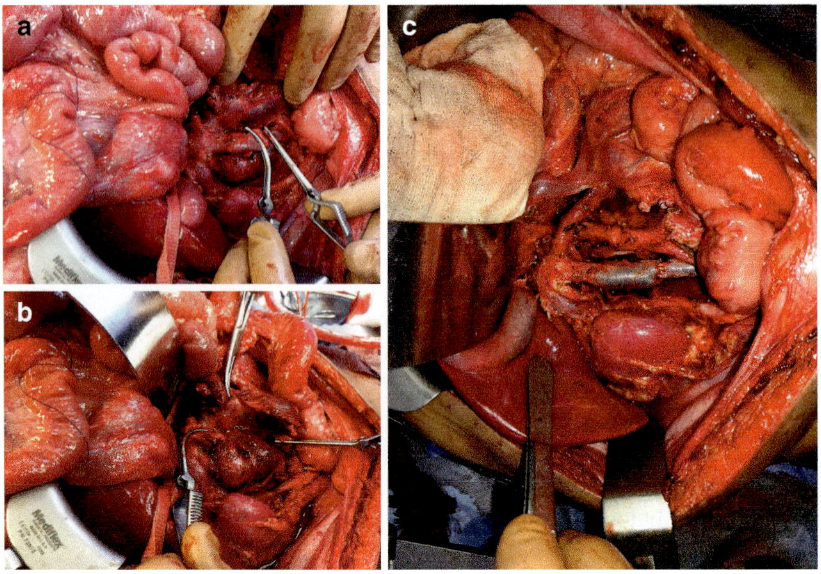

Fig. 32.13 Cut to flip technique; (**a**) the IVC is transected caudally. (**b**) The resultant exposure and facilitation of posterior dissection and dissection from aorta. (**c**) Reanastomosis of the IVC

If the tumor is infiltrating the posterior abdominal wall laterally, i.e., the musculature not the vertebral column, here lateral dissection might be very bloody and requiring too much traction on the tumor risking their rupture which is a thing to be avoided at any cost. To avoid this, it is highly recommended to change the position of the patient from supine to lateral position while doing the lateral/posterior dissection. The time and effort consumed to do so is a very good investment indeed and should not be refrained from.

32.3.1.6 Vena Cava Clamping

Clamping of the vena cava can have some significant hemodynamic effects. An already compromised lumen should lessen such effects. Infrahepatic clamps are almost systematically tolerated without any specific preparation. Suprahepatic clamps on the contrary need special consideration. A test-clamp should be put on the proximal control and the operation is to be paused for a while. When the anesthetist reassures that the clamp is well tolerated in terms of hemodynamic effects, handling the cava can then start. If signs of hemodynamic instability are observed, the clamp is to be released until necessary measures are implemented, and the test is repeated.

Measures to enhance tolerance of this clamp are known to anesthetists. Before test clamping it might be helpful to put the operating table in a head-down position for few minutes in order to allow pooling of the blood in the upper half of the body.

Unless readily accessible and clear, it is recommended to defer the top control of the cava after the bottom control and the Pringle's maneuver. In case the vena cava is injured during dissection in this relatively tight space, there will be an opportunity to lessen the bleeding by cross-clamping of the distal cava as well as occlusion of the Pringle's maneuver. If the repair can be done in these conditions, then well and good. If not, the hole is to be compressed and the liver returned back to rest on it. After which a sternotomy is to be performed and the intrapericardial cava is to be clamped. This is to be followed by returning back to the hole to get the necessary repair done.

Though total cross-clamps of suprahepatic vena cavas will eventually be tolerated by most if not all patients, it is to be mentioned that sometimes even the mere traction on the looped-around hepatic veins might cause considerable hypotension. Should hypotension happen unexplainably during surgery, it is recommended to have a look at the slings looping round the hepatic veins. Even when they look innocent, they might need to be loosened *completely or even removed, and the liver is to be returned back to the abdomen in the normal position.*

32.3.1.7 Vena Cava Grafting

Of the Threshold to Resect and Replace the Cava

In short, cavas that are easily dissectable from the tumor are to be dissected and left in place.

Adherent cavas will require harsh manipulation. They are not expected to perform better than the graft after this harsh manipulation; they will probably occlude anyway. In this case if there is a technical advantage of removing the cava in terms of blood loss or access and safety of dissection of other more important structures, namely, aorta and its branches, the surgical team is then advised to keep a low threshold to cross-clamp the cava and resect it. Please see section for lateral and posterior dissection.

Of the Best Caval Replacement Conduit

There is a reasonable sum of literature on the topic from which one can come out with valuable information about this issue [1, 2].

For small defects requiring patch graft, pericardial autografts serve as a good option as well as prosthetic grafts.

For full-circumference segment replacement, the body of literature present in the topic supports that PTFE is the conduit of choice. However, it is to be mentioned that not much Dacron grafts have been used for the purpose in the first place; those who have been used have performed as good.

In conclusion, if PTFE is available then it is reasonable to give it priority. However, if it is not available Dacron can be used instead.

The need for ring enhancement has been recommended by authors justified by the low pressure in the cava. However, it is to be remembered that the native cava is even of a more pliable wall than any graft. Therefore, ring-reinforced grafts are not to be considered a must unless for any reason the surgeon judges the presence of anatomical changes that will obviously compress the cava. An example of this is replacement of intrahepatic vena cava that required complete freeing from the central tendon.

Of the Implantation of a Single Renal Vein in the Graft

Caval resections above the level of renal veins would entail temporary interruption of renal vein and reimplantation into the graft (Fig. 32.8b rt.). This interruption might take time and is liable to postoperative thrombosis.

Risk on the remaining kidney can be assessed by various methods (Table 32.5). Temporary occlusion while observing urine output and observing the kidney for color and turgidity changes indicates congestion. This can be supplemented by intraoperative Doppler and invasive pressure measurement of the occluded renal vein stump. The presence of high pressure indicates venous outflow obstruction. Not much of this situation is written about in literature to conclude the figures that indicates absolute safety of the kidney. If all parameters are normal after clamping, it is well understood that there should be no worry. Yet how far can we drift from normal in each parameter and still stay safe is yet to be determined in future work and publications. For now, the author recommends that if no change in the abovementioned parameters happens for 30 min, then it is reasonable to assume that the kidney is having efficient collaterals. This is not very surprising as a tumor that requires resection of the cava must have narrowed its lumen and hence stimulating the collaterals development. If the parameters drift from normal, it will be left to the surgeon and radiologist to make a decision about the possible impact of this abnormality. It is recommended to have the Doppler done by a radiologist experienced in kidney transplant. His input will be based on experience from a close setting.

Table 32.5 Assessment of efficiency of collateral venous circulation

Assessment of efficiency of collateral venous circulation
1. Cross-clamping test and observing urine output, turgidity, and color
2. Doppler assessment during cross-clamping
3. Venous stump pressure

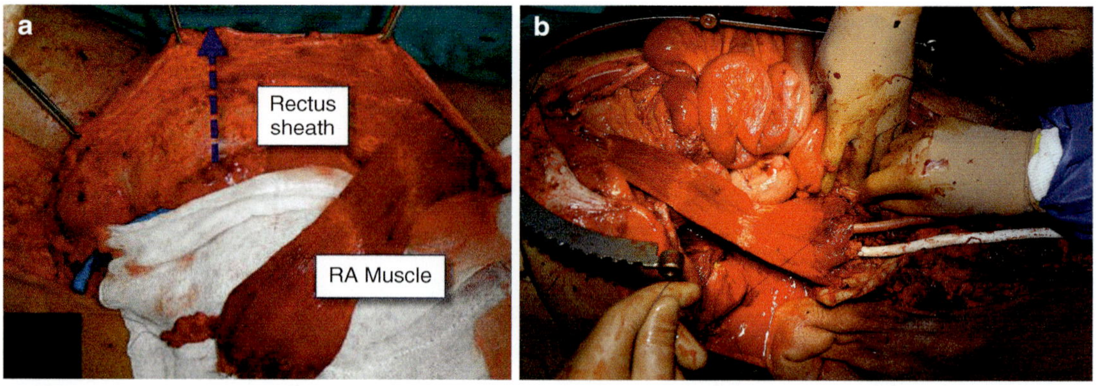

Fig. 32.14 (**a**) The rectus abdominis muscle (RA muscle) extracted from within the sheath before making the transverse extension of the wound marked by the blue dotted arrow. (**b**) Intra-abdominal placement of the muscle to cover suture lines. Here to cover the proximal anastomosis of a PTFE graft to iliac vessels as well as an inferior vena cava suture line after resection of huge abdominal mass invading abdominal wall and extending to groin

It is important to note that, while doing the assessment of efficiency of the collateral venous circulation of the kidney, the kidney is not to be mobilized or dissected for the purpose of better visualization. It should and it is always possible to do so while the kidney is still in place and not dissected. Mobilization and dissection can lead to disturbance of collaterals.

Of the Need for Muscle Cover for the Repaired Cava

The field after resection of these tumors is usually peritoneum-void leaving the repaired cava in contact with bowel. None of the authors who investigated the topic have reported the use of routine muscle cover. None reported enteric-caval fistulas as well.

Based on the author's personal experience as well as others, perhaps it is reasonable to say that if there is no concomitant bowel anastomosis, then there is no need for routine muscle cover.

If there is one, then separation of the suture lines by omentum or muscle should be the rule unless it is very difficult to attain. The muscle of choice in this situation would be the rectus abdominis muscle superiorly based or inferiorly based according to the situation. This is important to plan ahead before the incision since bilateral transverse incision will cut through the muscle bilaterally. In this situation the procedure can start by raising the muscle from within the sheath before making the transverse cut (Fig. 32.14). Careful interpretation of the scans should inform about the need for bowel resection. Bowel resections away from caval suture lines need not be taken into consideration.

32.3.1.8 Inviting an Old Technique: Vena Caval Compartmentalization

Nothing in the surgeons' pocket to guard against thrombosis of the harshly treated cavas other than anticoagulation and hemodilution. The use of anticoagulation should be balanced against the risk of bleeding specially in the first postoperative day after a surgery with an extensive raw area.

Guarding against pulmonary embolism in a setting where anticoagulation might be contraindicated is a call for a vena caval filter. Placing a filter preoperatively requires awareness of its presence during surgery. Maneuvering the cava risks the dislodgement of the filter. If taking this caution is not preferred or if filters are not available, resorting to an old technique can be an alternative, which is compartmentalization of the cava by three to five polypropylene sutures [3, 4]. Figure 32.15 demonstrates the technique.

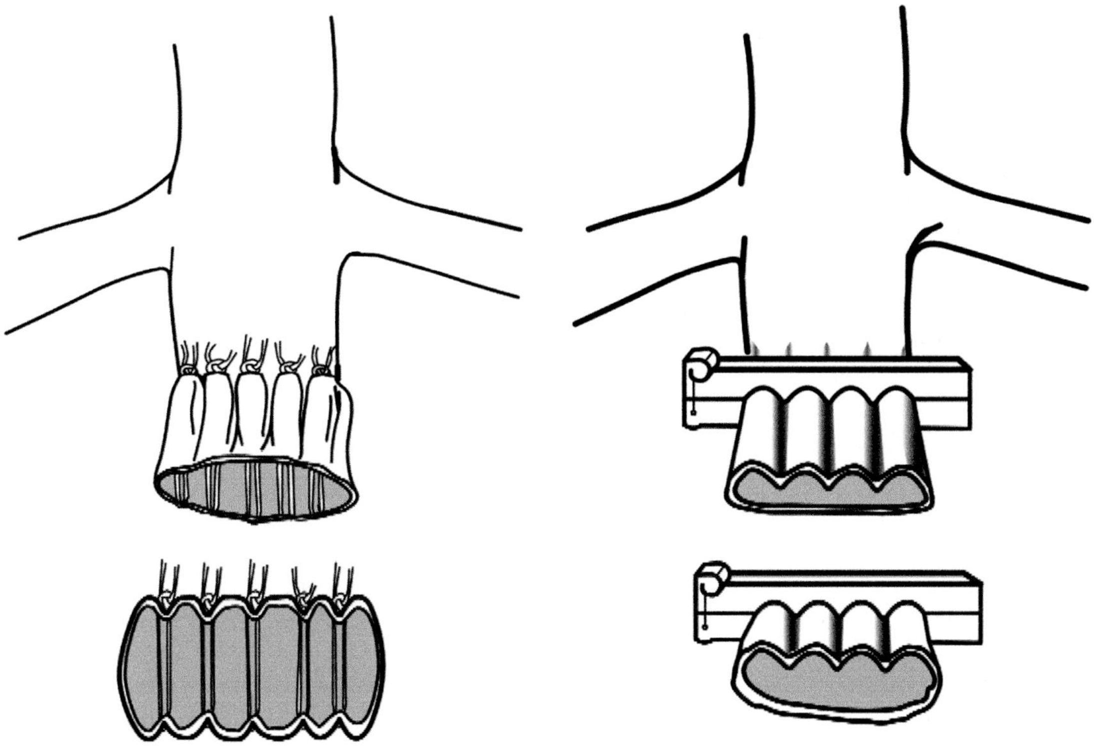

Fig. 32.15 Vena cava compartmentalization by plication technique using interrupted polypropylene sutures or by application of a specialized clip

32.3.2 Adjunctive Techniques

This section presents three adjunctive techniques that can be used. They are not basic components. Their place and indication are explained.

- Shunting and intraoperative balloon occlusion
- The use of cell savers
- In situ perfusion and ex vivo surgery

32.3.2.1 Shunting and Intraoperative Balloon Occlusion

Shunting the vena cava is a procedure that is usually required for trauma setting rather than for resection of tumors. Its application is particularly of usage for retrohepatic vena cava and intrahepatic vena cava. Shunting is not a maneuver to stop the bleeding. Vascular exclusion of the liver is the procedure that is intended for lessening of the bleeding; shunting is an adjunct to the vascular exclusion that allows flow from the lower body to reach the rt. atrium during the vascular exclusion. It is used when the vascular exclusion results in significant hypotension. It maintains a decent venous return for a patient who has already lost a significant amount of blood. The aforementioned scenario is not the usual case for vena cava-related tumor surgery. However, still it might happen. The options for shunting are veno-venous bypass or direct shunting by cuffed endotracheal tube of appropriate size [5, 6].

Balloon occlusion on the other hand is a method to stop bleeding. A Moore-Pilcher balloon is inserted through the femoral vein and advanced to the retrohepatic vena cava. Inflation of the balloon occludes the cava as well as the entry of the hepatic veins [5].

If inadvertent trauma to cava occurs or is expected, shunting might be still utilized in tumor surgery the same way it takes place in trauma.

In such a situation it is might be more accessible to introduce the shunt from a more caudal segment of the vena cava in a field with regular anatomy rather than from the rt. atrium.

Table 32.6 Maneuvers to prevent air embolism in low pressure cavas

1. Direct manual sealing of the injury
2. Rush to the top control first before bottom control and porta hepatis control
3. Valsalva maneuver by anesthetist
4. Filling the field with saline solution with a rt. shoulder uptilt to prevent saline from pouring out

Table 32.7 Signs of low pressure in cava

1. Direct measurement of CVP reflects pressure in cava if the patient is lying flat
2. Absence of profuse bleeding from caval injury
3. Brisk venous pulsations in the vena cava

It is helpful to do the vascular exclusion in the following sequence: clamping the porta hepatis first and squeezing the liver manually to push the blood out to the hepatic veins followed by caval distal control and finally caval proximal suprahepatic control.

If the caval pressure is low, one should either do direct manual sealing of the injury, rush to the top control first before bottom control and porta hepatis control, perform Valsalva maneuver, or fill the field with saline solution all aiming at preventing air embolism (Table 32.6). Patients who do *not* bleed profusely from an injured cava are the ones of concern, for this indicates that the pressure in the cava is low, and therefore the possibility of sucking air is more likely. Table 32.7 lists signs of low caval pressure and therefore higher probability of air embolism.

32.3.2.2 The Use of Cell Savers

As is the case with surgery for any form of malignant disease, the use of cell savers is controversial. Investigators found that the probability of presence of malignant cells in the scavenged blood is relatively high [7, 8].

Two integral questions are still not completely answered: do these cells have the capacity to become metastases? If they do, is this risk more than the risks associated with allogenic blood transfusion? It is out of the scope of this text to discuss this literature in thoroughness. This has been tackled comprehensively in transfusion literature [9].

Since the issue is not finally resolved by transfusion specialists, surgeons therefore need to make their choice. What relates here is that in very few occasions the use of cell savers will be found necessary should the abovementioned strategies be entertained. It might be helpful to have it in the operating room for very special situations or for use after taking the tumor out. The use of cell savers while the tumor is still in is a matter of judgment and choice of the operating team which entails knowledge of the pathology, natural history of the disease being handled, and indeed the patient and his preferences. It will be a choice between permitting blood loss with its consequences—particularly the need for allogenic transfusion—in one side and the risk of permitting malignant cells of an unknown potential to get through to the blood stream.

32.3.2.3 In Situ Perfusion and Ex Vivo Surgery

Ex vivo resections are indicated for hepatic segment of vena cava. They entail complete extraction of the liver altogether with the IVC and indeed the tumor followed by bench surgery. This will require liver wash by an organ preservation solution (e.g., HTK solution) and cooling for the length of bench surgery. This technique has been more widely used and described by authors involved in management of *Echinococcus granulosus* infestation of the liver than in patients with malignancy in general. They reported liver bench time of 360 min well tolerated by the liver [10–12].

An alternative is in situ perfusion; in this technique only a caval segment is divided proximal and distal and the liver extruded from the abdomen yet the porta hepatis is left uncut and used—while in place—to flush the liver with preservation solution which is flushed out of the liver through the cut caval ends and sucked out of the field. It obtains a bloodless caval and liver dissection along with a better access to hepatic veins confluence area. After resection, these can be replanted in the native cava or to a graft according to the situation.

Ex vivo resections for tumoral surgery have been utilized by some authors with promising results [13].

The author would see ex vivo surgery as the future of cancer surgery not only to decrease blood loss and improve accessibility but also there might be an oncological advantage for this technique. Most of retroperitoneal resections entail dissection of important structures. Ex vivo surgery will enable these dissections to be done on the bench, and hence minimizing tumoral spillage should rupture or capsule breaches occur while trying to dissect intimate important structures.

32.3.3 Special Situations

- Off-pump excision of cavo-atrial junction thrombi
- Advocating staging and multiple sittings surgery: merits and philosophy of

32.3.3.1 Off-Pump Excision of Cavo-atrial Junction Thrombi

Cavo-atrial junction thrombus approached by heart bypass is widely described in the literature. "Vena cava freeing" technique described earlier can be applied up to this segment enabling such excisions to take place off-pump. This avoids cannulation and heparinization. This requires the following maneuvers (Fig. 32.16):

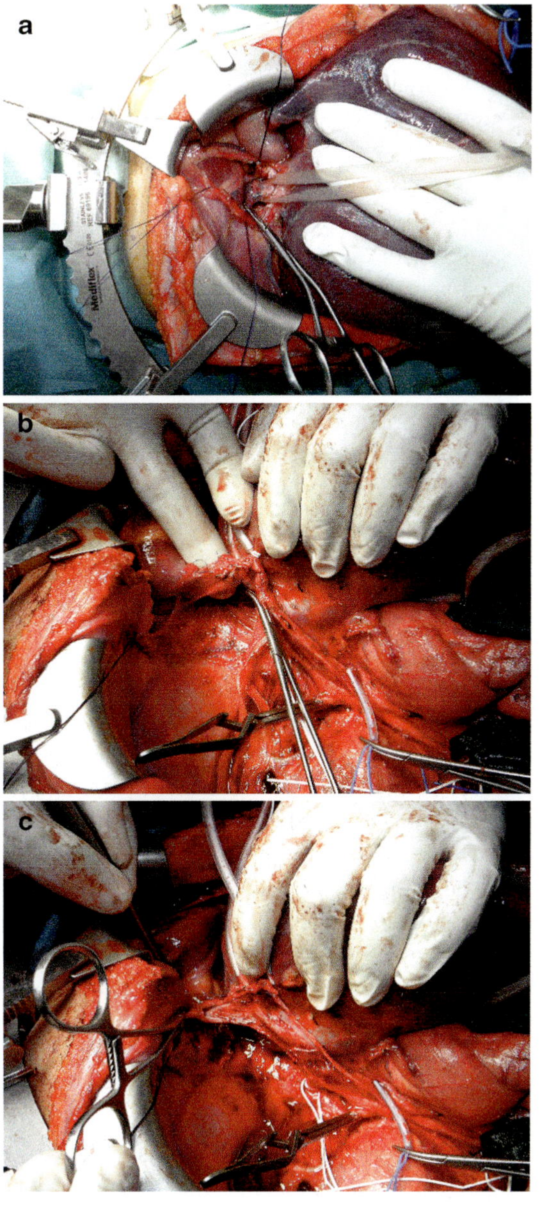

Fig. 32.16 (**a**) Exposure without sternotomy. Vena cava exposed yet not freed as necessary. (**b**) With sternotomy and vena cava completely freed denoted by the surgeon's finger passing behind the whole length of the suprahepatic cava from the heart to liver. (**c**) Vena cava clamped and opened. Note that freeing enabled placing the Satinsky clamp in a manner obtaining an extra centimeter in cranial direction by sliding cranially over the cavo-atrial junction now clamping on a bit of the atrial wall. This enabled rising over the top of the cavo-atrial junction thrombus off-pump

1. Division of the central tendon of the diaphragm longitudinally from sternum to few millimeters above the suprahepatic vena cava cut then encircles the cava leaving a cuff of central tendon on the caval wall.
2. This cut will lead the surgeon to the pericardial cavity seamlessly without much awareness of cutting the pericardium as a separate layer owing to the adherence of the pericardium to the central tendon in this area. The heart is protected from injury by cutting the central tendon-pericardium in the same manner that one cuts the peritoneum while entering the abdomen, pulling on a small bit between two artery forceps and making a small snip till entry takes place. This can be

started in the sternal side of the cut or even better halfway between the sternum and cava. The surgeon should be able to examine the span of the presumed cut and feel where the heart pokes the least while pulsating, and this spot is probably a favored spot for making the entry snip. The region near the cava is better avoided for the initial entry as the central tendon here fans and merges with cava and will make entry to the pericardial sac awkward.
3. Ligation of inferior phrenic vessels.
4. Freeing the cava posteriorly from the crus of the diaphragm (described earlier).
5. A low threshold to perform a sternotomy with or without manubriotomy.

32.3.3.2 Advocating Staging and Multiple Sittings Surgery: Merits and Philosophy Of

One thing about lengthy surgeries and surgeries that entails hemodynamic shifts is that they require a patient with a good physiological reserve. Several methods in medicine are in use to preoperatively assess the physiological reserve of different organ systems in a rather objective way.

In any surgery, patient's physiological status gets monitored minute by minute. The monitors in current practice offer you a panoramic view of this minute, yet they do not offer an eye on integral questions: "How much of the aforementioned physiological reserve is in action to offer the figures on the monitor? How much is still left in the reserves? For how long will they be able to do the required compensation to keep the physiological figures the way they are on the monitor?"

For instance, a mobile phone with a battery full will open up and do the call. When only 4% charge; it will still open up and do the call. Only when the call lasts long will the difference between the two shows up. One will continue and the other will *shut down* in the middle of the call.

We do not have the "% of battery charge" display in any medical monitor, and therefore it is sometimes difficult to tell when will the physiological reserve "shut down." We only have our experience with these kinds of procedures correlated to some rough parameters like age range and preoperative assessment abovementioned. Simple factors like inadequate thermal control inside the O.R. can drain a patient's reserve far faster than expected.

Most of vascular and cardiac surgeries are "one go" surgeries in which you cannot but have it all in one sitting.

The case for resection surgery in oncovascular practice is different. The strategy abovementioned allows staging of the procedure in more than one sitting. It is an approach in which one can pull out in the middle of it—say after the first two phases—in one sitting and defer the others a week later. One other way of drawing the line between the sittings is the use a certain time interval for the sitting. A range of 4 h of anesthesia and operative time in these surgeries is a good landmark after which the wounds are closed in an extra hour and the patient transferred to the ward or ICU. The author recommends as well that the team takes a break in the middle of the sitting, an "obligatory" break in a sense.

By the author's direct observation, patients have been explored up to 10 days after the initial sitting, and the field was as exact as was left and even clearer. The concern about getting adhesions in such an interval is not true.

Add to this the value of giving the surgical team an opportunity to custom a more detailed plan to the second sitting after having the opportunity to acquire the givens learned in the first.

It is reasonable to assume that if the team is coming out of the surgery drained, then probably the patient is in jeopardy. An unnecessary one indeed, given the opportunity to stage the surgery. Loosing such an opportunity is such a waste.

There is nearly no cost paid for such staging. Proper information fed to the patient about this plan obviates the inconvenience of having to do two or three surgeries. It is all about anticipation. When anticipated it is well accepted.

It is not about doing "a heroic" surgery; it is about making "a heroic" surgery regular.

This has been the author's practice in multiple occasions. It has never been regretted. What has been regretted—in fact—is not doing so, when it has been listened to the monitors portraying that the patient's physiology is doing well and that the operation can carry on.

To make this clearer we all know that the adrenal gland is critical in stress. Its store of adrenaline and cortisol is key in these situations. As well, the liver glycogen is the source of energy. Current monitoring devices and techniques offers absolutely no idea about how much of these have been used and how much is left. This is a frontier to anesthesia and critical care medicine indeed.

In between the sessions, it is advisable to institute TPN. This should supply the building blocks for the reserves that one wishes to replenish.

Staging has been practiced and praised by different authors in similar situations [14, 15].

32.4 Critical Note on Postoperative Care and Specific Complications

32.4.1 Anticoagulation

Anticoagulation has been commented on earlier in the section "Inviting an old technique: Vena cava compartmentalization." Hemodilution and hydration are as relevant as anticoagulant drugs and should be sought with focus. Hematocrit is to be kept between 25 and 30%. Blood transfusion should be kept to the minimum need.

32.4.2 Monitoring

The standard monitoring applies. Add to this a specific requirement.

For tumors that require dissection around the superior mesenteric artery (SMA) and in pediatric population who require "mobile evisceration" of the small bowel in the manner described, the occurrence of superior mesenteric artery thrombosis is a possibility. It is a deadly pathology and somehow silent. It does *not* necessarily reflect on *clinical and vital signs* with the gravity that calls for immediate exploration. Serum lactate has to be monitored closely with a *low threshold* for exploration. It is critical therefore to keep the patient volume replaced properly to avoid conflicting interpretation of high serum lactate and metabolic acidosis. These will commonly be attributed to general hypoperfusion. A well-perfused patient who still has acidosis and high lactate is one who is harboring a locally ischemic tissue somewhere in his body. The abdomen is a high-profile suspect.

When "mobile evisceration" of small bowel is utilized, it might be of value to stitch back the rt. colon to the paracolic gutter and the root of small bowel to retroperitoneum to prevent twisting over the SMA now acting as the only support.

The use of monitoring ileostomy (closed loop) for the first 48 h is to be considered in situations where SMA has been handled roughly.

It is left to reader to place these adjuncts as appropriate guided by (1) magnitude of bowel mobilization and SMA dissection and (2) efficiency of postoperative hemodynamic management and monitoring in each given setup.

This complication has been encountered by the author in pediatric population. The message is that the presence of a background disease in the vessel is not a necessity at all. Still in healthy vessels an eye has to be kept and the diagnosis entertained.

If a patient is diagnosed with the condition—specially in pediatric population with small vessels—instead of accessing the SMA directly, it is recommended to access the SMA through a transverse aortic arteriotomy opposite to SMA takeoff. This is a convenient access for thrombectomy, flushing, and thrombolytic therapy injection, the repair of which is more accessible and less likely to invite thrombosis in itself (Fig. 32.17).

32.5 Perioperative Mortalities and Oncological Outcome

32.5.1 Perioperative Mortalities

The author's experience with the application of the abovementioned strategies and techniques is given here. These series are not all published to the moment. The results are given here to draw some light to the perioperative outcome. Sixty-five patients in different centers have been

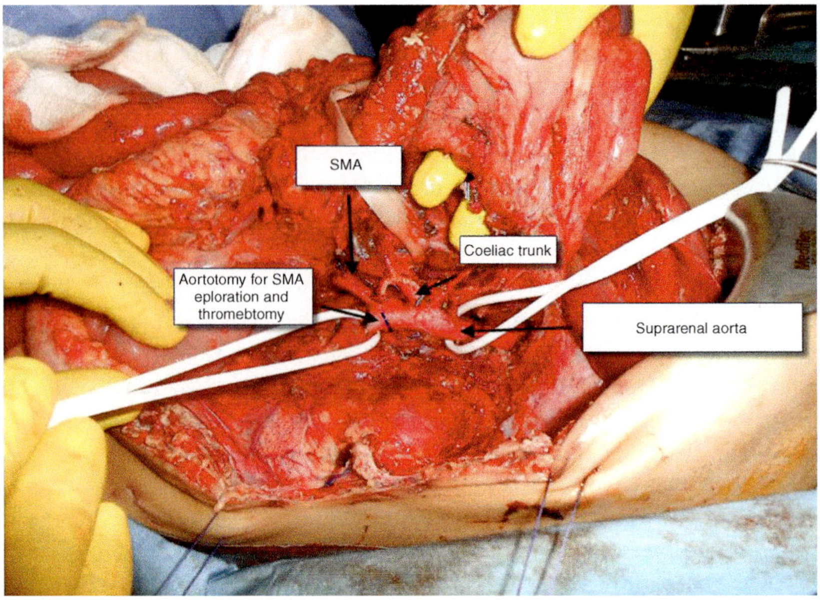

Fig. 32.17 Access to SMA and SMA thrombectomy through transverse aortic arteriotomy opposite to SMA origin (shown by dotted line)

managed, 35 of which were vena caval thrombi and 30 had centrally located retroperitoneal tumors encasing either cava alone *or cava and aorta*. One of the former 35 died. Three of the latter 30 died perioperatively which makes a perioperative mortality rate of 6.1%. Significant morbidities include a single patient with postoperative renal vein thrombosis and ATN that resolved with exploration, thrombectomy, and supportive medical treatment without the need for dialysis.

32.5.2 Oncological Outcome

Each of the case reports and series present in literature encompass a variety of tumors in terms of anatomical origin, stage, and histopathology [1, 2, 16–23]. It is not applicable therefore to release a survival rate for the entity "vena cava-related tumors." What brought them together is the need for application of a unified technical approach. Each of which is expected to follow—in terms of survival—the same figures that are expected for their counterparts of the same histopathology and tumor biology, etc.

For instance, a neuroblastoma encasing the cava will follow the same rules that govern survival in neuroblastoma in general which is, in this occasion, the risk stratification in common use putting into effect an interplay between five different factors that includes tumor stage, N-myc amplification, and others.

Should the decision to operate or not is to be based on the expected oncological outcome; this will need to be made patient by patient with proper patient counseling.

This abovementioned concept has been put to test and investigated by authors in the field of pancreatic adenocarcinoma. Matched results have been found when patients who required arterial resection along with the pancreaticoduodenectomy are matched to retrospective controls who did not require vascular resection [24].

32.6 Reproducing the Service and the Making of the Oncovascular Surgeons and Service

In a dedicated future publication, the author intends to address this topic in detail. For now, a note on the basic concepts that will be introduced is going to be mentioned and these are:

First: This is a *hybrid technique* between oncology, vascular, microvascular, and transplantation surgeries.

Second: The system proposed to produce these oncovascular surgeons is intended—contrary to presumption—*not* to be labor intensive or extended over a long duration. It is intended to be an economic model of surgical education and "training." Our current models are wasteful somehow, and it is to be admired that our medicine is still incomplete, and therefore we have to find a way to get people to learn it fast and economically to give them space, energy, and fund to look for real breakthroughs and look after their social life. That is what medicine is all about, to get people back to their social life healthy, isn't it? Medical practitioners are part of this.

32.7 Summary

- This is a unified approach to retroperitoneal tumors involving central structure in the abdomen, namely, cava, aorta, and their tributaries and branches.
- The procedure passes through four phases in a particular order.
- The phases put in this sequence allow staging, decrease blood loss, and enable management of different technical situations being it contact, infiltration, encasement, or intraluminal tumoral extension.
- Posterior dissection might require change of position of the patient.
- Posterior dissection might require cutting the cava, flipping it, and anastomosing it after resection.
- No need for cell savers in most cases.
- Tumors up to cavo-atrial junction can be removed off-pump.
- When liver resection is required, ex vivo resection or in situ perfusion can be used.
- One will never regret:
  - Staging the procedure
  - Bigger access, particularly sternotomy
  - Caval resection and replacement
- It is not about doing a heroic surgery; it is about making a heroic surgery regular and reproducible in different setups.
- Three points are yet to be made sharp in the future research:
  - How safe or unsafe are cell savers
  - *For now use to the minimum indications.*
  - Minimum parameters that indicates the efficiency of the collateral venous circulation of the kidney
  - *For now* Doppler *by a kidney transplant radiologist is the current best option.*
  - Oncological outcome for specific tumor types
  - *For now base decisions on the results of their counterparts in other anatomical locations.*

Acknowledgments The author would like to thank Dr. Hussein Khairy for his integral role in the development of the author's oncovascular surgery practice.

Thanks to Mr. Mark Tyrell for his key contribution in providing the concept of "vena cava-related tumors" and for his pushing forward to publish it.

Thanks to Mr. Morad Sallam for the time he offered providing opinion, liaising, and facilitating the publication.

Thanks to Mr. Mohamed Shahm, Mrs. Heba Eldeeb and Ms. Anna Boriak for their efforts doing the diagrammatic representation.

References

1. Hardwigsen J, Baque P, Crespy B, Moutardier V, Delpero JR, Le Treut YP. Resection of the inferior vena cava for neoplasms with or without prosthetic replacement. Ann Surg. 2000;233(2):242–9.
2. Silva E, Pedro LM, Moutinho M, Amorim P, Evangelista A, Ortiz S, López D, e Fernandes JF. Leiomyosarcoma of level II inferior vena cava; an original solution for bilateral renal vein reconstruction. Angiol Cir Vasc. 2016;12(1):55–61.
3. Eklof BGH. Deep venous thrombosis and pulmonary embolism. In: Chant ADB, Barros D'Sa AAB, editors. Emergency vascular practice. London: Arnold; 1997. p. 135–50.
4. Criado E, Johnson G Jr. Prevention of pulmonary emboli. In: Jamieson CW, Yao JST, editors. Rob and Smith's operative surgery; vascular surgery. London: Chapman and Hall Medical; 1994. p. 593–600.
5. Burch JM, Franciose RJ, Moore EE. Trauma. In: Schwartz SI, Tom Shires G, Spencer FC, Daly JM,

Fischer JE, Galloway AC, editors. Principles of surgery. Singapore: McGraw Hill; 1999. p. 190.
6. Demetriades D. Abdominal vascular injuries. In: Rutherford RB, Cronenwett JL, Glovicizki P, Wayne Johnston K, Krupski WC, et al., editors. Rutherford vascular surgery. Philadelphia: Elsevier Saunders; 2005. p. 1040–2.
7. Waters JH, Donnenberg AD. Blood salvage and cancer surgery: should we do it? Transfusion. 2009;49(10):2016–8.
8. Catling S, Williams S, Freites O, Rees M, Davies C, Hopkins L. Use of leucocyte filter to remove tumour cells from intraoperative cell salvage blood. Anaesthesia. 2008;63:1332–8. [PubMed: 19032302] 15.
9. Hansen E, Wolff N, Knuechel R, Ruschoff J, Hofstaedter F, Taeger K. Tumor cells in blood shed from the surgical field. Arch Surg. 1995;130:387–93.
10. Wen H, Dong J-H, Zhang J-H, Zhao J-M, Shao Y-M, Duan W-D, Liang Y-R, Ji X-W, Tai Q-W, Tuerganali A, Li T. Ex vivo liver resection followed by autotransplantation for end-stage hepatic alveolar echinococcosis. Chin Med J. 2011;124(18):2813–2817 2813.
11. Jianyong L, Jingcheng H, Wentao W, Lunan Y, Jichun Z, Bing H, Ding Y. Ex vivo liver resection followed by autotransplantation to a patient with advanced alveolar echinococcosis with a replacement of the retrohepatic inferior vena cava using autogenous vein grafting: a case report and literature review. Medicine (Baltimore). 2015;94(7):e514.
12. Hemming AW, Chari RS, Cattral MS. Ex vivo liver resections. Can J Surg. 2000;43(3):222–4.
13. Kato T, Lobritto SJ, Tzakis A, Raveh Y, Sandoval PR, Martinez M, Granowetter L, Armas A, Brown RS Jr, Emond J. Multivisceral ex vivo surgery for tumors involving celiac and superior mesenteric arteries. Am J Transplant. 2012;12(5):1323–8.
14. Zhang A-Q, Xue M, Wang D-J, Nie W-P, Xu D-B, Guan X-M. Two-stage resection of a disseminated mixed endometrial stromal sarcoma and smooth muscle tumor with intravascular and intracardiac extension. Taiwan J Obstet Gynecol. 2015;54:776–9.
15. Mohd Ariff S, Joehaimey J, Ahmad Sabri O, Abdul Halim Y. Two-stage surgery for a large cervical dumbbell tumourin neurofibromatosis 1: a case report. Malays Orthop J. 2011;5(3):24–7.
16. Vladov NN, Mihaylov VI, Belev NV, Mutafchiiski VM, Takorov IR, Sergeev SK, Odisseeva EH. Resection and reconstruction of the inferior vena cava for neoplasms. World J Gastrointest Surg. 2012;4(4):96–101.
17. Kobayashi T, Miura K, Ishikawa H, Soma D, Zhang Z, Yuza K, Hirose Y, Takizawa K, Nagahashi M, Sakata J, Kameyama H, Kosugi S, Wakai T. Successful re-resection for locally recurrent retroperitoneal liposarcoma at four years after ex vivo tumor resection and autotransplantation of the liver: a case report. Transplant Proc. 2016;48:1215–7.
18. Berumen J, Hemming A. Vascular reconstruction in hepatic malignancy. Surg Clin N Am. 2016;96: 283–98.
19. Goto H, Hashimoto M, Akamatsu D, Shimizu T, Miyama N, Tsuchida K, Tajima Y, Ohuchi N. Surgical resection and inferior vena cava reconstruction for treatment of the malignant tumor: technical success and outcomes. Ann Vasc Dis. 2014;7(2):120–6.
20. Castelli P, Caronno R, Piffaretti G, Tozzi M, Lomazzi C, Dionigi G, Boni L, Dionigi R. Surgical treatment of malignant involvement of the inferior vena cava. Int Semin Surg Oncol. 2006;3:19.
21. Sarkar R, Eilber FR, Gelabert HA, Quinones-Baldrich WJ. Prosthetic replacement of the inferior vena cava for malignancy. J Vasc Surg. 1998;28:75–83.
22. Bower TC, Nagorney DM, Cherry KJ Jr, Toomey BJ, Hallett JW, Panneton JM, Gloviczki P. Replacement of the inferior vena cava for malignancy: an update. J Vasc Surg. 2000;31:270–81.
23. Shen Z-J, Zhou X-L, Yu Y-L, Li M. One case of leiomyosarcoma of the inferior vena cava treated with radical resection and vascular reconstruction. Vasc Med. 2005;10:225–7.
24. Bachellier P, Rosso E, Lucescu I, Oussoultzoglou E, Tracey J, Pessaux P, Ferreira N, Jaeck D. Is the need for an arterial resection a contraindication to pancreatic resection for locally advanced pancreatic adenocarcinoma? A case-matched controlled study. J Surg Oncol. 2011;103(1):75–84.

33 Aortic Infection with Visceral Artery Involvement in the Endovascular Era: Treatment Options

Francesco Speziale, Pasqualino Sirignano, Laura Capoccia, Wassim Mansour, Alessandro d'Adamo, and Carlo Filippo Porreca

33.1 Introduction

In 1885, Osler described the infected peripheral aneurysms which result from endocarditis embolism for the first time [1]. Since then, the term "mycotic" has been used, in an inexact way, to identify all infected aneurysms. Theoretically, different clinical and physiopathological conditions could lead to mycotic aneurysms. Bacterial seeding can occur in normal arteries by contiguity from a nearby infectious outbreak or through vessel wall damage (e.g., atherosclerosis), with possible dangerous evolutions (perforation, suppuration, aneurysm, pseudoaneurysm), describing the typical microbial arteritis [2, 3]. Iatrogenic wall damage due to medical interventions (e.g., endovascular treatment) [4–6] or drug abuse [7–11] with an inadvertent intra-arterial injection gives rise to a local vascular infection followed by the development of a pseudoaneurysm. Bacteria could be found in the thrombus of degenerative aneurysms, even in the absence of clinical signs of infections, suggesting that a preexisting degenerative (atherosclerotic) aneurysm can be in any moment colonized by hematogenous or contiguous spread [3, 12, 13]. Last, but not least, in cases of endocarditis, septic emboli can occlude *vasa vasorum*, leading to ischemia, infection, and degeneration of the arterial wall, which develops a typical multiloculated aneurysms [1].

The diagnosis of infected aortic aneurysms is based on clinical findings and imaging features and should be made as soon as possible because sepsis and rupture frequently develop afterward [3, 14]. However, most patients are often asymptomatic or present nonspecific symptoms such as malaise and subjective fevers. In other cases, concomitant dyspnea; chest, back, or abdominal pain; nausea; gastrointestinal bleed; and jaundice, when associated with the finding of a pulsatile mass with or without associated cellulitis [9, 11, 15, 16], leukocytosis, and elevated erythrocyte sedimentation rates, should raise suspicion.

Blood cultures have been reported to be positive in approximately 75% of cases. Therefore, blood cultures alone are not sufficiently sensitive to rule out the diagnosis [7, 17]. The bacteriologic spectrum is very extensive, but *Staphylococcus* [18, 19], especially methicillin-resistant *S. aureus* [20–22], and *Salmonella* species [23] are the most common etiologic agents involved. Less frequently infected aneurysms are caused by *Streptococcus* species [8], fungal pathogens (*Candida* [24], *Cryptococcus* [25], *Aspergillus* [26]), and *Treponema pallidum*

F. Speziale (✉) · P. Sirignano · L. Capoccia
W. Mansour · A. d'Adamo · C. F. Porreca
Vascular and Endovascular Surgery Division, Department of Surgery "P Stefanini", Policlinico Umberto I, "Sapienza" University of Rome, Rome, Italy
e-mail: francesco.speziale@uniroma1.it

© Springer Nature Switzerland AG 2019
Y. Tshomba et al. (eds.), *Visceral Vessels and Aortic Repair*,
https://doi.org/10.1007/978-3-319-94761-7_33

[27–30]. Gram-negative infections are less common but more virulent than Gram-positive, due to the release of alkaline proteinase with many kinds of elastase that lead to vascular wall necrosis, graft disruption, and stump hemorrhage after reconstruction [3, 31].

Among imaging modalities, computed tomography angiography (CTA) is reasonable as the gold standard for diagnosis of infected aneurysms. The typical appearance is a saccular aneurysm or pseudoaneurysm with an absent or minimal calcification. Periaortic collections, intramural air, and soft tissue infiltration are other common radiographic findings [32, 33]. Moreover, rapidly enlarging or rapidly evolving aneurysms are highly suggestive of infection [34–37].

Additionally, ultrasound and arterial duplex can be used for initial diagnosis [11], while positron emission tomography (PET) [38–40], magnetic resonance imaging, magnetic resonance angiography [41, 42], and indium 111-labeled white blood cell scanning [43–45] could be useful to confirm the primary suspicions.

Every vessel may be involved, and patients are often immunosuppressed by their underlying condition [2, 3, 6, 11, 46–52]. For all these reasons, the multidisciplinary approach seems to be the best strategy to manage this complex condition. The approach should comprise an antibiotic strategy, surgical management, and optimal timing for surgical intervention.

Infected aneurysms still represent a big challenge for modern surgeons, despite the great strides that have been made in vascular surgery over the past decades. Antibiotic therapy alone is not enough to eradicate the problem, and so traditional surgery represents the mainstay of therapy, even carrying a significant morbidity and mortality rate [53–56]. Recently endovascular treatment has shown new ways to approach this kind of disease, like primary treatment or bridging therapy. However, invasive hemodynamic monitoring [57] and catheter-based procedures [4–6] have opened a door on the development of vascular infectious disease.

Antibiotic therapy should be initiated as soon as possible, initially as broad-spectrum and then culture-direct, and continued after surgical treatment. The duration of the course of antibiotics is variable, sometimes to lifelong courses, but in any case, no less than 6 weeks of intravenous therapy [58, 59]. Traditional infected aneurysm treatment consists of open surgical repair with resection of the infected segment, extensive local debridement, and in situ or extra-anatomic bypass [53–56].

Obviously, it depends on the location and extent of the infection, as well as patient comorbidities. Oderich et al. [17] reported the following distribution of infected aneurysms: infrarenal aorta (40%), distal thoracic aorta (16%), thoracoabdominal segment (16%), paravisceral aorta (13%), juxtarenal aorta (11%), and pararenal aorta (4%). In case of thoracic or thoracoabdominal involvement, in situ reconstruction with a homograft or antibiotic-treated prosthetic graft is the preferred treatment, with special consideration to spinal cord perfusion protection during this repair [60]. In case of infected abdominal aorta, repair can be achieved either with in situ reconstruction or by carrying out an extra-anatomic bypass [55]. If the juxtarenal or visceral aortic segments are involved, in situ repair is recommended [61], via neoaortoiliac system (NAIS) with the autogenous femoral-popliteal vein, cryopreserved arterial or venous homografts, or antibiotic-treated prosthetic grafts [49, 50, 62–68], and reimplantation of involved arteries or visceral debranching is mandatory. In particular, the most affected site is the superior mesenteric artery (SMA) [69–71], followed by the celiac artery and its branches. However, usually only a single segment is involved.

Although open repair is the established treatment, it is associated with a high morbidity-mortality rate, ranging from 10 to 44% [53–56]. Unfavorable outcomes generally result from performing major surgery in patients already debilitated by sepsis and/or massive bleeding together with having significant comorbidities. Endovascular aneurysm repair (EVAR) was first reported by Semba et al. [72], and over the past decade [17–19, 73–78], many reports of successful endovascular stent grafts for infected aortic aneurysms have been reported, as an alternative to conventional in managing infected aneurysms, especially in patients who are considered poor surgical candidates.

Improved endovascular techniques and materials brought into focus the use of endografts alone or in combination with open repair and hybrid approach [79–81].

While feasible, the implantation of an endograft within an infected area is highly controversial. In such cases, infective aortic tissue is not removed, and controversy remains not only regarding the persistence of an established local infection [82] but also with regard to the long-term durability of the endograft. Furthermore, in such patients, long-term or even lifelong antibiotic treatment may be inevitable.

33.2 Literature Review

As mentioned above, infected aortic aneurysms involving visceral aortic branches are, fortunately, not common; however, even in an antibiotic era, related mortality is still very high, and they are considered to be one of the most challenging problems faced by vascular specialists [83, 84].

Consistent with conventional infrarenal mycotic aneurysm, antibiotic treatment alone has been reported to have a mortality rate as high as 90% [85]. Historically, the preferred treatment option was surgery, even in these fields [84–86]. However, the surgical treatment of infections involving the juxtarenal or paravisceral aorta is complex; complicated and modern surgical outcomes are disappointing with mortality rates over 40% [17, 54]. For these reasons, over the years, many authors have reported a plethora of alternative, less invasive, hybrid, or endovascular approach. Here, several cases of infectious aneurysms involving visceral branches are reported, with particular attention to treatment strategies and relative results [80, 81, 87–94].

Visceral artery involvement in mycotic aneurysm was of course described long before the endovascular era began, and several different open surgical solutions have been proposed to preserve patency and eradicate infection.

In 1986, Reddy and coworkers described a case of a 7 cm saccular mycotic aneurysm that developed in the suprarenal abdominal aorta in a severely atherosclerotic 63-year-old man. At that time the infection was presumed to originate from a hematogenous inoculation of an atherosclerotic plaque. During intervention, a right axillo-bifemoral artery bypass graft was performed along with autotransplantation of the left kidney to the left common iliac vessels, and the suprarenal aorta was ligated, excised, and widely debrided. After 6 months, patient experimented a sudden occlusion of graft requiring thrombectomy for limb salvage and to preserve renal function. After a further 2-month period, an elective thoracic aorta to bilateral iliac artery bypass was successfully undertaken. Unfortunately, the patient suffered a fatal myocardial infarction at 2 weeks from surgery. Upon autopsy, a well-perfused nephrosclerotic kidney, healed aortic ligation, and no graft infections were found [87]. A few years later, in 1989, James reported a 13-year follow-up for a relatively similar patient, confirming the potential role of this kind of surgical approach [88].

Such reports and relatively good results, although probably affected by the so-called publication bias, justified the widespread use of open surgical solution even when the endovascular era was established.

In 2007, Itatani and collaborators described treatment performed to a 66-year-old man, presenting with back pain, high fever, and constipation and with a suprarenal infected abdominal aortic aneurysm involving the visceral vessels [89]. Blood cultures revealed *Bacteroides melaninogenicus*. The patient was successfully treated by an ex situ arterial reconstruction. After establishing temporary bypass from the right axillar artery to the right external iliac artery, the right renal artery, SMA, and common hepatic artery were bypassed from the right iliac artery using a Dacron graft, and the artery proximal to each anastomosis was ligated. These procedures were performed with an ascending colon and the second portion of the duodenum reflecting toward left side. The left renal artery was bypassed from the left external iliac artery using Dacron graft reflecting a descending colon, left kidney, spleen, and pancreas tail toward the right. Keeping the visceral blood flow through a temporary bypass graft from the right axillary artery, the abdominal aorta was cross-clamped between the supraceliac aorta and bilateral external and internal iliac arteries. Aneurysm wall excision and retroperitoneal space lavage were carried out. Aortic trunk reconstruction was performed using a different Dacron graft from the aorta at the diaphragm to bilateral terminal common iliac arteries with the body twisting left side to separate the graft from the infected field. In addition, omental flap was packed into the space where the aneurysm was situated. The patient had good recovery and no evidence of recurrent infection at a 31-month follow-up [89].

Dubois, in 2010, reported the first case series of 44 consecutive mycotic aneurysms, treated from 1990 to 2008 [90]. Among those patients, nine presented a juxtarenal aneurysm and two a thoracoabdominal aneurysm. Urgent surgery was performed in 18 cases (40.9%). Revascularization was achieved by in situ reconstruction in 37 patients (84.1%), while extra-anatomic reconstruction was performed in six patients (13.6%), reserving this approach to more compromised patients. One patient was treated with a combined in situ and extra-anatomic reconstruction. In 32 patients (72.7%), a transperitoneal approach to the mycotic aneurysm was performed. In 11 patients (25%), the access was retroperitoneal. A retroperitoneal approach was preferred when reimplantation or bypass of the visceral arteries was planned. In one case (2.3%), EVAR was performed. In patients with an extra-anatomic reconstruction, axillo-bifemoral reconstruction was performed in five cases (83.3%). One patient (16.7%) underwent a bilateral axillo-femoral bypass. In all of these patients, a resection of the mycotic aneurysm and a transfixion of the aortic stump with a nonabsorbable running suture and coverage by omentoplasty were carried out, followed by a debridement of all surrounding infected tissue. This second-stage procedure took place at a mean of 2 days after the extra-anatomic reconstruction. In 36 patients with an in situ repair, reconstruction to the iliac arteries was performed in 16 patients (44.4%) and to the femoral arteries in 6 patients (16.7%). Fourteen patients (38.9%) were treated with an aorto-aortic tube interposition. In 10 patients (27.8%), a Dacron graft was used, while in 13 patients (36.1%), silver-impregnated Dacron graft was used. In 18 (78.3%) of these, 23 patients were treated with a prosthetic graft. A homograft was used in eight cases (22.2%). In five patients (13.9%), an autologous deep vein was used for in situ reconstruction. Despite a such large series, only few patients required visceral or renal artery procedures. In seven patients (15.9%), visceral and renal arteries had to be reimplanted, while in five patients (11.4%), a bypass to the visceral or renal arteries was constructed. Resection of the mycotic aneurysm and rigorous debridement of all infected tissue was carried out in 43 patients (97.7%), and healing was supported by an omentoplasty in 30 cases (68.2%). Despite all reported adjunctive techniques in surgical management of infected aneurysms, in the Dubois series, in-hospital mortality was 22.7%, 50% in the extra-anatomic reconstruction group, and 18.9% in the in situ repair group. One-third (33.3%) of patients presenting with a ruptured aneurysm died in the perioperative period. Out of the 34 surviving patients, 12 patients (27.3%) died after hospital discharge and 3 (8%) showed reinfection [90].

Moving from reported good, but still unsatisfactory, results of open surgical treatment, in more recent years, several authors have proposed a "less invasive" hybrid or totally endovascular approach.

In the same year, Soule et al. reported a successful hybrid treatment to treat a 69-year-old man presenting symptomatic sacciform aneurysm of the abdominal aorta involving visceral arteries [80]. The patient's blood cultures were positive for *Escherichia coli*. CTA showed a sacciform aneurysm developed on the right side of the suprarenal aorta. The right aortic defect wall was almost punctiform measuring 17 mm in diameter and was located near the SMA origin, 18 mm above the renal arteries. The celiac trunk itself did not originate from the aortic pseudoaneurysm. However, the aneurysmal sac extended above the level of the celiac trunk. To avoid surgical risk associated with open surgical repair, the authors decided to exclude the celiac pseudoaneurysm by endograft implantation, as well as visceral debranching. A prosthetic bypass between the left common iliac artery and the hepatic artery with prepancreatic tunnel was performed, associated with direct reimplantation of SMA in the prosthesis. The infrarenal aortic wall approached to perform visceral bypass was normal. The celiac trunk and SMA area were slightly inflammatory without pus, and both their stumps were oversewn without difficulty. The graft was covered with an omentum flap. Then, a 30-mm diameter, 40-mm-length aortic endoprosthesis was implanted to exclude the pseudoaneurysm. Intraprocedural angiogram showed complete exclusion of the pseudoaneurysm and patency of all visceral vessels, without endoleak. At an 18-month follow-up, the patient remained asymptomatic without inflammatory syndrome. Enhanced CT showed complete shrinkage of the aneurysmal sac and patency of ilio-hepatic bypass and visceral arteries, in absence of graft migration or evidence of reinfection [80].

Kan, 1 year later, reported a series of 12 patients (three thoracic, two thoracoabdominal, and seven abdominal aortic aneurysms) in order to assess the supposed efficacy and outcome of EVAR for infected aneurysms with an adjunctive antibiotic treatment strategy [81]. All patients had positive blood culture reports showing *Salmonella* (ten cases), *Staphylococcus* (one case), and *Streptococcus* spp. (one case). In their experience six patients had ruptured aneurysms, and five received emergency EVAR. One patient received concomitant laparotomy for visceral vessel (right hepatic artery, SMA, and renal artery) bypass graft surgery. Three patients underwent CT-guided percutaneous drainage and one mini-laparotomy for open debridement due to persistent fever, preserving the implanted endografts. No hospital deaths occurred, while one patient (treated by TEVAR for thoracic aneurysm) died 8 months after the procedure. All other patients were well, with no evidence of EVAR graft infection, at a mean follow-up of 23.6 months (range 2–48 months) [81].

Over the years, despite the emerging role of endovascular surgery, open reconstruction has continued to perform with favorable results as in a very interesting East-European experience [91]. Petrunic et al. described a very rare and interesting case of patient with ruptured suprarenal aortic aneurysm, involving origins of visceral and renal arteries, associated with spondylodiscitis and an abscess of the left psoas muscle. After an initial medical management with antibiotics, the patient was submitted to open repair. Thoraco-phreno-laparotomy with medial visceral rotation was employed for the operative approach. A bifurcated silver-impregnated Dacron graft was used for a bypass from the uninvolved descending thoracic aorta to the uninvolved portions of the celiac trunk and SMA. The aneurysm was then opened, and a rupture of the posterior wall of 3 cm in length was identified. The aneurysm and surrounding fibrotic and necrotic tissues were debrided. Curettage of the adjacent vertebral body and disk was also performed. The resected aneurysm was replaced with a cryopreserved homograft of 25 mm in diameter. Renal arteries were reimplanted within the homograft using short silver-impregnated Dacron grafts of 8 mm in diameter. Cultures were positive for *Staphylococcus* species and *Propionibacterium* species. No recurrence of infection or other complications were evident at a 7-month follow-up [91].

Almost contemporarily, a completely different approach was proposed by Flis [92] and Reijnen [93]: both of whom suggested a role for multilayer flow-modulator stent in mycotic paravisceral aneurysms. Of note, it has been postulated that the absence of graft material provided the opportunity for the stent to remain in situ for life even in an infected field [93].

The first patient was a 50-year-old man admitted to hospital for rapid onset of intractable abdominal pain and high fever. Computed tomographic scan showed two different juxtarenal saccular aneurysms of abdominal aorta suggestive for an infectious etiology. The patient was treated with multilayer flow-modulating stent implantation in order to preserve renal and visceral artery patency. Follow-up imaging showed aneurysm exclusion and complete sac shrinkage 1 year after procedure. After 24 months, the patient was in a generally good state of health, with no recurrence of infection [92].

In accordance with the previously described paper, Reijnen presents a case of a *Salmonella serotype enteritidis*-induced rapidly expanding aortic pseudoaneurysm with a penetrating ulcer treated with a multilayer stent implantation. At 18 months of follow-up, the patient was in good clinical condition, with no infection-related signs or symptoms. CTA and 2-deoxy-2-[F18]-fluoro-d-glucose positron emission tomography/computed tomography showed a stable, mostly thrombosed aneurysm, with adequate perfusion of the side branches and no signs of recurrent or persistent infection [93].

Despite those encouraging results, recently Houston experience "rediscovered" the role of open surgery and direct visceral artery reconstruction for a mycotic aneurysm [94]. Coselli and his group described the case of a 60-year-old woman who presented with a 2-month history of back pain, associated with nausea and unintended weight loss. CT scans revealed a saccular aneurysm of the thoracoabdominal aorta, together with occlusion of the celiac artery. At hospital admission, blood and urine cultures were negative. An open Crawford extent III thoracoabdominal aneurysm repair was performed, with reimplantation of the celiac trunk using a prefabricated single-branched graft. During surgery, the opened aortic wall, visually suggestive for infection, was debrided. Intraoperative culture was positive for *Streptococcus pneumoniae*. After more than 17 months from repair, the patient was alive and free from infection [94].

In conclusion, from the few and fragmentary data in literature, it emerges that there is no unanimous consensus on the treatment of infected aortic aneurysms involving visceral vessels.

Facing this rare and difficult condition, each center must make a case-by-case choice on the intervention that feels more effective and safe. This is often based on their own experience and also on the patients' clinical and anatomical characteristics.

33.3 Personal Experience

Although our center has always been dedicated to diagnosis and treatment of primary and secondary aortic infections [95–98], in the last 8 years at Vascular and Endovascular Surgery of "La Sapienza" University of Rome, only two cases of aortic infections with visceral branch involvement have been observed and treated.

Those two cases, which are completely different in terms of clinical presentation and the surgical strategy adopted, are reported briefly.

33.3.1 Case 1

An 18-year-old female patient was admitted to our department with a history of recurrent fever, headache, lower back pain, and renovascular hypertension (250/130 mmHg). Her medical history was silent. Blood samples were normal. CTA revealed a partially thrombosed visceral abdominal aortic pseudoaneurysm with severe SMA stenosis and left renal artery occlusion. Broad-spectrum intravenous antibiotic therapy was initiated.

Due to the patient's young age, clinical presentation, and recent medical history, open surgical repair was performed in order to remove the infected aneurysm and restore all vessel patency.

Via the seventh intercostal space, the visceral pseudoaneurysm extending from the celiac trunk origin to the under renal abdominal aorta was reached. The entire aorta was found surrounded by an inflammatory tissue. A direct in situ aortic reconstruction with a 14-mm Dacron graft was performed, associated with a direct revascularization of all visceral arteries (Dacron graft for celiac trunk, SMA, and right renal artery; PTFE for preoperative occluded left renal artery).

Postoperative course was complicated by prolonged intensive care unit for multiorgan failure. Repeated blood cultures were always negative. The patient was discharged on the 27th postoperative day in a good general condition, in good clinical condition with an absence of fever, or other symptoms. Antibiotic therapy was maintained for a year following surgery. A two-year follow-up CT showed good patency of the aorta and visceral arteries with an absence of any complication (Fig. 33.1).

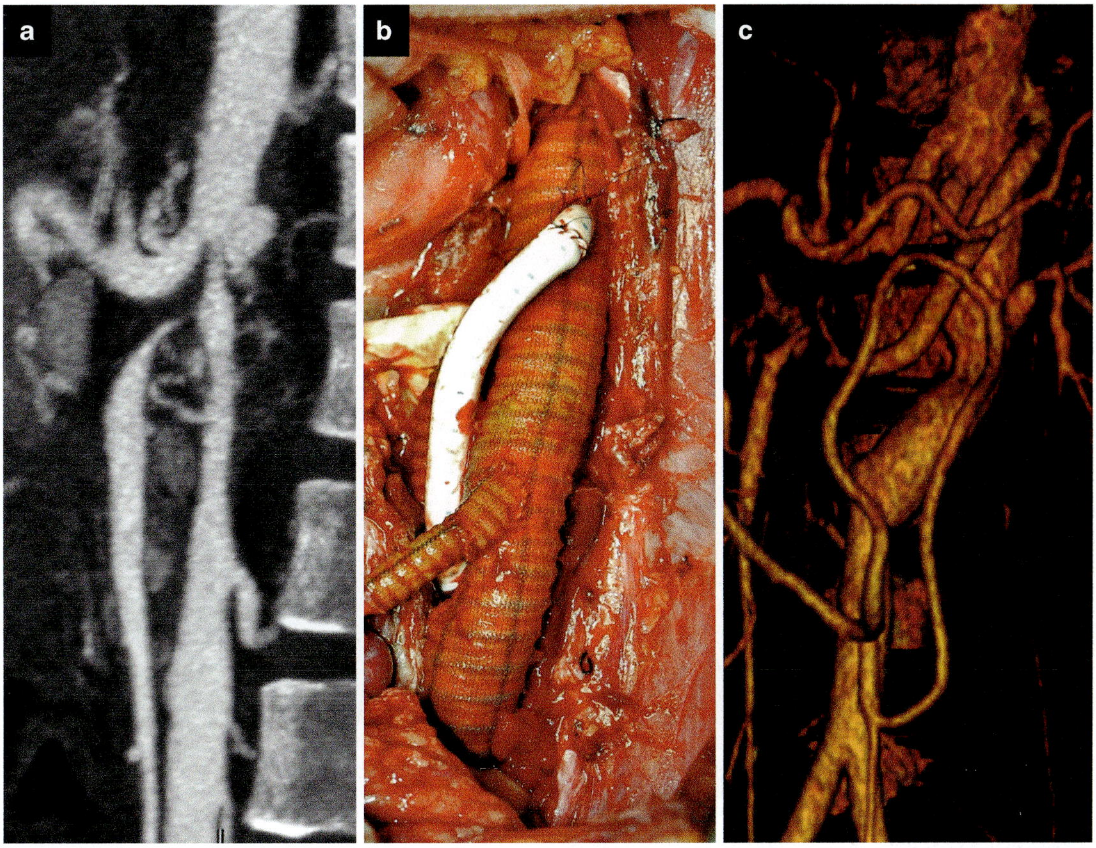

Fig. 33.1 (**a**) Preoperative multiplanar CT reconstruction showing the pseudoaneurysm associated with a narrowed aortic lumen, severe stenosis at SMA origin, and left renal artery occlusion; (**b**) intraoperative finding after extensive debridement and in situ aortic reconstruction; (**c**) postoperative CT 3D reconstruction, showing good patency of all visceral arteries

33.3.2 Case 2

An 81-year-old man was admitted to our emergency department for fever and severe anemia. His medical history was significant for mild hypertension, paroxysmal atrial fibrillation and a previous endovascular infrarenal aneurysm repair (Medtronic Endurant, 28-20-140 mm), and tobacco abuse. Physical examination revealed a palpable, pulsatile mass in the upper abdomen.

Blood test results showed hemoglobin (8.8 g/dL), peripheral white blood cells (18,500/μL), C-reactive protein (27,700 μg/L), and erythrocyte sedimentation rate (100 mm/h). Transthoracic echocardiogram revealed no evidence of endocarditis or vegetation. CTA showed the patency of the previous implanted endoprosthesis, the presence of a type IA endoleak, and a contained rupture of the visceral aorta surrounded by a nonspecific tissue with contrast enhancement. Blood culture revealed the presence of *Salmonella* spp.

The patient underwent an exclusion of the contained rupture of the paravisceral aorta and correction of the type IA endoleak by implanting two proximal aortic extensions (W.L Gore & Ass., Gore C-Tag 40-40-10 mm) with selective visceral artery stenting (W.L Gore & Ass., Viabhan peripheral endograft). Celiac trunk (9 × 100), SMA (9 × 100), and right renal artery (7 × 150 mm) were stented on a chimney fashion, while the left

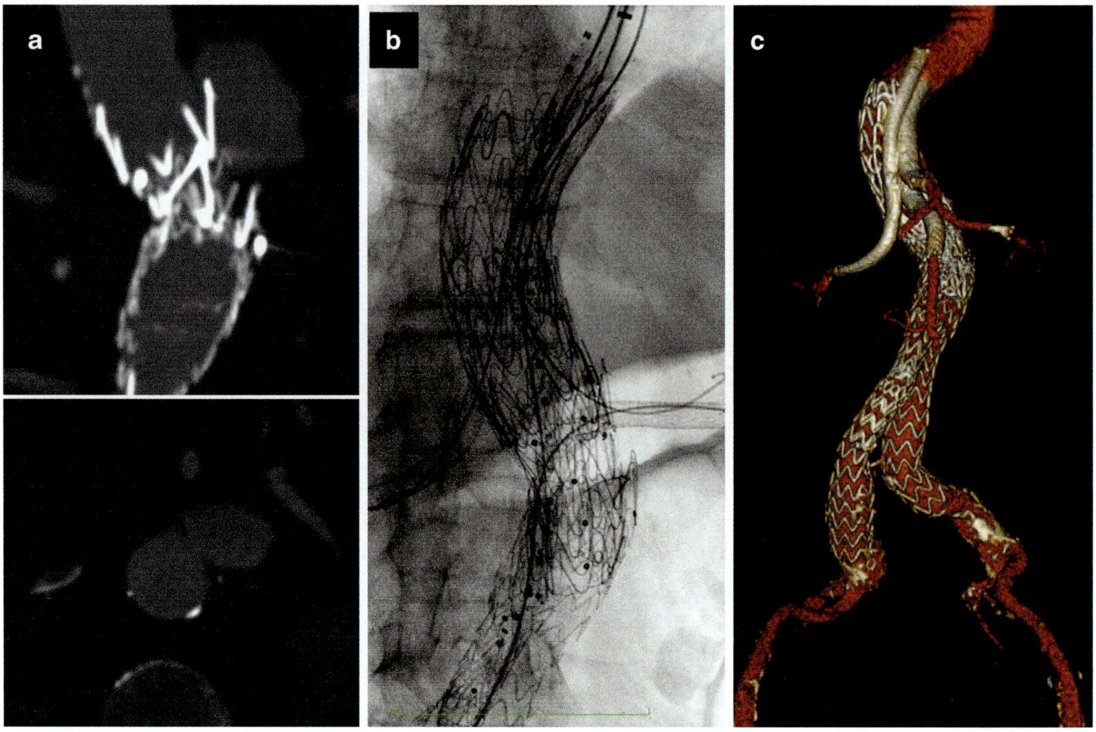

Fig. 33.2 (**a**) Preoperative sagittal and axial CT images showing the mycotic at renal arteries level, just above the implanted endograft; (**b**) intraoperative finding with all devices in place (3 chimney, 1 periscope); (**c**) postoperative CT 3D reconstruction, showing patency of all the implanted graft, complete aneurysm exclusion, and no sign of recurrent infection

renal (7 × 100 mm) was treated by periscope technique. Completion angiography showed patency of all the visceral vessels, absence of any type of endoleak, and complete exclusion of the contained aortic rupture.

The postoperative course was uneventful, and blood cultures were negative. The patient was discharged on the 18th postoperative day under levofloxacin and ceftriaxone. No evidence of recurrent infection was evident at 18-month follow-up CT scan (Fig. 33.2).

References

1. Osler W. The Gulstonian lectures, on malignant endocarditis. BMJ. 1885;1(1262):467–70.
2. Revell S. Primary mycotic aneurysms. Ann Intern Med. 1945;22(3):431–40.
3. Jarrett F, Darling RC, Mundth ED, et al. Experience with infected aneurysms of the abdominal aorta. Arch Surg. 1975;110(11):1281–6.
4. Baker WH, Moran JM, Dorner DB. Infected aortic aneurysm following arteriography. J Cardiovasc Surg. 1979;20(4):373–7.
5. Eshaghy B, Scanlon PJ, Amirparviz F, et al. Mycotic aneurysm of brachial artery. A complication of retrograde catheterization. JAMA. 1974;228(12):1574–5.
6. Samore MH, Wessolossky MA, Lewis SM, et al. Frequency, risk factors, and outcome for bacteremia after percutaneous transluminal coronary angioplasty. Am J Cardiol. 1997;79(7):873–7.
7. Anderson CB, Butcher HR Jr, Ballinger WF. Mycotic aneurysms. Arch Surg. 1974;109(5):712–7.
8. Johnson JR, Ledgerwood AM, Lucas CE. Mycotic aneurysm. New concepts in therapy. Arch Surg. 1983;118(5):577–82.
9. Padberg F, Hobson R 2nd, Lee B, et al. Femoral pseudoaneurysm from drugs of abuse: ligation or reconstruction? J Vasc Surg. 1992;15(4):642–8.
10. Patel S, Johnston KW. Classification and management of mycotic aneurysms. Surg Gynecol Obstet. 1977;144(5):691–4.
11. Reddy DJ, Smith RF, Elliott JP Jr, et al. Infected femoral artery false aneurysms in drug addicts: evolution of selective vascular reconstruction. J Vasc Surg. 1986;3(5):718–24.

12. Sommerville RL, Allen EV, Edwards JE. Bland and infected arteriosclerotic abdominal aortic aneurysms: a clinicopathologic study. Medicine. 1959;38:207–21.
13. Bennett DE, Cherry JK. Bacterial infection of aortic aneurysms. A clinico-pathologic study. Am J Surg. 1967;113(3):321–6.
14. Reddy DJ, Shepard AD, Evans JR, et al. Management of infected aortoiliac aneurysms. Arch Surg. 1991;126(7):873–9.
15. Mundth ED, Darling RC, Alvarado RH, et al. Surgical management of mycotic aneurysms and the complications of infection in vascular reconstructive surgery. Am J Surg. 1969;117(4):460–70.
16. Patel KR, Semel L, Clauss RH. Routine revascularization with resection of infection femoral pseudoaneurysms from substance abuse. J Vasc Surg. 1988;8(3):321–8.
17. Oderich GS, Panneton JM, Bower TC, et al. Infected aortic aneurysms: aggressive presentation, complicated early outcome, but durable results. J Vasc Surg. 2001;34(5):900–8.
18. Kan CD, Lee HL, Yang YJ. Outcome after endovascular stent graft treatment for mycotic aortic aneurysm: a systematic review. J Vasc Surg. 2007;46:906–12.
19. Clough RE, Black SA, Lyons OT, et al. Is endovascular repair of mycotic aortic aneurysms a durable treatment option? Eur J Vasc Endovasc Surg. 2009;37:407–12.
20. Zetola N, Francis JS, Nuermberger EL, et al. Community-acquired meticillin-resistant Staphylococcus aureus: an emerging threat. Lancet Infect Dis. 2005;5(5):275–86.
21. Utsumi T, Ohtsuka M, Uchida E, et al. Abdominal aortic pseudoaneurysm caused by prolonged methicillin-resistant Staphylococcus aureus sepsis. Int J Cardiol. 2008;5(5):294–5.
22. Karkos CD, Burnett C, Buckely H, et al. Mycotic common iliac artery aneurysm complicating methicillin-resistant Staphylococcus aureus bacteremia: an unusual cause of ureteric obstruction. Ann Vasc Surg. 2005;19(6):904–8.
23. Reddy DJ. Infected aortic aneurysms: recognition and management. Semin Vasc Surg. 1988;1:174–81.
24. Deitch JS, Plonk GW, Hagenstad C, et al. Cryptococcal aortitis presenting as a ruptured mycotic abdominal aortic aneurysm. J Vasc Surg. 1999;30(1):189–92.
25. Mostovych M, Johnson L, Cambria RP. Aortic sepsis from an appendiceal abscess. Cardiovasc Surg. 1994;2(1):67–9.
26. Mestres C, García I, Khabiri E, et al. Multiple mycotic aortic aneurysms in a drug addict. Asian Cardiovasc Thorac Ann. 2002;10(2):196.
27. Ernst CB, Campbell HC Jr, Daugherty ME, et al. Incidence and significance of intra-operative bacterial cultures during abdominal aortic aneurysmectomy. Ann Surg. 1977;185(6):626–33.
28. Murphy DP, Glazier DB, Krause TJ. Mycotic aneurysm of the thoracic aorta caused by clostridium septicum. Ann Thorac Surg. 1996;62(6):1835–7.
29. Sailors DM, Eidt JF, Gagne PJ, et al. Primary Clostridium septicum aortitis: a rare cause of necrotizing suprarenal aortic infection. A case report and review of the literature. J Vasc Surg. 1996;23(4):714–8.
30. Smith FC, Rees E, Elliott TS, et al. A hazard of immunosuppression: Aspergillus niger infection of abdominal aortic aneurysm. Eur J Vasc Surg. 1994;8(3):369–71.
31. Geary KJ, Tomkiewicz ZM, Harrison HN, et al. Differential effects of a gram-negative and a gram-positive infection on autogenous and prosthetic grafts. J Vasc Surg. 1990;11(2):339–45; discussion 346-347.
32. Lee WK, Mossop PJ, Little AF, et al. Infected (mycotic) aneurysms: spectrum of imaging appearances and management. Radiographics. 2008;28:1853–68.
33. Macedo TA, Stanson AW, Oderich GS, et al. Infected aortic aneurysms: imaging findings. Radiology. 2004;231:250–7.
34. Gomes MN, Schellinger D, Hufnagel CA. Abdominal aortic aneurysms: diagnostic review and new technique. Ann Thorac Surg. 1979;27(5):479–88.
35. Gomes MN, Choyke PL. Infected aortic aneurysms: CT diagnosis. J Cardiovasc Surg. 1992;33(6):684–9.
36. Lee MH, Chan P, Chiou HJ, et al. Diagnostic imaging of salmonella-related mycotic aneurysm of aorta by CT. Clin Imaging. 1996;20(1):26–30.
37. Rozenblit A, Bennett J, Suggs W. Evolution of the infected abdominal aortic aneurysm: CT observation of early aortitis. Abdom Imaging. 1996;21(6):512–4.
38. Spacek M, Stadler P, Bělohlávek O, et al. Contribution to FDG-PET/CT diagnostics and post- operative monitoring of patients with mycotic aneurysm of the thoracic aorta. Acta Chir Belg. 2010;110(1):106–8.
39. Bonekamp D, Smith JD, Aygun N. Avid FDG uptake in a rapidly enlarging common carotid artery mycotic aneurysm, mimicking lymphadenopathy. Emerg Radiol. 2009;16(5):383–6.
40. Davison JM, Montilla-Soler JL, Broussard E, et al. F-18 FDG PET-CT imaging of a mycotic aneurysm. Clin Nucl Med. 2005;30(7):483–7.
41. Moriarty JA, Edelman RR, Tumeh SS. CT and MRI of mycotic aneurysms of the abdominal aorta. J Comput Assist Tomogr. 1992;16(6):941–3.
42. Walsh DW, Ho VB, Haggerty MF. Mycotic aneurysm of the aorta: MRI and MRA features. J Magn Reson Imaging. 1997;7(2):312–5.
43. Brunner MC, Mitchell RS, Baldwin JC, et al. Prosthetic graft infection: limitations of indium white blood cell scanning. J Vasc Surg. 1986;3(1):42–8.
44. Chen P, Lamki L, Raval B. Indium-111 leukocyte appearance of salmonella mycotic aneurysm. Clin Nucl Med. 1994;19(7):646–8.
45. Van der Wall H, Palmer A, Thomas M, et al. Bone and leukocyte scintigraphy of a complicated case of ruptured mycotic aneurysm of the aorta. A case history. Angiology. 1994;45(4):315–9.
46. Wilson SE, Van Wagenen P, Passaro E Jr. Arterial infection. Curr Probl Surg. 1978;15(9):1–89.
47. Lewis D. Embolomycotic aneurisms. JAMA. 1909;53(22):1808–14.

48. Monson RC, Alexander RH. Vein reconstruction of a mycotic internal carotid aneurysm. Ann Surg. 1980;191(1):47–50.
49. Noel AA, Gloviczki P, Cherry KJ Jr, et al. Abdominal aortic reconstruction in infected fields: early results of the United States cryopreserved aortic allograft registry. J Vasc Surg. 2002;35(5):847–52.
50. Vogt PR, Brunner-LaRocca HP, Lachat M, et al. Technical details with the use of cryopreserved arterial allografts for aortic infection: influence on early and midterm mortality. J Vasc Surg. 2002;35(1):80–6.
51. Reid M. Studies on abnormal arteriovenous communications, acquired and congenital: report of a series of cases. Arch Surg. 1925;10(2):601–38.
52. Akers DL, Fowl RJ, Kempczinski RF. Mycotic aneurysm of the tibioperoneal trunk: case report and review of the literature. J Vasc Surg. 1992;16(1):71–4.
53. Moneta GL, Taylor LM, Yeager RA, et al. Surgical treatment of infected aortic aneurysm. Am J Surg. 1998;175:396–9.
54. Fillmore AJ, Valentine RJ. Surgical mortality in patients with infected aortic aneurysms. J Am Coll Surg. 2003;196:435–41.
55. Müller BT, Wegener OR, Grabitz K, et al. Mycotic aneurysms of the thoracic and abdominal aorta and iliac arteries: experience with anatomic and extra-anatomic repair in 33 cases. J Vasc Surg. 2001;33:106–13.
56. Hsu R, Tsay YG, Wang SS, et al. Surgical treatment for primary infected aneurysm of the descending thoracic aorta, abdominal aorta, and iliac arteries. J Vasc Surg. 2002;36(4):746–50.
57. Soderstrom CA, Wasserman DH, Ransom KJ, et al. Infected false femoral artery aneurysms secondary to monitoring catheters. J Cardiovasc Surg. 1983;24(1):63–8.
58. Chan FY, Crawford ES, Coselli JS, et al. In situ prosthetic graft replacement for mycotic aneurysm of the aorta. Ann Thorac Surg. 1989;47(2):193–203.
59. Crawford ES. Diseases of the aorta including an atlas of angiographic pathology and surgical techniques. Baltimore, MD: Williams & Wilkins; 1984.
60. Malouf JF, Chandrasekaran K, Orszulak TA. Mycotic aneurysms of the thoracic aorta: a diagnostic challenge. Am J Med. 2003;115(6):489–96.
61. Pasic M, Carrel T, Vogt M, et al. Treatment of mycotic aneurysm of the aorta and its branches: the location determines the operative technique. Eur J Vasc Surg. 1992;6:419–23.
62. Pasic M, Carrel T, Tönz M, et al. Mycotic aneurysm of the abdominal aorta: extra-anatomic versus in situ reconstruction. Cardiovasc Surg. 1993;1(1):48–52.
63. Koskas F, Plissonnier D, Bahnini A, et al. In situ arterial allografting for aortoiliac graft infection: a 6-year experience. Cardiovasc Surg. 1996;4(4):495–9.
64. Knosalla C, Weng Y, Yankah AC, et al. Using aortic allograft material to treat mycotic aneurysms of the thoracic aorta. Ann Thorac Surg. 1996;61(4):1146–52.
65. Pagano D, Guest P, Bonser RS. Homograft replacement of thoraco-abdominal aorta for a leaking mycotic aneurysm. Eur J Cardiothorac Surg. 1996;10(5):383–5.
66. Vogt PR, von Segesser LK, Goffin Y, et al. Eradication of aortic infections with the use of cryopreserved arterial homografts. Ann Thorac Surg. 1996;62(3):640–5.
67. Vogt PR, Brunner-La Rocca HP, Carrel T, et al. Cryopreserved arterial allografts in the treatment of major vascular infection: a comparison with conventional surgical techniques. J Thorac Cardiovasc Surg. 1998;116(6):965–72.
68. McCready RA, Brunner-La Rocca HP, Carrel T, et al. Arterial infections in the new millenium: an old problem revisited. Ann Vasc Surg. 2006;20(5):590–5.
69. Lorelli DR, Cambria RA, Seabrook GR, et al. Diagnosis and management of aneurysms involving the superior mesenteric artery and its branches. A report of four cases. Vasc Endovasc Surg. 2003;37(1):59–66.
70. Messina LM, Shanley CJ. Visceral artery aneurysms. Surg Clin N Am. 1997;77(2):425–42.
71. Fong A, Navuluri R. Infected superior mesenteric artery aneurysm. Semin Interv Radiol. 2016;33(1):61–4.
72. Semba CP, Sakai T, Slonim SM, et al. Mycotic aneurysms of the thoracic aorta: repair with use of endovascular stent-grafts. J Vasc Interv Radiol. 1998;9:33–40.
73. Lee KH, Won JY, Lee DY, et al. Stent graft treatment of infected aortic and arterial aneurysms. J Endovasc Ther. 2006;13:338–45.
74. Patel HJ, Williams DM, Upchurch GR, et al. Late outcomes of endovascular aortic repair for the infected thoracic aorta. Ann Thorac Surg. 2009;87:1366–72.
75. Ting AC, Cheng SW, Ho P, et al. Endovascular stent graft repair for infected thoracic aortic pseudoaneurysms—a durable option? J Vasc Surg. 2006;44:701–5.
76. Zhou T, Guo D, Chen B, et al. Endovascular stent-graft repair of mycotic aneurysms of the aorta: a case series with a 22-month follow-up. World J Surg. 2009;33:1772–8.
77. Tiesenhausen K, Hessinger M, Tomka M, et al. Endovascular treatment of mycotic aortic pseudoaneurysms with stent grafts. Cardiovasc Intervent Radiol. 2008;31:509–13.
78. Hsu RB, Lin FY. Infected aneurysm of the thoracic aorta. J Vasc Surg. 2008;47:270–6.
79. Jones KG, Bell RE, Sabharwal T, et al. Treatment of mycotic aortic aneurysms with endoluminal grafts. Eur J Vasc Endovasc Surg. 2005;29:139–44.
80. Soule M, Javerliat I, Rouanet A, et al. Visceral debranching and aortic endoprosthesis for a suspected mycotic pseudoaneurysm of the abdominal aorta involving visceral arteries. Ann Vasc Surg. 2010;24:825.e13–6.
81. Kan CD, Yen HT, Kan CB, et al. The feasibility of endovascular aortic repair strategy in treating infected aortic aneurysms. J Vasc Surg. 2012;55:55–60.
82. Sharif MA, Lee B, Lau LL, et al. Prosthetic stent graft infection after endovascular abdominal aortic aneurysm repair. J Vasc Surg. 2007;46:442–8.

83. Kritpracha B, Premprabha D, Sungsiri J, et al. Endovascular therapy for infected aortic aneurysms. J Vasc Surg. 2011;54(5):1259–65.
84. Gibbons CP. What is the best treatment for primary infected aortic aneurysms? Eur J Vasc Endovasc Surg. 2011;42(5):625–6.
85. Soravia-Dunand VA, Loo VG, Sali IE. Aortitis due to Salmonella: report of 10 cases and comprehensive review of the literature. Clin Infect Dis. 1999;29(4):862–8.
86. Forbes LT, Harding GE. Endovascular repair of Salmonella infected abdominal aortic aneurysm: a word of caution. J Vasc Surg. 2006;44(1):198–200.
87. Reddy DJ, Lee RE, Oh HK. Suprarenal mycotic aortic aneurysm: surgical management and follow-up. J Vasc Surg. 1986;3(6):917–20.
88. James EC. Suprarenal mycotic aortic aneurysm: surgical management and follow-up. J Vasc Surg. 1989;10(3):359–60.
89. Itatani K, Miyata T, Komiyama T, et al. An ex-situ arterial reconstruction for the treatment of an infected suprarenal abdominal aortic aneurysm involving visceral vessels. Ann Vasc Surg. 2007;21(3):380–3.
90. Dubois M, Daenens K, Houthoofd S, et al. Treatment of mycotic aneurysms with involvement of the abdominal aorta: single-centre experience in 44 consecutive cases. Eur J Vasc Endovasc Surg. 2010;40(4):450–6.
91. Petrunic M, Mestrovic T, Loncaric Y, et al. In situ repair of a mycotic suprarenal aortic aneurysm using a cryopreserved aortic homograft and visceral debranching in a patient with spondylodiscitis and left psoas muscle abscess. Ann Thorac Cardiovasc Surg. 2013;19(5):394–8.
92. Flis V, Matela J, Breznik S, et al. Treatment of primary infected juxtarenal aortic aneurysm with the multilayer stent. Vasc Endovasc Surg. 2013;47(7):561–5.
93. Reijnen MM, van Sterkenburg SM. Treatment of a Salmonella-induced rapidly expanding aortic pseudoaneurysm involving the visceral arteries using the Cardiatis multilayer stent. J Vasc Surg. 2014;60(4):1056–8.
94. Dolapoglu A, de la Cruz KI, Coselli JS. Management of a mycotic thoracoabdominal aortic aneurysm involving the celiac artery. Tex Heart Inst J. 2016;43(6):528–30.
95. Fiorani P, Speziale F, Calisti A, et al. Endovascular graft infection: preliminary results of an international enquiry. J Endovasc Ther. 2003;10(5):919–27.
96. Ducasse E, Calisti A, Speziale F, et al. Aortoiliac stent graft infection: current problems and management. Ann Vasc Surg. 2004;18(5):521–6.
97. Menna D, Capoccia L, Sirignano P, et al. Infective etiology affects outcomes of late open conversion after failed endovascular aneurysm repair. J Endovasc Ther. 2015;22(1):110–5.
98. Capoccia L, Speziale F, Menna D, et al. Preliminary results from a national enquiry of infection in abdominal aortic endovascular repair (registry of infection in EVAR—R.I.EVAR). Ann Vasc Surg. 2016;30:198–204.

34 Management of Aortic Infections: Role of Open Surgery and the Value of Multidisciplinary Team Approach

Morad Sallam, Oliver Lyons, and Tommaso Donati

34.1 Introduction

Aortic graft infection is known to be a very complex and challenging pathology, whether it is a surgical graft or an endograft, and despite of all the recent surgical and medical advances, it still carries a significant risk of morbidity and mortality. Since the first aortic endograft was inserted by Volodos and colleagues in Ukraine, the use of endografts in aortic disease has increased dramatically [1–3]. The majority of early endograft explantations were performed for complications in device insertion and deployment and persistent endoleak causing sac expansion. Stent infection was first reported in 1993 and is now thought to occur in 1–4% of endografts, resulting in major morbidity, mortality and economic cost [4–10]. It is unclear whether or not the incidence of endograft infection is increasing, but the use of endografts in infected fields such as mycotic aneurysms or aorto-enteric fistulae will result in an ongoing case load [6, 11–13]. There are few data available to guide management, and clinical approaches to this complex condition differ widely with variable outcomes, but consensus diagnostic criteria have been defined [14]. Large multicentre retrospective analyses have been performed using the Swedish vascular dataset and in France and the USA [9, 11, 12, 15]. Multicentre prospective data collection is underway by the Management of Aortic Graft Infection Collaboration (www.gsttbrc.com/MAGIC) [14, 16].

No aortic endoprosthesis is designed to ever be removed, and doing so presents several unique challenges to the vascular surgeon. As yet there are no methods for percutaneous endograft removal, and therefore open surgery is mandatory and entails all of the major operative risks that the initial endovascular repair was designed to avoid. This is of particular concern for infection affecting the visceral segment. Whilst some endografts are removed electively or urgently, the patient may also present with haemorrhage through an aorto-enteric, aorto-bronchial or aorto-cutaneous fistula, and disease affecting the visceral segment will frequently involve these a fistula [17]. Proximal and distal control is usually sought beyond the anatomic limits of devices which are often positioned just distal to important arterial branches, for example, the renal,

M. Sallam (✉)
Vascular Surgeon, Guy's and St Thomas' NHS Foundation Trust London, London, UK

King's College London, London, UK
e-mail: morad.sallam@gstt.nhs.uk

O. Lyons
Vascular Surgery, Academic Department of Vascular Surgery, School of Cardiovascular Medicine & Sciences, BHF Centre of Research Excellence, St Thomas' Campus, King's College London and King's Health Partners, London, UK

T. Donati
Vascular Surgeon, Guy's and St Thomas' NHS Foundation Trust London, London, UK

© Springer Nature Switzerland AG 2019
Y. Tshomba et al. (eds.), *Visceral Vessels and Aortic Repair*,
https://doi.org/10.1007/978-3-319-94761-7_34

subclavian or carotid arteries. Several devices incorporate active fixation with hooks, barbs or anchors to secure the device to the aortic wall preventing migration; these and any bare stent may become incorporated into the wall and make removal difficult. In the setting of infection, it is necessary to remove additional devices such as internal iliac artery embolisation coils if these are within the infected field. Thus complex surgery is required in patients who may have been deemed unfit for open surgical management of their original disease. It is usually not necessary to remove extra-anatomic grafts, for example, those used to de-branch the arch or a femoral-femoral crossover graft, if these are remote from the operating field and well incorporated into the tissues. Once the main device and other infected prosthetic materials have been removed, the arterial circulation must be reconstructed, and in the case of infection, this should not involve placing new prosthetic material in the infected field. Previously this has been by axillobifemoral bypass, but attention has moved towards in situ reconstruction using biological materials [18–25].

34.2 Diagnosis of Aortic Prosthetic Infection

A high index of suspicion is required for diagnosis because the clinical presentation can be varied and occur at any time after graft insertion [10]. A detailed history and examination are essential not just for aortic graft infection (AGI) diagnosis but also determining aetiology and associated features (such as spinal osteomyelitis, visceral fistulae) that must also be managed [26]. Mycotic aneurysms may remain occult for many months. Conversely, because the morbidity and mortality of graft explantation (or even lifelong antimicrobial therapy) are so great, a high degree of certainty is required in AGI diagnosis. Most clinical series on aortic graft infection and mycotic aneurysms have reported their diagnostic criteria as being a combination of 'clinical, radiological and microbiological' features but have always been vague about how these have been applied [15, 27]. Historically, the way in which these three groups of factors should be combined has not been addressed, hindering conglomeration of data and precluding future trial design [5, 28–31]. Consensus diagnostic criteria for the *suspicion* and *diagnosis* of AGI have now been published, allowing consistent diagnosis in future studies and guiding the investigation of suspected AGI (Fig. 34.1) [14]. Aortic graft infection (AGI) is *suspected* in a patient with any isolated major criterion or minor criteria from two of the three categories: clinical/surgical, radiological or laboratory. AGI is *diagnosed* in the presence of a single major criterion, plus any other criterion (major or minor) from another category. Note that where microbiological investigations identify potential 'contaminant' organisms (e.g. coagulase-negative staphylococci, propionibacteria, corynebacteria and other skin commensals), a minimum of (1) two intraoperative specimens, (2) two blood cultures or (3) one intraoperative specimen plus one blood culture must be positive with an indistinguishable organism in each sample based on antibiograms or a recognised typing method, e.g. pulsed-field electrophoresis. These criteria have subsequently been utilised in the diagnosis of mycotic aneurysms [20].

34.3 The Role of 18F-FDG PET/CT and Labelled Leucocytes

Most AGI is suspected based on CT angiography [14, 32]. Both 18F-FDG PET/CT and SPECT-CT allow accurate localisation of sites of inflammation, and these investigations are invaluable in the diagnostic workup of AGI, both in the confirmation of AGI (as part of the diagnostic criteria) and in their ability to identify occult non-aortic infection or other causes of inflammation (e.g. vasculitis), thereby preventing unnecessary surgery [33–47]. MRI may have a very limited role [48, 49].

The 18F-FDG uptake in both normal aorta and in aneurysmal (untreated) aorta has been well defined in a large number of patients, with an upper limit of SUV_{max} of 3.8 [14]. Others have suggested a high degree of sensitivity and specificity in the diagnosis of aortic graft infection using SUV_{max} cutoffs between 3.8 and 8, and further work is required in this area. The positive predictive value of PET/CT may be improved by

	CLINICAL / SURGICAL	RADIOLOGY	LABORATORY
MAJOR CRITERIA	• Pus (confirmed by microscopy) around graft or in aneurysm sac at surgery • Open wound with exposed graft or communicating sinus • Fistula development e.g. aorto-enteric or aorto-bronchial • Graft insertion in an infected site e.g. fistula, mycotic aneurysm or infected pseudoaneurysm	• Peri-graft fluid on CT scan ≥ 3 months after insertion • Peri-graft gas on CT scan ≥ 7 weeks after insertion • Increase in peri-graft gas volume demonstrated on serial imaging	• Organisms recovered from an explanted graft • Organisms recovered from an intra-operative specimen • Organisms recovered from a percutaneous, radiologically-guided aspirate of peri-graft fluid
MINOR CRITERIA	• Localized clinical features of AGI e.g. erythema, warmth, swelling, purulent discharge, pain • Fever ≥38°C with AGI as most likely cause	• Other e.g. suspicious peri-graft gas/fluid/soft tissue inflammation; aneurysm expansion; pseudoaneurysm formation; focal bowel wall thickening; discitis/osteomyelitis; suspicious metabolic activity on FDG PET/CT; radiolabelled leukocyte uptake	• Blood culture(s) positive and no apparent source expect AGI • Abnormally elevated infalmmatory markers with AGI as most likely cause e.g. ESR, CRP, white cell count

Fig. 34.1 Diagnostic criteria for aortic graft infection. Aortic graft infection (AGI) is *suspected* in a patient with any isolated major criterion or minor criteria from two of the three categories: clinical/surgical, radiological or laboratory. AGI is *diagnosed* in the presence of a single major criterion, plus any other criterion (major or minor) from another category. *CT*, computed tomography; *FDG*, fluorodeoxyglucose; *PET*, positron emission tomography; *ESR*, erythrocyte sedimentation rate; *CRP*, C-reactive protein. Reproduced from Lyons et al., Eur J Vasc Endovasc Surg (2016) 52, 758–763

combining a SUV_{max} cutoff with visual scoring of the uptake pattern [50]. The normal limits of 18F-FDG uptake in the early period after endograft deployment or open surgical repair have not been clearly defined, and this remains a limitation to the use of 18F-FDG [51]. Several attempts to develop infection-specific PET tracers are underway [52]. All these diagnostic imaging techniques require further validation in a prospective study enrolling patients diagnosed according to standardised criteria. 18F-FDG PET/CT may continue to play an important role in monitoring the response to antimicrobial therapy once AGI has been diagnosed.

34.4 Decision-Making

In 2016 the AHA published guidelines on the management of vascular graft infections, mycotic aneurysms and endovascular infections [10]. In general these recommendations are based on a low level of evidence and are not specific to the aorta. The evidence base for the advice to make management decisions based on microbial growth, and for the duration of antimicrobial therapy, is particularly lacking. Little guidance is given on the complexities of managing the visceral segment (Fig. 34.2).

34.5 Medical Management

Detailed investigation and antimicrobial therapy will not be discussed here [53]. Multidisciplinary management involving interventional radiology, infectious diseases/microbiology and nuclear medicine (all with an interest in AGI management) is essential to guide appropriate investigation and ongoing antimicrobial therapy in all patients. We discuss all patients with suspected or confirmed AGI in a vascular infection

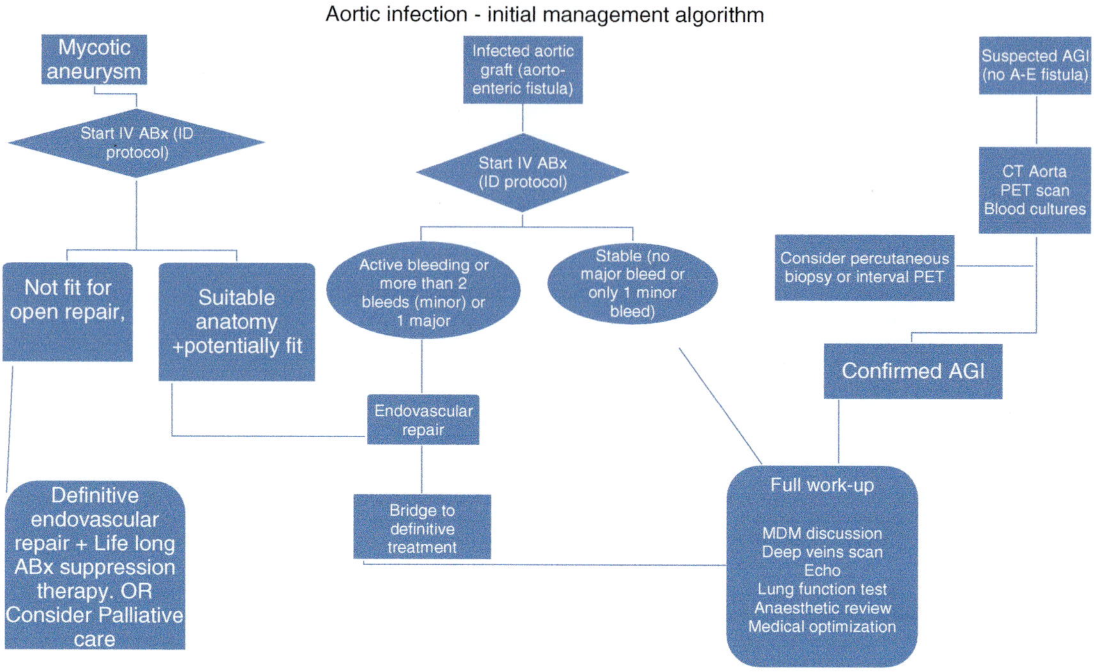

Fig. 34.2 Aortic infection initial management algorithm

multidisciplinary team meeting. Rifampicin-soaking implanted grafts may reduce infection rates in preclinical models [54]. We recommend trying to send at least three separate peripheral blood cultures before the start of antimicrobial therapy if an aortic infection is suspected. Unfortunately the diagnosis of prosthetic infection is often delayed, and many patients presenting to us have received antimicrobial therapy without adequate cultures. Further blood cultures should still be obtained. Broad-spectrum cover is almost always mandated at this stage unless a certain organism has been confirmed. We add antifungal therapy for all suspected and confirmed enteric fistula, due to the inevitable fungal contamination from the gastrointestinal tract. Once a source and an organism have been identified, the protocol should be targeted accordingly in order to minimise harm from antimicrobial therapy. There is low-quality evidence for the route and duration of antimicrobial therapy, but it is important to note the persistence of deaths with sepsis following the endovascular treatment of mycotic aneurysms and deaths from haemorrhage (local sepsis, disease extension) when infected endografts are not explanted [11, 19].

34.6 Endograft Bridging in Aorto-enteric Fistulae

In our experience of using endografts for haemorrhage control in the setting of AGI, infection persisted despite ongoing antimicrobial therapy, and all patients had died of their aortic disease within 2 years of follow-up [19]. We now therefore proceed to explantation of infected grafts wherever the patient's condition allows. We frequently use an endograft as a bridging tool, mainly to stabilise patients who present with bleeding from an aorto-enteric/aorto-bronchial fistula or rapidly expanding mycotic aneurysm. The main aim is to 'separate bleeding from sepsis' giving a chance to prepare and optimise the patient for a major operation as well as allow sufficient time for planning further management strategies.

34.7 The Role of Percutaneous Drainage and Irrigation

Aspiration may be performed for diagnostic purposes, but a *drain* should not be placed unless AGI has been confirmed [14, 55]. When time allows, drainage of collections can lead to resolution of overt sepsis (but not cure of infection) and may improve the outcome of subsequent surgery [56]. Management of AGI without explantation likely carries a far higher mortality than with explantation in the medium term. In series with longer follow-up, the mortality from leaving infected prostheses in situ can approach 100% [9, 19]. In selected patients who are deemed unfit for explantation, conservative measures such as antibiotic therapy and percutaneous drainage of pus and irrigation of the aneurysm sac may be appropriate [57–61]. Irrigation of the native aneurysm sac (in the proven absence of endoleak) or an abscess cavity with povidone-iodine or antimicrobials has been described [62–64].

34.8 Open Surgery for Visceral Segment Infection

34.8.1 Aim of Treatment

Primary aortic infection (termed a mycotic aneurysm) is associated with aortic dilatation and early rupture, whilst aortic graft infection carries a grave prognosis in the medium term [19, 65]. The main goal of treatment is to prevent death from haemorrhage. We define 'cure' as persistent eradication of infection with no need for lifelong suppressive antibiotic therapy.

Our current protocol for aortic infections considers radical surgery in the form of complete graft explantation and in situ anatomical reconstruction with a biological graft as the treatment of choice for any patient deemed to be fit enough for this operation (Fig. 34.3). The components of operative management should include:

- Excision of all infected artery and synthetic material
- Debridement of infected/necrotic tissue (source control, e.g. aorto-enteric fistula) and drainage of related collections
- Tissue sampling for microbial culture and/or PCR
- Arterial reconstruction (ideally anatomical and autologous)
- Source control (aorto-enteric fistula)

Achieving all of the above can be very challenging and certainly involves significant physiological insult with an associated inflammatory response from surgical trauma. If tolerated by the patient, the control of sepsis is achieved faster, and cure (without the need for long-term antimicrobial therapy) is feasible.

With the increased complexity of surgery resulting from infections involving the visceral segment, these aims may frequently be unachievable. The only viable option may be to temporise with an endovascular graft and lifelong suppressive antimicrobial therapy.

34.8.2 Treatment Options

- Open surgery
- Endovascular
- Lifelong antimicrobial suppressive therapy
- Short-term palliative care

34.8.3 Open Surgery

Most of the published series describing aortic graft infection suggest that 'cure' cannot be achieved without full explantation of infected grafts. Mycotic aneurysms are a different pathology to fistulae, and there may well be a chance of cure with antimicrobial therapy with an endovascular graft remaining in situ [11, 66]. This may relate the duration or preoperative antimicrobial therapy and pre-deployment 'control of sepsis', but data are inconclusive [11]. The difficulty remains in predicting the patients in whom we can safely stop antimicrobial therapy once the mycotic aneurysm has been treated,

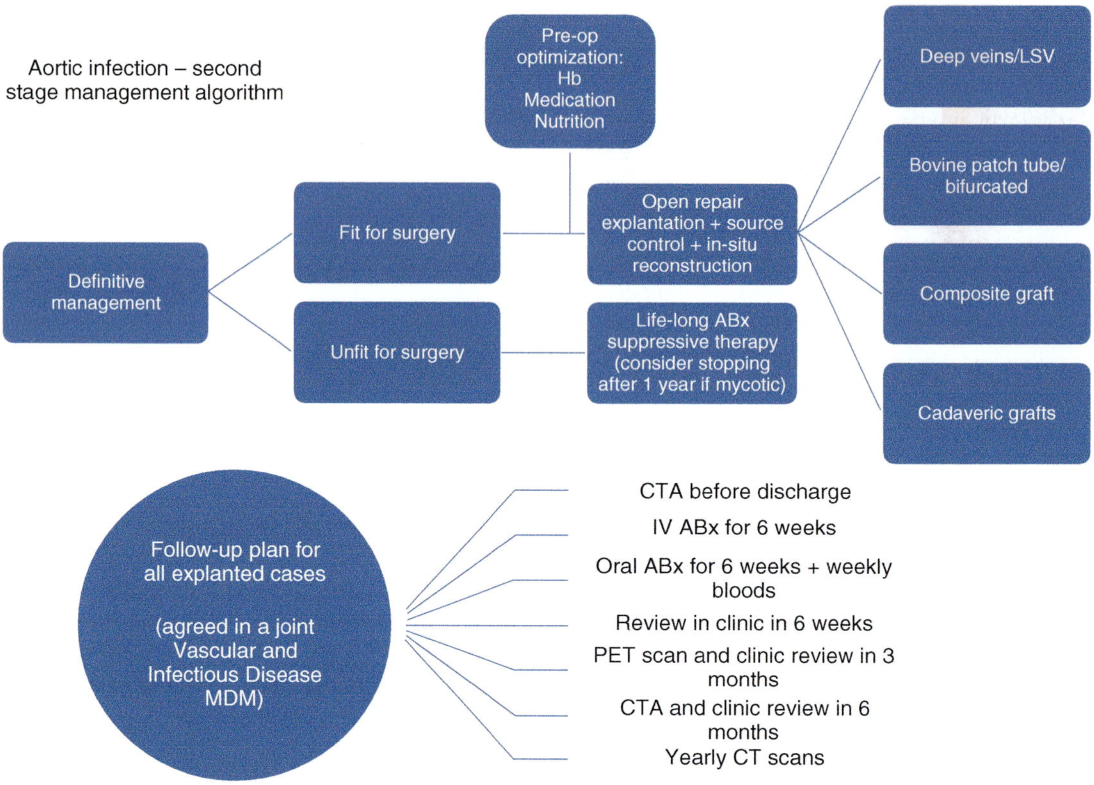

Fig. 34.3 Aortic infection second stage management

and 18F-FDG PET/CT may play an important role. The long-term outcomes of this approach remain questionable [11, 12].

34.8.3.1 Perioperative Planning Considerations

We cannot emphasise enough the importance of thorough planning in these cases. Planning is a fundamental part of the operation, required in order to achieve good outcomes. The patient's condition may deteriorate rapidly, and we suggest that these plans should be in place shortly after the patient's initial emergency presentation.

34.8.3.2 Damage Control Plan

A damage control plan allows the team to prepare well for the definitive management and to get the patient to be ready for such a major intervention. Patients may be haemodynamically unstable at presentation (or may become unstable) due to the combination of sepsis and haemorrhage. A plan to stop any bleeding, whether this is a ruptured aorta or an aorto-enteric/aorto-bronchial fistula, should always be in place. Endovascular intervention is the best option for this, and unless it has been agreed that it will be the definitive option, the aim here is to temporise the bleeding, and so endograft deployment should be planned to avoid making the complex open repair more difficult (Fig. 34.4).

Endografts are very effective in the thoracic segment. Covering one or more of the visceral arteries with a chimney or snorkel technique may be required, but we would advise to do this only when it's the only way to control haemorrhage. We would consider keeping the visceral stents as proximal as possible in the target vessel origin to

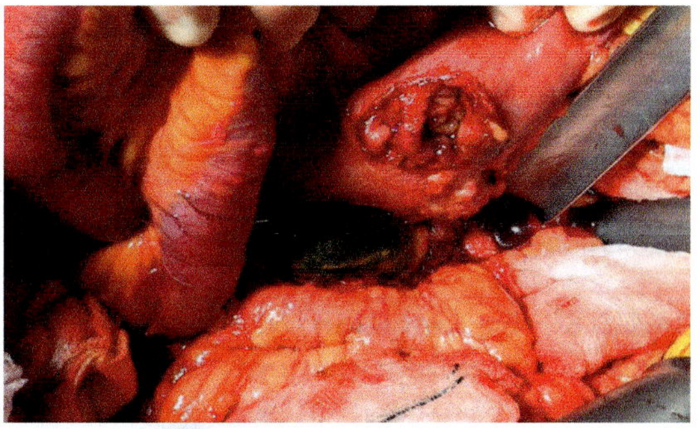

Fig. 34.4 Source control. An aorto-enteric fistula has been disconnected

facilitate future explantation. Since the aim here is to control the bleeding temporarily, long-term durability is not an issue, and the more aorta is covered, the more complex the next step will be. Consideration should be given to sites of aortic and visceral artery clamping during subsequent operations.

34.8.3.3 Preoperative Optimization Plan

This should include the preoperative workup and investigations as well as a nutrition plan and any other cardiorespiratory intervention or medical optimization to improve fitness. Some patients may require temporary filtration during that period. Anaesthetic and intensive care team involvement is valuable when it comes to the operative planning.

34.8.3.4 Intraoperative Plan

Graft explantation and aortic reconstruction are complex surgical procedures and the pathologies encountered are heterogeneous. Although the general concepts and stages of the procedure can to an extent be standardised, the details can make all the difference. For example, a failure to perform adequate debridement of *all* infected tissues may render the entire operation pointless (relative to a nonoperative management). In our experience, spending time in planning and discussing the technical details of various steps and bailout options have never been a waste of time and may highlight further risks, which may require rediscussion within the multidisciplinary team.

Involvement of the visceral segment significantly increases the complexity of these procedures. In a frail patient, open surgical procedures may be considered futile, and other alternatives including long-term suppressive therapy or indeed short-term palliation should be considered.

The following stages of this operation can be considered as separate entities for the sake of detailed planning; however, eventually there will be overlap and cross implications when it comes to the execution of the plan intraoperatively.

34.8.3.5 Access

This should be planned with consideration not only of the steps of the present operation but also bailout options and potential future operations. If at all possible, a single position for the whole procedure should be sought, avoiding the need for intraoperative repositioning. This may not always be possible. We recommend a very generous access incision from the beginning, keeping in mind access to easy vascular control (mainly the proximal), the need for cardiopulmonary bypass (full or left heart) and the possibility of enteric fistula, which will need to be disconnected and dealt with.

If the thoracic aorta is involved, we prefer a standard left thoracolaparotomy, whilst if the affected segment is totally abdominal, we tend to use a rooftop incision with a transperitoneal approach and left visceral rotation. This incision gives good access for supracoeliac control, both iliac arteries and very good exposure for the bowel, and it is very well tolerated. The incision cannot easily be extended, and if there is doubt about the proximal control, a thoracolaparotomy would be the incision of choice.

34.8.3.6 Control

Although the general concepts of aortic surgery apply here, a few extra considerations need to be kept in mind. The use of endovascular 'bridging' techniques has helped significantly in making exposure and control much more predictable, which reflects on the overall outcome. Temporary stenting allows full access and usually full preparation of the surgical field without significant blood loss or need for aortic cross clamping, thereby shortening the visceral ischaemia time.

It is very important to note that the healthy aortic wall may be further from the diseased region than is evident on the preoperative CT scan, i.e. the normal diameter aortic adjacent to mycotic aneurysms may be infected and unable to hold sutures (or endografts). The extent of infected artery can progress very quickly, and what was previously a healthy zone for clamping can become weakened in the days between the scan and the operation. A CT scan within a week of surgery is ideal and sometimes just preoperative if in doubt of any progression.

Adhesions and obliterated tissue planes may mandate more generous control, at least initially, and clamps can subsequently be moved closer to the reconstruction area once explantation has been completed, in order to reduce the visceral ischaemia time.

Particular consideration must be given to endovascular stent grafts with suprarenal fixation, which typically extends for a few centimetres and across the origins of the visceral vessels up to coeliac origin. We usually use two proximal clamp sites, one for the explantation and then a second more distal clamp for the reconstruction [67–73].

If the distal control site is the iliac arteries, then balloon endoclamping may save a lot of time and the hassle of difficult dissection and avoid iliac vein injuries. It is particularly helpful when the right iliac artery is not easily accessible in a left thoracolaparotomy.

34.8.3.7 Specific Considerations for Thoracic Aorta

If the thoracic aorta is involved, then a thoracotomy will be required; we recommend cardiopulmonary bypass to be used in these cases whether a left heart bypass or a deep hypothermic circulatory arrest, depending on the extent of repair and the site of the proximal clamp. A short shunt bypass or a right axillobifemoral bypass could also be used to allow distal and visceral perfusion as an alternative but less controlled technique, and the use of cardiopulmonary bypass is recommended.

34.8.3.8 Explantation and Debridement

Once the proximal and distal control sites are fully dissected and ready for clamping, following a brief rehearsal of the following steps with the team, the dissection should now extend distally towards the affected segment of the aorta aiming at trying to identify visceral vessel origins from the outside and also take some samples for microbiology. In some cases this would allow moving the proximal clamp a bit distal or at least prepare the second clamp space to minimise the visceral ischaemia time (Fig. 34.5).

34.9 Techniques of Reconstruction

There are many techniques described in the literature for reconstruction, and although using an in situ biological graft is our preferred option, sometimes it is deemed to be too complex, risky or not feasible; hence, other options of reconstruction should be considered. Regardless of the reconstruction material chosen, continued infection (sometimes termed 'reinfection') is a significant problem in a proportion of patients [74, 75].

A very important decision to be made ideally in the preoperative planning stage is whether the visceral vessels will be reconstructed with a visceral patch or separate branches, which could be tailored within the graft or made separately as an extra-anatomical bypass. The backup of selective visceral perfusion should also be considered. If on cardiopulmonary bypass selective visceral perfusion techniques can be used, and if not a shunt bypass at least to the SMA allows more time to reconstruct the visceral segment.

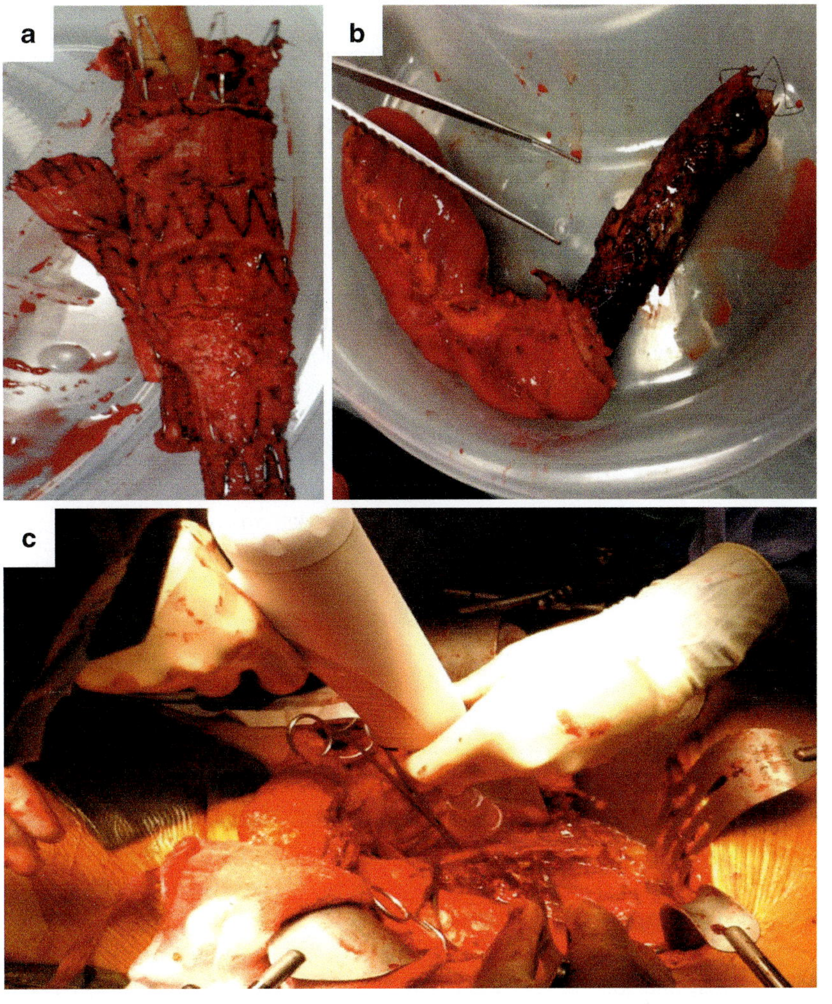

Fig. 34.5 Explanted aortic grafts. (**a**) Explanted endograft with suprarenal fixation. A large intraluminal Foley catheter was used for proximal supracoeliac endoclamping during explantation. (**b**) An aortic endograft has been removed en bloc with a section of duodenum containing duodenal stents (initially placed to treat radiation-induced strictures). (**c**) Extensive pulse lavage of the operative site after debridement of all infected tissues

34.9.1 Extra-anatomic

Right axillobifemoral bypass has always been the most popular option; the ease of the procedure and being away from the infected field made it the gold standard for a period of time; however, sometimes with visceral segment involvement, other options have to be considered [18]. Ascending to infrarenal is a more complex option; however, it allows direct jump grafts to revascularise the visceral vessels. Separate bypasses from the iliac arteries to any of the visceral vessels or hepato-/spleno-renal bypass could also be considered.

Bowel perfusion is of paramount importance, and at least one of the superior mesenteric or coeliac arteries should be perfused as soon as possible.

34.9.2 Deep (Femoral) Veins

Using one or two (panelled) femoral veins is our current preferred option for reconstruction of the aorta (type 4, supra- and juxtarenal); the versatility of the graft, resistance to infection and being autologous make it a very good option. It is time-consuming and adds potential complications of the vein harvest to the procedure (Fig. 34.6) [21].

34.9.3 Spiral Vein Reconstruction

Spiral reconstruction entails using a small calibre vein to create a larger diameter graft to match the aortic diameter. By stitching the longitudinally

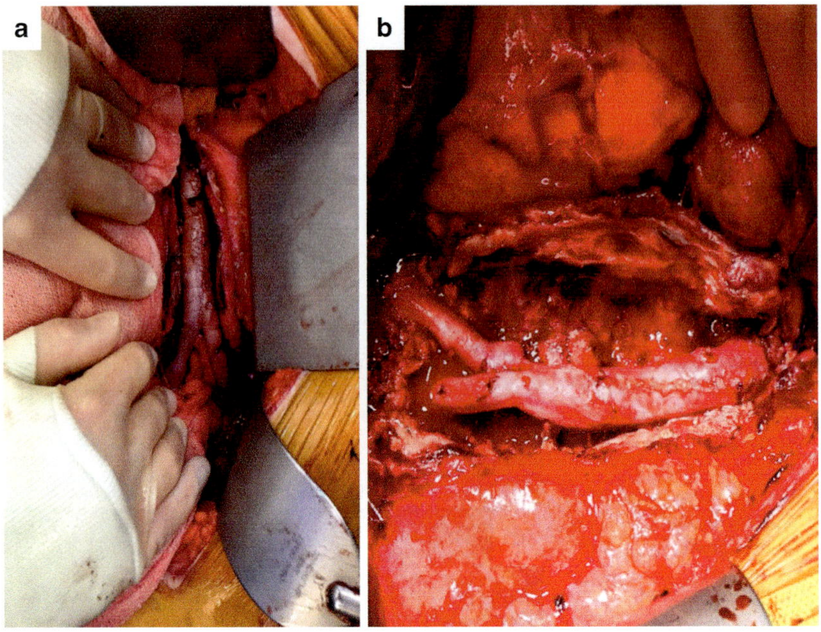

Fig. 34.6 Bifurcated NAIS. (**a**, **b**) Bifurcated neo-aorto-iliac system using superficial femoral veins for in situ reconstruction through transperitoneal and retroperitoneal approaches

spatulated vein in a spiral manner, any diameter can be created; however, this is usually time-consuming with a very long suture line and in visceral segment reconstruction that is less than ideal.

34.9.4 Cryopreserved Human Allografts

Cryopreserved homografts have been an option for the last few decades and have gained more popularity recently with comparable results to deep veins graft in some recent series [76, 77]. Due to calibre match, it's usually the preferred option in the thoracic aorta. Visceral jump grafts can be constructed using a femoropopliteal arterial homograft or native long saphenous or femoral vein.

34.9.5 Rifampicin-Bonded Grafts

There is some evidence that rifampicin-bonded or rifampicin-soaked grafts may allow reasonable outcomes in the medium term [78, 79].

34.9.6 Bovine Pericardial Tube Grafts

This is a relatively new technique and entails an off-label use of the bovine pericardial patches to make a tube [20, 80]. The technique is gaining in popularity as a reconstruction option. It offers a readily available 'off the shelf' solution that can be constructed on the bench to the required diameter and configuration even before the start of the operation. There are a few published reports showing good short-term outcome; however, long-term outcomes are yet to be assessed [20].

34.9.7 Endograft Preserving Techniques

The literature is plagued by small series with relatively short-term follow-up, but some successes have been reported without endograft explantation [81]. Washout, debridement, continuous irrigation and omental wrap techniques are some of the available tools; however, the long-term outcomes remain highly dubious, and we recommend keeping this option as a last resort [82].

34.9.8 Postoperative Care

This can be a long in-hospital journey, and in many cases, the early postoperative days require multi-organ support. Ideally the early postoperative period should be in an intensive care unit, with continuous multidisciplinary team input. The combination of sepsis, major surgical trauma and potentially bleeding can only be tolerated with very prompt and comprehensive postoperative care. Acute kidney injury and cardiorespiratory complications are not uncommon and need to be managed expectantly. If there are any doubts of bleeding, ongoing sepsis or bowel malperfusion, we recommend a very low threshold for early imaging or even re-exploration.

Long-term antimicrobial treatment is a fundamental part of the postoperative care; the details of the antimicrobial treatment are beyond the scope of this chapter.

34.10 Conclusion

Aortic graft infection is fatal in the medium term without explantation and either in situ or extra-anatomic reconstruction. In the visceral segment, this carries a substantial morbidity and mortality; many patients will be unfit for surgical repair, and so optimal multidisciplinary therapy (with the aim of suppression of infection) may remain the mainstay of treatment for many. By definition AGI is suspected when mycotic aneurysms are treated with endografts (a graft placed in an infected field). With appropriate antibiotics cover not all cases progress to reach the diagnostic criteria for AGI, and survival without explant of the graft in the medium term has been shown to be feasible in undetermined groups. Long term outcomes are yet to be assessed and deaths with sepsis do occur. Importantly and towards development of evidence-based clinical guidelines that are presently lacking, the development of diagnostic criteria for AGI provides a consistent diagnostic standard, essential for future clinical trial design and meaningful comparison between diagnostic and therapeutic strategies. Working on developing management strategies using a multidisciplinary team approach could have a positive impact on surgical outcomes. A special focus must be placed on reducing the incidence of aortic graft infection [83].

Acknowledgement Vascular Infection Multidisciplinary team at Guy's and St Thomas' NHS Foundation Trust

Rachel Bell Consultant Vascular Surgeon

Nicholas Price Consultant in Infectious Diseases

Dan Taylor Consultant Anaesthetist

References

1. Volodos NL, Shekhanin VE, Karpovich IP, Troian VI, Gur'ev Iu A. A self-fixing synthetic blood vessel endoprosthesis. Vestn Khir Im I I Grek. 1986;137(11):123–5.
2. Volodos NL, Karpovich IP, Shekhanin VE, Troian VI, Iakovenko LF. A case of distant transfemoral endoprosthesis of the thoracic artery using a self-fixing synthetic prosthesis in traumatic aneurysm. Grudn Khir. 1988;6:84–6.
3. Parodi JC, Palmaz J, Barone HD. Transfemoral intraluminal graft implantation for abdominal aortic aneurysms. Ann Vasc Surg. 1991;5:491–9.
4. Chalmers N, Eadington DW, Gandanhamo D, Gillespie IN, Ruckley CV. Case report: infected false aneurysm at the site of an iliac stent. Br J Radiol. 1993;66(790):946–8.
5. Hobbs SD, Kumar S, GL G-S. Epidemiology and diagnosis of endograft infection. J Cardiovasc Surg. 2010;51(1):5–14.
6. Numan F, Gulsen F, Solak S, Cantasdemir M. Management of endograft infections. J Cardiovasc Surg. 2011;52(2):205–23.
7. O'Connor S, Andrew P, Batt M, Becquemin JP. A systematic review and meta-analysis of treatments for aortic graft infection. J Vasc Surg. 2006;44(1):38–45.
8. Setacci C, De Donato G, Setacci F, Chisci E, Perulli A, Galzerano G, Siringano P. Management of abdominal endograft infection. J Cardiovasc Surg. 2010;51(1):33–41.
9. Smeds MR, Duncan AA, Harlander-Locke MP, Lawrence PF, Lyden S, Fatima J, Eskandari MK, Vascular Low-Frequency Disease Consortium. Treatment and outcomes of aortic endograft infection. J Vasc Surg. 2016;63(2):332–40.
10. Wilson WR, Bower TC, Creager MA, Amin-Hanjani S, O'Gara PT, Lockhart PB, Darouiche RO, Ramlawi B, Derdeyn CP, Bolger AF, Levison ME, Taubert KA, Baltimore RS, Baddour LM, American Heart Association Committee on Rheumatic Fever E, Kawasaki Disease of the Council on Cardiovascular

Disease in the Y, Council on C, Stroke N, Council on Cardiovascular R, Intervention, Council on Cardiovascular S, Anesthesia, Council on Peripheral Vascular D, and Stroke C. Vascular graft infections, mycotic aneurysms, and endovascular infections: a scientific statement from the American Heart Association. Circulation. 2016;134(20):e412–e60.

11. Sorelius K, Mani K, Bjorck M, Sedivy P, Wahlgren CM, Taylor P, Clough RE, Lyons O, Thompson M, Brownrigg J, Ivancev K, Davis M, Jenkins MP, Jaffer U, Bown M, Rancic Z, Mayer D, Brunkwall J, Gawenda M, Kolbel T, Jean-Baptiste E, Moll F, Berger P, Liapis CD, Moulakakis KG, Langenskiold M, Roos H, Larzon T, Pirouzram A, Wanhainen A, European MAAc. Endovascular treatment of mycotic aortic aneurysms: a European multicenter study. Circulation. 2014;130(24):2136–42.
12. Sorelius K, Wanhainen A, Furebring M, Bjorck M, Gillgren P, Mani K, Swedish Collaborator Group for Mycotic Abdominal Aortic A. Nationwide study of the treatment of mycotic abdominal aortic aneurysms comparing open and endovascular repair. Circulation. 2016;134(23):1822–32.
13. Cernohorsky P, Reijnen MM, Tielliu IF, van Sterkenburg SM, van den Dungen JJ, Zeebregts CJ. The relevance of aortic endograft prosthetic infection. J Vasc Surg. 2011;54(2):327–33.
14. Lyons OT, Baguneid M, Barwick TD, Bell RE, Foster N, Homer-Vanniasinkam S, Hopkins S, Hussain A, Katsanos K, Modarai B, Sandoe JA, Thomas S, NM P. Diagnosis of aortic graft infection: a case definition by the Management of Aortic Graft Infection Collaboration (MAGIC). Eur J Vasc Endovasc Surg. 2016;52(6):758–63.
15. Chaufour X, Gaudric J, Goueffic Y, Khodja RH, Feugier P, Malikov S, Beraud G, Ricco JB, Collaborators A. A multicenter experience with infected abdominal aortic endograft explantation. J Vasc Surg. 2017;65(2):372–80.
16. Hinchliffe RJ, Powell JT. The value of registries for rare diseases: bacterial or mycotic aortic aneurysm. Circulation. 2014;130(24):2129–30.
17. Jones KG, Bell RE, Sabharwal T, Aukett M, Reidy JF, Taylor PR. Treatment of mycotic aortic aneurysms with endoluminal grafts. Eur J Vasc Endovasc Surg. 2005;29(2):139–44.
18. Blaisdell FW, Hall AD, Lim RC Jr, Moore WC. Aorto-iliac arterial substitution utilizing subcutaneous grafts. Ann Surg. 1970;172(5):775–80.
19. Lyons OT, Patel AS, Saha P, Clough RE, Price N, Taylor PR. A 14-year experience with aortic endograft infection: management and results. Eur J Vasc Endovasc Surg. 2013;46(3):306–13.
20. Weiss S, Tobler EL, von Tengg-Kobligk H, Makaloski V, Becker D, Carrel TP, Schmidli J, Wyss TR. Self made Xeno-pericardial aortic tubes to treat native and aortic graft infections. Eur J Vasc Endovasc Surg. 2017;54(5):646–52.
21. Heinola I, Kantonen I, Jaroma M, Alback A, Vikatmaa P, Aho P, Venermo M. Editor's choice - treatment of aortic prosthesis infections by graft removal and in situ replacement with autologous femoral veins and fascial strengthening. Eur J Vasc Endovasc Surg. 2016;51(2):232–9.
22. Harlander-Locke MP, Harmon LK, Lawrence PF, Oderich GS, McCready RA, Morasch MD, Feezor RJ, Vascular Low-Frequency Disease C, Zhou W, Bismuth J, Pevec WC, Correa MP, Jim J, Ladowski JS, Kougias P, Bove PG, Wittgen CM, White JV. The use of cryopreserved aortoiliac allograft for aortic reconstruction in the United States. J Vasc Surg. 2014;59(3):669–74.
23. Weymann A, Ruhparwar A, Karck M. Management of abdominal stent graft infection with cryopreserved aortic allograft. Asian Cardiovasc Thorac Ann. 2016;24(9):904.
24. Oderich GS, Bower TC, Cherry KJ Jr, Panneton JM, Sullivan TM, Noel AA, Carmo M, Cha S, Kalra M, Gloviczki P. Evolution from axillofemoral to in situ prosthetic reconstruction for the treatment of aortic graft infections at a single center. J Vasc Surg. 2006;43(6):1166–74.
25. van Zitteren M, van der Steenhoven TJ, Burger DH, van Berge Henegouwen DP, Heyligers JM, Vriens PW. Spiral vein reconstruction of the infected abdominal aorta using the greater saphenous vein: preliminary results of the Tilburg experience. Eur J Vasc Endovasc Surg. 2011;41(5):637–46.
26. Evans TJ, Lyons OT, Brown A, Price N, Bell RE, Sallam M. Mycotic aneurysm following a dog bite: the value of the clinical history and molecular diagnostics. Ann Vasc Surg. 2016;32:130–e5.
27. Setacci C, Chisci E, Setacci F, Ercolini L, de Donato G, Troisi N, Galzerano G, Michelagnoli S. How to diagnose and manage infected endografts after endovascular aneurysm repair. Aorta. 2014;2(6):255–64.
28. Williamson MR, Boyd CM, HR S. Prosthetic vascular graft infections: diagnosis and treatment. Crit Rev Diagn Imaging. 1989;29(2):181–213.
29. Rossi P, Arata FM, Salvatori FM, Bezzi M, Speziale F, Lauri D, Sbarigia E. Prosthetic graft infection: diagnostic and therapeutic role of interventional radiology. J Vasc Interv Radiol. 1997;8(2):271–7.
30. FitzGerald SF, Kelly C, Humphreys H. Diagnosis and treatment of prosthetic aortic graft infections: confusion and inconsistency in the absence of evidence or consensus. J Antimicrob Chemother. 2005;56(6):996–9.
31. Valentine RJ. Diagnosis and management of aortic graft infection. Semin Vasc Surg. 2001;14(4):292–301.
32. Orton DF, LeVeen RF, Saigh JA, Culp WC, Fidler JL, Lynch TJ, Goertzen TC, McCowan TC. Aortic prosthetic graft infections: radiologic manifestations and implications for management. Radiographics. 2000;20(4):977–93.
33. Fiorani P, Speziale F, Rizzo L, De Santis F, Massimi GJ, Taurino M, Faraglia V, Fiorani L, Baiocchi P, Santini C, et al. Detection of aortic graft infection with leukocytes labeled with technetium 99m-hexametazime. J Vasc Surg. 1993;17(1):87–95. discussion -6

34. Bruggink JL, Glaudemans AW, Saleem BR, Meerwaldt R, Alkefaji H, Prins TR, Slart RH, Zeebregts CJ. Accuracy of FDG-PET-CT in the diagnostic work-up of vascular prosthetic graft infection. Eur J Vasc Endovasc Surg. 2010;40(3):348–54.
35. Modrall JG, Clagett GP. The role of imaging techniques in evaluating possible graft infections. Semin Vasc Surg. 1999;12(4):339–47.
36. Liberatore M, Iurilli AP, Ponzo F, Prosperi D, Santini C, Baiocchi P, Rizzo L, Speziale F, Fiorani P, Colella AC. Clinical usefulness of technetium-99m-HMPAO-labeled leukocyte scan in prosthetic vascular graft infection. J Nucl Med. 1998;39(5):875–9.
37. Saleem BR, Berger P, Vaartjes I, de Keizer B, Vonken EJ, Slart RH, de Borst GJ, Zeebregts CJ. Modest utility of quantitative measures in (18)F-fluorodeoxyglucose positron emission tomography scanning for the diagnosis of aortic prosthetic graft infection. J Vasc Surg. 2015;61(4):965–71.
38. Speziale F, Calisti A, Zaccagnini D, Rizzo L, Fiorani P. The value of technetium-99m HMPAO leukocyte scintigraphy in infectious abdominal aortic aneurysm stent graft complications. J Vasc Surg. 2002;35(6):1306–7.
39. Spacek M, Belohlavek O, Votrubova J, Sebesta P, Stadler P. Diagnostics of "non-acute" vascular prosthesis infection using 18F-FDG PET/CT: our experience with 96 prostheses. Eur J Nucl Med Mol Imaging. 2009;36(5):850–8.
40. Fukuchi K, Ishida Y, Higashi M, Tsunekawa T, Ogino H, Minatoya K, Kiso K, Naito H. Detection of aortic graft infection by fluorodeoxyglucose positron emission tomography: comparison with computed tomographic findings. J Vasc Surg. 2005;42(5):919–25.
41. Tokuda Y, Oshima H, Araki Y, Narita Y, Mutsuga M, Kato K, Usui A. Detection of thoracic aortic prosthetic graft infection with 18F-fluorodeoxyglucose positron emission tomography/computed tomography. Eur J Cardiothorac Surg. 2013;43(6):1183–7.
42. Lauwers P, Van den Broeck S, Carp L, Hendriks J, Van Schil P, Blockx P. The use of positron emission tomography with (18)F-fluorodeoxyglucose for the diagnosis of vascular graft infection. Angiology. 2007;58(6):717–24.
43. Keidar Z, Engel A, Hoffman A, Israel O, Nitecki S. Prosthetic vascular graft infection: the role of 18F-FDG PET/CT. J Nucl Med. 2007;48(8):1230–6.
44. Tegler G, Sorensen J, Bjorck M, Savitcheva I, Wanhainen A. Detection of aortic graft infection by 18-fluorodeoxyglucose positron emission tomography combined with computed tomography. J Vasc Surg. 2007;45(4):828–30.
45. Stadler P, Bilohlavek O, Spacek M, Michalek P. Diagnosis of vascular prosthesis infection with FDG-PET/CT. J Vasc Surg. 2004;40(6):1246–7.
46. Balink H, Reijnen MM. Diagnosis of abdominal aortic prosthesis infection with FDG-PET/CT. Vasc Endovasc Surg. 2007;41(5):428–32.
47. Chrapko BE, Chrapko M, Nocun A, Stefaniak B, Zubilewicz T, Drop A. Role of 18F-FDG PET/CT in the diagnosis of inflammatory and infectious vascular disease. Nucl Med Rev Cent East Eur. 2016;19(1):28–36.
48. Shahidi S, Eskil A, Lundof E, Klaerke A, Jensen BS. Detection of abdominal aortic graft infection: comparison of magnetic resonance imaging and indium-labeled white blood cell scanning. Ann Vasc Surg. 2007;21(5):586–92.
49. Spartera C, Morettini G, Bafile G, Di Cesare E, Alagia G, Ventura M. Diagnostic imaging techniques in vascular graft infection. Eur J Vasc Endovasc Surg. 1997;14:24–6.
50. Sah BR, Husmann L, Mayer D, Scherrer A, Rancic Z, Puippe G, Weber R, Hasse B, Cohort V. Diagnostic performance of 18F-FDG-PET/CT in vascular graft infections. Eur J Vasc Endovasc Surg. 2015;49(4):455–64.
51. Keidar Z, Pirmisashvili N, Leiderman M, Nitecki S, Israel O. 18F-FDG uptake in noninfected prosthetic vascular grafts: incidence, patterns, and changes over time. J Nucl Med. 2014;55(3):392–5.
52. Weinstein EA, Ordonez AA, DeMarco VP, Murawski AM, Pokkali S, MacDonald EM, Klunk M, Mease RC, Pomper MG, Jain SK. Imaging Enterobacteriaceae infection in vivo with 18F-fluorodeoxysorbitol positron emission tomography. Sci Transl Med. 2014;6(259):259ra146.
53. Seifert H. The clinical importance of microbiological findings in the diagnosis and management of bloodstream infections. Clin Infect Dis. 2009;48(Suppl 4):S238–45.
54. McDougal EG, Burnham SJ, Johnson G Jr. Rifampin protection against experimental graft sepsis. J Vasc Surg. 1986;4(1):5–7.
55. Cunat JS, Haaga JR, Rhodes R, Bekeny J, El Yousef S. Periaortic fluid aspiration for recognition of infected graft: preliminary report. AJR Am J Roentgenol. 1982;139(2):251–3.
56. Belair M, Soulez G, Oliva VL, Laperriere J, Gianfelice D, Blair JF, Sarrazin J, Therasse E. Aortic graft infection: the value of percutaneous drainage. AJR Am J Roentgenol. 1998;171(1):119–24.
57. Hart JP, Eginton MT, Brown KR, Seabrook GR, Lewis BD, Edmiston CE Jr, Towne JB, Cambria RA. Operative strategies in aortic graft infections: is complete graft excision always necessary? Ann Vasc Surg. 2005;19(2):154–60.
58. Blanch M, Berjon J, Vila R, Simeon JM, Romera A, Riera S, Cairols MA. The management of aortic stent-graft infection: endograft removal versus conservative treatment. Ann Vasc Surg. 2010;24(4):554 e1–5.
59. Lawrence PF. Conservative treatment of aortic graft infection. Semin Vasc Surg. 2011;24(4):199–204.
60. Morris GE, Friend PJ, Vassallo DJ, Farrington M, Leapman S, Quick CR. Antibiotic irrigation and conservative surgery for major aortic graft infection. J Vasc Surg. 1994;20(1):88–95.
61. Wakefield TW, Schaberg DR, Pierson CL, Bouffard JA, Petry NA, Nolan KD, Spaulding SA, Whitehouse WM Jr, Stanley JC. Treatment of established pros-

thetic vascular graft infection with antibiotics preferentially concentrated in leukocytes. Surgery. 1987;102(1):8–14.
62. Saleem BR, Berger P, Zeebregts CJ, Slart RH, Verhoeven EL, van den Dungen JJ. Periaortic endograft infection due to *Listeria monocytogenes* treated with graft preservation. J Vasc Surg. 2008;47(3):635–7.
63. Pryluck DS, Kovacs S, Maldonado TS, Jacobowitz GR, Adelman MA, Charles HC, Clark TW. Percutaneous drainage of aortic aneurysm sac abscesses following endovascular aneurysm repair. Vasc Endovasc Surg. 2010;44(8):701–7.
64. Numan F, Gulsen F, Cantasdemir M, Solak S, Arbatli H. Percutaneous treatment of an infected aneurysmal sac secondary to aortoesophageal fistula with a history of stent-graft treatment for thoracic aortic aneurysm. Cardiovasc Intervent Radiol. 2012;35(3):690–4.
65. Rosbotham JL, Brice GW, Child AH, Nunan TO, Mortimer PS, Burnand KG. Distichiasis-lymphoedema: clinical features, venous function and lymphoscintigraphy. Br J Dermatol. 2000;142(1):148–52.
66. Clough RE, Black SA, Lyons OT, Zayed HA, Bell RE, Carrell T, Waltham M, Sabharwal T, Taylor PR. Is endovascular repair of mycotic aortic aneurysms a durable treatment option? Eur J Vasc Endovasc Surg. 2009;37(4):407–12.
67. Krysa J, Taylor P. Explantation of aortic infrarenal stent graft. Ann R Coll Surg Engl. 2012;94(5):365–6.
68. Shibutani S, Obara H, Ono S, Kakefuda T, Kitagawa Y. Complete removal of infected abdominal aortic stent-graft with suprarenal fixation. Ann Vasc Surg. 2011;25(7):980.e7–10.
69. Brinster CJ, Fairman RM, Woo EY, Wang GJ, Carpenter JP, Jackson BM. Late open conversion and explantation of abdominal aortic stent grafts. J Vasc Surg. 2011;54(1):42–6.
70. Usatii A, Payne W, Santilli S. Removal of an infected aortic endograft and open aortic reconstruction: technical remarks. Ann Vasc Surg. 2013;27(5):679–83.
71. Chaufour X, Segal J, Lebas B, Le Gall M, Galley J. Comparative analysis of the results of the conventional surgical treatment of the juxtarenal and suprarenal abdominal aorta. Ann Vasc Surg. 2017;38:e25–e6.
72. May J, White GH, Harris JP. Techniques for surgical conversion of aortic endoprosthesis. Eur J Vasc Endovasc Surg. 1999;18(4):284–9.
73. Sternbergh WC 3rd, Conners MS 3rd, Money SR. Explantation of an infected aortic endograft with suprarenal barb fixation. J Vasc Surg. 2003;38(5):1136.
74. Debus ES, Diener H. Reconstructions following graft infection: an unsolved challenge. Eur J Vasc Endovasc Surg. 2017;53(2):151–2.
75. Charlton-Ouw KM, Sandhu HK, Huang G, Leake SS, Miller CC 3rd, Estrera AL, Azizzadeh A, Safi HJ. Reinfection after resection and revascularization of infected infrarenal abdominal aortic grafts. J Vasc Surg. 2014;59(3):684–92.
76. Minga Lowampa E, Holemans C, Stiennon L, Van Damme H, Defraigne JO. Late fate of cryopreserved arterial allografts. Eur J Vasc Endovasc Surg. 2016;52(5):696–702.
77. Heo SH, Kim YW, Woo SY, Park YJ, Kim DK, Chung DR. Recent results of in situ abdominal aortic reconstruction with cryopreserved arterial allograft. Eur J Vasc Endovasc Surg. 2017;53(2):158–67.
78. Uchida N, Katayama A, Tamura K, Miwa S, Masatsugu K, Sueda T. In situ replacement for mycotic aneurysms on the thoracic and abdominal aorta using rifampicin-bonded grafting and omental pedicle grafting. Ann Thorac Surg. 2012;93(2):438–42.
79. Oderich GS, Bower TC, Hofer J, Kalra M, Duncan AA, Wilson JW, Cha S, Gloviczki P. In situ rifampin-soaked grafts with omental coverage and antibiotic suppression are durable with low reinfection rates in patients with aortic graft enteric erosion or fistula. J Vasc Surg. 2011;53(1):99–106. 7 e1–7; discussion –7
80. Dulbecco E, Camporrotondo M, Blanco G, Haberman D. In situ reconstruction with bovine pericardial tubular graft for aortic graft infection. Rev Bras Cir Cardiovasc. 2010;25(2):249–52.
81. Calligaro KD, Veith FJ, Yuan JG, Gargiulo NJ, Dougherty MJ. Intra-abdominal aortic graft infection: complete or partial graft preservation in patients at very high risk. J Vasc Surg. 2003;38(6): 1199–205.
82. Kloppenburg GTL, van de Pavoordt E, de Vries JPM. Endograft-preserving therapy of a patient with Coxiella burnetii-infected abdominal aortic aneurysm: a case report. J Med Case Rep. 2011;5:565.
83. Allegranzi B, Zayed B, Bischoff P, Kubilay NZ, de Jonge S, de Vries F, Gomes SM, Gans S, Wallert ED, Wu X, Abbas M, Boermeester MA, Dellinger EP, Egger M, Gastmeier P, Guirao X, Ren J, Pittet D, Solomkin JS, Group WHOGD. New WHO recommendations on intraoperative and postoperative measures for surgical site infection prevention: an evidence-based global perspective. Lancet Infect Dis. 2016;16(12):e288–303.

Large-Vessel Vasculitides: Takayasu Arteritis and Giant Cell Arteritis

35

Giulio Cavalli, Giacomo De Luca, and Lorenzo Dagna

35.1 Takayasu Arteritis

35.1.1 Clinical Features

Takayasu arteritis (TA) is a chronic, large-vessel granulomatous vasculitis of unknown etiology, which primarily affects the aorta and its primary branches ("aortic arch syndrome") [1]. TA chiefly affects young women: patients are female in 80–90% of cases, and the age of onset is typically before 40 years, with a mean age at diagnosis between 25 and 30 years. It has a worldwide distribution, with peak prevalence in Asian countries (0.004% in Japan versus 4.7 cases per million in the UK).

The etiology of TA is largely obscure [2]. A genetic predisposition for the immune-mediated process is postulated, but disease pathogenesis and natural history are poorly understood. The histologic hallmark of TA is granuloma formation and transmural infiltration with inflammatory cells, eventually leading to a marked thickening of the walls of affected arteries. Despite remarkable variability in disease expression, the initial vascular lesions frequently occur in the left middle or proximal subclavian artery (Fig. 35.1). As the disease progresses, the left common carotid, vertebral, brachiocephalic, right middle or proximal subclavian artery, right carotid, vertebral arteries, and aorta may also be affected. The abdominal aorta and pulmonary arteries are involved in approximately 50% of patients. Vascular inflammation may be localized to a portion of the thoracic or abdominal aorta and branches or may extensively involve the entire vessels. The inflammatory process within the

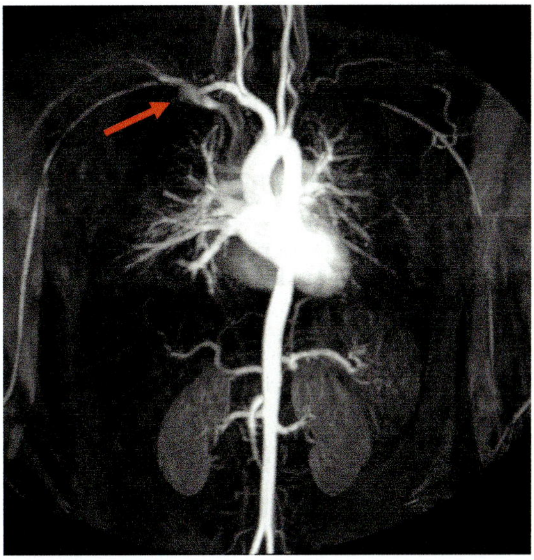

Fig. 35.1 CMR angiography in large-vessel vasculitides. Contrast-enhanced magnetic resonance angiography coronal plane showing diffuse luminal irregularities without significant stenosis and marked right subclavian wall thickening up to 25 mm (arrowheads) with intense contrast enhancement

G. Cavalli · G. De Luca · L. Dagna (✉)
Unit of Immunology, Rheumatology, Allergy and Rare Diseases, San Raffaele Hospital and University, Milan, Italy
e-mail: dagna.lorenzo@hsr.it

© Springer Nature Switzerland AG 2019

Y. Tshomba et al. (eds.), *Visceral Vessels and Aortic Repair*,
https://doi.org/10.1007/978-3-319-94761-7_35

vessel can lead to narrowing, occlusion, or dilation of involved portions of the arteries, which cause a wide variety of symptoms.

Clinical presentation is highly variable and varies from nonspecific constitutional symptoms without clinical or imaging evidence of arterial occlusive disease (pre-pulseless stage) to symptoms attributable to arterial stenosis, aneurysm, and occlusion (pulseless stage) [3]. At time of disease onset, the clinical picture tends to be subacute, for example, with nonspecific constitutional symptoms (i.e., fatigue, malaise, night sweats, weight loss, fever) and arthralgia. This elusive clinical picture often causes a remarkable delay in diagnosis, ranging from months to years, during which vascular disease likely progresses. Although vascular involvement is often asymptomatic at presentation, it later becomes clinically apparent as dilation, narrowing, or occlusion of arteries develops, resulting in a broad spectrum of vascular symptoms including limb cyanosis and claudication, lightheadedness or other symptoms of reduced blood flow, vascular bruits, arterial pain and tenderness (i.e., carotidynia), and neurovascular hypertension. The pulseless phase is characterized by vascular insufficiency manifesting as arm or leg claudication and neurological symptoms due to decreased blood flow to the brain. Rare but alarming complications of TA include ocular involvement in form of various degrees of visual field defects, coronary artery aneurysms, as well as rupture of aneurysms in other sites [4].

35.1.2 Diagnosis

TA should be suspected in a young patient, chiefly woman, who has constitutional symptoms, hypertension, diminished or absent pulses, and/or arterial bruits. At physical examination, accurate measurements of blood pressure and palpation of pulses may reveal asymmetric or discordant findings. Absent or weak peripheral pulses are most common at the level of the radial arteries and led to the usual definition of "pulseless disease." Vascular bruits or a murmur consistent with aortic valve insufficiency are common.

There are no gold standard imaging or laboratory tests with adequate sensitivity or specificity for the diagnosis of TA [5]. Testing for inflammatory markers such as the erythrocyte sedimentation rate (ESR) and the acute-phase reactant C-reactive protein (CRP) indicates the presence of a systemic inflammatory process; however, normal values may occasionally be observed and should not unequivocally rule out a diagnosis of TA. Anemia often accompanies the earliest inflammatory stages of the disease. In most cases, the diagnosis is based on suggestive clinical features and specific imaging findings of the aorta and/or its branches. In these regards, TA is sometimes incidentally suspected upon findings of arterial disease at imaging obtained for other clinical indications or revealed when vasculitis is observed on histologic examination of surgically removed arteries.

Imaging studies of the arterial tree are essential for ascertaining the diagnosis of TA and for determining the extent and severity of vascular involvement [6].

Preferred techniques are magnetic resonance angiography (MRA) and computed tomography angiography (CTA), which allow for evaluation of the arterial lumen. MRA use circumvents the risks of exposure to radiation and iodinated contrast of CTA; since periodic re-evaluations can be anticipated, MRA is the preferred technique. Imaging of the vasculature of the chest, abdomen, head and neck, or other areas by MRA or CTA demonstrates smoothly tapered luminal narrowing or occlusion, which may sometimes be accompanied by circumferential thickening of the vessel wall. The characteristic finding on contrast angiography is the presence of "skip lesions," where stenosis or aneurysms alternate with normal vessels. FDG-PET can help in diagnosing an active inflammation, providing additional information apart from vessel anatomy and patency, and thus resulting particularly useful in monitoring disease activity during follow-up [7] (Fig. 35.2).

Conditions that should be considered in the differential diagnosis of TA include other diseases which can feature large-vessel vasculitis or aortitis, such as giant cell (temporal) arteritis,

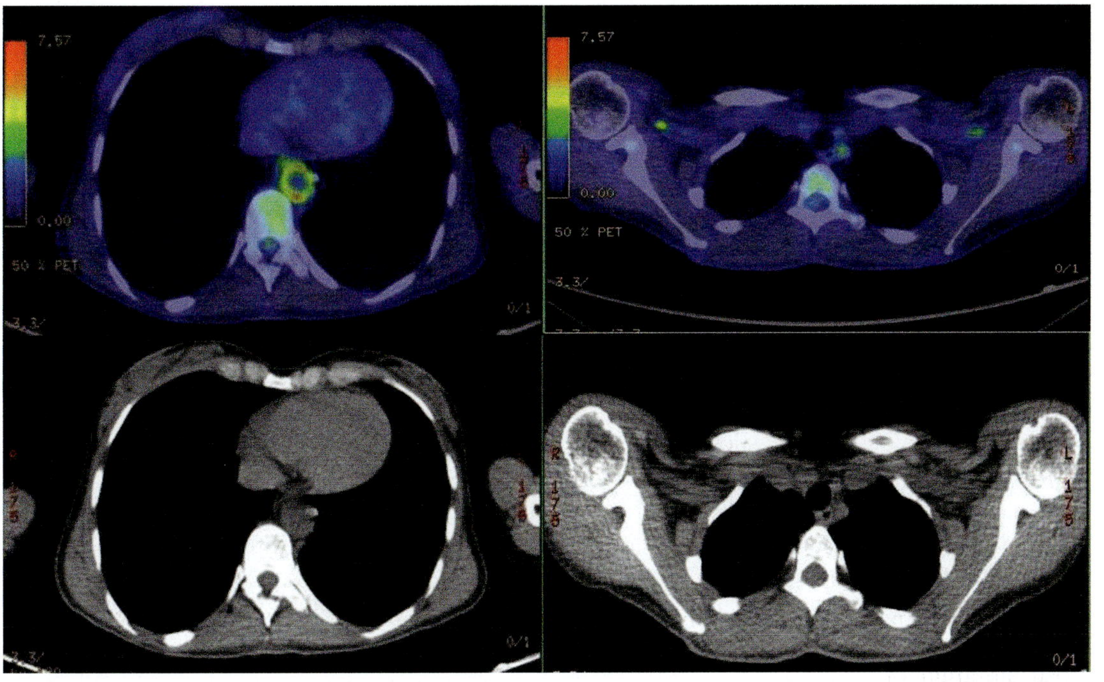

Fig. 35.2 CT/F-FDG-PET in large-vessel vasculitides (Takayasu arteritis). CT/PET showing FDG uptake in the thoracic aorta and in both subclavian arteries

Cogan's syndrome, Behçet's syndrome, relapsing polychondritis, infectious aortitis, atherosclerosis, fibromuscular dysplasia, and genetically determined causes of aneurysms such as Ehlers-Danlos syndrome, IgG4-related disease, and spondyloarthropathies.

35.1.3 Treatment

TA is a chronic, relapsing, and progressive disease requiring long-term immunosuppression [8].

Glucocorticoids The cornerstone of therapy for TA is glucocorticoids. High-dose glucocorticoids effectively control systemic inflammation and related clinical manifestations (fever, arthritis or arthralgia, normochromic anemia, and elevated acute-phase reactants) in the majority of cases and can arrest or fully revert the progression of vascular inflammation and damage of TA. In early cases, arterial stenosis may reverse, and ischemic symptoms may improve remarkably upon corticosteroid treatment. On the other and, in later disease stages, fibrous damage may develop and be poorly responsive to treatment.

A daily dose of 45–60 mg of prednisone (0.5–1 mg/Kg) is typically considered an adequate starting dosing for adults of average size. A single morning is convenient and preferred, as divided doses are associated with an increased number of adverse reactions.

Gradual tapering when symptoms and laboratory analyses related to the inflammatory process have improved follows this loading steroid dose. Long-term, low-dose prednisone therapy may be necessary to prevent progression of arterial stenoses. Glucocorticoids can be discontinued if the disease enters prolonged remission, but the dose should be increased if flares occur. Supplementation with calcium and vitamin D, as well as prophylactic use of an oral bisphosphonate, is recommended to prevent glucocorticoid-related osteoporosis, since duration and cumulative dose of treatment cannot be predicted at time of initiation.

Evaluation of Disease Activity and Response to Treatment Assessing residual disease activity and response to treatment is a challenging task, given the lack of specific laboratory tests or validated tools for assessing disease activity. Clinical evaluations include monitoring of constitutional or vascular symptoms and levels of acute-phase reactants (ESR and CRP). Efforts aimed at developing a quantitative clinical assessment instrument are undergoing. The Indian Takayasu Clinical Activity Score (ITAS 2010) and a composite ITAS-A, which also includes acute-phase reactants (ESR or CRP), are currently used for research purposes and provide a quantitative score of clinical disease activity for patient monitoring [9].

Imaging techniques provide some aid in evaluating disease activity and response to treatment. CTA, MRA, and FDG-PET can be used.

Glucocorticoid-Resistant Disease Approximately, one-half of all TA patients exhibit chronically active disease and vascular inflammation refractory to treatment with glucocorticoids. These patients normally benefit from the adjunctive use of immunosuppressant medications. Drugs used in the management of TA include methotrexate, azathioprine, leflunomide, and mycophenolate mofetil [8]. In small open-label studies, the use of these medications in association with glucocorticoids was generally associated with a significant reduction in disease activity scores, acute-phase reactants, and glucocorticoid use. More sparse evidence and limited experience indicate that mycophenolate mofetil and cyclophosphamide may have some value as steroid-sparing agents in patients with TA refractory to conventional therapy. There is currently no evidence to clearly privilege any of these drugs over others. Comparative randomized trials can hardly be conceived and populated, given the small size of patient in individual centers.

Pharmacologic blockade of pro-inflammatory cytokines with monoclonal antibodies represents a promising option for difficult-to-treat patients. Experience with antitumor necrosis factor (TNF)-alpha agents infliximab or etanercept in TA is limited, but available evidence point at a role for these agents in the management of difficult-to-treat patients. Emerging evidence indicates that blockade of interleukin (IL)-6 with tocilizumab may also be effective in TA; of note, this drug exhibited remarkable efficacy in a larger number of patients with giant cell arteritis [10].

Revascularization Despite medical treatment, irreversible arterial stenosis or significant ischemic symptoms may develop in late cases and necessitate treatment with percutaneous transluminal angioplasty, bypass grafts, or other surgeries. In general, surgical treatments yield better outcomes than endovascular interventions. In a long-term follow-up study of 106 Japanese patients who required surgical revascularization, survival to hospital discharge was 89% and overall survival 73%. Of note, aneurysms at sites of anastomosis eventually developed in 13.8% of long-term survivors, requiring lifelong surveillance for the development of this complication.

Percutaneous angioplasty and stenting are burdened with frequent postoperative complications, the most common of which is restenosis, occurring in 77% of angioplasty procedures, as opposed to 34% of surgical bypasses. Nevertheless, angioplasty may be preferred in the event of lesions amenable to catheter-based dilation. Stenosis or occlusions affecting sizeable tracts of an artery, as well as heavy scarring of vessels, may reduce both the feasibility and the success rate of percutaneous revascularization [11].

Of note, a state of active inflammation prior to or after revascularization is associated with poor outcomes, regardless of procedure modality. Complications include graft detachment or restenosis, new arterial lesions, and development of progressive symptomatic disease. It is thus crucial that disease activity is controlled with adequate immunosuppressive treatment prior to or – in case of urgent revascularization – at least following a procedure [12].

Aortic Valve Surgery Progressive aortic regurgitation (AR) may develop when the ascending aorta is involved. This complication may require surgical valve replacement or repair. The state of inflammation and fragility of affected walls make this surgery more challenging than usual. In a large series of 90 patients (63 undergoing aortic valve replacement and 27 undergoing composite graft repair), in-hospital mortality was 5.5%, and 15-year survival was 76%; the long-term outcome after surgery seemed comparable between these two approaches [13].

35.1.4 Prognosis

The development of TA marks the onset of a severe, chronic disease in the most productive years of life. Vascular involvement tends to be progressive, and disease activity may vary over time leading to occasional exacerbations of the inflammatory process; however, spontaneous remissions also rarely occur as the disease may eventually burn out.

The short-term prognosis of TA is generally favorable, with several follow-up studies reporting a 5-year survival rate of 80–90%. The overall mortality has declined over time such that the 15-year survival rate has increased from 82.9% for patients diagnosed between 1957 and 1975 to 96.5% for those diagnosed from 1976 to 1990. However, the 15-year survival rate may drop to 40–70% in those TA patients with a progressive course and major complications, including retinopathy, hypertension, aortic regurgitation, and aneurysms. In these subsets of patients, more aggressive medical and/or surgical therapy is warranted to prevent an unfavorable outcome [14].

35.2 Giant Cell Arteritis

35.2.1 Clinical Features

Giant cell arteritis (GCA), or Horton's disease, is a systemic vasculitis of unknown etiology. GCA is historically classified as a large-vessel vasculitis chiefly involving the cranial arteries, typically the temporal artery ("temporal arteritis") [15]. However, GCA exhibits a larger disease spectrum also including idiopathic aortitis and small-medium vessel involvement. The disease, indeed, may also involve the aorta and carotid, subclavian, iliac arteries and the superficial temporal, ophthalmic, occipital, vertebral, posterior ciliary, and proximal vertebral arteries. Given this lesion distribution, GCA may cause a variety of systemic, neurologic, and ophthalmologic complications.

The incidence of GCA peaks between age 70 and 80 years, and the disease occurs with greater frequency in females ((female-to-male ratio 3.7:1) and in Nordic countries. GCA virtually never occurs before the age of 50, making GCA the most common systemic vasculitis in adults with a reported incidence of 0.5–27 cases per 100,000 people aged 50 years or older [16, 17].

GCA is often associated with polymyalgia rheumatica (PMR), an inflammatory condition characterized by inflammatory pain in the shoulder and hip girdles. PMR occurs in about 50% of patients with GCA, and GCA may develop in about 15% of patients with PMR [18]. Musculoskeletal symptoms in addition to those of PMR can be observed in a minority of patients.

The onset of GCA may be either abrupt or insidious, and clinical presentation is highly variable from mild constitutional symptoms to complete visual loss [19]. Prodromal constitutional symptoms such as anorexia, fatigue, low-grade fever, malaise, myalgia, night sweats, weight loss, and nonproductive cough may herald the disease. A common presentation is the onset of temporal or occipital headache in a patient without a history of headaches or a new, unusual complaint in a patient with a history of chronic headache [18, 20].

Jaw claudication is also common and highly predictive, and it is reported as fatigue or discomfort of the jaw muscles upon prolonged chewing or speaking; it is due to ischemia of the maxillary artery supplying the masseter muscles. Involvement of other branches of the external carotid artery may result in many other extracranial GCA symptoms, including maxillary and dental pain, facial swelling, throat pain, and tongue pain.

Visual symptoms are a common, feared manifestation of GCA [21]. Transient monocular (and, rarely, binocular) impairment of vision can be an early manifestation of GCA. Patients typically note an abrupt partial field defect or temporary curtain effect in the field of vision of one eye. Transient episodes of blurred vision are usually reversible, but sudden and painless irreversible loss of vision may occur if treatment is not started promptly [22]. Permanent loss of vision in GCA results from anterior ischemic optic neuropathy (80% of cases), central or branch retinal arterial occlusion, posterior ischemic optic neuropathy, or, rarely, posterior cerebral ischemia [23]. Loss of vision may be partial or complete and unilateral or bilateral. Once established, visual loss is rarely reversible. Before the advent of glucocorticoid treatment, the prevalence of visual complications was high. Increasing awareness by physicians of the symptoms of GCA and advances in diagnostic techniques over the past 20 years have also contributed to a substantial decline in the frequency of permanent visual loss.

GCA can also affect the central nervous system [24]: involvement of the vertebral arteries can cause vertigo, ataxia, dysarthria, homonymous hemianopsia, or bilateral cortical blindness; bilateral vertebral artery involvement can cause rapidly progressive brain stem and/or cerebellar neurologic deficits. Stroke is uncommon but may derive from involvement of vertebrobasilar or internal carotid arteries.

GCA can also involve extracranial arteries, chiefly the aorta and its major proximal branches, especially in the upper extremities: the subclavian arteries distal to the emergence of the vertebral arteries and extend through the axillary arteries to the proximal brachial arteries. Arterial bruits, diminished or absent pulses, arm claudication, and cold intolerance are possible complaints. Patients with these peripheral presentations of GCA are usually younger at diagnosis and have fewer cranial symptoms. Complications include aortic aneurysms and dissection, particularly affecting the thoracic aorta, as well as stenosis, occlusion, and ectasia of large arteries. While these complications occur in a minority of GCA patients, subclinical or clinical aortitis is commonly detected at imaging [25, 26].

As incidence of aortic aneurysms in GCA increases over time, especially in male smokers, ongoing clinical vigilance is warranted. Imaging modalities for diagnosing large-vessel involvement in GCA include color Doppler ultrasonography, CT or CT with angiography (CTA), MRI or MR angiography (MRA), and FDG-PET or PET with CT.

35.2.2 Diagnosis

The diagnosis of GCA should be considered in a patient over the age of 50 years with new headaches, abrupt onset of visual disturbances (especially transient monocular visual loss), jaw claudication, unexplained constitutional symptoms, and inflammatory manifestations including fever, anemia, elevated ESR, and/or CRP. A current or prior diagnosis of polymyalgia rheumatica strengthens the predictive value of any of these findings.

At physical examination, the temporal or other cranial arteries can be tender or thickened. Bruits may be heard on auscultation of the carotid or supraclavicular areas: over the axillary, brachial, or femoral arteries. Murmurs over the abdominal aorta and of aortic regurgitation may reveal the development of an aortic aneurysm.

The laboratory hallmark of GCA is an elevation in ESR and CRP levels. The ESR usually exceeds 50 mm/h but may be normal in 7–20% of patients with GCA; thus, a normal ESR does not rule out GCA. CRP is typically elevated. Combined assessment of ESR and CRP provides a remarkable sensitivity for the diagnosis of GCA [27, 28].

The definite diagnosis of GCA is based on histopathology on temporal artery biopsy. Histologic confirmation should be obtained almost without exception in patients with clinically suspected GCA, since glucocorticoid treatment is prolonged and often complicated. A positive temporal artery biopsy has 100% specificity; however, sensitivity is relatively low (15–87%) due to a "skip lesion" pattern of disease involvement, with normal intervening segments [29]. For this reason, large (5 cm) and occasionally bilateral specimens should be obtained. In the setting of a high diagnostic suspicion for GCA, scheduling of the biopsy should not interfere with initiation of glucocorticoid therapy due to concerns for possible catastrophic sight loss [30].

Color Doppler ultrasonography of the temporal artery has emerged as a promising alternative or complement to temporal artery biopsy, with a specificity of 80–100% when a dark halo surrounds the vessel ("halo sign") [31]. This key diagnostic feature is believed to represent vessel wall edema.

The following are classification criteria for GCA issued by the American College of Rheumatology in 1990 [32]:

- Age 50 years or older
- New-onset localized headache or localized head pain
- Temporal artery tenderness to palpation or decreased pulsation
- ESR of 50 mm/h or higher
- Positive arterial biopsy results (vasculitis characterized by mononuclear infiltration or granulomatous inflammation, usually with multinucleated giant cells)

The presence of three or more criteria yields a diagnostic sensitivity of 93.5% and specificity of 91.2%.

35.2.3 Treatment

Immunosuppressive Treatment The mainstay of treatment for GCA is high-dose corticosteroids. For patients in whom the diagnostic suspicion of GCA is high, especially those with recent vascular complications such as visual loss, therapy should be started promptly, even before the diagnosis is confirmed. A temporal artery biopsy should be obtained as soon as possible, but treatment should not be delayed while awaiting biopsy.

For GCA not complicated by ischemic organ damage (i.e., visual loss), treatment is started at a single glucocorticoid dose equivalent to 40–60 mg of prednisone [33]. However, in the setting of visual loss, damage may be irreversible if treatment is delayed beyond 48 h, and intravenous pulse methylprednisolone (1000 mg intravenously each day for 3 days, followed by oral therapy with 1 mg/kg per day) is recommended. High-dose prednisone should be continued at the starting dose for 2–4 weeks, followed by tapering by approximately 10% of the total daily dose each 1 or 2 weeks. After achieving a daily dose of 10 mg, the prednisone taper should be slowed substantially, so that patients remain on progressively lower doses for 9 to 12 months. The risk of disease flare increases as the daily prednisone dose declines. Supplementation with calcium, vitamin D, bisphosphonate therapy, antimicrobial prophylaxis, and initiation of a proton pump inhibitor or histamine H2-receptor antagonist should be considered. Low-dose aspirin in association to corticosteroids decreases the risk of cranial ischemic complications (visual loss, transient ischemic attacks, or stroke).

Oral corticosteroid therapy is required for months to years with careful follow-up and periodic laboratory evaluations with ESR and CRP: recurrence of inflammation is common in GCA and necessitates an escalation of corticosteroid dose and/or a second-line therapy. Immunomodulatory therapy may be considered in patients experiencing relapsing inflammation despite high doses of corticosteroids or those with corticosteroid-induced complications. Emerging evidence for adjunctive suitable steroid-sparing agents such as methotrexate and the anti-IL-6 tocilizumab is encouraging and may lead to a more mainstream role for these therapies among patients with GCA [34].

Surgery Despite medical treatment, irreversible arterial stenosis or significant ischemic symptoms may develop in late stages in rare cases and necessitate treatment with percutaneous transluminal angioplasty, bypass grafts, or other surgeries. A surgical approach is rarely needed in GCA with extracranial involvement. Moreover, when endovascular revascularization procedures and open surgical treatment for aneurysms and dissections are necessary, results are not always favorable and relapses are common. Given the elderly population of patients with GCA, comorbidities often limit surgical interventions [25].

35.2.4 Prognosis

The prognosis of untreated GCA is extremely poor: serious disability may occur from blindness, or death may result from myocardial infarction, stroke, or dissecting aortic aneurysm. However, in most treated patients, GCA tends to have a self-limited course over several months to several years and may not adversely affect overall survival. Evidence is emerging that overall mortality in GCA patients is at best slightly higher than expected in relation to general population mortality data, but GCA is associated with an increase in morbidity and mortality specifically related to aortic aneurysm or other cardiovascular causes [35].

Glucocorticoid therapy can eventually be reduced and discontinued in the majority of patients. The burden of morbidity from steroid therapy is significant and includes diabetes mellitus, hypertension, osteoporosis, steroid myopathy, steroid psychosis, and immunosuppression-related infections.

References

1. Arend WP, et al. The American College of Rheumatology 1990 criteria for the classification of Takayasu arteritis. Arthritis Rheum. 1990;33(8):1129.
2. Weyand CM, Goronzy JJ. Medium- and large-vessel vasculitis. NEJM. 2003;349(2):160.
3. Mason JC. Takayasu arteritis--advances in diagnosis and management. Nat Rev Rheumatol. 2010;6(7):406–15.
4. Serra R, et al. Updates in pathophysiology, diagnosis and management of Takayasu arteritis. Ann Vasc Surg. 2016;35:210–25.
5. Kim E, et al. Takayasu arteritis: challenges in diagnosis and management. Heart. 2017;104(7):558–65.
6. Alibaz-Oner F, et al. Update on Takayasu's arteritis. Presse Med. 2015;44:e259–65.
7. Barra L, et al. Imaging modalities for the diagnosis and disease activity assessment of Takayasu's arteritis: a systematic review and meta-analysis. Autoimmun Rev. 2018;17(2):175–87.
8. Keser G, et al. What is new in management of Takayasu arteritis? Presse Med. 2017;46:e229–35.
9. Misra R, et al. Development and initial validation of the Indian Takayasu Clinical Activity Score (ITAS2010). Rheumatology (Oxford). 2013;52:1795–801.
10. Abisror N, et al. Tocilizumab in refractory Takayasu arteritis: a case series and updated literature review. Autoimmun Rev. 2013;12:1143–9.
11. Kazibudzki M, et al. New endovascular techniques for treatment of life-threatening Takayasu arteritis. Adv Interv Cardiol. 2016;12:171–4.
12. Saadoun D, et al. Retrospective analysis of surgery versus endovascular intervention in Takayasu arteritis: a multicenter experience. Circulation. 2012;125:813–9.
13. Matsuura K, et al. Surgical treatment of aortic regurgitation due to Takayasu arteritis: long-term morbidity and mortality. Circulation. 2005;112(24):3707.
14. Schmidt J, et al. Diagnostic features, treatment, and outcomes of Takayasu arteritis in a US cohort of 126 patients. Mayo Clin Proc. 2013;88(8):822.
15. Jennette JC, et al. 2012 revised international Chapel Hill consensus conference nomenclature of vasculitides. Arthritis Rheum. 2013;65(1):1–11.
16. Goodwin JS. Progress in gerontology: polymyalgia rheumatica and temporal arteritis. J Am Geriatr Soc. 1992;40(5):515–25.
17. Gonzalez-Gay MA, et al. Epidemiology of giant cell arteritis and polymyalgia rheumatica. Arthritis Rheum. 2009;61(10):1454.
18. Gonzalez-Gay MA, et al. Giant cell arteritis: disease patterns of clinical presentation in a series of 240 patients. Medicine (Baltimore). 2005;84(5):269.
19. Buttgereit F, et al. Polymyalgia rheumatica and giant cell arteritis: a systematic review. JAMA. 2016;315(22):2442–58.
20. Myklebust G, Gran JT. A prospective study of 287 patients with polymyalgia rheumatica and temporal arteritis: clinical and laboratory manifestations at onset of disease and at the time of diagnosis. Br J Rheumatol. 1996;35(11):1161–8.
21. González-Gay MA, et al. Visual manifestations of giant cell arteritis. Trends and clinical spectrum in 161 patients. Medicine (Baltimore). 2000;79(5):283–92.
22. Salvarani C, et al. Risk factors for visual loss in an Italian population-based cohort of patients with giant cell arteritis. Arthritis Rheum. 2005;53(2):293–7.
23. Soriano A, et al. Visual loss and other cranial ischaemic complications in giant cell arteritis. Nat Rev Rheumatol. 2017;13:476–84.
24. Gonzalez-Gay MA, et al. Strokes at time of disease diagnosis in a series of 287 patients with biopsy-proven giant cell arteritis. Medicine (Baltimore). 2009;88(4):227–35.

25. Lensen KD, et al. Extracranial giant cell arteritis. Neth J Med. 2016;74(5):182–92.
26. Nuenninghoff DM, et al. Incidence and predictors of large-artery complication (aortic aneurysm, aortic dissection, and/or large-artery stenosis) in patients with giant cell arteritis: a population-based study over 50 years. Arthritis Rheum. 2003;48:3522–31.
27. Weyand CM, Goronzy JJ. Clinical practice: giant-cell arteritis and polymyalgia rheumatica. N Engl J Med. 2014;371(1):50–7.
28. Gonzalez-Gay MA, et al. Giant cell arteritis: laboratory tests at the time of diagnosis in a series of 240 patients. Medicine (Baltimore). 2005;84(5):277.
29. Niederkohr RD, Levin LA. A Bayesian analysis of the true sensitivity of a temporal artery biopsy. Invest Ophthalmol Vis Sci. 2007;48(2):675–80.
30. Jakobsson K, et al. The effect of clinical features and glucocorticoids on biopsy findings in giant cell arteritis. BMC Musculoskelet Disord. 2016;17(1):363.
31. Dejaco C, et al. EULAR recommendations for the use of imaging in large vessel vasculitis in clinical practice. Ann Rheum Dis. 2018;77:636–43.
32. Hunder GG, et al. The American College of Rheumatology 1990 criteria for the classification of giant cell arteritis. Arthritis Rheum. 1990;33:1122–8.
33. Dasgupta B, et al. BSR and BHPR guidelines for the management of giant cell arteritis. Rheumatology (Oxford). 2010;49:1594–7.
34. Dejaco C, et al. Giant cell arteritis and polymyalgia rheumatica: current challenges and opportunities. Nat Rev Rheumatol. 2017;13:578–92.
35. Hill CL, et al. Risk of mortality in patients with giant cell arteritis: a systematic review and meta-analysis. Semin Arthritis Rheum. 2017;46(4):513–9.

Visceral Artery Involvement in Takayasu Patients: Treatment Options

36

Laurent Chiche

Takayasu arteritis (TA) is a chronic non-specific inflammatory arteritis which affects large and medium caliber arteries, predominantly the aorta and its main visceral branches. Its cause remains unknown. The disease mostly occurs in young patients during the second or third decade and has been now identified in both genders and many ethnic and racial groups worldwide. It is a lifetime affection with recurrence and progression of symptoms related to occlusive of aneurysmal complications. When vessel inflammation leads to wall thickening, fibrosis, stenosis, and thrombus formation, symptoms reflect end-organ ischemia. More acute inflammation can destroy the arterial media and lead to aneurysm formation. The coexistence of occlusive and aneurysmal lesions is highly evocative of the diagnosis of Takayasu arteritis.

Whether isolated or more frequently associated to aortic occlusive or aneurysmal lesions, lesions of visceral arteries may be responsible for specific symptoms. Although commonly encountered in thoracoabdominal aortic occlusive disease, renovascular hypertension may also be directly related to severe renal artery stenosis. Less frequently, due to the usual development of collateral circulation, occlusive lesions of the main intestinal arteries may lead to the occurrence of chronic or acute mesenteric ischemia.

This chapter aims to describe the specific involvement of visceral arteries during Takayasu arteritis and the current treatment options.

36.1 Involvement of Visceral Arteries

The vast majority of occlusive aortic lesions, especially when they affect the interrenal or abdominal aorta, coexists with lesions of visceral, namely, renal or intestinal, arteries. These lesions may be occlusive and aneurysmal or may associate a post-stenotic dilatation distal to a tight stenosis.

Involvement of renal arteries during Takayasu arteritis might be diagnosed in 40–60% of patients submitted to systematic angiography. Lesions are more frequently occlusive and bilateral. Occlusive lesions of the renal arteries are usually located at the level of their ostia or close to it. Most of the time, they do not extend distal to the first 2 cm of the main renal trunk. In that situation, they represent a direct extension of aortic lesions, whereas more distal and extending lesions may occur independently of aortic occlusive disease. In rare cases, they may affect the hilar division branches of the artery. During their progression, these lesions may lead to renal atrophy following complete occlusion of the

L. Chiche (✉)
Department of Vascular Surgery, Pitie-Salpetriere University Hospital, Paris, France
e-mail: laurent.chiche@aphp.fr

© Springer Nature Switzerland AG 2019
Y. Tshomba et al. (eds.), *Visceral Vessels and Aortic Repair*,
https://doi.org/10.1007/978-3-319-94761-7_36

renal artery. In more favorable cases, the occlusion remains located to a short segment of the artery, and blood supply to the kidney is provided by a rich collateral network issued from adrenal, lumbar, and ureteral arteries. This providential development of collaterals preserves the viability of the kidney and allows to consider an adapted revascularization in the absence of renal atrophy. A part from post-stenotic dilatations, there are rare cases of true fusiform or sacciform aneurysms of the renal arteries.

Hypertension is the main revealing symptom of renal artery involvement in the Takayasu disease. Most of the times, it is uncontrolled hypertension despite intensive medical therapy. Alternatively, hypertension may be caused by a severe aortic coarctation and then predominates at the level of the upper limbs, while femoral pulses are absent unless an extensive collateral network has already developed. Hypertension may be difficult to diagnose in case of bilateral subclavian or axillary artery stenosis. Sometimes, lesions of renal arteries are depicted by the imaging workup in the absence of renovascular hypertension.

Intestinal arteries are frequently involved in Takayasu disease. The superior mesenteric artery (SMA) is the most frequently diseased. The lesions are similar to that observed at the level of the renal arteries. They may include short ostial and paraostial stenoses or more frequently long lesions of the arterial trunk. Therefore, occlusive lesions of the SMA are usually longer than atherosclerotic lesions. In case of a single involvement of this artery, blood supply is coming from the celiac artery via peripancreatic anastomoses. In case of combined celiac artery involvement, an ascending Riolan artery provides an efficient supply to the intestine and supramesocolic organs. This artery may also develop and provide the unique blood supply to the lower limbs in case of severe stenoses or complete occlusion of the infrarenal aorta. Subsequent overflow may be responsible for the development of aneurysms of this collateral vessels.

Acute and chronic intestinal ischemia are rare during Takayasu disease. In most cases, the extensive development of a rich collateral network precludes the occurrence of intestinal symptoms, even in case of multiple occlusions of intestinal arteries.

36.2 Preoperative Workup

CT scan appears to be the most relevant preoperative imaging technique. At the acute phase of the disease, CT scan may depict the severity of the arteritis which typically appears as a wall thickening preexisting to any vessel stenosis of dilatation. Preoperative corticosteroid therapy may reduce this thickening. At the chronic stage of the disease, CT scan may depict circumferential aortic wall calcifications with potential extension toward the visceral arteries. CT angiogram provides an accurate workup of renal and intestinal vessels and of their main branches. Distal arterial runoff supplying the kidneys and the intestine is also addressed by CT angiogram. Measurement of the long axis of the kidney and evaluation of the corticomedullary index are easily done.

TEP scan is probably the most accurate examination to predict the intensity of periarteritis, both at the level of the aorta and at the level of the visceral arteries. TEP scan is essential to estimate the inflammatory status of the disease before attempting to a direct surgical revascularization [1].

Digitalized angiography is now rarely indicated since the accuracy of CT angiogram is excellent. The technique may remain useful in case of distal extension of occlusive lesions of the renal or intestinal arteries, less accessible to CT angiogram. Selective catheterization of renal or intestinal arteries may help to diagnose precisely the development of collaterals and the distal extension of stenotic lesions.

36.3 Treatment Indications

The goal of the treatment of Takayasu arteritis is to relieve inflammation in the arteries and to prevent potential complications related to end-organ ischemia. Even with early detection and treatment, Takayasu arteritis may be challenging to manage, although recent advancements in medical and surgical treatments, including endovascular procedures, have improved the prognosis of patients with Takayasu arteritis [1]. Biological inflammation at the time of revascularization increases the likelihood of postoperative complications in patients with Takayasu arteritis. Therefore, first-line treatment is immunosuppression, primarily with corticosteroids. With glucocorticoid treatment, remissions may occur in 40–60% of all patients. About 40% of all steroid-resistant patients respond to the addition of cytotoxic agents. Approximately only 20% of all patients are resistant to any kind of medical treatment [1]. Therefore, aggressive medical and surgical treatment is required for patients suffering from major complications and a progressive disease course.

Severe hypertension should always be medically addressed before surgery. Several medical treatments may sometimes be associated to obtain a significant decrease in blood pressure level. Renal percutaneous arterial angioplasty may temporarily help to decrease blood pressure in order to schedule a short-delayed more complete surgical repair.

In most cases, lesions of visceral arteries during Takayasu arteritis are surgically treated in combination to aortic repair, either for occlusive or for aneurysmal abdominal or thoracoabdominal aortic lesions [2]. The surgical approach is thus mainly designed according to aortic patterns of lesions, given that (right) renal and distal intestinal arteries are best approached by midline laparotomy than by isolated thoracophrenolumbotomy. Techniques of open revascularization of visceral arteries are numerous. They should take into account the type and extension of the visceral arterial involvement and the estimated technique of aortic revascularization.

Direct reimplantation of visceral arteries into the native aorta is rarely indicated. Most frequently, visceral artery lesions are not limited to the ostia, and they extend distally, thus precluding the opportunity of such a revascularization. Thickening of the aortic wall confers also a high risk of anastomotic intimal hyperplasia.

Transaortic visceral artery endarterectomy is technically hazardous, if not impossible, due to the severity of aortic wall involvement and to the frequent distal extension of visceral artery lesions.

Bypasses are the most appropriate technique of revascularization for visceral artery involvement during Takayasu disease. They offer a treatment for severe and long occlusive lesions of both renal and intestinal arteries. In this specific young population, we advocate the use of autografts rather than prosthetic (Dacron or PTFE) grafts. Given the frequent late deterioration and dilation of venous autografts, we recommend the use of arterial autografts and especially the harvesting of the superficial artery (or sometimes the internal iliac artery). Superficial femoral artery autograft is often a congruent conduit which provides excellent long-term anatomical and hemodynamic outcomes.

The proximal anastomosis is rarely made on a healthy segment of the native abdominal aorta or iliac arteries, due to potential future involvement of these arteries by an evolutive disease. Distal thoracic aorta, if healthy, may be at the origin of the bypass which thus takes an anterograde conformation. In rare cases, mainly in patients already approached at the level of the descending or abdominal aorta, bypasses can be proximally implanted into the ascending aorta with good long-term results [3]. Less frequently, due to potential secondary evolution of the intestinal arteries, bypasses to the renal arteries may originate from the splenic, the hepatic, or the superior mesenteric arteries [4]. In these last alternatives, it is mandatory to assess precisely the absence of aortic lesions proximal to the level of the renal arteries, in order to avoid a secondary deterioration of the inflow intestinal vessel. Therefore, redo surgery is probably the most appropriate condition for such extra-anatomic bypasses to the renal arteries.

The most reliable origin of a bypass to the visceral arteries in Takayasu disease is certainly an aortic prosthesis. The proximal anastomosis of an arterial or venous autograft should be done after excision of a small circle of the prosthesis, in order to avoid future hyperplasia and development of an anastomotic stenosis. A prosthetic excision far larger from the native diameter of the autograft exposes to secondary disruption of the anastomosis, especially when venous grafts are used, and may lead to acute or chronic formation of an anastomotic false aneurysm.

Intestinal arteries are quite easy to treat with an anterograde bypass. The right renal artery may be revascularized from the infradiaphragmatic segment of a ventral aorta (bypass originating from the ascending aorta), with the graft thus positioned behind the hepatic pedicle. The right renal artery is less easy to approach during a dorsal aortic revascularization (bypass originating from the descending thoracic aorta). In this case, it is better to bypass from the lower abdominal segment of the prosthesis with the graft positioned behind the duodenum of the inferior vena cava as it would be done during an isolated right aortorenal bypass. Bypasses to the left renal artery are sometimes difficult to position due to the relatively short distance separating the dorsal aortic prosthesis from the hilum of the left kidney. Direct left renal artery reimplantation into the prosthesis is an alternative to short bypasses or to long bypasses running laterally to the aortic prosthesis. If necessary, left renal bypass may originate from the superior mesenteric artery or from a bypass to this artery.

Renal autotransplantation may be indicated in case of distal occlusive or aneurysmal lesions, extending to the hilar branches, and in case of homolateral multiple and diseased renal arteries [5]. Renal autotransplantation is also useful in case of intense periarterial fibrosis which renders the surgical exposure of the renal artery and its branches particularly difficult. Autotransplantation allows ex situ repair of complex and often distal lesions with the use of an arterial autograft. The heterotopic transposition has our preference, and the kidney is thus replaced in the iliac fossa, the graft being proximally anastomosed to the iliac artery or to a prosthesis. Thanks to renal autotransplantation, our indications of primary nephrectomy are now limited to severe and nonreversible parenchymatous kidney lesions, to small kidneys (long axis less than 7 cm) with non-accessible lesions of the distal arterial branches, or to infarcted kidneys following a failed attempt to revascularization. Primary nephrectomy may also be indicated in combination of contralateral renal revascularization, in case of severe renovascular hypertension complicating an ipsilateral renal infarction.

Given the usual good physical status of young patients with Takayasu disease, we often advocate a single-stage revascularization of both aortic and visceral artery lesions. More complex revascularizations may also include the simultaneous treatment of lesions of the supra-aortic trunks. Logically, supra-aortic trunks are first treated when patients are deemed at high risk for a single-stage procedure.

36.4 Surgical Results

As they are the more frequent symptomatic lesions among visceral artery lesions in Takayasu disease, results of renal artery revascularization are the easiest to analyze. Previous data from our institution, published by Kieffer et al. [4], showed satisfactory early and long-term outcome in 24 patients with Takayasu arteritis who underwent surgery for renal artery stenosis. Renal artery revascularization was unilateral in 46% and bilateral in 54%. During the 61.3-month follow-up, repeated renal artery revascularization was required in only four patients. Hypertension was cured in 63%, improved in 31%, and unchanged in 6%. We also reported [5] a series of 26 renal autotransplantations in 19 Takayasu patients and demonstrated that hypertension normalized or improved in 89% of patients who survived the procedure. On the basis of this experience, we have progressively made renal autotransplantation the procedure of choice for treatment of patients with Takayasu disease with renovascular lesions that would be difficult to dissect because of the inflammatory nature of the disease or extensive occlusive lesions of distal branches. We now also advocate renal autotransplantation in patients with aortic lesions that are not sufficiently severe to warrant reconstruction but that would interfere with aortorenal or iliorenal bypass or direct reimplantation. In this regard, it should be noted that thickening of the aortic wall is almost always associated with involvement of the hepatic, mesenteric, and splenic arteries, thus excluding their use for bypass inflow. Overall postoperative morbidity, especially represented by pulmonary complications, is linked mainly to the extent of the operative exposure that is necessary to achieve single-stage reconstruction of thoracoabdominal aorta and renal involvement, which we advocate in young patients.

36.5 The Endovascular Alternative

Balloon angioplasty and stenting are now currently proposed to treat involvement of visceral arteries during Takayasu disease [6–9]. Stent indications are residual stenosis of more than 30% of the native diameter, significant dissection following angioplasty, and distal lesions. Due to the fibrotic nature of the arterial lesion, endovascular treatment is in most reports considered technically successful if the arterial lumen after treatment is less than 30% residual stenosis. Similar to surgery, endovascular repair is recommended at a time of quiescent Takayasu arteritis disease to avoid early and late arterial complications. In our opinion, endovascular procedures are best used as a temporary alternative to improve rapidly severe renovascular hypertension or subacute or acute mesenteric ischemia. Nevertheless, several studies have shown enthusiastic results of renal angioplasty in renovascular hypertension caused by Takayasu arteritis. Tyagi et al. [8] reported a 44.2% cure rate and an improvement rate of 48.4% but with a 13.5% restenosis rate. Sharma et al. [9] reported that angioplasty was beneficial in 89% of patients and their restenosis rate was 16%. In these studies, the follow-up period was about 2 years only. In a more recent series [6] with a longer average follow-up period of 5 years, rates of restenosis were 9% after angioplasty and 62.5% in the setting up of a stent. Renal artery patency rates were 100%, 90.9%, and 90.9% in angioplasty alone; the rates of primary permeability by the introduction of a stent were 62.5%, 37.5%, and 37.5% and assisted permeability 87.5%, 75%, and 50% at 1, 3, and 5 years, respectively.

In conclusion, in the treatment of visceral arteries involved by Takayasu arteritis, surgery remains an effective and durable alternative, especially for patients with associated aortic pathologies and in case of failure of first-line endovascular treatment. The establishment of a stent should probably be reserved for the failure of plain balloon angioplasty.

References

1. Saadoun D, Lambert M, Mirault T, et al. Retrospective analysis of surgery versus endovascular intervention in Takayasu arteritis. A multicenter experience. Circulation. 2012;125:813–9.
2. Brami P, Chiche L, Kieffer E, et al. Maladie de Takayasu: traitement chirurgical. In: Kieffer E, Godeau P, editors. Maladies non athéroscléreuses de l'adulte. Paris: AERCV; 1994. p. 309–22.
3. Chiche L, Kieffer E. Use of the ascending aorta as bypass inflow for treatment of chronic intestinal ischemia. J Vasc Surg. 2005;41:457–61.
4. Kieffer E, Piquois A, Bertal A, Blétry O, Godeau P. Reconstructive surgery of the renal arteries in Takayasu's disease. Ann Vasc Surg. 1990;4:156–65.
5. Chiche L, Kieffer E, Sabatier J, Colau A, Koskas F, Bahnini A. Renal autotransplantation for vascular disease: late outcome according to etiology. J Vasc Surg. 2003;37:353–61.
6. Khinjo H, Kafa A. The results of treatment in renal artery stenosis due to Takayasu disease: comparison between surgery, angioplasty, and stenting. A monocentrique retrospective study. G Chir. 2015;36:161–5.
7. Dong ZJ, Li SH, Lu XC. Percutaneous transluminal angioplasty for renovascular hypertension in arteritis: experience in China. Radiology. 1987;162:477–9.
8. Tyagi S, Singh B, Kaul UA, et al. Balloon angioplasty for renovascular hypertension in Takayasu's arteritis. Am Heart J. 1993;125:1386–93.
9. Sharma S, Gupta H, Saxena A, et al. Results of renal angioplasty in nonspecific aortoarteritis (Takayasu disease). J Vasc Interv Radiol. 1998;9:429–35.

Printed by Printforce, the Netherlands